FUNDAMENTALS SUCCESS
A Course Review Applying Critical Thinking to Test Taking

PATRICIA M. NUGENT, RN, MA, MS, EdD
Professor Emeritus
Nassau Community College
Garden City, New York
Private Practice—President of Nugent Books, Inc.

BARBARA A. VITALE, RN, MA
Associate Professor
Nassau Community College
Garden City, New York

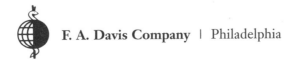
F. A. Davis Company | Philadelphia

F. A. Davis Company
1915 Arch Street
Philadelphia, PA 19103

Printed in the United States of America

Last digit indicates print number: 10 9 8 7 6 5 4

Publisher: Robert Martone
Developmental Editor: Alan Sorkowitz
Cover Designer: Louis J. Forgione

As new scientific information becomes available through basic and clinical research, recommended treatments and drug therapies undergo changes. The authors and publisher have done everything possible to make this book accurate, up to date, and in accord with accepted standards at the time of publication. The authors, editors, and publisher are not responsible for errors or omissions or for consequences from application of the book, and make no warranty, expressed or implied, with regard to the contents of the book. Any practice described in this book should be applied by the reader in accordance with professional standards of care used with regard to the unique circumstances that may apply in each situation. The reader is advised always to check product information (package inserts) for changes and new information regarding dose and contraindications before administering any drug. Caution is especially urged when using new or infrequently ordered drugs.

Library of Congress Cataloging-in-Publication Data

Nugent, Patricia Mary, 1944-
    Fundamentals success : a course review applying critical thinking to test taking / Patricia Nugent, Barbara A. Vitale.
        p. ; cm.
        ISBN 10: 0-8036-1056-4   ISBN 13: 978-0-8036-1056-9
    1. Nursing—Examinations, questions, etc. 2. Critical thinking—Examinations, questions, etc. I. Vitale, Barbara Ann, 1944- II. Title.
    [DNLM: 1. Nursing—Examination Questions. 2. Problem Solving—Examination Questions. WY 18.2 N967f 2003]
RT41.N83 2003
610.73—dc21
                                                                            2003053076

Dedicated to

Joseph Vitale
and
Neil Nugent

For their love and support,
particularly during the production of this book

A Message to Nursing Instructors

Following the resounding success of our book titled *TEST SUCCESS: Test-Taking Techniques for Beginning Nursing Students*, we have heard the same comment from students. **"More questions. We want more questions!"** In addition, the main comment we have heard from nursing faculty members is **"How can we help our students to think critically?"** In the spring of 2003 the National Council of State Boards of Nursing announced that Alternate Item Formats would be included on NCLEX examinations. Both students and faculty are asking, **"What are these questions going to look like?"** This book addresses these felt needs.

The entire premise of this book is based on the beliefs that:

- People use critical thinking all the time in their daily lives
- Nurses continue to use critical thinking in their professional lives
- People can enhance their critical thinking skills
- Students can use critical thinking skills when taking a nursing examination

Chapter 1, Fundamentals of Critical Thinking Related to Test Taking: the RACE Model, discusses the topic of critical thinking in relation to everyday living and introduces the Helix of Critical Thinking. **The Helix of Critical Thinking** schematically represents the cognitive and personal competencies involved in critical thinking. This model is then discussed relative to the cognitive processes used in nursing (the nursing process, problem solving, decision-making, diagnostic reasoning, and the scientific method). Maximizing your critical thinking abilities is presented in the context of personal competencies that foster critical thinking. Information related to being positive, reflective, inquisitive, and creative are explored, and strategies to overcome barriers to the development of these competencies are interwoven throughout the discussion. The application of critical thinking applied to test taking begins with a brief overview of educational domains, components of a multiple-choice test question, and the cognitive levels of nursing questions. Finally, the main ingredient of this textbook is presented – The RACE Model. The **RACE Model** is a formula for using critical thinking when answering multiple-choice questions on a nursing examination. The theoretical framework of the RACE Model is explained and then applied to three sets of sample test items that span the cognitive domains of knowledge, comprehension, application, and analysis. This illustrates the increasing complexity of critical thinking required as the difficulty of questions increase in relation to the same nursing content.

This book contains 1225 questions that reflect a depth and breadth that comprehensively address the content commonly included in a fundamentals of nursing curriculum. They have been clustered by chapter into the related domains of: Chapter 2—Nursing Within the Context of Contemporary Health Care; Chapter 3—Psychosociocultural Nursing Care; Chapter 4—Essential Components of Nursing Care; and Chapter 5—Basic Human Needs and Related Nursing Care. Chapter 6, Alternate Question Formats, presents information regarding the new NCLEX item formats introduced in April 2003 by the National Council of State Boards of Nursing. Formats include questions that require test takers to fill in the blanks, identify multiple answers, perform a mathematical calculation, or respond to a question in relation to a graphic image, picture, or chart/table.

Questions for inclusion were selected considering content validity and the results of an elaborate field-testing process that included statistical item analyses and focus groups with student nurses to ensure quality questions. Every question in the book has rationales for the correct and incorrect answers. These questions can be used to apply the **RACE Model** to answering the questions, practice test taking, and study or review nursing content. Each section of questions in Chapters 2 through 5 is preceded by a list of keywords commonly associated with the content included in that area. Knowing the definition of these words and understanding information, concepts, and principles associated with these words will build a theoretical base for answering the questions in the content area. In addition, a Glossary of over 250 English words commonly encountered on nursing examinations is included in the back of the book for consideration by the reader. Familiarity with these words will refocus the challenge of a nursing examination away from the form of the test and back to the nursing content of the test.

Our goals were to produce more quality fundamentals of nursing questions and to design a model to assist nursing students to use critical thinking strategies when taking a nursing test. We believe we have attained our goals. However, only nursing students' and faculty members' responses to the book will determine if we have really achieved these goals.

Many people with F. A. Davis were essential to the production of this book. We especially want to thank Bob Martone, Publisher for Nursing, whose skills of listening, focusing, and prodding were instrumental to the progression of an idea into a manuscript. He shared our enthusiasm for this project throughout the publishing process without losing his sense of humor, and we value his knowledge and friendship. We gratefully acknowledge Alan Sorkowitz, of Alan Sorkowitz Editorial Services, for his valuable recommendations and editorial expertise that helped turn a manuscript into a book and clarify its unique benefits. Thanks also go to the entire F.A. Davis staff, and to Al Beringer of Maryland Publishing Services, who competently transformed our manuscript into a book.

Field-testing was essential to the development of quality multiple-choice nursing questions. We are grateful to Jean Hassett and Claudia Iannucci for their invaluable assistance in scheduling field-testing sessions, which required perseverance and attention to detail. Special recognition goes to all the nursing students that participated in field-testing sessions and focus groups for their commitment to excellence and generosity in sharing their time, energy, and intellects. Jordan Achilli, Creative Director, Hi Fidelity Design Products, turned our abstract thoughts into computer graphic art. We appreciate him for his expertise, patience, and professionalism. We acknowledge the interest and support we received from other nursing faculty, particularly Dr. MaryAnn Hellmer-Saul who listened and provided emotional encouragement. Finally, but most importantly, we would like to thank our husbands Neil and Joseph for their love, support, senses of humor, enthusiasm for life, and their attempts to keep our compulsive natures under control.

Patricia M. Nugent

Barbara A. Vitale

A Message to Nursing Students

Following the popularity of our book titled *TEST SUCCESS: Test-Taking Techniques for Beginning Nursing Students*, we conducted focus groups with nursing faculty and nursing students to determine what were their additional perceived needs. Nursing faculty was concerned about assisting students with developing intellectual reasoning skills and supporting students' personal qualities that promote effective inquiry. **"HOW CAN WE HELP OUR STUDENTS TO THINK CRITICALLY?"** Although beginning nursing students alluded to the concerns identified by faculty, their greatest concern was the need for more fundamentals-of-nursing questions with which to practice test taking. **"WE WANT MORE FUNDAMENTALS OF NURSING QUESTIONS!"** No book existed that applied critical thinking to answering fundamentals of nursing multiple-choice questions and provided questions that focused only on fundamentals of nursing curriculum content. This book, containing 1225 questions, was written to fill this void.

In the spring of 2003, the National Council of State Boards of Nursing announced that Alternate NCLEX Item Formats would be included on NCLEX after April 2003. Both students and faculty are asking, **"WHAT ARE INNOVATIVE QUESTIONS GOING TO LOOK LIKE?"** At the date of publication, no other textbook for beginning nursing students included information regarding Alternate NCLEX Item Formats or provided sample practice questions of Alternate NCLEX Item Formats. An entire chapter (Chapter 6) in *Fundamentals Success* was designed to fill this void.

If you are similar to the average nursing student, you read assigned chapters in your textbook and articles in nursing journals, review your classroom notes, complete computer instruction programs related to nursing content, practice nursing skills in a simulated laboratory, and apply in the clinical area what you have learned. All of these activities are excellent ways for you to expand and strengthen your theoretical base and become a safe practitioner of nursing. However, they may not be enough for you to be successful when taking a nursing examination. You need to practice test taking as early as possible in your program of study and with questions appropriate for your level of nursing education. In addition, you must be aware of, strengthen, and expand your cognitive competencies (intellectual reasoning skills) and personal competencies (individual attitudes or qualities) reflected in **The Helix of Critical Thinking**, and then utilize these components of critical thinking when answering nursing questions.

In this book, we discuss personal competencies and present the RACE Model to provide you with a blueprint for applying critical thinking to answering multiple-choice questions in nursing. **The components of the RACE Model are:**

R—**R**ecognize what information is in the stem.
A—**A**sk, What is the question asking?
C—**C**ritically analyze the options in relation to the question asked in the stem.
E—**E**liminate as many options as possible.

The theoretical framework of the RACE Model is explained and then applied to three sets of sample test questions that span the cognitive domains of knowledge, comprehension, application, and analysis. This illustrates for you the increasing complexity of critical thinking required as the difficulty of questions increases in relation to the same nursing content. In addition, the book contains 1200 multiple-choice questions organized into 24 content areas commonly included in a fundamentals of nursing curriculum. When answering these questions you can use critical thinking by applying the RACE model and practice test taking. When examining the rationales for the correct and incorrect answers you can review fundamentals of nursing content and identify what you still need to study.

For your personal development, each of the fundamentals of nursing content areas is preceded by a list of key words, nursing/medical terminology, concepts, principles, or information associated with the topics presented. In addition, a glossary of 250 English words commonly found in nursing multiple-choice questions is included at the end of the textbook. Familiarity with these words will refocus the challenge of a nursing examination away from defining the words in a test question and back to the theoretical content being evaluated in the test question.

WHY YOU SHOULD READ THIS TEXTBOOK: FEATURES AND BENEFITS

FEATURES	BENEFITS
Questions with formats other than multiple-choice questions	These questions will: Expose you to the new types of question formats that appear on NCLEX examinations. Allow you to practice nursing questions that incorporate multiple answers, fill in the blanks, graphic illustrations, tables/charts, and pictures. Reduce anxiety concerning alternate item formats you will be confronted with on NCLEX.
Key word lists at the beginning of each content chapter that include vocabulary, concepts, nursing/medical terminology, principles, and information	These words encourage you to focus on the critical components of a topic of study. Understanding these critical components expands your theoretical base and provides a strong foundation for more advanced concepts.
Glossary that identifies and defines ordinary English words that appear frequently in nursing examinations	Familiarity with these words reduces the challenge of a test question because you can center your attention on the theoretical content presented in the question.
A discussion of maximizing your critical thinking abilities including the attitudes and qualities of successful critical thinkers and strategies to overcome barriers to critical thinking	This discussion provides a basis for a self-assessment in relation to these qualities and introduces strategies that you can use to overcome barriers to your critical thinking. This discussion should motivate you to maintain a positive mental attitude and be reflective, inquisitive, and creative when thinking.
The RACE Model is introduced and applied to a variety of sample questions.	These concrete examples model the critical thinking processes involved when answering increasingly complex multiple-choice questions in nursing. This facilitates the imitation or emulation of the critical thinking activities used in the examples when you are confronted with answering a multiple-choice question in nursing. Ultimately, when you can

	critically analyze a question and answer it correctly, you will feel empowered and your test anxiety will decrease.
1225 quality fundamentals of nursing questions	These questions allow you to practice test taking and apply the use of critical thinking via the use of the RACE model. This should increase your critical thinking skills, promote your self-confidence, build your stamina when taking tests, and reduce test anxiety.
Rationales for the correct and incorrect answers for every question	Reviewing the rationales for every question will: Reinforce what you know—This increases trust in your ability and promotes a sense of security. Teach you new information—This increases your knowledge and builds self-confidence. Identify what you still need to learn—This focuses and prioritizes your study activities so that the return on your effort is maximized.

To increase your knowledge of fundamentals of nursing theory and experience success on nursing examinations, it is important for you to use this book—*Fundamentals Success: A Course Review Applying Critical Thinking to Test Taking*. Although this book is valuable for all nursing students regardless of their level of nursing education, it is essential for beginning nursing students. The related knowledge, attitudes, and skills that you develop early in your fundamental nursing courses influence your present and future educational performance. A house will stand and survive only when it is built on a strong foundation. The same concept can be applied to your nursing education. The components of a strong foundation in nursing are a comprehensive understanding of the fundamentals of nursing theory, well-developed critical thinking abilities, and an inventory of strategies for successful test taking.

Another textbook that you may find helpful to maximize your success when preparing for and taking examinations in nursing is *Test Success: Test-Taking Techniques for Beginning Nursing Students* (Authors: Nugent & Vitale, Publisher: F.A. Davis). This book focuses on empowerment, critical thinking, study techniques, the multiple-choice question, the nursing process, test-taking techniques, testing formats other than multiple-choice questions, and computer applications in education and evaluation. It also contains over 700 fundamentals of nursing questions with test-taking techniques and rationales for correct and incorrect answers for each question. Three simulated tests are included to mimic testing situations, and demonstrate progress in learning.

We are firm believers in the old sayings, "You get out of it what you put into it!" and "Practice makes perfect!" The extent of your learning, the attitudes you develop, and the skills you acquire depend on the energy you are willing to expend. It is our belief that if you give this book your best effort you will strengthen and expand your theoretical foundation of fundamentals of nursing and your critical thinking abilities in testing situations. We expect your efforts to be rewarded with success on your nursing examinations!

Contents

Fundamentals of Critical Thinking Related to Test Taking: The RACE Model

1

INTRODUCTION

The purpose of this book is to impress upon you that you already use critical thinking in your everyday life. Since you already use critical thinking, you should be able to apply the same thinking to your professional life. This book will help you to:

- Enhance your critical thinking abilities when studying.
- Employ critical thinking skills when taking a nursing examination.

HYSTERICAL PERSPECTIVES

To prepare for writing this chapter I did what all writers should do. I performed a detailed search of the literature about critical thinking, I reviewed all the significant materials that related to test taking or nursing practice, and I wrote an outline for a comprehensive discussion of critical thinking in relation to nursing examinations. The introductory section of the chapter was to be titled The Historical Perspective of Critical Thinking. When I typed the chapter heading and reread it, I had written "Hysterical" instead of "Historical." Having a relatively good sense of humor and the ability to laugh at myself, my response was peals of laughter. I realized that this was a Freudian slip! Loosely defined, a *Freudian slip* occurs when unconscious mental processes result in a verbal statement that reflects more accurately the true feelings of the speaker than does the originally intended statement. Being a true believer in the statement that *all behavior has meaning*, I could not continue until I explored why I wrote what I wrote.

When I looked up the word *hysterical* in the dictionary, its definition was *an uncontrollable outburst of emotion*, or *out of control* and *extremely comical or hilarious*. Associating the word hysterical to the concept of critical thinking raised 2 thoughts. Am I overwhelmed, frantic, and out of control when considering the relationship between critical thinking and nursing, or do I find this relationship funny, comical, and hilarious? If you feel overwhelmed, frenzied, or out of control when considering critical thinking, carefully read the section in this chapter titled *Be Positive: You Can Do It!* When I personalized the word to my own experiences, I recalled that when I believe that something is funny my internal communication is "Isn't that hysterically funny?" So, now I was faced with the task of exploring why I thought reviewing the historical perspective of critical thinking was so funny or why it could be overwhelming. I actually spent several hours pursuing this goal. At the completion of this process, I arrived at three conclusions:

- The words *critical thinking* are just buzz words. Critical thinking is a skill that we all possess uniquely, and we use this skill routinely in all the activities of our daily living. It is funny to profess that critical thinking is something new and different.
- Who cares about the historical perspectives of critical thinking! Information about the abstract topic of critical thinking must be presented in a manner that the information learned today can be implemented tomorrow.
- Feelings of being overwhelmed can be conquered because critical thinking abilities can be enhanced.

Definition of Critical Thinking

As I sat back and reflected on my morning's work in relation to Alfaro-LeFevre's (1995) definition of critical thinking, I recognized and appreciated the fact that I had been thoroughly involved with critical thinking. I had:

- Engaged in purposeful, goal-directed thinking.
- Aimed to make judgments based on evidence (fact) rather than conjecture (guess-work).
- Employed a process based on principles of science (e.g., problem solving, decision making).
- Used strategies (e.g., metacognition, reflection, Socratic questioning) that maximized my human potential and compensated for problems caused by human nature.

Critical thinking is a cognitive strategy by which you reflect on and analyze your thoughts, actions, and decisions. Critical thinking is often integrated into traditional linear processes. Linear processes usually follow a straight line, with a beginning and a product at the end. Some linear-like processes, such as the nursing process, are considered cyclical because they repeat themselves. Some formal reasoning processes include:

- **Problem Solving**—involves identifying a problem, exploring alternative interventions, implementing selected interventions, and arriving at the end product, which is a solution to the problem.
- **Decision Making**—involves carefully reviewing significant information, using methodical reasoning, and arriving at the end product, which is a decision.
- **Diagnostic Reasoning**—involves collecting information, correlating the collected information to standards, identifying the significance of the collected information, and arriving at the end product, which is a conclusion or nursing diagnosis.
- **The Scientific Method**—involves identifying a problem to be investigated, collecting data, formulating a hypothesis, testing the hypothesis through experimentation, evaluating the hypothesis, and arriving at the end product, which is acceptance or rejection of the hypothesis.
- **The Nursing Process**—involves collecting information (Assessment), determining significance of information and making a nursing diagnosis (Diagnosis), identifying goals, expected outcomes, and planning interventions (Planning), and implementing nursing interventions (Intervention), assessing the patient's response to interventions and comparing the actual to expected outcomes (Evaluation), and arriving at the end product, which is meeting a person's needs.

Each of these methods of manipulating and processing information incorporates critical thinking. They all are influenced by intellectual standards such as focused, methodical, deliberate, logical, relevant, accurate, precise, clear, comprehensive, creative, and reflective. It is helpful to incorporate critical thinking into whatever framework or structure works for you.

The purpose of this discussion was to impress on you that you:

- Use critical thinking in your personal life.
- Will continue to use critical thinking in your professional life.
- Should enhance your critical thinking abilities when studying.
- Can employ critical thinking skills when taking a nursing examination.

In an attempt to make the abstract aspects of critical thinking more concrete, we have schematically represented our concept of thinking by the Helix of Critical Thinking. In Figure 1-1 the Helix of Critical Thinking has been unwound and enlarged so that the components of the cognitive competencies and personal competencies can be viewed easily. The cognitive competencies are the intellectual or reasoning processes employed when thinking. The personal competencies are the characteristics or attitudes of the individual thinker. These lists of competencies represent the cognitive abilities or personal qualities commonly associated with critical thinkers. No one possesses all of these competencies, and you may identify competencies that you possess that are not on these lists. The lists are not all-inclusive. Make lists of your own cognitive and personal competencies. Your lists represent your repertoire or inventory of thinking skills. As you gain knowledge and experience, your lists will expand. The more cognitive and personal competencies you possess, the greater your potential to think critically.

The Helix of Critical Thinking (Fig. 1-2) demonstrates the integration of cognitive competencies and personal competencies essential to thinking critically. Not all of these competencies are used in every thinking situation. You can pick or choose from them as from a smorgasbord when you are confronted with situations that require critical thinking. Initially you may have to stop and consciously consider what cognitive competencies (intellectual skills) or personal competencies (abilities, attitudes) to use. As you gain knowledge and experience and move toward becoming an expert critical thinker, the use of these competencies becomes second nature. The Helix will contract or expand depending on the competencies you utilize in a particular circumstance. In addition, there is constant interaction among cognitive competencies, among personal competencies, and between cognitive competencies and personal competencies.

The interactive nature of the Helix of Critical Thinking and the Nursing Process is demonstrated in Figure 1-3. The Nursing Process is a dynamic, cyclical process in which each phase interacts with and is influenced by the other phases of the process. The Nursing Process provides a precise framework in which purposeful thinking occurs. Critical thinking is an essential component within, between, and among the phases of the Nursing Process. Different combinations of cognitive and personal competencies may be used during the different phases of the Nursing Process.

The interactive nature of the Helix of Critical Thinking and the Problem-Solving Process is demonstrated in Figure 1-4. The Problem-Solving Process is a dynamic, linear process that has a beginning and an end, with a resolution of the identified problem. The Problem-Solving Process provides a progressive step-by-step method in which goal-directed thinking occurs. Critical thinking is an essential component within and between the steps of the Problem-Solving Process. Different combinations of cognitive and personal competencies may be used during the different steps of the Problem-Solving Process.

MAXIMIZE YOUR CRITICAL THINKING ABILITIES

Be Positive: You Can Do It!

Assuming responsibility for the care one delivers to a patient and desiring a commendable grade on a nursing examination raise anxiety because a lot is at stake: to keep the patient safe; to achieve a passing grade; to become a nurse ultimately; and to support one's self-esteem. The most important skill that you can learn to help you achieve all of these goals is to be an accomplished critical thinker. We use critical thinking skills every day in our lives when we explore, "What will I have for breakfast?" "How can I get to school from my home?" and "Where is the best place to get gas for my car?" Once you recognize that you are *thinking* critically already, it is more manageable to *think* about *thinking* critically. If you feel threatened by the idea of critical thinking then you must do something positive to confront the threat. You need to be disciplined and to work at increasing your sense of control, which contributes to confidence! YOU CAN DO IT!

OVERCOME BARRIERS TO A POSITIVE MENTAL ATTITUDE

Supporting a positive mental attitude requires developing discipline and confidence. **Discipline** is defined as self-command or self-direction. The disciplined person will work in a planned manner, explore all options in an organized and logical way, check for accuracy, and seek excellence. When you work in a planned and systematic

Cognitive Competencies	Personal Competencies
Dissect	Tolerant of ambiguity
Modify	Think independently
Analyze	Perseverance
Interpret	Self-confident
Examine	Open-minded
Correlate	Accountable
Synthesize	Courageous
Recall facts	Imaginative
Investigate	Disciplined
Categorize	Committed
Summarize	Inquisitive
Understand	Motivated
Demonstrate	Risk taker
Self-examine	Confident
Translate data	Reflective
Query evidence	Objective
Make inferences	Authentic
Manipulate facts	Assertive
Present arguments	Intuitive
Establish priorities	Rational
Make generalizations	Creative
Compare and contrast	Humble
Determine significance	Curious
Determine implications	Honest
Determine consequences	Moral

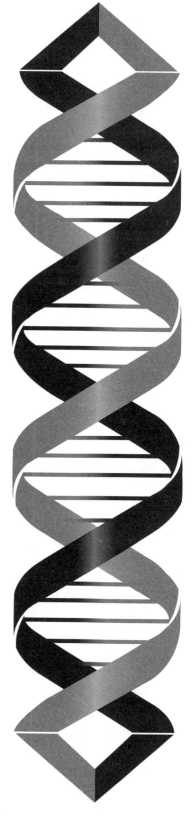

Figure 1–1. The Helix of Critical Thinking schematically elongated to demonstrate the components of cognitive competencies and personal competencies. The more cognitive competencies and personal competencies a person possesses, the greater the potential the person has to think critically.

Figure 1–2. The Helix of Critical Thinking demonstrates the interwoven relationship between cognitive competencies and personal competencies essential to thinking critically. Throughout the thinking process there is constant interaction among cognitive competencies, among personal competencies, and between cognitive and personal competencies.

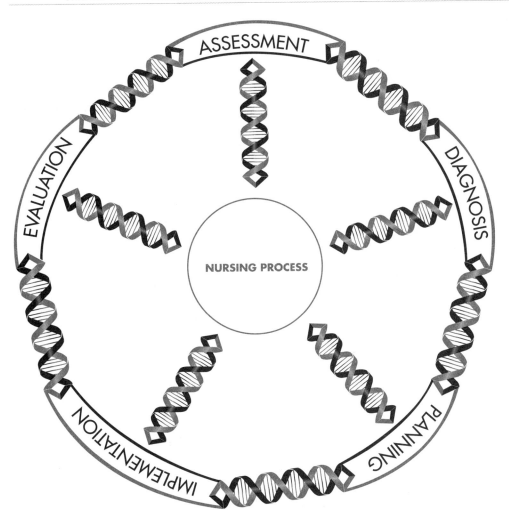

Figure 1–3. The interactive nature of the Helix of Critical Thinking within the Nursing Process. The Nursing Process is a dynamic, cyclical process in which each phase interacts with and is influenced by the other phases of the process. Critical thinking is an essential component within, between, and among phases of the Nursing Process. Different combinations of cognitive and personal competencies may be used during the different phases of the Nursing Process.

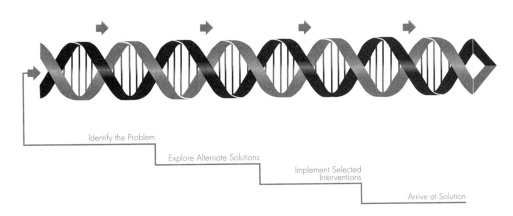

Figure 1–4. The interactive nature of the Helix of Critical Thinking within the Problem-Solving Process. The Problem-Solving Process is a dynamic, linear process that has a beginning and end, with the resolution of the identified problem. Different combinations of cognitive and personal competencies may be used during the different steps of the Problem-Solving Process.

manner with conscious effort, you are more organized, and therefore more disciplined. Disciplined people generally have more control over the variables associated with an intellectual task. Effective critical thinkers are disciplined, and discipline helps to develop confidence.

Confidence is defined as poise, self-reliance, or self-assurance. Confidence increases as one matures in the role of the student nurse. Understanding your strengths and limitations is the first step to increasing confidence. When you know your strengths you can draw on them and when you know your limitations you know when it is time to seek out the instructor or another resource to help you in your critical thinking. Either way, you are in control! For example, ask the instructor for help in critically analyzing a case study, share with the instructor any concerns you have about a clinical assignment, and seek out the instructor in the clinical area when you feel the need for support. Failing to use your instructor is like putting your head in the sand. Learning needs must be addressed, not avoided. Although your instructor is responsible for your clinical practice and for stimulating your intellectual growth as a nursing student, you are the consumer of your nursing education. As the consumer, you must be an active participant in your own learning by ensuring that you get the assistance and experiences you need to build your abilities and confidence. When you increase your theoretical and experiential knowledge base, you will increase your sense of control, which ultimately increases your confidence. This applies not just to beginning nursing students but every level of practice because of the explosion in information and technology. When you are disciplined you are more in control, when you are more in control you are more confident, and when you are more confident you have a more positive mental attitude.

Be Reflective: You Need to Take One Step Backward before Taking Two Steps Forward!

Reflection is the process of thinking back or recalling a situation or event to rediscover its meaning. It helps you to seek and understand the relationships among information, concepts, and principles and to apply them in future clinical or testing situations. Reflection can be conducted internally as quiet thoughtful consideration, in a one-on-one discussion with an instructor or another student, or in a group.

As a beginning nursing student, you are just starting to develop an experiential background from the perspective of a health care provider. However, you have a wealth of experiences, personal and educational, that influence your development as a professional nurse. Your personal experiences include activities such as using verbal and written communication, delegating tasks to family members or coworkers, setting priorities for daily activities, using mathematics when shopping or balancing a checkbook, etc. A nursing program of study incorporates courses from a variety of other disciplines such as anatomy and physiology, chemistry, physics, psychology, sociology, reading, writing, mathematics, informatics, etc. Every single experience is a potential valuable resource for future learning. Recognize the value of "the you" you bring to your nursing education and incorporate it into your reflective processes.

Engaging in reflection is a highly individualized mental process. One form of reflection is writing a journal. A **journal** is an objective and subjective diary of your experiences. It is a chronicle that includes cognitive learning, feelings, and attitudes, and requires you to actively develop skills related to assessing, exploring the meaning of critical incidents, documenting, developing insights into thoughts and actions that comprise clinical practice, and evaluating. Journal writing is a rich resource that provides a written record of where you have been, where you are, and where you are going. It helps you to incorporate experiences into the development of your professional being. After an examination, explore your feelings and attitudes regarding the experience. Be honest with yourself. Did you prepare adequately for the test? Did you find the content harder or easier than content on another test? Were you anxious before, during, or after the test and, if so, was it low, medium, or high? What would a low score or high score on the test mean to you? When you were confronted with a question that you perceived as difficult, how did you feel and how did you cope with the feeling? You do not necessarily have to ask yourself all of these questions. You should ask yourself those questions that have meaning for you.

Another form of reflection is making **mental pictures** of information under consideration one day for recall in the future. For example, when caring for a patient who has Parkinson's disease, compare the patient's adaptations to the classic adaptations associated with the disease. Then make a visual picture of this patient's classic adaptations in your mind. Visualize the pill-rolling tremors, mask-like face, drooling, muscle rigidity, etc. so that in the future you can recall the visual picture rather than having to remember a memorized list of symptoms.

Retrospective (after the event) reflection involves seeking an understanding of relationships between previously learned information and the application of this information in patient-care situations or testing experiences. This type of reflection helps you to judge your personal performance against standards of practice. A self-assessment requires the willingness to be open to identifying one's successful and unsuccessful interventions, strengths and weaknesses, and knowledge and lack of knowledge. The purpose of retrospective reflection is not to be judgmental or to second-guess decisions but rather to learn from the situation. The worth of the reflection depends on the abilities that result from it. When similar situations arise in subsequent clinical practice, previous actions that were reinforced or modified can be accessed to have a present successful outcome.

A *clinical postconference* is an example of retrospective reflection. Students often meet in a group (formally or informally) after a clinical experience to review the day's events. During the discussion students have an opportunity to explore feelings and attitudes, consider interventions and alternative interventions, assess decision making and problem solving skills, identify how they and other students think through a situation, etc. You can also review your own thinking when reviewing a patient experience by speaking aloud what you were thinking. For example,

> "When I went into the room to take my postoperative patient's vital signs I realized that the patient had an IV in the right arm. I knew that if I took a blood pressure in the arm with an IV it could interfere with the IV so I knew I had to take the blood pressure in the left arm. When I looked at my patient, he looked very pale and sweaty. I got a little nervous but I continued to get the other vital signs. I put the thermometer in the patient's mouth and started to take his pulse. It was very fast and I knew that this was abnormal so I paid special attention to its rhythm and volume. It was very thready but it was regular. The temperature and respirations were within the high side of the normal range." A beginning nursing student may immediately respond by saying, "I don't know what is going on here so I better take this information to my instructor." A more advanced student might say, "What could be happening? Maybe the patient is bleeding or has an infection. I think I should inform my instructor but I'll inspect the incision first."

When you review an experience like this example, you can identify your thinking skills. Taking the blood pressure in the left arm and assessing the rate, rhythm, and volume of the pulse were habits because you did not have to figure out a new method when responding to the situation. Remembering the normal range for the various vital signs used the thinking skill of total recall because you memorized and internalized the normal values. Determining further assessments after obtaining the vital signs required inquiry. You collected and analyzed information and did not take the vital sign results at just face value. You recognized abnormalities and gaps in information, collected additional data, considered alternative conclusions, and identified alternative interventions.

Another example of retrospective reflection is reviewing an examination. When reviewing each question determine why you got a question wrong in relation to one of the following three factors.

- I did not understand what the question was asking because of the English or medical vocabulary used in the question.
- I did not know or understand the content being tested.
- I knew the content being tested but I did not apply it correctly in the question.

When a limited English or medical vocabulary prevents you from answering a question correctly, you must spend time expanding this foundation. A list of English words that appear repeatedly in nursing examinations is included in a glossary at the end of this textbook. In addition, nursing/medical keyword lists have been included in each content area in this textbook. You can use these word lists to review key terminology used in nursing-related topics. To expand your vocabulary, keep English and medical dictionaries at your side when studying and look up new words, write flash cards for words you need to learn, and explore unfamiliar words that confront you on tests.

When you answered a question incorrectly because you did not understand the content, make a list so that you can design a study session devoted to reviewing this information. This study session should begin with a brief review of what you do know about the topic (5 minutes or less). The majority of your efforts should be devoted to studying what you identified as what you need to know. You should do this after reviewing every test. This exercise is based on the axiom *strike while the iron is hot*. The test is over, so your anxiety level is reduced and how nursing-related content is used in a test question is fresh in your mind. Study sessions that are goal directed tend to be more focused and productive.

When you know the content being tested but have applied the information incorrectly, it is an extremely frustrating experience. However, do not become deflated. It is motivating to recognize that you actually know the content! Your next task is to explore how to tap your knowledge successfully. Sometimes restating or summarizing what the question is asking places it into your own perspective, which helps to clarify the content in relation to the test question. You can also view the question in relation to specific past experiences or by reviewing the information in two different textbooks to obtain different views on the same content. Another strategy to reinforce your learning is to use the left page of your notebook for taking class notes and leave the facing page blank. After an examination, use the blank page to make comments to yourself about how the content was addressed in test questions or add information from your textbook to clarify class notes. How to review thinking strategies in relation to cognitive levels of nursing questions is explored later in this chapter.

Examine your test-taking behaviors. For example, if you consistently changed your initial answers on a test, it is wise to explore what factors influenced you to change your answers. In addition, determine how many questions were converted to either right or wrong answers. The information you collect from this assessment should influence your future behaviors. If you consistently changed correct answers to incorrect answers, you need to examine the factors that caused you to change your answers. Maybe you should even leave your eraser at home in the future. If you changed incorrect answers to correct answers, you should identify what mental processes were used to arrive at your second choice so that you can use them the first time you look at a question.

Reflection is an essential component of all learning. How can you know where you are going without knowing where you have been? Therefore, to enhance your critical thinking abilities you must TAKE ONE STEP BACKWARDS BEFORE TAKING TWO STEPS FORWARD!

OVERCOME BARRIERS TO EFFECTIVE REFLECTION

Reflecting on your knowledge, strengths, and successes is easy, but reflecting on your lack of knowledge, weakness, and mistakes takes courage and humility. **Courage** is the attitude of confronting anything recognized as dangerous or difficult without avoiding or withdrawing from the situation. Courage is necessary because when people look at their shortcomings they tend to be judgmental and are their own worst critics. This type of negativity must be avoided because it promotes defensive thinking, interferes with the reception of new information, and limits self-confidence.

Humility is having a modest opinion of one's own abilities. Humility is necessary because it is important to admit your limitations. Only when you identify what you do and do not know can you make a plan to acquire the knowledge necessary to be successful on nursing examinations and practice safe nursing care. Arrogance or a "know it all" attitude can interfere with maximizing your potential. For example, when reviewing examinations with students, the students that benefit the most are the ones who are willing to listen to their peers or instructor as to why the correct answer is correct. The students who benefit the least are the ones who consistently and vehemently defend their wrong answers. A healthy amount of inquiry, thoughtful questioning, and not accepting statements at their face value are important critical thinking competencies; however, a self-righteous or obstructionist attitude more often than not impedes, rather than promotes, learning.

Be Inquisitive: If You Don't Go There, You'll Never Get Anywhere!

Inquiry means to question or investigate. The favorite words of inquisitive people are: *what*, *where*, *when*, and most importantly *how* and *why*; *if … then*; and *it depends*. When studying, ask yourself these words to delve further into a topic under consideration. Below are examples as illustrations.

- You raise the head of the bed when a patient is short of breath. You recognize that this intervention will facilitate respirations. Ask yourself the question, "*How* does this intervention facilitate respirations?" The answer could be, "Raising the head of the bed allows the abdominal organs to drop by gravity, which reduces pressure against the diaphragm, which in turn permits maximal thoracic expansion."
- You insert an indwelling urinary catheter and are confronted with the decision as to where to place the drainage bag. Ask yourself *what* questions. "*What* will happen if I place the drainage bag on the bed frame?" The answer could be, "Urine will flow into the drainage bag by gravity." "*What* will happen if I place the drainage bag on an IV pole." The answer could be, "Urine will remain in the bladder because the IV pole is above the level of the bladder and fluid does not flow up hill, and if there is urine in the bag it will flow back into the bladder."
- When palpating a pulse you should use gentle compression. Ask yourself the question, "*Why* should I use gentle compression?" The answer could be, "Gentle compression allows you to feel the pulsation of the artery and prevents excessive pressure on the artery that will cut off circulation and thus obliterate the pulse."
- The textbook says that in emergencies nurses should always assess the airway first. Immediately ask, "*Why* should I assess the airway first?" There may be a variety of answers. "In an emergency, follow the ABCs of assessment which always begins with airway. Maslow's Hierarchy of Needs identifies that physiologic needs should be met first. Because an airway is essential for the passage of life-sustaining gases in and out of the lung." Although all of these responses answer the question why, only the last answer really provides an in-depth answer to the *why* question. If your response to the original *why* question still raises a *why* question, you need to delve deeper. "*Why* do the ABCs of assessment begin with airway?" "Why should physiologic needs be met first?"
- When talking with a patient about an emotionally charged topic, the patient begins to cry. You are confronted with a variety of potential responses. Use the method of *if … then* statements. *If … then* thinking links an action to a consequence. For example, if I remain silent, then the patient may refocus on what was said. If I say, "You seem very sad?" then the patient may discuss the feelings being felt at the time. If I respond with an open-ended statement, then the patient may pursue the topic in relation to individualized concerns. After you explore a variety of courses of action with the *if … then* method, you should be in a better position to choose the most appropriate intervention for the situation.
- You will recognize that you have arrived at a more advanced level of critical thinking when determining that your next course of action is based on the concept of *It depends*. For example, a patient suddenly becomes extremely short of breath and you decide to administer oxygen during this emergency. When considering the amount and route of delivery of the oxygen, you recognize that *it depends*. You need to collect more data. You need to ask more questions such as, "Is the patient already receiving oxygen? Does the patient have a chronic obstructive pulmonary disease?

Is the patient a mouth breather? What other adaptations is the patient exhibiting?" The answers to these questions will influence your choice of interventions.

When exploring the *how, what, where, when, why, if … then,* and *it depends* methods of inquiry, you are more likely to arrive at appropriate inferences, assumptions, and conclusions that will ensure safe, effective nursing care.

These same techniques of inquiry can be used when practicing test taking. Reviewing textbooks that have questions with rationales is an excellent way to explore the reasons for correct and incorrect answers. When answering a question, state why you think your choice is the correct answer and why you think each of the other options is an incorrect answer. This encourages you to focus on the reasons why you responded in a certain way in a particular situation. It prevents you from making quick judgments (choice of correct versus incorrect answers) before exploring the rationales for your actions. After you have done this, compare your rationales to the rationales for the correct and incorrect answers in the textbook. Are your rationales focused, methodical, deliberate, logical, relevant, accurate, precise, clear, comprehensive, creative, and reflective? This method of studying not only reviews nursing content but it fosters critical thinking and applies critical thinking to test taking.

During or after the review of an examination these techniques of inquiry also can be employed, particularly with those questions you got wrong. Although you can conduct this review independently, it is more valuable to review test questions in a group. Your peers and the instructor are valuable resources that you should use to facilitate your learning. Different perspectives, experiential backgrounds, and levels of expertise can enhance your inquiry. Be inquisitive. IF YOU DON'T GO THERE, YOU'LL NEVER GET ANYWHERE.

OVERCOME BARRIERS TO BEING INQUISITIVE

Effective inquiry requires more than just a simplistic, cursory review of a topic. Therefore, critical thinkers must have curiosity, perseverance, and motivation. **Curiosity** is the desire to learn or know and is a requirement to delve deeper into a topic. If you are uninterested in or apathetic about a topic, you are not going to go that extra mile. Sometimes you may have to "psych yourself up" to study a particular topic. Students frequently say they are overwhelmed by topics such as fluid and electrolytes, blood gases, or chest tubes. As a result, they develop a minimal understanding of these topics and are willing to learn by trial and error in the clinical area or surrender several questions on an examination. Never be willing to let a lack of knowledge be the norm because this results in incompetence, and never give away credits on an examination! Overcome this attitude by maximizing your perseverance.

Perseverance means willingness to continue in some effort or course of action despite difficulty or opposition. Critical thinkers never give up until they obtain the information that satisfies their curiosity. To perform a comprehensive inquiry when studying requires time. Make a schedule for studying at the beginning of the week and adhere to it. This prevents procrastination later in the week when you will prefer to rationalize doing something else and postpone studying. In addition, studying an hour a day is more effective than studying 7 hours in one day. Breaks between study periods allow for the processing of information, and they provide time to rest and regain focus and concentration. The greatest barrier to perseverance is a deadline. When working under a time limit you may not have enough time to process and understand information. The length of time to study for a test depends on the amount and type of content to be tested and how much previous studying has been done. If you study 2 hours every day for 2 weeks during a unit of instruction, a 1-hour review may be adequate for an examination addressing this content. If you are preparing for a comprehensive examination for a course at the end of the semester, you may decide to study 3 hours a night for 1 to 2 weeks. If you are studying for the NCLEX-RN you may decide to study 2 hours a day for 3 months. Only you can determine how much time you need to study or prepare for a test. Perseverance can be enhanced by the use of motivation strategies.

Motivation strategies inspire, prompt, encourage, instigate, or enthuse you to act.

For example, divide the information to be learned into segments and set multiple short-term goals for studying. After you reach a goal, cross it off the list. Also, this is the time to use incentives. Reward yourself after an hour of studying. Think about how proud you will be when you earn an excellent grade on the examination. Visualize yourself walking down the isle at graduation or working as a nurse during your career. Incentives can be more tangible; e.g., having a beverage, reading a book for 10 minutes, playing with your children, or doing anything that strikes your fancy. You need to identify the best pattern of studying that satisfies your needs, use motivation techniques to increase your enthusiasm, and then draw on your determination to explore in depth the *how, what, where, when,* and *whys, If ... then,* and *it depends* of nursing practice.

Be Creative: You Must Think Outside the Box!

A **creative** person is imaginative, inventive, innovative, resourceful, original, and visionary. To find solutions beyond common, predictable, and standardized procedures or practices you must be creative. Creativity is what allows you to be yourself and individualize the nursing care you provide to each patient. With the explosion of information and technology, the importance of thinking creatively will increase in the future because the "old" ways of doing things will be inadequate. Nor are any two situations or people ever alike. Therefore, YOU MUST THINK OUTSIDE THE BOX!

OVERCOME BARRIERS TO CREATIVITY

To be creative you must be open-minded, have independence of thought, and be a risk-taker. It is difficult to think outside the box when you are not willing to color outside the lines! Being **open-minded** requires you to consider a wide range of ideas, concepts, and opinions before framing an opinion or making judgments. You need to identify your opinions, beliefs, biases, stereotypes, and prejudices. We all have them to one extent or another, so do not deny them. However, they must be recognized, compartmentalized, and placed on a "back burner." Unless these attitudes are placed in perspective, they will interfere with creative thinking. In every situation you need to remain open to all perspectives, not just your own. When you think that your opinion is the only right opinion, you are engaging in egocentric thinking. Egocentric thinking is based on the belief that the world exists or can be known only in relation to the individual's mind. This rigid thinking creates a barrier around your brain that obstructs the inflow of information, imaginative thinking, and the outflow of innovative ideas. An example of an instance in which you have been open-minded is one in which you have changed your mind after having had a discussion with someone else. The new information convinced you to think outside of your original thoughts and opinions.

Independence of thought means the ability to consider all the possibilities and then arrive at an autonomous conclusion. To do this you need to feel comfortable with ambiguity. Ambiguous means having two or more meanings and is therefore being uncertain, unclear, indefinite, and vague. For example, a nursing student may be taught by an instructor to establish a sterile field for a sterile dressing change by using the inside of the package of the sterile gloves. When following a sterile dressing change procedure in a clinical skills book, the directions may state to use a separate sterile cloth for the sterile field. When practicing this procedure with another student, the other student may open several 4×4 gauze packages and leave them open as their sterile fields. As a beginning nursing student, this is difficult to understand because of a limited relevant knowledge base and experiential background. Thinking frequently is concrete and follows rules and procedures, is black and white, or is correct or incorrect. It takes knowledge and experience to recognize that you have many options and may still follow the principles of sterile technique. One nursing faculty member loves to say, "There is more than one road to Philadelphia!"

To travel a different path requires taking risks. Risk in the dictionary means the chance of injury, damage, or loss. However, **risk-taking** in relation to nursing refers to considering all the options, eliminating potential danger to a patient, and acting in a reasoned, logical, and safe manner when implementing unique interventions. Being creative requires intellectual stamina and a willingness to go where no one has been before. Risk-takers tend to be leaders, not followers. The greatest personal risk of creativity is the blow to the ego when confronted with failure. However, you must recognize that throughout your nursing career you will be faced with outcomes that are successful as well as those that are unsuccessful. How you manage your feelings with regard to each, particularly those that are unsuccessful, will influence your willingness to take future creative risks. Successful outcomes build confidence. If appropriately examined unsuccessful outcomes should not be defeating or prevent future creativity. The whole purpose of evaluation in the nursing process is to compare and contrast patient outcomes with expected outcomes. If expected outcomes are not attained, the entire process must be re-examined and than re-performed. You must recognize that:

* unsuccessful outcomes do occur
* unsuccessful outcomes are not a reflection on your competence
* the number of successful outcomes far out-number the unsuccessful outcomes

When you accept these facts, then you may feel confident to take risks with your creativity.

CRITICAL THINKING APPLIED TO TEST TAKING

Educational Domains

Nursing as a discipline includes three domains of learning—affective, psychomotor, and cognitive. The **affective domain** is concerned with attitudes, values, and the development of appreciations. An example of nursing care in the affective domain is the nurse quietly accepting a patient's statement that there is no God without imposing personal beliefs on the patient. The **psychomotor domain** is concerned with manipulative or motor skills related to procedures or physical interventions. An example of nursing care in the psychomotor domain is the nurse administering an intramuscular injection to a patient. The **cognitive domain** is concerned with recall, recognition of knowledge, comprehension, and the development and application of intellectual skills and abilities. An example of nursing care in the cognitive domain is the nurse clustering collected information and determining its significance. When discussing the application of critical thinking to test taking, the focus will be on the cognitive domain.

Components of a Multiple-Choice Question

A multiple-choice question is called an **item**. Each item has two parts. The **stem** is the part that contains the information that identifies the topic and its parameters and then asks a question. The second part consists of one or more possible responses, which are called **options**. One of the options is the **correct answer** and the others are wrong answers (called **distractors**).

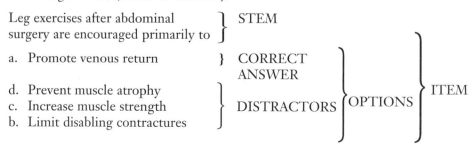

Leg exercises after abdominal surgery are encouraged primarily to — STEM

a. Promote venous return — CORRECT ANSWER

d. Prevent muscle atrophy
c. Increase muscle strength
b. Limit disabling contractures — DISTRACTORS — OPTIONS — ITEM

Cognitive Levels of Nursing Questions

Questions on nursing examinations reflect a variety of thinking processes that nurses use when caring for patients. These thinking processes are part of the cognitive domain and they progress from the simple to the complex, from the concrete to the abstract, and from the tangible to the intangible. There are four types of thinking processes represented by nursing questions.

- **Knowledge Questions** - the emphasis is on recalling remembered information.
- **Comprehension Questions** - the emphasis is on understanding the meaning and intent of remembered information.
- **Application Questions** - the emphasis is on remembering understood information and utilizing the information in new situations.
- **Analysis Questions** - the emphasis is on comparing and contrasting a variety of elements of information.

THE RACE MODEL: THE APPLICATION OF CRITICAL THINKING TO MULTIPLE-CHOICE QUESTIONS

Answering a test question is like participating in a race. Of course, you want to come in first and be the winner. However, the thing to remember about a race is that success is not just based on speed but also on strategy and tactics. The same is true about success on nursing examinations. Although speed may be a variable that must be considered when taking a timed test so that the amount of time spent on each question is factored into the test strategy, the emphasis on RACE is the use of critical-thinking techniques to answer multiple-choice questions. The **RACE Model** presented below is a critical-thinking strategy to use when answering nursing multiple-choice questions. If you follow the **RACE Model** every time you examine a test question, its use will become second nature. This methodical approach will improve your abilities to critically analyze a test question and improve your chances of selecting the correct answer.

The **RACE Model** has four steps to answering a test question. The best way to remember the four steps is to refer to the acronym **RACE.**

R - **R**ecognize what information is in the stem.
- **R**ecognize the key words in the stem
- **R**ecognize who the client is in the stem
- **R**ecognize what the topic is about

A - **A**sk what is the question asking?
- **A**sk what are the key words in the stem that indicate the need for a response
- **A**sk what the question is asking me to do

C - **C**ritically analyze the options in relation to the question asked in the stem.
- **C**ritically scrutinize each option in relation to the information in the stem
- **C**ritically identify a rationale for each option
- **C**ritically compare and contrast the options in relation to the information in the stem and their relationships to one another.

E - **E**liminate as many options as possible.
- **E**liminate one option at a time.

The following discussion explores the **RACE Model** in relation to the thinking processes represented in multiple-choice nursing questions. Thoughtfully read several times the *Cognitive Requirements* under each type of question (Knowledge, Comprehension, Analysis, and Application). This content is important to understand to apply the critical thinking strategies inherent in each cognitive level question as you apply the **RACE Model**. In addition, 3 sets of sample test questions are presented to demonstrate the increasing complexity of thinking reflected in the various levels focusing on specific fundamentals of nursing content.

Knowledge Questions: Remember Information!

COGNITIVE REQUIREMENTS

Knowledge is information that is filed or stored in the brain. It represents the elements essential to the core of a discipline. In nursing, this information consists of elements such as terminology and specific facts including steps of procedures, phenomena, normal laboratory values, classifications, and the ranges of vital signs. When using this information it requires no alteration from one use or application to another because it is concrete. The information is recalled or recognized in the form in which it was learned originally. This information is the foundation of critical thinking. You must have adequate, accurate, relevant, and important information on which to base your more theoretical, abstract thinking in the future.

Beginning nursing students find knowledge level questions the easiest because they require just the recall or regurgitation of information. Information may be memorized, which involves repeatedly reviewing information to place it and keep it in the brain. Information also can be committed to memory through repeated experiences with the information. Repetition is necessary because information is forgotten quickly unless reinforced. When answering knowledge level questions you either know the information or you don't. The challenge of answering knowledge questions is defining what the question is asking and tapping your knowledge. See the textbook *TEST SUCCESS: Test-Taking Techniques for Beginning Nursing Students*, F.A. Davis publishers, for specific study techniques related to knowledge level questions.

APPLICATION OF THE RACE MODEL TO KNOWLEDGE QUESTIONS

1. What is the classification of the medication docusate sodium (Colace)?
   a. Diuretic
   b. Laxative
   c. Bronchodilator
   d. Antihypertensive

RACE:

Recognize key words (highlighted). **R**ecognize who the client is. **R**ecognize what the topic is about.	What is the **classification** of the drug **docusate sodium (Colace)**? There is no client in this question. The classification of the drug docusate sodium (Colace).
Ask what the question is asking.	It is asking you to identify **what the classification of docusate sodium (Colace) is**.
Critically analyze options in relation to the question.	This question does not require complex understanding, comparative analysis or application skills, it only requires recall of information about docusate sodium (Colace). **Rationales:** a. Diuretics are medications that increase urine secretion. Docusate sodium (Colace) is not a diuretic. **b. Laxatives are medications that promote the elimination of fecal material. Docusate sodium (Colace) is a laxative.** c. Bronchodilators are medications that dilate the bronchi of the lungs. Docusate sodium (Colace) is not a bronchodilator. d. Antihypertensives are medications that reduce the blood pressure. Docusate sodium (Colace) is not an antihypertensive.
Eliminate incorrect options.	Because a, c, and d are not the name of the classification of docusate sodium (Colace) they can be eliminated.

2.   What is the description of the interviewing technique of paraphrasing?
     a. Asking the patient to repeat what was just said
     b. Condensing a discussion into an organized review
     c. Restating what the patient has said using similar words
     d. Asking goal-directed questions concentrating on key concerns

RACE:

Recognize key words (high-lighted). **R**ecognize who the client is. **R**ecognize what the topic is about.	What is the **description** of the interviewing technique of **paraphrasing**? There is no client in this question. The interviewing technique of paraphrasing.
Ask what the question is asking.	The question is asking you **what is the description of paraphrasing**.
Critically analyze options in relation to the question.	To answer this question you must know the definition or characteristic of paraphrasing. It is information that you must recall from your memory. You do not have to know other interviewing skills or their descriptions and characteristics to answer this question. **Rationales**: a. Asking a patient to repeat what was just asked is known as clarifying, not paraphrasing. b. Reviewing a discussion is known as summarizing, not paraphrasing. c. **Paraphrasing or restating is an interviewing skill where the nurse listens for a patient's basic message and then repeats the contents of the message in similar words. This validates information from the patient without changing the meaning of the statement and provides an opportunity for the patient to hear what was said.** d. Asking goal-directed questions concentrating on key concerns is known as focusing, not paraphrasing.
Eliminate incorrect options.	Options a, b, and d are not examples of paraphrasing and can be eliminated.

3.   What is another name for a decubitus ulcer?
     a. Skin tear
     b. Pressure ulcer
     c. Surface abrasion
     d. Penetrating wound

RACE:

Recognize key words (high-lighted). **R**ecognize who the client is. **R**ecognize what the topic is about.	What is **another name** for **decubitus ulcer**? There is no client in this question. The names for decubitus ulcers.
Ask what the question is asking.	The question is asking you to identify **what is another name for decubitus ulcer**.
Critically analyze options in relation to the question.	To answer this question you must know the alternate name for a decubitus ulcer. It is information you must recollect from your memory. You do not have to know the description or characteristics of other types of wounds to answer this question.

continued

RACE: *continued*

	Rationales:
	a. A skin tear is a break in the continuity of thin, fragile skin caused by friction or shearing force.
	b. A pressure ulcer is impaired skin (reddened area, sore, or lesion characterized by sloughing of tissue) over a bony prominence caused by pressure that interferes with the delivery of oxygen to body cells.
	c. An abrasion is the scraping or rubbing away of the superficial layers of the skin.
	d. A penetrating wound occurs when a sharp object pierces the skin and injures underlying tissues.
Eliminate incorrect options	Options a. c, and d are not other names for a decubitus ulcer and can be eliminated.

Comprehension Questions: Understand Information!

COGNITIVE REQUIREMENTS

Comprehension is the ability to understand that which is known. To be safe practitioners, nurses must understand information such as reasons for nursing interventions, physiology and pathophysiology, consequences of actions, and responses to medications. To reach an understanding of information in nursing you must be able to translate information into your own words to personalize its meaning. Once information is rearranged in your own mind, you must interpret the essential components for their intent, corollaries, significance, implications, consequences, and conclusions in accordance with the conditions described in the original communication. The information is manipulated within its own context without being used in a different or new situation.

Beginning nursing students generally consider comprehension level questions slightly more difficult than knowledge level questions, but less complicated than application and analysis level questions. Students often try to deal with comprehension level information by memorizing the content. For example, when studying local adaptations to an infection, students may memorize the following list: heat, erythema, pain, edema, and exudate. Although this can be done, it is far better to understand why these adaptations occur. Erythema and heat occur because of increased circulation to the area. Edema occurs because of increased permeability of the capillaries. Pain occurs because the accumulating fluid in the tissue presses on nerve endings. Exudate occurs because of the accumulation of fluid, cells, and other substances at the site of infection. The mind is a wonderful machine, but unless you have a photographic memory lists of information without understanding often become overwhelming and confusing. The challenge of answering comprehension questions is understanding information. See the textbook *TEST SUCCESS: Test-Taking Techniques for Beginning Nursing Students* for specific study techniques related to comprehension level questions.

APPLICATION OF THE RACE MODEL TO COMPREHENSION QUESTIONS

1. The medication docusate sodium (Colace) facilitates defecation by:
   a. Softening the stool
   b. Forming a bulk residue
   c. Irritating the intestinal wall
   d. Dilating the intestinal lumen

RACE:

Recognize key words (highlighted). **R**ecognize who the client is.	The medication **docusate sodium (Colace) facilitates defecation by:** There is no client.

Recognize what the topic is about.	The drug docusate sodium (Colace) and how it works.
Ask what the question is asking.	The question is asking you **how and why does docusate sodium (Colace) facilitate defecation?**
Critically analyze options in relation to the question.	The words in the stem that indicates that this is a comprehension level question is **facilitates**. To answer this question you need to recall and **understand how or why** docusate sodium (Colace) works in the body to promote defecation. You need to scrutinize each option to identify whether the description in the option correctly **explains how or why** docusate sodium (Colace) works to facilitate defecation. Defecation is the consequence of taking Colace. **Rationales:** a. **Docusate sodium (Colace) softens and delays the drying of feces by lowering the surface tension of water permitting water and fat to penetrate the feces.** b. Bulk-forming laxatives, such as psyllium hydrophilic mucilloid (Metamucil) increase the fluid, gaseous, or solid bulk in the intestines. c. Irritants or stimulants, such as Bisacodyl (Dulcolax), irritate the intestinal mucosa or stimulate intestinal wall nerve endings, which precipitates peristalsis. d. Large volume enemas, not medications, enlarge the lumen of the intestine, which precipitates peristalsis.
Eliminate incorrect options.	Options b, c, and d do not accurately describe the therapeutic action of docusate sodium (Colace) and can be eliminated.

2. The interviewing technique of paraphrasing promotes communication because it:
   a. Requires patients to defend their point of view
   b. Limits patients from continuing a rambling conversation
   c. Allows patients to take their conversation in any desired direction
   d. Offers patients an opportunity to develop a clearer idea of what they said

RACE:

Recognize key words (highlighted). Recognize who the client is. Recognize what the topic is about.	The interviewing technique of **paraphrasing promotes communication because it:** There is no client. The interviewing technique of paraphrasing and how it works.
Ask what the question is asking.	The question is asking you **how and why does paraphrasing promote communication?**
Critically analyze options in relation to the question.	The word in the stem that **indicates** that this is a comprehension level question is **promotes**. It requires you to **understand how or why** paraphrasing works rather than just recall information. What is the consequence of paraphrasing? You need to scrutinize each option to identify whether the description in the option correctly **explains how or why** paraphrasing works to promote communication. **Rationales:** a. This describes the results of *challenging statements* that usually are barriers to communication.

continued

RACE: *continued*

	b. This describes one purpose of the interviewing skill of *focusing*, which is the use of questions or statements to center on one concern mentioned within a wordy, confusing conversation. c. This is the purpose of open-ended questions or statements. **d. Paraphrasing involves actively listening for patient concerns that are then restated by the nurse in similar words. This intervention conveys that the nurse has heard and understood the message and gives the patient an opportunity to review what was said.**
Eliminate incorrect options.	Options a, b, and c do not accurately describe how paraphrasing works to promote communication and can be eliminated.

3. Turning patients every 2 hours prevents pressure ulcers because:
    a. Relieving weight on the capillaries allows oxygen to reach body cells
    b. Moving promotes muscle contractions that increase the basal metabolic rate
    c. Keeping the extremities dependent allows blood to flow to distal cells by gravity
    d. Dropping of the abdominal organs by gravity relieves pressure against the diaphragm

RACE:

Recognize key words (highlighted). **R**ecognize who the client is. **R**ecognize what the topic is about.	**Turning** patients every 2 hours **prevents pressure ulcers because:** The patient is the client. How turning a patient every two hours prevents pressure ulcers.
Ask what the question is asking.	The question is asking you to **explain how and why turning a patient prevent a pressure ulcer?**
Critically analyze options in relation to the question.	The word in the stem that indicates that this is a comprehension level question is **prevents**. It requires you to **understand how or why** turning a patient relieves pressure and prevents a pressure ulcer rather than just recall information. What is the consequence of turning patients every 2 hours? You need to scrutinize each option to identify whether the description in the option correctly **explains how or why** turning a patient relieves pressure and prevents a pressure ulcer. Rationales: a. **Capillary beds are compressed and blood flow is obliterated with excessive external pressure (12 to 32 mmHg). Changing position removes the weight of the body off dependent areas permitting blood to flow through the capillaries supporting gaseous exchange at the cellular level.** b. Muscle contraction expends energy that raises the basal metabolic rate; however, this is unrelated to the development of pressure ulcers. c. Blood flow to the extremities will increase when they are kept below the level of the heart; however, this is unrelated to the development of pressure ulcers. d. Relieving pressure against the diaphragm by abdominal organs allows for greater thoracic expansion; however, this is unrelated to the development of pressure ulcers.

Eliminate incorrect options.	The options b, c, and d do not accurately explain how turning relieves pressure thereby preventing a pressure ulcer and can be eliminated.

Application Questions: Use Information!

COGNITIVE REQUIREMENTS

Application is the ability to use known and understood information in new situations. It requires more than just understanding information because you must demonstrate, solve, change, modify, or manipulate information in other than its originally learned form or context. In application questions you are confronted with a new situation that requires you to recall information and manipulate the information from within a familiar context to arrive at abstractions, generalizations, or consequences regarding the information that can be used in the new situation to solve the problem and answer the question. Application questions require you to make rational, logical judgments that result in a course of action.

Beginning nursing students frequently find these questions challenging because they require a restructuring of understood information into abstractions, commonalities, and generalizations, which are then applied to new situations. You do this all the time. Although there are parts of your day that are routine, every day you are exposed to new, challenging experiences. The same concept holds true for application questions. In application questions you will be confronted by situations that you learned about in a book, experienced personally, relived through other students' experiences, or never heard about or experienced before. In addition, this will happen throughout your entire nursing career. The challenge of answering application questions is going beyond rules and regulations and using information in a unique, creative way. See the textbook *TEST SUCCESS: Test-Taking Techniques for Beginning Nursing Students* for specific study techniques related to application level questions.

APPLICATION OF THE RACE MODEL TO APPLICATION QUESTIONS

1. A patient complains about not having had a bowel movement in three days. Which classification of drugs would be most helpful in relieving this problem?
    a. Diuretics
    b. Laxatives
    c. Bronchodilators
    d. Antihypertensives

RACE:

Recognize key words (highlighted). **R**ecognize who the client is. **R**ecognize what the topic is about.	A patient complains about **not having a bowel movement in three days.** Which **classification** of **drug** is **most helpful** in **relieving** this problem? The patient is the client. A patient who has not had a bowel movement in three days and needs a drug from a classification of drugs that will be the most helpful in facilitating defecation.
Ask what the question is asking.	The question is asking **which classification of drugs is most helpful in facilitating defecation.**
Critically analyze options in relation to the question.	The words in the stem that indicate that this is an application question are **most helpful in relieving**. Application questions require more complex mental processes than comprehension level questions to answer the question.

continued

RACE: *continued*

	Application questions require you to: manipulate recalled and understood information in other than its original form or context; apply this information to the new situation presented in the stem; and as a result, make a logical, rational judgment by choosing an option that solves the problem identified in the stem. To choose which classification of drugs would be most helpful in relieving this patient's problem, you must know that a patient who has not had a bowel movement in three days may be constipated, the therapeutic action and outcome of various classifications of drugs, and which classification of drugs would be helpful in relieving constipation. **Rationales:** a. Diuretics are medications that increase urine output. They are prescribed for people who retain excessive fluid. b. **Laxatives are medications that promote the elimination of fecal material. They are prescribed to prevent or treat constipation.** c. Bronchodilators are medications that dilate the bronchi of the lungs. They are prescribed for patients who have difficulty breathing. d. Antihypertensives are medications that reduce the blood pressure. They are prescribed for people who have high blood pressure (hypertension).
Eliminate incorrect options.	Options a, c, and d can be eliminated because they are not drug classifications that will facilitate defecation and the ultimate relief of this patient's constipation.

2. A patient scheduled for major surgery says, "I don't know if I can go through with this surgery." The nurse responds, "You'd rather not have surgery now?" Which interviewing technique was used by the nurse?
   a. Focusing
   b. Reflection
   c. Paraphrasing
   d. Clarification

RACE:

Recognize key words (highlighted). **R**ecognize who the client is. **R**ecognize what the topic is about.	A patient scheduled for major surgery says, **"I don't know if I can go through with this surgery."** The nurse responds, **"You'd rather not have surgery now?"** Which **interviewing technique was used** by the nurse? The patient is the client. The name of a specific interviewing technique that repeats basically what the patient is saying.
Ask what the question is asking.	The question is asking, what interviewing technique is being used by the nurse when the nurse says in response to the patient, "You'd rather not have surgery now?"
Critically analyze options in relation to the question.	The words in the stem that indicate that this is an application question are **was used**. Application questions require more complex mental processes than comprehension level questions to answer the question.

	Application questions require you to: manipulate recalled and understood information in other than its original form or context; apply this information to the new situation presented in the stem; and as a result, make a logical, rational judgment by choosing an option that solves the problem identified in the stem. To identify which technique was used by the nurse you have to understand the elements of a paraphrasing statement and you need to be able to recognize a paraphrasing statement when it is used. Although it is helpful to understand the elements of the other interviewing techniques because it will help you eliminate incorrect options, it is not necessary to answer the question as long as you are able to understand and recognize a paraphrasing statement. Once you identify the technique being portrayed, you can choose the correct answer. **Rationales:** a. This example is not focusing because the patient's statement was short and contained one message that was reiterated by the nurse. Focusing is used to explore one concern among many statements made by the patient. b. This example is not reflection because the nurse's statement is concerned with the content, not the underlying feeling, of the patient's statement. Reflective technique focuses on feelings. **c. The nurse used paraphrasing because the patient's and nurse's statements contain the same message but they are expressed with different words.** d. This example is not clarification. Clarification is when the nurse says something like, "I'm not quite sure that I know what you mean when you say you would rather not have surgery now." The nurse is asking the patient to further explain what is meant in the patient's statement.
Eliminate incorrect options.	Options a, b, and d can be eliminated because these techniques are different from the technique portrayed in the nurse's response in the stem.

3. The nurse would recognize that a patient on prolonged bed rest may be developing a pressure ulcer when the skin over a bony prominence appears:
    a. Red
    b. Blue
    c Black
    d. Yellow

RACE:

Recognize key words (highlighted).	The nurse would recognize that a patient may be developing a **pressure ulcer** when the **skin** over a bony prominence **reveals**:
Recognize who the client is. **R**ecognize what the topic is about.	The patient is the client. Early signs and symptoms of a pressure ulcer.
Ask what the question is asking.	Which early adaptation would indicate a pressure ulcer caused by immobility?

continued

RACE: *continued*

Critically analyze options in relation to the question.	The words in the stem that indicate that this is an application question are **recognize** and **developing pressure ulcer**.
	Application questions require more complex mental processes than comprehension level questions to answer the question.
	Application questions require you to: manipulate recalled and understood information in other than its original form or context; apply this information to the new situation presented in the stem; and as a result, make a logical, rational judgment by choosing the option that is the correct answer.
	To answer this question you have to understand how and why pressure can cause a pressure ulcer and know the common early adaptations that indicate the formation of a pressure ulcer.
	Although it would be helpful to know what is happening when the skin reflects each of the colors indicated so that you can eliminate incorrect answers, it is not necessary to answer the question.
	Rationales:
	a. **Erythema is a red discoloration generally caused by local vasodilation in an attempt to bring more oxygen to the area.**
	b. Cyanosis is a bluish color caused by an increased amount of deoxygenated hemoglobin associated with hypoxia, not pressure.
	c. Eschar generally appears black and is the scab or dry crust that result from the death of tissue.
	d. Jaundice is a yellow-orange color caused by increased deposits of bilirubin in tissue, not a response to pressure.
Eliminate incorrect options.	Options b, c, and d are not early signs or symptoms of a pressure ulcer and are incorrect answers. They can be eliminated.

Analysis Questions: Scrutinize Information!

COGNITIVE REQUIREMENTS

Analysis is the separation of an entity into its constituent parts and examination of their essential features in relation to each other. Analysis questions assume that you know, understand, and can apply information. It now asks you to engage in higher-level critical thinking strategies. To answer analysis level questions you first must examine each element of information as a separate entity. Secondly, you need to dissect, examine, and investigate the differences among the various elements of information. In other words, you must compare and contrast information. Thirdly, you must analyze the structure and organization of the compared and contrasted information to arrive at a conclusion or answer. Analysis questions often ask you to set priorities and in the stem use words such as *first, initially, best, priority,* and *most important.*

Beginning nursing students find analysis level questions the most difficult to answer. Analysis questions demand scrutiny of individual elements of information. Sometimes students do not remember or understand basic information. Analysis questions require identification of differences among elements of information. Sometimes students cannot discriminate among the various elements of information. Analysis questions involve exploration of the relationship among elements of information. Sometimes students cannot identify the structural or organizational relationship of elements of information. The challenge of answering analysis questions is performing a complete analysis of all the various elements of information and their interrelationships without over-analyzing or "reading into" the question. See the textbook *TEST SUCCESS: Test-Taking Techniques for Beginning Nursing Students* for specific study techniques related to analysis level questions.

APPLICATION OF THE RACE MODEL TO ANALYSIS QUESTIONS

1. A frail, malnourished older adult has been experiencing constipation. The nurse anticipates that the physician will most likely order:
   a. Bisacodyl (Dulcolax)
   b. Docusate sodium (Colace)
   c. Mineral oil (Haley's M-O)
   d. Magnesium hydroxide (Milk of Magnesia)

RACE:

Recognize key words (high-lighted). **R**ecognize who the client is. **R**ecognize what the topic is about.	A **frail, malnourished older adult** has been experiencing **constipation**. The nurse anticipates that the **physician will most likely order**: The patient is the client. Medications for constipation for a debilitated older adult.
Ask what the question is asking.	Which cathartic or laxative is the least likely to cause problems in a debilitated older adult?
Critically analyze options in relation to the question.	Analysis questions often ask you to set priorities as indicated by the words **most likely order** in the stem of this question. Analysis questions require more complex mental processes than comprehension and application level questions to answer the question. Analysis level questions require you to: examine each element of information as a separate entity: dissect, examine, and investigate the differences and commonalities among the various elements; and compare and contrast them to seek understanding about their interrelationship to each other and arrive at an answer to the question. This question requires you to: understand that frail, malnourished older adults have minimal compensatory reserve in various body systems to manage responses to cathartics and laxatives; know the physiologic action, outcome, side effects, and toxic effects of all four medications presented in the stem; contrast and compare the drugs and the risks they pose in the older adult to arrive at which drug would be the least risky drug. The least risky drug is the one the physician is most likely to order. **Rationales:** a. Dulcolax irritates the intestinal mucosa, stimulates nerve endings in the wall of the intestines, and causes rapid propulsion of waste from the body. Dulcolax is not the best choice of a laxative for an older adult because it can cause intestinal cramps, fluid and electrolyte imbalances, and irritation of the intestinal mucosa. **b. Colace permits fat and water to penetrate feces and softens stool. Of all the options, Colace has the fewest side effects in older adults.**

continued

RACE: *continued*

	c. Mineral oil lubricates feces in the colon; however, it can inhibit the absorption of fat-soluble vitamins and is not the best laxative for an older adult. d. Milk of Magnesia (MOM) draws water into the intestine by osmosis, which stimulates peristalsis. It is contraindicated for an older adult because it can cause fluid and electrolyte imbalances and inhibit absorption of fat-soluble vitamins.
Eliminate incorrect options.	Options a, c, and d are more potent than the correct answer and therefore are least likely to be ordered to relieve constipation in a debilitated older adult.

2. The mother of a terminally ill child says, "Who would have thought that I would have such a sick child." The best initial response by the nurse would be:
   a. "How do you feel right now?"
   b. "What do you mean by sick child?"
   c. "Life is not fair to do this to a child."
   d. "It's hard to believe that your child is so sick."

RACE:

Recognize key words (highlighted). **R**ecognize who the client is. **R**ecognize what the topic is about.	The mother of a terminally ill child says, **"Who would have thought that I would have such a sick child."** The **best initial response** by the nurse would be: The mother is the client. Interviewing skills the nurse can use when initially responding to a statement by the mother of a sick child.
Ask what the question is asking.	Which is an example of the best interviewing skill to use when initially responding to a statement made by the mother of a sick child?
Critically analyze options in relation to the question.	Analysis questions often ask you to set priorities as indicated by the words **best initial response** in the stem of this question. Analysis questions require more complex mental processes than comprehension and application level questions to answer the question. Analysis level questions require you to: examine each element of information as a separate entity: dissect, examine, and investigate the differences and commonalities among the various elements; and compare and contrast them to seek understanding about their interrelationship to each other and arrive at an answer to the question. To answer this question you need to: identify which interviewing techniques are portrayed in the statements in each option; understand how and why each interviewing skill works; compare and contrast the pros and cons of each technique if used in this situation; identify which technique would be the most supportive, appropriate, and best initial response by the nurse. **Rationales:** a. Direct questions cut off communication and should be avoided b. This response focuses on the seriousness of the child's illness, which is not the issue raised in the mother's statement.

	c. This statement reflects the beliefs and values of the nurse, which should be avoided. **d. This is a declarative statement that paraphrases the mother's beliefs and feelings. It communicates to the mother that the nurse is attentively listening and invites the mother to expand on her thoughts if she feels ready.**
Eliminate incorrect options.	Options a, b, and c can be eliminated because they are not the best initial response by the nurse of the options offered.

3. The patient with the greatest risk for developing a pressure ulcer is:
    a. An older adult on bed rest
    b. A toddler learning to walk
    c. A thin young woman in a coma
    d. An emotionally unstable middle-aged man

RACE:

Recognize key words (highlighted). **R**ecognize who the client is. **R**ecognize what the topic is about.	The patient with the **greatest risk** for **developing** a **pressure ulcer** is: The patient is the client. Identifying risk factors for pressure ulcers and who would be at most risk.
Ask what the question is asking.	The question is asking which patient in the various age groups is at the greatest risk for a pressure ulcer?
Critically analyze options in relation to the question.	Analysis questions often ask you to set priorities as indicated by the words **greatest risk** in the stem of this question. Analysis questions require more complex mental processes than comprehension and application level questions to answer the question. Analysis level questions require you to: examine each element of information as a separate entity; dissect, examine, and investigate the differences and commonalities among the various elements; and compare and contrast them to seek understanding about their interrelationship to each other and arrive at an answer to the question. To answer this question you need to: know what are the major risk factors that contribute to the development of a pressure ulcer; what are the risk factors for pressure ulcer development in all four of the specific categories of the lifespan represented in the options; and assign a level of risk to each of the individuals identified in the options in comparison to each of the other individuals. Once you have completed this intellectual analysis, you will have identified the individual at greatest risk. **Rationales:** a. Although the skin of older adults is vulnerable to the development of pressure ulcers because of decreased subcutaneous fat, reduced thickness and vascularity of the dermis, and decreased sebaceous gland activity, older adults are still capable of changing position and moving around in bed, which relieve pressure on integumentary tissue.

continued

RACE: *continued*

	b. A toddler learning to walk is not immobile. In addition, the skin of toddlers usually has adequate circulation, subcutaneous tissue and hydration and is supple. A toddler may fall and develop bruises (contusions) or scrapes (abrasions), not pressure ulcers. **c. Of the options offered, this person is the most vulnerable for developing a pressure ulcer. A thin person has little protective subcutaneous fat over bony prominences, and a person in a coma is immobile and unable to move or turn purposefully. Immobility results in prolonged pressure, which interferes with the oxygen supply to body cells.** d. Middle-aged men usually do not exhibit the effects of aging on the integumentary system. In addition, emotionally unstable people are able to move and change positions, which permits circulation to the cells of the skin.
Eliminate incorrect options.	Individuals presented in options a, b, and d are at less of a risk than a thin person who is immobile for the development of pressure ulcers. Options a, b, and d can be eliminated.

SUMMARY

Thinking about thinking is more strenuous than physical labor. A physical task is always easier if you use the right tool. This concept is true also for mental labor. The **RACE Model** is a tool that provides a methodical format to apply critical thinking to answering multiple-choice questions in nursing. As with any tool, it takes practice and experience to perfect its use. Therefore, you are encouraged to use the **RACE Model** when practicing test taking or reviewing examinations.

Nursing within the Context of Contemporary Health Care

2

Theory-Based Nursing Care

KEYWORDS

The following words include English vocabulary, nursing/medical terminology, concepts, principles, or information relevant to content specifically addressed in the chapter or associated with topics presented in it. English dictionaries, your nursing textbooks, and medical dictionaries such as *Taber's Cyclopedic Medical Dictionary* are resources that can be used to expand your knowledge and understanding of these words and related information.

Actualization
Adaptation
Adaptive capacity
Beliefs
Carl Jung
Compensatory reserve
Conceptual framework
Critical time
Defense mechanism
Developmental task
Ego differentiation
Erik Erikson—Personality
   Development
Fixation

Free association
Gordon's Functional Health
   Patterns
Health
Health belief
Health-illness continuum
Holistic health
Homeostasis
Human behavior
Illness-wellness continuum
Instinctual drive
Jean Piaget
Kübler-Ross—Stages of Grieving
Libido

Maslow's Hierarchy of Basic Human
   Needs
Model
Moral development
Multiplicity of stressors
Paradigm
Philosophy of nursing
Secondary stressor
Sigmund Freud
Stress
Stressor
Theory
Values
Wellness

QUESTIONS

1. The statement that supports why a nurse must be aware of the patient's perception of health is that the nurse can:
   a. Identify the patient's needs based on Maslow's Hierarchy of Basic Human Needs
   b. Provide more meaningful assistance to help the patient regain a state of health
   c. Help the patient prevent the occurrence of human responses to disease
   d. Choose a place for the patient along the health-illness continuum

2. One of the most serious outcomes of prolonged periods of stress is:
   a. Difficulty sleeping
   b. Impaired immunity
   c. Increased muscle tension
   d. Decreased intestinal peristalsis

3. Which statement reflects Kübler-Ross's stage of denial in the grief process?
   a. "Why did this have to happen to me now?"
   b. "My daughter will live with my sister after I am gone."
   c. "Maybe they mixed up my records with someone else's."
   d. "How could this happen when I quit smoking and drinking?"

4. The word that best describes adaptive capacity is:
   a. Change
   b. Etiology
   c. Remission
   d. Compliance

5. Maslow's theory helps the nurse to identify the patient's:
   a. Problem that has top priority
   b. Developmental level
   c. Coping patterns
   d. Health beliefs

6. Which concept is reflective of the work of Sigmund Freud?
   a. Human nature is essentially irrational
   b. An instinctual drive is the underlying stimulus for human behavior
   c. Universal moral principles are internalized as standards of behavior
   d. Moral development is based on concepts of caring and responsibility

7. Which is most important when preparing a child for the death of a grandparent?
   a. Wait until the child asks a question about the situation
   b. Encourage the child to participate in mourning rituals
   c. Begin at the child's level of understanding
   d. Praise the child for being strong

8. A basic principle associated with Sigmund Freud and his work is that:
   a. Not all emotional or psychological events are understandable
   b. Defense mechanisms are used to protect one's self-esteem
   c. The Id is the part of the psyche that imposes a conscience
   d. The conscious mind is unrelated to human behavior

9. The most common human response to an emotional stressor is:
   a. Anger
   b. Denial
   c. Anxiety
   d. Depression

10. Which statement best reflects the relationship between stress and adaptation?
    a. Stressors usually cause maladaptive responses
    b. Addressing an adaptation will in turn limit the stressor
    c. Stress and adaptation are intertwined in a cyclic relationship
    d. The ability to adapt to stress is solely dependent on the nature of the stressor

11. Which word describes a level of health toward the wellness end of the illness-wellness continuum?
    a. Signs
    b. Disability
    c. Symptoms
    d. Awareness

12. Which psychodynamic theorist believed that an infant seeking pleasure through oral gratification is important to psychosocial growth?
    a. Sigmund Freud
    b. Erik Erikson
    c. Jean Piaget
    d. Carl Jung

13. According to Maslow's Hierarchy of Needs theory, a person who is no longer aware of a need has:
    a. Experienced emotional and physical health
    b. Had the need met to one's level of satisfaction
    c. The ability to achieve one's role performance expectations
    d. Moved toward the healthy end of the health-illness continuum

14. The word that best describes adaptive capacity is:
   a. Treatment
   b. Flexible
   c. Threat
   d. Illness

15. Which is a physiological adaptation to stress?
   a. Slow, bounding pulse
   b. Delayed response time
   c. Inability to concentrate
   d. Rapid, shallow breathing

16. The person who would have the hardest time coping would be the patient who is:
   a. Waiting for the results of a biopsy
   b. Unable to control the course of illness
   c. Experiencing a multiplicity of stressors
   d. Going to have to relocate to a nursing home

17. A nurse inadvertently commits a medication error without the knowledge of other nursing team members. According to Freud what part of the personality guides the nurse to initiate an incident report?
   a. Id
   b. Ego
   c. Libido
   d. Superego

18. A true statement about adaptation is that adaptations:
   a. Depend on the nature of the stressor
   b. Are secondary stressors ultimately
   c. Can be conscious or unconscious
   d. Are maladaptive responses

19. When considering Kübler-Ross's Stages of Grieving, in what stage would a patient with terminal cancer be if the patient is willing to try new therapies?
   a. Denial
   b. Bargaining
   c. Depression
   d. Acceptance

20. Which level need in Maslow's Hierarchy of Needs is met when the nurse provides a resident in a nursing home a choice about which color shirt to wear?
   a. Physiologic
   b. Self-esteem
   c. Safety and Security
   d. Love and Belonging

21. Which classification of stress is a pressure ulcer?
   a. Microbiological
   b. Developmental
   c. Physiological
   d. Physical

22. Which nursing intervention would best support a problem in the Role-Relationship Pattern category of Gordon's Functional health patterns?
   a. Assessing a family member's readiness to provide care in the home
   b. Referring a patient to a self-help group to learn colostomy care
   c. Teaching the patient self-care in preparation for going home
   d. Seeking assistance from a spiritual advisor

23. Which action by the nurse in the occupational setting reflects the fourth level need according to Maslow?
   a. Provides emergency care for injury
   b. Determines demands on employees' physical health
   c. Complies with Worker's Compensation Act requirements
   d. Identifies an employee's maladaptation to stress associated with a new role

24. The phrase that best reflects the concept of stress is:
    a. Natural process
    b. Specific response
    c. Defense mechanisms
    d. Compensatory reserve

25. Which is an example of a secondary stressor?
    a. Pain
    b. Cold weather
    c. Death of a spouse
    d. Ingested microorganisms

26. Which is an example of a health belief?
    a. Eating foods that are low in fat
    b. Accepting positive results of diagnostic tests
    c. Concluding that illness is the result of being bad
    d. Respecting a patient's decision regarding therapeutic treatment

27. According to Maslow's Hierarchy of Needs theory, which level need should be met just before self-esteem needs can be met?
    a. Safety
    b. Belonging
    c. Physiologic
    d. Self-actualization

28. Which statement best reflects a principle common to all theories of health, wellness, and illness?
    a. A sense of well-being is synonymous with health
    b. People are able to control factors that affect health
    c. Many variables influence a person's perception of health
    d. Being able to meet the demands of one's role is necessary for health

29. Maslow's Hierarchy of Needs helps the nurse to:
    a. Determine which patient need requires nursing attention first
    b. Organize data according to functional health patterns
    c. Keep a patient's problems from getting worse
    d. Identify the safety needs of a patient

30. Which social stressor possesses the greatest risk for developing illness?
    a. Change in marital status
    b. Teenage motherhood
    c. Single parent family
    d. Living on the street

31. Which is an example of an adaptation to a physiologic stressor?
    a. A sunburn after being outside all day
    b. Diarrhea after eating contaminated food
    c. Shortness of breath when walking up a hill
    d. A rapid heart rate during a final examination

32. According to Maslow, which behavior would least describe a person who is self-actualized? A person who:
    a. Is autonomous
    b. Has the ability to problem solve
    c. Is able to see the good in others
    d. Has an external locus of control

33. A concept basic to the health-illness continuum is that:
    a. A person can be both healthy and ill at the same time on the continuum
    b. There is no distinct boundary between health and illness along the continuum
    c. When variables are in balance a person is in the exact center of the continuum
    d. Actualization must be achieved to be placed on the healthy end of the continuum

34. A nurse completes a difficult day at work and feels satisfaction in performing well and helping others. According to Freud, this feeling of satisfaction is associated with what part of the personality?
    a. Ego
    b. Libido
    c. Fixation
    d. Superego

35. Which person would be considered healthy when referring to the Role Performance Model of Health?
    a. Coach who continues to coach after becoming a paraplegic
    b. Coal miner who retires after having acquired black lung disease
    c. Policeman who begins selling alarm systems after being shot while on duty
    d. Brick layer who takes a leave of absence while recovering from hernia surgery

36. Freedom from which situation demonstrates a safety and security need in Maslow's Hierarchy of Basic Human Needs?
    a. Pain
    b. Hunger
    c. Ridicule
    d. Loneliness

37. Which stressful life event has the greatest potential to contribute to stress related illness?
    a. Retirement
    b. Pregnancy
    c. Adoption
    d. Divorce

38. The word that best describes adaptive capacity is:
    a. Safety
    b. Health
    c. Restore
    d. Imbalance

39. Which action most reflects dysfunctional grieving?
    a. Being continuously angry three months after the death of a parent
    b. Displaying clinical symptoms of depression after one year
    c. Remarrying within six months after the death of a spouse
    d. Keeping a deceased child's room unchanged for years

40. Which is a developmental stressor?
    a. Illness
    b. Divorce
    c. Relocation
    d. Menopause

41. Love and belonging needs associated with Maslow's Hierarchy of Needs are related to which of Gordon's Functional Health Patterns?
    a. Values-belief pattern
    b. Role-relationship pattern
    c. Cognitive-perceptual pattern
    d. Sexuality-reproductive pattern

42. Which level need in Maslow's Hierarchy of Needs is supported when the nurse tapes the patient's get well cards to the wall where the patient can see them?
    a. Physiologic
    b. Self-esteem
    c. Safety and Security
    d. Love and belonging

43. The word that best describes adaptive capacity is:
    a. Role
    b. Cope
    c. Stimuli
    d. Energy

44. A basic principle associated with Sigmund Freud and his work is that:
    a. The reality principle reflects man's need for immediate gratification
    b. Defense mechanisms are a common means of conscious coping
    c. No human behavior is accidental
    d. The Id controls the personality

45. A concept that nurses need to recognize about health is that:
    a. Perceptions of health vary among cultures
    b. To be considered healthy a person needs to be productive
    c. There must be an absence of illness for a person to be considered healthy
    d. An underlying consensus exists among theorists about the definition of health

46. What is most closely associated with the concept of adaptation?
    a. Flexible process seeking holistic balance
    b. Mechanism that is under conscious control
    c. Failure to maintain homeostasis of body systems
    d. Response to negative, rather than positive, stressors

47. Freud believed that conflicts that arise from inner impulses are dealt with through:
    a. Free association
    b. Ego differentiation
    c. Developmental tasks
    d. Defense mechanisms

48. Which statement by a dying patient in an intensive care unit reflects Kübler-Ross's stage of depression in the grief process?
    a. "I can't bear not to be here for my daughter's wedding."
    b. "I wrote a letter to be read by my daughter on the day of her wedding."
    c. "I only need to get a little stronger so I can go to my daughter's wedding."
    d. "I don't care if I die as long as I live long enough to see my daughter married."

49. Which level need in Maslow's Hierarchy of Needs is supported when the nurse moves a patient's recliner closer to the nurses' station so the patient can be monitored?
    a. Self-esteem
    b. Physiologic
    c. Belonging
    d. Safety

50. An immobilized patient develops a pressure ulcer. What type of stressor precipitated the ulcer?
    a. Psychological
    b. Physiological
    c. Chemical
    d. Physical

ANSWERS AND RATIONALES

1. a. A patient's perceptions are part of the data that must be collected before the nurse can establish the priority of the patient's needs. Maslow's Hierarchy of Basic Human Needs helps the nurse to determine the patient's needs in order of priority based on the collected data.
   b. Health perception reflects a person's knowledge, behavior, and attitudes regarding illness, disease prevention, health promotion, and what constitutes a healthy lifestyle. An assessment of these factors captures the uniqueness of each individual and is essential data that must be considered before a nursing diagnosis can be made and a plan formulated.
   c. A healthy lifestyle can promote health and prevent some illness or even minimize complications; however, understanding a person's perceptions of health without action will not prevent human responses to disease.
   d. Only a patient, not a nurse, can choose a patient's place along the health-illness continuum. How people perceive themselves is subjective and is influenced by their own attitudes, values, and beliefs.

2. a. Difficulty sleeping is a common adaptation to stress, but it is not life threatening. Although it can contribute to fatigue, it is not as serious a concern as one of the other options offered.
   b. Impaired immunity is a serious threat caused by prolonged periods of stress. Stressors elevate blood cortisone levels, which decrease anti-inflammatory responses, deplete energy stores, lead to a state of exhaustion, and decrease resistance to disease.
   c. This is a physiologic indicator of stress. However, it is not as serious a concern as one of the other options offered.
   d. When stressed, the patient's parasympathetic nervous system precipitates a decrease in intestinal peristalsis. Constipation is a concern, but it is not as serious as one of the other options offered.

3. a. This statement characterizes the anger, not denial, stage in the grieving process. During the anger stage the person may vent hostile feelings or displace these feelings on others through acting out behaviors.
   b. This statement characterizes the bargaining, not denial, stage of the grieving process. During bargaining the person may put personal affairs in order, visit friends and relatives, and make final living arrangements for surviving family members.
   c. This statement characterizes the denial stage of the grieving process. During denial the person is not ready to believe that the loss is happening. In denial, the person may isolate one's self from reality or repress the discussion about the loss.
   d. This statement characterizes the anger, not denial, stage of the grieving process. During the anger stage the person may question, "Why me when I did everything right?"

4. a. Adaptive capacity refers to the quality and quantity of resources one can draw on to regain balance after one is threatened. This process requires an individual to change consciously or unconsciously in the physical, emotional, mental, or spiritual dimension in an effort to achieve balance or homeostasis.
   b. Etiology refers to the stressor or threat to homeostasis that stimulates a person to draw upon personal resources within the physical, emotional, mental, or spiritual dimension. Adaptive capacity refers to a person's potential or lack of potential to respond to a stress or threat.
   c. Remission refers to the abatement or lessening of intensity of the symptoms of a disease or illness, not adaptive capacity.
   d. Compliance refers to adherence to an established therapeutic action plan, not adaptive capacity.

5. a. Patient problem/needs can be ranked in order of ascending importance according to how important they are for survival using Maslow's Hierarchy of Needs as a framework. Maslow identifies five levels of human needs. A person must meet lower-level needs before addressing higher-level needs. Physiologic needs are first level needs: air, food, water, sleep, shelter etc.; safety and security needs are second; love and belonging needs are third; self-esteem needs are fourth; and self-actualization is the fifth level need.
   b. Erikson's Developmental Theory is designed to identify a patient's developmental level, not Maslow's Hierarchy of Needs.
   c. Maslow's Hierarchy of Needs is not designed to identify a person's coping patterns in response to illness.
   d. Rosenstock's and Becker's Health Belief Models identify the relationship between health beliefs and the use of preventive actions to promote health, not Maslow's Hierarchy of Needs.

6. a. Freud's Theory of Personality Development does not include the thought that human nature is essentially irrational. Piaget believed that humans are rational, not irrational, and that a person's goal is to master the environment.
   b. Freud believed that libidinal or instinctual drives are the underlying stimulus for human behavior in an attempt to gain pleasure or satisfaction through the mouth, anus, or genitals.
   c. Freud's Theory of Personality Development does not include the concept of universal moral principles internalized as standards of behavior. He believed that the Superego is the center of the conscience monitoring and influencing the behavior of the Ego.
   d. Carol Gilligan, not Sigmund Freud, described the importance of not overlooking the concepts of caring and responsibility in moral development.

7. a. This is not a healthy way to deal with childhood grieving. Children are very perceptive and capable of recognizing that something is wrong, but, may not know what questions to ask. By avoiding discussing the loss with the child, the child may feel afraid, lonely, or even abandoned.
   b. The child's age, level of understanding, feelings, and fears will determine how much the child should engage in mourning rituals. Children should not be

forced to attend mourning rituals nor should they be pushed aside in an attempt to protect them from pain because this can lead to feelings of abandonment, fear, or loneliness.

c. **Beginning at the child's level of understanding is essential when preparing a child for the death of a grandparent. Because there is such a difference regarding how children of different ages view the concept of death, it is important to first assess the child's level of understanding.**

d. No one should be told how to feel or behave when it comes to reacting to loss. Expression of diverse feelings is essential if a child is to cope with the loss of the grandparent or develop positive coping strategies to deal with loss later as an adult.

8. a. Freud believed that the underlying stimulus for all behavior was sexuality; therefore, all behavior can be explained and understood.

b. **Defense mechanisms are unconscious coping patterns that deny, distort, or reduce awareness of a stressful event in an attempt to protect the Ego from anxiety. People tend to act in ways that support their self-esteem or how they feel about themselves. Anxiety, being a threat to self-esteem, stimulates the use of defense mechanisms to protect the Ego.**

c. The Superego, not the Id, is the part of the psyche that imposes a conscience. The Id is the source of instinctive and unconscious urges seeking self-gratification.

d. Freud believed that all behavior has meaning and that behavior is directly related to unconscious as well as conscious motivation.

9. a. Although anger may be identified as an adaptation to stress, it is not the most common response to stress. Anger is more commonly and classically seen in Kübler-Ross's second emotional stage of dying/grieving.

b. Denial is more commonly seen in Kübler-Ross's first emotional stage of dying/grieving, not as the most common response to stress.

c. **Anxiety is the most common response to all new experiences that serve as an emotional threat.**

d. Depression is an extreme response to prolonged stress and is not the most common human response to stress.

10. a. Stress can cause a change in a person's balanced state which can cause positive or negative responses. When an adaptation is maladaptive it reflects ineffective coping, which leads to illness. However, adaptations that result in a balanced state or promote personal growth are considered positive responses.

b. Adaptations do not limit stressors, but are responses to stressors. Internal or external stimuli (stressors) precipitate a positive or negative response (adaptation) that attempts to restore balance. If balance is not achieved, the stress continues resulting in disease/illness.

c. **Adaptation occurs as a response to a stressor. It is an ongoing process that is constant and dynamic and is essential to physical, psychosocial, spiritual and emotional well-being.**

d. The nature of a stressor is only one factor that influences a person's ability to adapt. Adaptations are an attempt to seek balance and are based on many variables which include a person's available physiological, psychosocial, spiritual, and emotional resources as well as interactive factors, not just the nature of the stressor.

11. a. According to Travis and Ryan's illness/wellness continuum, *Signs* is the first step to the left of center or worsening state of health, not towards the right, which is the *high-level wellness* end of the continuum.

b. According to Travis and Ryan's illness/wellness continuum, *Disability* is the third and last step to the left of the neutral position and is closest to the *premature death* end of the continuum, not the right side, which is the *high-level wellness* end of the continuum.

c. According to Travis and Ryan's illness/wellness continuum, *Symptoms* is in the center of the left side moving towards the *premature death* end of the continuum, not the right side, which is the *high-level wellness* end of the continuum.

d. **According to Travis and Ryan's illness/wellness continuum the center is a neutral state, left of center moves towards *premature death* (which is the extreme left side of the continuum), and right of neutral moves toward *high-level wellness* (which is the extreme right side of the continuum). *Awareness* is the first step to the right of neutral moving towards *education*, then *growth*, and *high-level wellness* at the extreme right end. *Awareness* of the need to move towards *high-level wellness*, and not merely experiencing the absence of disease, is the first step in the process.**

12. a. **Sigmund Freud stressed the importance of instinctual human urges driving human behavior. Sucking, swallowing, chewing, and biting all give an infant pleasure, comfort, and a feeling of safety. If these needs are not met, the personality can become fixated at the oral stage. The adult may have difficulty trusting others and engage in dysfunctional behaviors such as drug abuse, smoking, overeating, alcoholism, and overdependent behavior.**

b. Erik Erikson does not focus on oral gratification but rather on the infant's need to achieve the task of developing trust versus mistrust. Erikson expands upon Freud's theory and emphasizes the importance of environment on personality development.

c. Jean Piaget's Cognitive Theory does not focus on oral gratification as being important to psychosocial growth. Piaget believed that humans are rational and that a person's goal is to master the environment. Mastery depends on a person's ability to assimilate, accommodate and adapt as one responds to new situations and knowledge.

d. Carl Jung created a model called Analytical Psychology that focused on introverted and extroverted personalities. He also developed the concept of *Persona*, what a person appears to others in contrast to what he or she actually is.

13. a. Because a particular need is met it does not mean that the person is physically or emotionally healthy. A person who is ill and in pain can be medicated for the pain. The person will no longer be aware of the pain because the need for comfort is met; however, the person will still be ill.
    b. **Maslow's Hierarchy of Needs ranks human needs in order of ascending importance, with the basic needs first, according to how important the needs are for survival. When a need is met to one's level of satisfaction the person is no longer aware of the need and can move on to the next level.**
    c. In spite of unmet needs many people are able to achieve the expectations they and others set regarding their role performance.
    d. Maslow's Hierarchy of Needs Model does not address where on a health-illness continuum a person is placed before or after a need is met. A person can have a need met and still be either healthy or ill somewhere along the continuum.

14. a. Treatment refers to actions designed to help the patient achieve homeostasis, not adaptive capacity.
    b. **A major component of adaptive capacity is the ability to be flexible in all realms of human dimension as a person seeks to regain homeostasis or balance. Adaptive capacity refers to the quality and quantity of resources one can draw on to regain balance after one is threatened.**
    c. The threat that a person perceives is the stressor, not the adaptation.
    d. Illness refers to a maladaptive response to a stressor, not to adaptive capacity.

15. a. While a bounding pulse is a physiological response to stress, a rapid pulse, not slow pulse, is a physiological response to the body's neurohormonal reaction to stress. During the alarm phase of the General Adaptation Syndrome the autonomic nervous system initiates the fight-or-flight response and releases large amounts of epinephrine and cortisone into the body which contribute to a rapid pulse.
    b. Level of alertness is considered a psychosocial, not physiological, response to stress. In addition, there is an increase, not a decrease, in response time as a result of an increase in alertness and energy associated with the alarm phase of the General Adaptation Syndrome.
    c. Concentration is considered a psychosocial, not physical, response to stress. Concentration and level of alertness are enhanced, not reduced, during the fight-or-flight response of the autonomic nervous system when large amounts of epinephrine and cortisone are released into the body.
    d. **Rapid, shallow breathing is a physiological adaptation associated with the flight-or-flight response of the autonomic nervous system when large amounts of epinephrine and cortisone are released into the body as a person perceives a threat.**

16. a. Although waiting for the results of a biopsy is stressful, it is not as stressful as one of the other options offered.
    b. Although being unable to control the course of illness is stressful, it is not as stressful as one of the other options offered.
    c. As the multiplicity of stressors increases the harder it is for a person to cope. As each stress is added, the accumulated impact is greater than just the sum of each individual stressor.
    d. Relocation is stressful whether it is voluntary or involuntary. However, it is not as stressful as one of the other options offered..

17. a. The Id would not guide a nurse to initiate an incident report because the Id is the source of instinctive and unconscious urges, not the center of the conscience.
    b. The Ego seeks compromise between the Id and the Superego and represents the psychologic aspect of the personality, not the center of the conscience.
    c. The Libido refers to the psychic energy derived from basic biological urges, not the center of the conscience.
    d. **The Superego monitors the Ego. The Superego is concerned with social standards, ethics, self criticism, moral standards, and conscience. If the nurse initiates an incident report it is the Superego that directs the achievement of ego-ideal behavior. If the nurse does not initiate an incident report it is the Superego that criticizes, punishes, and causes a sense of guilt.**

18. a. The General and Local Adaptation Syndromes involve automatic nonspecific responses that are not dependent on specific stressors. The body automatically responds in the same way physiologically regardless of the nature of the stressor.
    b. Although adaptations may become a secondary stressor, many do not.
    c. **Adaptations to stress are both conscious and unconscious. In the General and Local Adaptation Syndromes automatic physiologic responses are not under conscious control. Adaptations, such as behavioral responses, are often under conscious control.**
    d. Adaptations can be maladaptive and fail to help a person achieve balance or they can be positive and help a person achieve balance.

19. a. A patient in the denial stage of grieving refuses to believe that the event is happening and is unable to deal with practical problems such as trying new therapies.
    b. **A patient in the bargaining stage of grieving seeks to avoid the loss and will try new therapies to gain more time.**
    c. A patient in the depression stage of grieving usually will acknowledge the reality and inevitability of the impending loss, grieve the loss of present relationships and future experiences, and may stop all but palliative therapy.
    d. The patient in the acceptance stage of grieving comes to terms with the loss. The patient begins to detach from surroundings and supportive people and generally no longer has the emotional or physical energy to try new therapies.

20. a. This does not meet needs on the physiologic level of Maslow's Hierarchy of Needs. Physiologic needs are related to having adequate air, food, water, rest, shelter, and the ability to eliminate and regulate body temperature.
   b. **Choosing which color shirt to wear provides a person with the opportunity to make a choice and supports feelings of independence, competence, and self-respect, which all contribute to a positive self-esteem.**
   c. This does not meet needs on the safety and security level of Maslow's Hierarchy of Needs. Safety and security needs are related to being and feeling protected in the physiologic and interpersonal realms.
   d. This does not meet needs on the love and belonging level of Maslow's Hierarchy of Needs. Love and belonging needs are related to giving and receiving affection, attempting to avoid loneliness and isolation, and wanting to feel as though one belongs.

21. a. A pressure ulcer is not a microbiologic stressor. If an ulcer becomes infected, the organism causing the infection is a microbiologic stressor.
   b. A pressure ulcer is not a developmental stressor. Developmental stressors are stressors that a person is exposed to during the normal stages of growth.
   c. **Pressure is a physical stressor that stimulates adaptations that cause an ulcer. Once an ulcer is present, the ulcer becomes a secondary stressor and is considered physiologic in nature.**
   d. A pressure ulcer is not a physical stressor. The pressure that caused the ulcer is a physical stressor.

22. a. **This action would support achievement of a goal in the Role-Relationship category under the nursing diagnosis of Interrupted Family Process.**
   b. This action would support the achievement of a goal in the health perception/health management category under the nursing diagnosis, Health Seeking Behaviors or in the Cognitive-Perceptual category under the nursing diagnosis, Deficient Knowledge, not the Role-Relationship Pattern category.
   c. This action would support achievement of a goal in the Cognitive-Perceptual category under the nursing diagnosis, Deficient Knowledge, not the Role-Relationship category.
   d. This action would support the achievement of a goal in the Value-Belief category, not the Role-Relationship category.

23. a. Providing emergency care for an injury supports physiologic needs, a first-level need, according to Maslow's Hierarchy of Needs, not a fourth-level need, which is meeting self-esteem needs.
   b. Determining demands on employees' physical health is a physiologic need, a first-level need according to Maslow's Hierarchy of Needs, not a fourth-level need, which is meeting self-esteem needs.
   c. Complying with Worker's Compensation Act meets workers' safety and security needs, a second-level need according to Maslow's Hierarchy or Needs, not a fourth-level need, which is meeting self-esteem needs.
   d. A person's maladaptation to stress associated with a new work role is generally associated with

factors that impact on self-esteem, a fourth-level need according to Maslow's Hierarchy of Needs.

24. a. Stress is a natural, normal, and universal every day experience. Stressors continually stimulate a person either positively or negatively in a variety of human dimensions and are considered a part of the normal process of living.
   b. While responses to stress can be either general or local, both are nonspecific responses. Regardless of the nature of stressors people respond in the same characteristic pattern of physiologic events.
   c. Defense mechanisms, whether they are physiological or psychological in origin, are related to concepts associated with attempts to seek balance, not the nature of the stressor.
   d. Compensatory reserve refers to the body's ability to draw on homeostatic mechanisms that are activated automatically in the healthy individual when subjected to a stressor. Compensatory reserve refers to the process of adaptation, rather than the concept of stress.

25. a. **Pain initially is an adaptation to some previous primary stressor, threat, or stimuli. However, when pain stimulates additional responses in an effort to manage the pain, the pain becomes a secondary stressor.**
   b. Cold weather is a primary physical stressor, not an adaptation to some previous stressor or primary threat.
   c. Death of a spouse is a primary psychosocial stressor, not an adaptation to some previous stressor or primary threat.
   d. Ingested microorganisms is a primary microbiological stressor, not an adaptation to some previous stressor or primary threat.

26. a. Eating foods low in fat is a health practice, not a health belief. A health behavior, such as eating a low-fat diet, reflects the belief that preventive measures will minimize risk factors that contribute to disease/illness.
   b. Accepting positive results of diagnostic tests reflects a behavior in response to good news, rather than a behavior reflecting a health belief.
   c. **This is an example of a health belief. A health belief is a conviction or opinion that influences health care practices or decisions. If a person believes that illness is the result of being bad, the patient may feel the need to suffer in silence as a form of penance.**
   d. Respecting a patient's decision is not an example of a health belief. It reflects the nurse's acceptance of a patient as a unique individual and recognizes the patient's right to make personal choices about one's own health care.

27. a. Safety and security needs are not just before self-esteem needs on Maslow's Hierarchy of Needs. Safety and security needs are second-level needs and self-esteem needs are fourth-level needs.
   b. **Belonging and love needs are directly below self-esteem needs on Maslow's Hierarchy of Needs. Belonging and love are third-level needs and self-esteem needs are fourth-level needs.**

c. Physiologic needs are not just before self-esteem needs on Maslow's Hierarchy of Needs. Physiologic needs are first-level needs and self-esteem needs are fourth-level needs.

d. Self-actualization needs are after, not before, self-esteem needs on Maslow's Hierarchy of Needs Model. Self-actualization is a higher-level need then self-esteem needs, therefore, self-esteem needs need to be met before self-actualization needs.

28. a. Not all models of health agree with this view of health. For example, the Clinical Model has a narrow interpretation which views health as the absence of signs and symptoms of disease or injury. Well-being is a subjective perception of energy and vigor. A person able to carry out daily tasks, interact successfully with others, manage stress and emotions, strive for continued growth and who has meaning or purpose in life has a sense of well-being, regardless of the severity of disease or infirmity.

b. Not all definitions of health identify that a person is able to control factors that affect health. The Adaptive Model is one of the few that addresses a person's ability to use purposeful adaptive responses and processes in response to internal and external stimuli to achieve health.

c. **There is little consensus about any one definition of health, wellness, and illness. However, all definitions of health, wellness, and illness address the fact that there are a number of factors that influence health.**

d. Not all definitions of health define health in terms of an individual's ability to fulfill societal roles. For example, the Clinical Model views people from the perspective of a physiologic system with related functions with health being the absence of disease or injury.

29. a. **Maslow's Hierarchy of Needs can be used as a framework for setting priorities when establishing preferential order of nursing diagnoses as well as ordering planned nursing interventions. Maslow identifies five levels of human needs arranged in order of ascending importance related to survival. A person must meet lower-level needs before addressing higher-level needs.**

b. Data are grouped into significant categories based on Gordon's Functional Health Patterns, not Maslow's Hierarchy of Needs.

c. Maslow's Hierarchy of Needs is not designed to keep a patient's problems from getting worse. It identifies needs in order of ascending importance based on how important the needs are for survival.

d. Maslow's Hierarchy of Needs is not designed to identify safety needs of a patient. It identifies needs in order of ascending importance according to how important the needs are for survival. According to the hierarchy, physiologic needs should be met first and then safety needs.

30. a. A person with a changing marital status would experience several stressors but would probably not be at as great a risk for developing an illness as a person in one of the other options.

b. A teenage mother may experience several stressors but would probably not be at as great a risk to develop an illness as a person in one of the other options.

c. A single parent family may experience several stressors but would probably not be at as great a risk to develop an illness as a person in one of the other options.

d. **People living on the street would most likely have a multiplicity of stressors in many different categories that would place them at the greatest risk for developing an illness. For example, physiologic (poor nutrition and sleep patterns), physical (exposure to heat and cold), psychologic (fear of being a target for assault, robbery and abuse, lack of family support, and possible history of mental or emotional illness), economic (inadequate or no income), developmental (inability to complete developmental tasks), chemical (dependence on drugs, alcohol, and cigarettes), and microbiologic (exposure to pathogens from living on the street and not having access to adequate bathing and toileting environments).**

31. a. A sunburn is an adaptation to the ultraviolet rays of the sun which is a physical, not a physiologic, stressor. Once the person has a sunburn, the sunburn is a physiologic stressor.

b. Diarrhea after eating contaminated food is an adaptation to a microbiologic, not a physiologic, stressor.

c. **Shortness of breath is an adaptation to the physiologic stress of walking up a hill. The body is reacting via physiological mechanisms to take in more oxygen to meet the oxygen demand of cells when walking.**

d. The threat or stressor is the final examination, a psychologic, not a physiologic, stressor. The rapid heart rate during a final examination is a physiological adaptation to a psychosocial stressor.

32. a. Self-actualized people are autonomous, independent, self-directed, and governed from within.

b. Self-actualized people are accurate in predicting future events, highly creative, open to new ideas and have superior perception. All these qualities contribute to problem-solving abilities.

c. Self-actualized people are friendly and loving. They respect themselves and others and seek out the good in others.

d. **An external locus of control would least describe self-actualized people. People who are self-actualized strive to develop their maximum potential based on motivation from within, not in response to external rewards or recognition.**

33. a. Where people place themselves on the health-illness continuum is a self-perception of their status in relation to health and illness. From their perspectives they cannot be healthy and ill at the same time.

b. Health and illness are on opposite ends of the health-illness continuum and there is no distinct boundary between health and illness. Only a person can place her/himself somewhere along the health-illness continuum based on one's own perceptions about health, illness, and wellness.

    c. Variables, such as genetic makeup, race, gender, age, lifestyle, risk factors, culture, environment, standard of living, support system, spiritual beliefs, and emotional factors, may be in balance and individuals view themselves at the extremes of the continuum or they may be out of balance and view themselves in the center of the continuum.

    d. Only the Eudaemonistic Model of Health incorporates the concept of actualization or realization of a person's potential as the major component of a definition of health.

34. a. The Ego is associated with mediating instinctual drives, social prohibitions, and reality and is not concerned with self-satisfaction.

    b. The Libido refers to the psychic energy derived from basic biologic urges. Desire for sex, life, pleasure, and satisfaction are attributed to the Libido.

    c. Fixation is the inability of the personality to develop to the next stage as a result of unresolved anxiety and is not the source of the pleasure principle.

    d. The Superego monitors the Ego. The Superego is concerned with social standards, ethics, self criticism, moral standards, and conscience, not achievement of self-satisfaction.

35. **a. According to the Role-Performance Model of Health, as long as a person can perform work associated with societal roles, even if a person is clinically ill, the person is considered healthy. A coach who continues coaching, even though ill or disabled, is considered healthy in light of the Role-Performance Model of Health.**

    b. If a person retires because of illness the person has not met society's expectation in terms of role performance and, therefore, would be considered unhealthy in light of the Role-Performance Model of Health.

    c. A strict interpretation of the Role-Performance Model of Health would most likely describe a policeman who changes jobs because of a physical or emotional inability to continue as unhealthy. Even though the former policeman is still a wage earner, it is not in the same job.

    d. According to the Role-Performance Model of Health, a person who cannot fulfill responsibilities associated with one's job is considered sick. Therefore, a person who takes a leave of absence from work to recover is someone who is considered unhealthy in this model.

36. **a. According to Maslow's Hierarchy of Needs, freedom from pain is considered a safety and security need. Confusion occurs because other theorists such as R.A. Kalish believe that pain should be categorized along with adequate air, food, water, rest/sleep, shelter, elimination, and temperature regulation as a first level physiologic need.**

    b. According to Maslow's Hierarchy of Needs, freedom from hunger is considered a first level physiologic need, not a safety and security need.

    c. According to Maslow's Hierarchy of Needs, freedom from ridicule is associated with self-esteem needs, not safety and security needs.

    d. According to Maslow's Hierarchy of Needs, freedom from loneliness is associated with the need to feel loved and to belong, not to feel safe and secure.

37. a. According to the Social Readjustment Rating Scale by Holmes and Rahe, retirement is ranked 10th on the list of life events likely to cause stress related illness with a life-change-unit score of 45 out of 100. Retirement is considered less stressful than one of the other options offered.

    b. According to the Social Readjustment Rating Scale by Holmes and Rahe, pregnancy is ranked 12th on the list of life events likely to cause stress related illness with a life-change-unit score of 40 out of 100. Pregnancy is considered less stressful than two other options offered.

    c. According to the Social Readjustment Rating Scale by Holmes and Rahe, the gaining of a new family member is ranked fourteenth on the list of life events likely to cause stress related illness with a life-change-unit score of 39 out of 100. All of the other options are considered more stressful than gaining a new family member.

    d. According to the Social Readjustment Rating Scale by Holmes and Rahe, divorce is ranked second on the list of life events likely to cause stress related illness with a life-change-unit score of 73 out of 100. Only death of a spouse, ranked first on the scale with a score of 100, is considered more stressful than divorce.

38. a. Safety refers to a basic human need, not adaptive capacity.

    b. Health refers to a relative state of a person at a particular moment in time in the physical, emotional, spiritual, and mental dimension, not adaptive capacity.

    c. Restore refers to the return to a previous state or original condition. Adaptive capacity refers to the physical, emotional, mental and spiritual resources one can draw on to reestablish or restore one's previous state or original condition.

    d. Imbalance occurs when a person is threatened by a stressor. Adaptive capacity refers to the physical, emotional, mental, and spiritual resources one can draw on to seek to correct the imbalance and return to a state of homeostasis.

39. a. Being continuously angry three months after the death of a parent is within the realm of normal grieving behavior and is not dysfunctional. If a person was continuously angry after three years it would be considered dysfunctional grieving.

    b. Depression after one year is within the realm of normal grieving and is not uncommon, particularly if the relationship was meaningful, intense, or no one was able to fill the role of the deceased. If depression does not resolve within three years it would be considered dysfunctional grieving.

    c. Moving on with one's life is a sign of successful grieving. Mourning periods may be abbreviated if the loss is immediately replaced by another equally respected person or if the person experienced anticipatory grieving, which is grieving experienced before the death.

   d. Keeping a deceased child's room unchanged for years is outside normal limits of grieving and is dysfunctional. Often a person can get stuck in a stage of grieving and is unable to progress to the next stage. Keeping a room unchanged for years reflects an inability to face the reality of the loss or to deal with the feelings associated with the loss.

40. a. Illness is a physiological, not a developmental, stressor.
    b. Divorce is a psychological, not a developmental, stressor.
    c. Relocation is a psychological, not a developmental, stressor.
    d. Menopause is a normal stage of growth and development and therefore is a developmental stressor.

41. a. Love and belonging needs identified in Maslow's Hierarchy of Needs are not associated with Gordon's Value-Belief Patterns category. Nursing diagnoses found under Gordon's Value-Belief Patterns address topics such as spiritual distress and well-being, not love and belonging needs.
    b. Love and belonging needs identified in Maslow's Hierarchy of Needs are associated with Gordon's Role-Relationship Patterns category. Nursing diagnoses found under Gordon's Role-Relationship Patterns address topics such as social issues, loneliness, and relationships among family members and others.
    c. Love and belonging needs identified in Maslow's Hierarchy of Needs are not associated with Gordon's Cognitive-Perceptual Patterns category. Nursing diagnoses found under Gordon's Cognitive-Perceptual Patterns address topics such as comfort, confusion, conflict, knowledge deficit, disturbed thought processes and sensory perception, not love and belonging needs.
    d. Love and belonging needs identified in Maslow's Hierarchy of Needs are not associated with Gordon's Sexuality-Reproduction Patterns category. Nursing diagnoses found under Gordon's Sexuality-Reproduction Patterns address topics such as altered sexuality patterns and dysfunction, not love and belonging needs.

42. a. This does not support a patient's physiologic needs. Physiologic needs are related to having adequate air, food, water, rest, shelter, and the ability to eliminate and regulate body temperature.
    b. This does not support a patient's self-esteem needs. Self-esteem needs are met from within. It is how the patient feels about oneself.
    c. This does not support a patient's safety and security needs. Safety and security needs are related to being and feeling protected in the physiologic and interpersonal realms.
    d. Taping a patient's get well cards to the wall where the patient can see them supports the patient's need to feel loved and appreciated and

meets love and belonging needs according to Maslow's Hierarchy of Needs.

43. a. Role refers to a characteristic behavior in response to expectations of others or oneself and not adaptive capacity.
    b. Cope refers to an attempt to contend with or overcome some threat or stress which directly depends upon a person's potential or lack of potential to respond to a stress or threat. A person's potential or lack of potential to respond to a stress or threat is referred to as a person's adaptive capacity.
    c. Stimuli refers to the stressor portions of the stress and adaptation relationship, not the adaptation portion of the relationship. Adaptive capacity refers to the adaptation portion of the stress and adaptation relationship.
    d. Although all body activities require energy, including one's ability to adapt, one of the other three options is more clearly and directly related to the concept of adaptive capacity than is the word energy.

44. a. The reality principle is a learned Ego function whereby a person is able to delay the need for pleasure, not seek immediate gratification.
    b. Defense mechanisms are unconscious, not conscious, coping patterns that deny, distort, or reduce awareness of a stressful event in an attempt to protect the personality from anxiety.
    c. Freud believed that all behavior has meaning and called this theory *psychic determinism*. He believed that every psychic event is determined by prior events. Behavior, mental phenomenon, and even dreams are not accidental, but rather an expression of thoughts, feelings, or needs which have a relationship to the rest of a person's life.
    d. The Ego, not the Id, controls the personality. The Ego mediates the urges of the Id and the conscience of the Superego and is therefore the part of the psyche that controls the personality.

45. a. Every individual is influenced by family, ethnic, and cultural beliefs and values. These beliefs and values influence a person's lifestyle through how one perceives, experiences, and copes with health, illness, and disability. The nurse needs to assess the impact of a patient's cultural influences on the patient's health and health practices.
    b. Only in the Role-Performance Model of Health is productivity or performance of one's role a necessary component to be considered healthy. While important to understand, it is a narrow definition of health and fails to include the multitude of other factors that impact on a definition of health.
    c. Absence of disease or injury is the foundation of the Clinical Model of Health and fails to include the multitude of other factors that impact on a definition of health.
    d. Health cannot be easily measured or defined in common terms. There is no consensus on a definition of health, because health is unique to each individual and is based on personal expectations and values.

46. a. Adaptation is a response to stimuli that accommodates changes in the internal or external environment to preserve function. The process of adaptation is flexible, resilient, and responsive.
    b. The process of adaptation can be under conscious as well as unconscious control.
    c. Adaptations help to maintain homeostasis. If an adaptation is unsuccessful, then there is a failure to maintain homeostasis.
    d. Positive as well as negative events can be equally stressful. Events that are generally thought of as happy life events such as birth of a child, marriage, or move to a new home are stressful even though they are considered positive.

47. a. Free association, the free expression of thoughts or feelings just as they come to mind, is not a protective mechanism that is used in everyday life. It is a psychoanalytical technique used during therapy to lower a patient's defenses.
    b. R. Peck proposed three developmental tasks during old age. Ego Differentiation versus Work-Role Preoccupation is the developmental task associated with adjusting to retirement from meaningful work. Individuals need to replace work roles with new roles that are a source of self-esteem.
    c. Developmental Task Theory is attributed to R. J. Havighurst and is unrelated to Freud's Theory of Personality Development. According to Havighurst, developmental tasks associated with each age group are the source of conflict, not adaptations in an attempt to reduce anxiety.
    d. Defense mechanisms are unconscious coping techniques that deny, distort, or reduce awareness of a stressful event in an attempt to protect the Ego from anxiety.

48. a. This statement characterizes the depression stage in the grieving process. The person grieves over what will not happen.
    b. This statement characterizes the bargaining, not depression, stage in the grieving process. During bargaining, the person may make funeral plans, complete final arrangements regarding personal belongings, and write letters to family members to be read in the future.

    c. This statement characterizes the denial, not depression, stage in the grieving process. If one is in the intensive care unit and dying, it is unrealistic to believe that attendance at a daughter's wedding is a viable option.
    d. This statement characterizes the bargaining, not depression stage, in the grieving process and is an attempt to barter for more time. The patient is saying, "Yes me, but…"

49. a. This does not meet a patient's self-esteem needs. Self-esteem needs are met best when the nurse treats a patient with dignity and respect.
    b. This does not meet a patient's physiologic needs. Physiologic needs are met when the needs related to survival are supported.
    c. This does not meet a patient's love and belonging needs. Love and belonging needs are met when affection is given and received or when a person feels part of a group.
    d. When a patient is moved closer to the nurses' station so the patient can be monitored, safety and security needs are being met. The nurse's presence should give emotional comfort to the patient and will allow the nurse frequent opportunities to monitor and meet the patient's safety needs.

50. a. Pressure is not a psychological stressor. Psychological stressors are threats to one's values and beliefs, self-image, self concept, interpersonal relationships, or roles.
    b. Pressure is not a physiological stressor. Physiological stressors are disturbances in structure or function of any tissue, organ, system, or body part.
    c. Pressure is not a chemical stressor. Chemical stressors are drugs, poisons, and toxins.
    d. The force of pressure is a physical stressor. Pressure is the continuous force of a body part on a surface as a result of gravity compressing the tissue between the body part and the surface on which the body part is resting. This force is external to the body. The pressure ulcer which is the adaptation becomes a secondary stressor and is physiologic in nature.

Legal Issues

The following words include English vocabulary, nursing/medical terminology, concepts, principles, or information relevant to content specifically addressed in the chapter or associated with topics presented in it. English dictionaries, your nursing textbooks, and medical dictionaries such as *Taber's Cyclopedic Medical Dictionary* are resources that can be used to expand your knowledge and understanding of these words and related information.

Accountability
Accreditation
Act of commission/omission
Advanced directives
American Nurses Association
    Standards of Nursing Practice
Americans With Disabilities
    Act
Assault
Autonomy
Autopsy
Battery
Beneficence
Breach of Duty
Certification
Civil law
Code of Ethics
Collective bargaining
Common law
Confidentiality
Constitution of United States
Contract
Contractual relationship
Controlled Substance Acts
Controlled substances
Crime
Criterion (*pl.* criteria)
Death certificate
Defamation
Defendant
Defense
Dependent function
Disciplinary action

Do Not Resuscitate
Document
Duty
Ethics
Euthanasia
False imprisonment
Federal legislation
Fidelity
Fraud
Futility
Good Samaritan Law
Health Care Quality Improvement Act
Health Care Proxy
Incident Report
Incompetent
Independent function
Informed Consent
Interdependent function
Invasion of privacy
Joint Commission on Accreditation of
    Healthcare Organizations (JCAHO)
Justice
Liability
Libel
Licensure
Litigation
Living Will
Malpractice
National Council Licensing
    Examinations (NCLEX)
National League for Nursing
National League for Nursing
    Accrediting Commission

Negligence
Nonmaleficence
North American Nursing Diagnosis
    Association (NANDA)
Nurse Practice Act
Occupational Safety and Health Acts
Organ donation
Patient's Bill of Rights
Plaintiff
Professional liability insurance
Professional misconduct
Public law
Quality of life
Reciprocity
Registration
Res ipsa loquitur
Respondeat superior
Risk management program
Sigma Theta Tau
Slander
Standards of care
State Board of Nursing
State legislation
Statutory law
Sue
Supreme Court
Testify
Tort
Veracity
Voluntary
Will
Witness

1. Licensure of Registered Professional Nurses is required primarily to protect:
    a. Nurses
    b. Patients
    c. Common law
    d. Health care agencies

2. Which factor is unique to malpractice when comparing negligence and malpractice?
   a. The action did not meet standards of care
   b. The inappropriate care is an act of commission
   c. There is harm to the patient as a result of the care
   d. There is a contractual relationship between the nurse and patient

3. The main purpose of an Incident Report is to:
   a. Ensure that all parties have an opportunity to document what happened
   b. Help establish who is responsible for the incident
   c. Make data available for quality control analysis
   d. Document the incident on the patient's chart

4. When the nurse administers a drug that has PRN after the order, the nurse functions:
   a. Collegially
   b. Dependently
   c. Independently
   d. Interdependently

5. A main purpose of the American Nurses Association is to:
   a. Establish standards of nursing practice
   b. Recognize academic achievement in nursing
   c. Monitor educational institutions granting degrees in nursing
   d. Prepare nurses to become members of the nursing profession

6. The nurse says, "If you do not let me do this dressing change, I will not let you eat dinner with the other residents in the dining room." This is an example of:
   a. Assault
   b. Battery
   c. Negligence
   d. Malpractice

7. State legislatures are responsible for:
   a. Standardized care plans
   b. Enactment of Nurse Practice Acts
   c. Accreditation of educational nursing programs
   d. Certification in specialty areas of nursing practice

8. Which is specifically related to the doctrine of *respondeat superior*?
   a. Nurses must respond to the Supreme Court when they commit acts of malpractice
   b. Health care facilities are responsible for the negligent actions of the nurses that they employ
   c. Nurses are responsible for their actions when they have contractual relationships with patients
   d. The laws absolve nurses from being sued for negligence if they provide inappropriate care at the scene of an accident

9. When attempting to administer a 10:00 p.m. sleeping medication, the nurse assesses that the patient appears to be asleep. What should the nurse do?
   a. Hold the drug
   b. Notify the physician
   c. Awaken the patient and administer the drug
   d. Administer it later if the patient awakens during the night

10. Licensure of Registered Nurses in America is:
    a. Governed by each state
    b. Controlled by federal law
    c. Regulated by constitutional law
    d. Authorized by the American Nurses Association

11. The nurse causes harm to a hospitalized patient because of improper use of medical equipment. This is most specifically called:
    a. Battery
    b. Assault
    c. Negligence
    d. Malpractice

12. The role of the American Nurses Association Standards of Nursing Practice is to:
    a. Establish criteria for quality practice
    b. Define the philosophy of nursing practice
    c. Identify the legal definition of nursing practice
    d. Determine educational standards for nursing practice

13. Which patient is unable to give an informed consent for surgery?
    a. A 16-year-old boy who is married
    b. A 35-year-old woman who is depressed
    c. A 50-year-old woman who does not speak English
    d. A 65-year-old man who has received a narcotic for pain

14. When the nurse decides to give a partial bath instead of a complete bath the nurse is working:
    a. Dependently
    b. Independently
    c. Collaboratively
    d. Interdependently

15. What should the nurse do if when administering a medication to a confused patient the patient says, "This pill looks different from the one I had before."
    a. Ask what the other pill looked like
    b. Check the original medication order
    c. Explain the purpose of the medication
    d. Encourage the patient to take the medication

16. An Incident Report is completed primarily to:
    a. Record the event for future litigation
    b. Provide a basis for designing new policies
    c. Prevent similar situations from happening again
    d. Ensure accountability for the cause of the accident

17. What should the nurse do when the physician orders medication that is larger than the standard dose?
    a. Inform the supervisor
    b. Give the drug as ordered
    c. Call the physician to discuss the order
    d. Give the normal average dose and inform the physician

18. When the nurse works on a skin care team, the nurse is functioning:
    a. Dependently
    b. Independently
    c. Collaboratively
    d. Interdependently

19. What is the position of the American Nurses Association in relation to assisted suicide? Nurses should:
    a. Not participate in active euthanasia
    b. Participate based on their own value and belief system
    c. Participate when the patient is experiencing severe pain
    d. Not participate unless 2 physicians are consulted and the patient has had counseling

20. Which is responsible for ensuring that Registered Nurses are minimally qualified to practice nursing?
    a. Sigma Theta Tau
    b. State Boards of Nursing
    c. American Nurses Association
    d. Constituent Leagues of the National League for Nursing

21. The nurse gave the wrong patient an enema that resulted in dehydration and an electrolyte imbalance. The nurse could be sued for:
    a. Malpractice
    b. Battery
    c. Assault
    d. Libel

22. The nurse works interdependently when:
    a. Helping a patient choose high protein foods from the ordered diet
    b. Applying a dry sterile dressing to an abdominal incision
    c. Irrigating a feeding tube that appears obstructed
    d. Giving ice chips to a patient who is NPO

23. A nurse expert is called to testify in a lawsuit for professional nursing malpractice primarily to testify:
    a. About standards of nursing care as they apply to the facts in the case
    b. With regard to laws governing the practice of nursing
    c. To the appropriateness of the nursing diagnosis
    d. For the defense

24. When the nurse initiates a visit from a member of the clergy, the nurse functions:
    a. Interdependently
    b. Independently
    c. Dependently
    d. Collegially

25. Which protects the patient who is being asked to participate in a medical research study?
    a. Code of Ethics
    b. Informed Consent
    c. Nurse Practice Act
    d. Constitution of the United States

26. What is the most serious consequence associated with an ineffective bowel preparation before a colonoscopy?
    a. Discomfort
    b. Misdiagnosis
    c. Wasted expense
    d. Psychological stress

27. The physician's order states OOB. When the nurse moves the patient out of bed to a chair the nurse is working:
    a. Dependently
    b. Independently
    c. Collaboratively
    d. Interdependently

28. A patient suddenly has difficulty swallowing oral secretions. When the nurse suctions this patient to maintain a patent airway, the nurse functions:
    a. Collegially
    b. Dependently
    c. Independently
    d. Interdependently

29. Which of the following actions is the most important standard that should be met when a Registered Nurse functions as a Good Samaritan at the scene of an accident that has caused a person a life-threatening injury?
    a. Stay at the scene until another qualified person takes over
    b. Seek consent from the injured party before rendering assistance
    c. Implement every possible critical care intervention necessary to sustain life
    d. Insist on helping because a nurse is the best qualified person to provide care

30. Licensure of Registered Nurses is:
    a. Granted upon graduation from a nursing program
    b. A standard of the American Nurses Association
    c. Approved by the National League for Nursing
    d. Required by state law

31. The most common situation involving malpractice is:
    a. Medication errors
    b. False imprisonment
    c. Failure to prevent a fall
    d. Application of warm soaks

32. Which situation would require that an Incident Report be completed?
    a. A nurse left work early without reporting to the supervisor
    b. A patient did not receive a medication ordered by the physician
    c. A visitor ambulated a patient who should have been on bed rest
    d. A patient refused to go to physical therapy as ordered by the physician

33. When the nurse uses a straight catheter to obtain a urine specimen for culture and sensitivity, the nurse works:
    a. Interdependently
    b. Independently
    c. Dependently
    d. Collegially

34. When considering legal issues the term "contract" is to "liable" as "standard" is to:
    a. Rights
    b. Negligence
    c. Malpractice
    d. Accountable

35. An anxious patient repeatedly uses the call bell to get the nurse to come to the room. Finally the nurse says to the patient, "If you keep ringing, there will come a time I won't answer your bell." This is an example of:
    a. Slander
    b. Assault
    c. Battery
    d. Libel

36. The organization associated with the credentialing of hospitals is:
    a. NCLEX
    b. JCAHO
    c. ANA
    d. NLN

37. A Living Will is a document that:
    a. Instructs a physician to withhold/withdraw life-sustaining procedures if death is near
    b. Enables a person to request medication to end life in a humane and dignified manner
    c. Gives consent to perform life-sustaining medical intervention during an emergency
    d. Wills one's organs to help others who need a transplant to sustain life

38. Which action is unrelated to a State Nurse Practice Act?
    a. Setting guidelines for nurses' salaries in the state
    b. Establishing reciprocity for licensure between states
    c. Determining minimum requirements for nursing education
    d. Maintaining a list of nurses who can legally practice in the state

39. When changing a dry sterile dressing the nurse is working:
    a. Interdependently
    b. Collaboratively
    c. Independently
    d. Dependently

40. What should the nurse do first before administering a medication?
    a. Ensure that the medication is in the medication cart
    b. Determine the appropriateness of the medication
    c. Check the patient's identification armband
    d. Verify the physician's order for accuracy

41. Which is not verified when a nurse witnesses the signing of a consent for a procedure? That the patient:
    a. Signs the consent voluntarily in the presence of the nurse
    b. Is the person who signed the consent in front of the nurse
    c. Was explained the risks and benefits of the procedure by the nurse
    d. Appears alert and competent to give a consent as determined by the nurse

42. Which organization is responsible for ensuring that nursing schools in the United States meet standards of nursing education?
    a. National League for Nursing Accrediting Commission
    b. North American Nursing Diagnosis Association
    c. American Nurses Association
    d. Sigma Theta Tau

43. The patient's diet order is "clear liquids to regular as tolerated." When the nurse progresses the diet to full liquid the nurse is working:
    a. Dependently
    b. Independently
    c. Collaboratively
    d. Interdependently

44. Which is an example of slander?
    a. A volunteer telling another volunteer a patient's age
    b. A nurse telling a patient that another nurse is incompetent
    c. A Nursing Assistant telling a patient about another patient's diagnosis
    d. A Nurse Manager documenting a nurse's medication error in a performance appraisal

45. What should the nurse do first before giving an ordered preoperative medication?
    a. Check that the preoperative check list is completed
    b. Verify that the surgical consent is signed
    c. Ensure that an IV is in place
    d. Assess the vital signs

1. a. Licensure does not protect the nurse. Licensure grants an individual the legal right to practice as a Registered Nurse.
   b. **Licensure indicates that a person has met minimal standards of competency, thus protecting the public's safety.**
   c. Licensure does not protect common law. Common law comprises standards and rules based on the principles established in prior judicial decisions.
   d. Licensure does not protect health care agencies. The Joint Commission on Accreditation of Healthcare Organizations (JCAHO) determines if agencies meet minimal standards of health care delivery, thus protecting the public.

2. a. There is a violation of standards of care with both negligence and malpractice.
   b. Negligence and malpractice both involve acts of commission or omission.
   c. The patient must have sustained injury, damage, or harm with both negligence and malpractice.
   d. **Malpractice is misconduct performed in professional practice, where there is a contractual relationship between the patient and nurse, which results in harm to the patient.**

3. a. The nurse who identifies or creates the potential or actual harm completes the Incident Report. The report identifies the people involved in the incident, describes the incident, and records the date, time, location, actions taken, and other relevant information.
   b. Documentation should be as factual as possible and avoid accusations. Questions of liability are the responsibility of the courts.
   c. **Incidence reports help to identify patterns of risk so that corrective action plans can take place.**
   d. The report is not part of the patient's medical record and reference to the report should not be made in the patient's medical record.

4. a. Collegial or collaborative interventions are actions the nurse carries out in conjunction with other health team members.
   b. Dependent interventions are those activities carried out under a practitioner's direction and supervision.
   c. Independent interventions are those activities the nurse is licensed to initiate based on knowledge and expertise.
   d. **An interdependent intervention requires a practitioner's order associated with a set parameter. The parameter, such as *whenever necessary*, requires that the nurse use judgment in implementing the order.**

5. a. **The American Nurses Association has established Standards of Care and Standards of Professional Performance. These standards reflect the values of the nursing profession, provide expectations for nursing practice, facilitate the evaluation of nursing practice, and define the profession's accountability to the public.**
   b. Sigma Theta Tau, the international honor society of nursing, recognizes academic achievement.
   c. The National League for Nursing Accrediting Commission and State Education Departments monitor educational institutions granting degrees in nursing.
   d. Schools of Nursing (Diploma, Associate Degree, and Baccalaureate) educate individuals for entry into the practice of nursing.

6. a. **This statement is an unjust threat. Assault is the threat to touch another person unjustly.**
   b. This is not an example of battery. Battery is the actual willful touching of another person that may or may not cause harm.
   c. This is not an example of negligence. Negligence occurs when harm or injury is caused by an act of either commission or omission.
   d. This is not an example of malpractice. Malpractice is negligence by a professional person as compared to the actions of another professional person in a similar circumstance when a contract exists between the patient and nurse.

7. a. Nursing team members or an interdisciplinary team of health care providers write standardized care plans.
   b. **Every state has its own Nurse Practice Act that describes and defines the legal boundaries of nursing practice within the state.**
   c. The National League for Nursing Accrediting Commission is the major organization accrediting nursing education programs in the United States.
   d. The American Nurses Association and other specialty organizations offer certification in specialty areas in nursing practice.

8. a. This is unrelated to *respondeat superior*. Negligence and malpractice, which are unintentional torts, are litigated in local courts by civil actions between individuals.
   b. **The ancient legal doctrine *respondeat superior* means *let the master answer*. By virtue of the employer-employee relationship, the employer is responsible for the conduct of its employees.**
   c. Individual responsibility is unrelated to *respondeat superior*. A nurse can have an independent contractual relationship with a patient. When a nurse works for an agency the contract between the nurse and patient is implied. In both instances, the nurse is responsible for the care provided.
   d. This is unrelated to *respondeat superior*. Good Samaritan laws do not provide absolute immunity.

9. a. This would be a violation of the practitioner's order. Drug administration is a dependent nursing function.
   b. This is unnecessary.
   c. **Administering a medication is a dependent function of the nurse, and the order should be followed as written if the order is reasonable and prudent.**
   d. The drug should be administered as ordered, not at a later time.

10. a. **The power to grant licenses to professional health care providers is reserved for the states. An individual must meet minimum proficiency standards to receive a license, thus protecting the public.**

b. Nurse Practice Acts govern the practice of nursing and licensure, not federal law.

c. Nurse Practice Acts govern the practice of nursing and licensure, not constitutional law.

d. The American Nurses Association (ANA) is the national professional organization for nursing in the United States. It fosters high standards of nursing practice; it does not grant licensure.

11. a. This is not an example of battery. Battery is the purposeful, angry, or negligent touching of a patient without consent.

b. This is not an example of assault. Assault is an attempt or threat to touch another person unjustly.

c. This is not an example of negligence. Negligence occurs when the nurse's actions do not meet appropriate standards of care and result in injury to another.

d. **Malpractice is misconduct performed in professional practice that results in harm to another.**

12. a. **The ANA Standards of Clinical Nursing Practice describe the nature and scope of nursing practice and the responsibilities for which nurses are accountable.**

b. A philosophy incorporates the values and beliefs about the phenomena of concern to a discipline. The ANA Standards of Clinical Nursing Practice reflect, not define, a philosophy of nursing. Each nurse and nursing organization should define its own philosophy of nursing.

c. The laws of each state define the practice of nursing within the state.

d. Educational standards are established by accrediting bodies such as the National League for Nursing Accrediting Commission and State Education Departments.

13. a. Legally, individuals younger than 18 years old can provide informed consent if they are married, pregnant, parents, members of the military, or emancipated.

b. A depressed person is capable of making health care decisions until proven to be mentally incompetent.

c. This person can provide informed consent after interventions ensure that the person understands the facts and risks concerning the treatment.

d. **Narcotics depress the central nervous system including decision-making abilities. This person is considered functionally incompetent.**

14. a. The nurse does not need a practitioner's order to provide nursing care that is within the realm of nursing practice.

b. **Providing hygiene, an activity of daily living, is within the scope of nursing practice.**

c. The nurse does not need to collaborate with other health care professionals to provide nursing care.

d. The nurse does not need a practitioner's order, with or without a restriction, to implement nursing care that is within the realm of nursing practice.

15. a. This action by itself is unsafe because the patient is confused and the information obtained may be inaccurate.

b. **This is the safest intervention because it goes to the original source of the order.**

c. This intervention ignores the patient's concern. Although this ultimately may be done, it is not the priority action.

d. This action ignores the patient's statement and is unsafe without first obtaining additional information.

16. a. Although documentation of an incident may be used in a court of law, it is not the primary reason for an Incident Report.

b. This is not the primary reason for Incident Reports. New policies may or may not have to be written and implemented.

c. **Risk management committees use statistical data about accidents and incidents to identify patterns of risk and prevent future accidents and incidents.**

d. Although nurses are always accountable for their actions, accountability for the cause of an incidence is the role of the courts.

17. a. It is unnecessary to call the supervisor in this situation.

b. This would be unsafe for the patient and could result in malpractice.

c. **Nurses have a professional responsibility to know or investigate the standard dose for medications being administered. In addition, nurses are responsible for their own actions regardless of whether there is a written order. The nurse has a responsibility to question and/or refuse to administer an order that appears unreasonable.**

d. Changing a medication prescription is not within the scope of nursing practice.

18. a. Although some interventions by a skin care team are within the scope of nursing practice, others require a practitioner's order.

b. Many of the interventions performed by a skin care team require a practitioner's order and are therefore beyond the scope of independent nursing practice.

c. **Collaborative or collegial interventions are actions the nurse carries out in conjunction with other health team members. A skin care team works with other health care providers to meet a patient's needs.**

d. The nurse works interdependently when implementing a practitioner's order that requires the consideration of certain factors outlined in the original order. Some interventions of a skin care team are within the scope of nursing practice and some require a practitioner's specific order.

19. a. **Nursing actions must comply with the law and the law states that euthanasia is legally wrong. Euthanasia can lead to criminal charges of homicide or civil lawsuits for providing an unacceptable standard of care.**

b. A nurse's beliefs, values, or moral convictions should not be imposed on patients.

c. Compassion and good intentions are not an acceptable basis for actions beyond the scope of nursing practice.

d. These factors do not permit a nurse to be involved with euthanasia.

20. a. Sigma Theta Tau, the international honor society of nursing, recognizes academic achievement and leadership qualities, encourages high professional standards, fosters creative endeavors, and supports excellence in the profession of nursing.
    b. **The National Council of State Boards of Nursing is responsible for the NCLEX-RN examination; however, the licensing authority in the jurisdiction in which the graduate takes the examination verifies the acceptable score on the examination.**
    c. The American Nurses Association (ANA) is the national professional organization for nursing in the United States. It fosters high standards of nursing practice; it does not grant licensure.
    d. The National League for Nursing is committed to promoting and improving nursing service and nursing education.

21. a. **Malpractice is negligence by a professional person as compared to the actions of another professional person in a similar situation. Four elements must be proven: a professional relationship with the patient (duty); failure to meet a standard of care (breach of duty); patient must sustain harm, injury or damage (harm); and harm that directly results from the nurse's failure to follow standards of care (causation).**
    b. This is not an example of battery. Battery is the willful touching of a person (including their clothing or something they are carrying) that may or may not cause harm.
    c. This is not an example of assault. Assault is a threat or attempt to touch another person unjustly.
    d. This is not an example of libel. Libel is false communication about another by writing, print, or pictures.

22. a. **An interdependent intervention requires a practitioner's order associated with a set parameter. When the practitioner orders a specific diet, the nurse can teach the patient which foods on the diet are high in a particular nutrient.**
    b. This is an example of a dependent function of the nurse.
    c. This is an example of an independent function of the nurse.
    d. This is an example of a violation of a practitioner's order. This action could harm the patient and result in malpractice.

23. a. **The American Nurses Association Standards of Nursing Practice are authoritative statements by which the national organization for nursing describes the responsibilities for which its practitioners are accountable. An expert nurse is capable of explaining these standards as they apply to the situation under litigation. These professional standards are one criterion that helps a judge or jury determine if a nurse was negligent.**
    b. An expert nurse is not an expert in the law. The expert nurse's role is not to make judgments about the laws as they apply to the practice of nursing.

   c. A judge or jury, not the expert nurse, decides the appropriateness of behavior.
   d. A nurse expert can testify for either the prosecution or the defense.

24. a. The nurse does not need a physician's order to make a referral to a member of the clergy. An interdependent intervention requires a practitioner's order associated with a parameter.
    b. **The nurse is initiating the referral to the member of the clergy and is therefore working independently. Nurses are legally permitted to diagnose and treat human responses to actual or potential health problems.**
    c. This action is within the scope of nursing practice. The nurse does not need a physician's order to make a referral to a member of the clergy.
    d. The nurse can make a referral to a member of the clergy without collaborating with another professional health team member.

25. a. A code of ethics is the official statement of a group's ideals and values. It includes broad statements that provide a basis for professional actions.
    b. **Informed consent is an agreement by a client to accept a course of treatment or a procedure after receiving complete information necessary to make a knowledgeable decision.**
    c. Nurse Practice Acts define the scope of nursing practice; they are unrelated to informed consent.
    d The Constitution of the United States addresses broad individual rights and responsibilities. The rights related to nursing practice and patients include the rights of privacy, freedom of speech, and due process.

26. a. Although this could occur, it is not the most serious outcome of an inappropriate preparation for a colonoscopy.
    b. **Fecal material in the intestines can interfere with the visualization, collection, and analysis of data obtained through a colonoscopy, resulting in diagnostic errors.**
    c. A test may have to be cancelled or performed a second time if the patient has an ineffective bowel preparation. Although this is a serious consequence, it is not life threatening.
    d. Although this is a serious consequence, it is not life threatening.

27. a. **Determining the extent of activity desirable for a patient is within the physician's, not nurse's, scope of practice. Following activity orders is a dependent function of the nurse.**
    b. The responsibility to determine a patient's activity level is not within the legal scope of nursing practice.
    c. A physician works independently when determining a patient's desired activity level.
    d. The nurse is following the physician's order to get the patient OOB. There are no restrictions or parameters in relation to the order.

28. a. The nurse does not need to confer with another professional health team member to suction a patient's airway to maintain patency.

b. Suctioning a patient's airway routinely would require a physician's order.

c. Nurses are permitted legally to diagnose and treat human responses. Maintaining a patent airway in an emergency is within the scope of nursing practice.

d. An interdependent intervention is performed when the nurse suctions a patient's airway in the presence of the order *oropharyngeal suctioning PRN.*

29. a. **When a nurse renders emergency care, the nurse has an ethical responsibility not to abandon the injured person. The nurse should not leave the scene until the injured person leaves or another qualified person assumes responsibility.**

b. Depending on the injured person's physical and emotional status, the person may or may not be able to consent to care.

c. When a nurse helps in an emergency, the nurse is required to render care that is consistent with care that any reasonably prudent nurse would provide under similar circumstances. The nurse should not attempt interventions that are beyond the scope of nursing practice.

d. A nurse should offer assistance, not insist on assisting, at the scene of an emergency.

30. a. When a person graduates from a school of nursing the individual receives a diploma that indicates completion of a course of study; the diploma is not a license to practice nursing.

b. The ANA Standards of Professional Performance do not address licensure. They only indicate that a nurse should maintain current knowledge and competency.

c. The National League for Nursing promotes nursing service and nursing education, it is not involved with licensure.

d. **The Nurse Practice Act in a state stipulates the requirements for licensure within the state.**

31. a. **Administration of medications is a major area of potential liability for nurses. Medication errors often occur in relation to failure to question unclear medication orders; lack of knowledge about a medication; incorrect calculations; failure to identify the patient correctly; preparing the wrong concentration; administering a medication via the wrong route; and failure to identify nontherapeutic patient responses.**

b. The majority of malpractice does not involve false imprisonment, which is the restraining of an individual against the person's wishes.

c. The majority of malpractice does not involve patient falls. Most falls occur in patients' rooms when they are attempting to go to the bathroom unassisted.

d. The majority of malpractice does not involve burning a patient. Hot water bottles, heating pads, and solutions that are too hot for application cause most burns.

32. a. This action does not require an Incident Report. The nurse manager should discuss this behavior with the nurse and may document it in the nurse's personnel file.

b. **Not receiving an ordered medication may have the potential to cause harm. Therefore, an Incident or Adverse Occurrence Report should be completed to document the incident to add to the data so that similar situations can be prevented in the future.**

c. An Incident Report does not have to be completed in this instance. The incident should be documented in the patient's medical record.

d. An Incident Report is unnecessary in this situation. Patients have the right to refuse care; however, the patient's refusal of care and the reasons for the refusal should be documented in the patient's medical record.

33. a. An interdependent intervention requires a practitioner's order associated with a parameter. This order for a straight catheter to obtain a urine specimen is a directive without parameters.

b. Inserting a catheter into a body cavity without a physician's order is not within the scope of nursing practice and is not an independent function of the nurse.

c. **Dependent interventions are physician-prescribed therapies or treatments that a nurse is legally permitted to perform.**

d. Collegial or collaborative interventions are actions the nurse carries out in conjunction with other health team members.

34. a. Although patients have a right to receive care that meets appropriate standards, the word *right* does not have the same relationship to the word *standard* as the relationship between the words *contract* and *liable.*

b. The words *standards* and *negligence* do not have the same relationship as *contract* and *liable.* Negligence involves an act (of commission or omission) that a reasonably prudent person would not do.

c. The words *standards* and *malpractice* do not have the same relationship as *contract* and *liable.* Malpractice is negligence by a professional person.

d. *Liable* **means a person is responsible (accountable) for fulfilling a contract that is enforceable by law.** *Accountable* **means a person is responsible (liable) for meeting standards, which are expectations established for making judgments or comparisons.**

35. a. This is not an example of slander, which is a false spoken statement resulting in damage to a person's character or reputation.

b. **This is an example of assault. Assault is either a physical or verbal attack or unlawful threat causing a fear of harm. No actual contact is necessary for a threat to be an assault.**

c. This is not an example of battery, which is the unlawful touching of a person's body without consent.

d. This is not an example of libel, which is a false printed statement resulting in damage to a person's character or reputation.

36. a. In the United States, graduates of educational programs that prepare students to become Registered Professional Nurses must successfully complete the National Council Licensure Examination-RN (NCLEX-RN) as part of the criteria for licensure.

b. The Joint Commission of Accreditation of Healthcare Organizations (JCAHO) evaluates healthcare organizations' compliance with JCAHO standards. Accreditation indicates that the organization has the capabilities to provide quality care. In addition, federal and state regulatory agencies and insurance companies require JCAHO accreditation.

c. The American Nurses Association (ANA) is the national professional organization for nursing in the United States. Its purposes are to promote high standards of nursing practice and to support the educational and professional advancement of nurses.

d. The National League for Nursing (NLN) fosters the development and improvement of nursing education and nursing service.

37. a. A living will provides specific instructions about the care the person does or does not want to receive, including withholding or withdrawing life-sustaining procedures.

b. Euthanasia, the act of painlessly putting to death a person who is suffering, is against the law.

c. When an individual cannot provide written or oral consent (express consent) during an emergency, care is provided under the concept of *implied consent*.

d. Under the Uniform Anatomical Gift Act and the National Organ Transplant Act in the United States, an individual 18 years or older may donate all or part of their body for education, research, advancement of science, therapy or transplantation. Consent for organ donation usually is made via a signed organ donation card.

38. a. State Nurse Practice Acts define and regulate the practice of nursing within the state. The salary of nurses is determined through negotiations between nurses or their representatives, such as a union or a professional nursing organization, and the representatives of the agency in which they work.

b. A state's Nurse Practice Act determines the criteria for reciprocity for licensure.

c. A state's Nurse Practice Act stipulates minimum requirements for nursing education.

d A state's Nurse Practice Act defines the criteria for licensure within the state. The actual functions may be delegated to another official body such as a State Board of Nursing or State Education Department.

39. a. The changing of a dry sterile dressing would be an interdependent action by the nurse when the physician's order for wound care stated, *Dry Sterile Dressing PRN*.

b. In this situation, the nurse is not working with other health care professionals to implement a physician's order.

c. This intervention is not within the scope of nursing practice without a physician's order.

d. A nurse is not permitted legally to prescribe wound care. The nurse needs a practitioner's order to provide wound care.

40. a. Although this may be done as a time management practice, it is not the first step when preparing to administer a medication to a patient.

b. A nurse is legally responsible for the safe administration of medications; therefore, th should assess if a medication order is reasonabic. However, this is not the first step when preparing to administer a medication to a patient.

c. Although this action is essential for the safe administration of a medication to a patient, it is not the first step of this procedure.

d. The administration of medications is a dependent function of the nurse. The physician's order should be verified for accuracy. The order must include the name of the patient, the name of the drug, the size of the dose, the route of administration, and the number of times per day to be administered.

41. a. Consent must be given freely and without coercion, and the consent form is signed in the presence of the nurse.

b. The person receiving the treatment or a legally accepted alternative, such as the parent of a child, legal guardian, or spouse, must sign the consent form in front of the nurse.

c. It is the responsibility of the practitioner, not the nurse, to provide this information. Patients have a legal right to have adequate and accurate information to make knowledgeable decisions about their treatment.

d. If the nurse determines that a patient is incapable of signing a consent form because of an impaired decision-making ability, such as a lowered level of consciousness, confusion, or lack of touch with reality, the physician should be notified immediately.

42. a. The National League for Nursing Accrediting Commission (NLNAC) is an organization that appraises and grants accreditation status to nursing programs that meet predetermined structure, process, and outcome criteria.

b. The North American Nursing Diagnosis Association (NANDA) developed a constantly evolving taxonomy of nursing diagnoses to provide a standardized language that focuses on the patient and related nursing care.

c. The American Nurses Association (ANA) is the national professional organization for nursing in the United States. It does not accredit schools of nursing.

d. Sigma Theta Tau, the international honor society of nursing, recognizes academic achievement. It does not accredit schools of nursing.

43. a. This dietary order has parameters that exceed a simple dependent function of the nurse.

b. Prescribing a dietary order for a patient is outside the scope of nursing practice.

c. Collaborative or collegial interventions are actions the nurse carries out in conjunction with other health team members.

d. The physician's order implies a progression in the diet as tolerated. The nurse uses judgment to determine the time of this progression, which is an interdependent action.

44. a. This is a violation of the patient's right to confidentiality, not slander.

b. This is an example of slander. Slander is a false spoken statement resulting in damage to a person's character or reputation.

c. This is a violation of the patient's right to confidentiality, not slander.

d. This is not slander because it is a written, not spoken, statement and it documents true, not false, information.

45. a. Although this is done, it is not the priority.

b. The consent for surgery must be signed before preoperative medications are administered because they depress the central nervous system impairing problem solving and decision-making.

c. This is unnecessary. This can be done at any time during the preoperative phase or at the beginning of the intraoperative phase of surgery.

d. Although this is done, it is not the priority.

Management and Leadership

The following words include English vocabulary, nursing/medical terminology, concepts, principles, or information relevant to content specifically addressed in the chapter or associated with topics presented in it. English dictionaries, your nursing textbooks, and medical dictionaries such as *Taber's Cyclopedic Medical Dictionary* are resources that can be used to expand your knowledge and understanding of these words and related information.

Accountability
Accountable
Alternatives
Assignment
Bureaucratic
Case management
Change theory
Controlling
Consensus
Cooperation
Creative
Cyclical process
Decision
Delegate
Directing
Documentation
Efficiency
Empower
Feedback
Five Rights of Delegation
Flexible
Human resource management
Incentives

Job description
Leadership
Leadership styles - classic
    Autocratic – directive
    Democratic – participative, consultative
    Laissez-faire – nondirective, permissive
Leadership styles – contemporary
    Charismatic leadership
    Connective leadership
    Transactional leadership
    Transformational leadership
    Shared leadership
Linear process
Managers - types
    First-line managers
    Unit managers
    Middle managers
    Nurse executives
Motivation
Network
Organization

Performance evaluation
Power—types of
    Expert
    Influence
    Legitimate
    Referent
    Reward
Preceptor
Primary nursing
Problem solving
Productivity
Resistance
Resource
Resource management
Role model
Solution
Subordinate
Systems theory
Table of Organization
Time management
Trial and error

1. Which type of leadership style would be most appropriate when a nurse manager is informed that a large number of patients will be admitted in response to a terrorist attack?
   a. Collaborative
   b. Authoritarian
   c. Laissez-faire
   d. Democratic

2. To overcome resistance to change, the most important action by the Nurse Manager would be to:
   a. Identify the reason for the resistance
   b. Modify the objectives to appeal to more key people
   c. Emphasize the positive consequences of the change
   d. State clearly and concisely the purpose of the change

3. Leadership's major focus is on:
   a. Inspiring people
   b. Creating change
   c. Controlling others
   d. Producing a product

4. The primary difference between effective leaders and managers is that managers have:
   a. Vision
   b. Charisma
   c. Confidence
   d. Responsibility

5. A Registered Nurse on a patient care unit delegates a component of patient care to an unlicensed Nursing Assistant. The person most responsible for the safe performance of the care is the:
   a. Head Nurse who is in charge of the unit
   b. Nursing Assistant assigned to provide the care
   c. Nurse who delegated the care to the Nursing Assistant
   d. Nursing Care Coordinator who is the supervisor for the unit

6. Which situation is most reflective of the saying, *A stitch in time saves nine*?
   a. Obtaining the vital signs for the patients on the unit at the same time
   b. Collecting equipment for a procedure before entering the room
   c. Delegating some interventions to the Licensed Practical Nurse
   d. Documenting the nursing care given every two hours

7. The Registered Nurse delegates a procedure to a Licensed Practical Nurse. This act of delegation is used primarily to:
   a. Create change
   b. Establish a network
   c. Improve productivity
   d. Transfer accountability

8. When providing feedback to a subordinate who needs a change in behavior, the best intervention by nurse would be to:
   a. Be assertive
   b. Explore alternatives
   c. Identify the unacceptable behavior
   d. Document the content of the counseling session

9. Which leadership style generally works best when the staff is personally and professionally mature and motivated?
   a. Directive
   b. Autocratic
   c. Democratic
   d. Laissez-faire

10. Which assignment would be most appropriate for a Registered Nurse?
    a. Taking the pulse of a patient with a dysrhythmia
    b. Applying a condom catheter on a patient who is incontinent
    c. Changing the linen on an occupied bed for a comatose patient
    d. Transferring a patient from a bed to a chair with a mechanical lift

11. The main purpose of achieving a consensus when making a decision within a group is to:
    a. Explore possible alternative solutions
    b. Demonstrate that staff members are flexible
    c. Facilitate cooperative effort toward goal achievement
    d. Ensure the use of effective autocratic decision making

12. When the Nurse Manager evaluates the performance of a subordinate, which management function is being implemented by the Nurse Manager?
    a. Planning
    b. Directing
    c. Controlling
    d. Organizing

13. Which of the "Five Rights of Delegation" is associated with ensuring that the intervention can be legally implemented by the assigned individual? The right:
    a. Communication
    b. Feedback
    c. Person
    d. Task

14. Which is most related to systems theory?
    a. End result
    b. Linear format
    c. Trial and error
    d. Cyclical process

15. An accurate assessment drives the rest of the steps of the nursing process. Which management function drives effective management?
    a. Planning
    b. Directing
    c. Controlling
    d. Organizing

16. The nurse works independently when:
    a. Limiting fluids when a patient has an order for 1000-cc fluid restriction
    b. Assigning another nurse to administer medications
    c. Irrigating a patient's wound with normal saline
    d. Applying a warm soak on an infiltrated IV site

17. Which leadership style is used when the Nurse Manager makes out the daily assignment of subordinates and continually monitors their activities and decisions?
    a. Authoritarian
    b. Bureaucratic
    c. Laissez-faire
    d. Democratic

18. Which is most basic for a nurse new to a management position?
    a. An understanding of when to be confrontational
    b. Strong interpersonal communication skills
    c. Knowledge of the role of a change agent
    d. Recognition by peers as a leader

19. Which type of power is being used when a Unit Manager mentors a new Unit Manager as part of orientation to the position?
    a. Influence
    b. Coercive
    c. Referent
    d. Expert

20. There are "Five Rights of Delegation," right task, right person, right communication, right time, and right:
    a. Preceptor
    b. Feedback
    c. Route
    d. Place

21. To overcome resistance to change, the Nurse Manager must first:
    a. Ensure that the planned change is within the current beliefs and values of the group
    b. Provide incentives to encourage commitment to the change
    c. Implement change in small steps rather than large steps
    d. Use informational power to ensure that goals are met

22. Which specimen collection should a Registered Nurse delegate to a Licensed Practical Nurse rather than an unlicensed Nursing Assistant?
    a. Sputum for cytology
    b. Urine for specific gravity
    c. Stool for presence of ova and parasites
    d. Wound drainage for culture and sensitivity

23. A Nurse Manager who values the importance of positive role modeling will:
    a. Counsel subordinates who fail to meet expectations
    b. Hold team meetings to review rules of the agency
    c. Follow the policies and procedures of the agency
    d. Review job descriptions with employees

24. When considering leadership styles an "autocratic" leader is to "authoritarian" as a "democratic" leader is to:
    a. Directive
    b. Permissive
    c. Oppressive
    d. Consultative

25. A nursing care delivery model based on case management is:
    a. Primary nursing
    b. Critical pathways
    c. Diagnostic Related Groups
    d. Patient classification system

26. Which statement is most significant in relation to the concept of change theory in the health care environment?
    a. Weigh the risks and benefits
    b. The stages of change are predictable
    c. Change in activity results in positive outcomes
    d. A large change is easier to adapt to than multiple smaller changes

27. When working within a nursing team, which intervention should a Registered Nurse perform rather than an unlicensed Nursing Assistant?
    a. Measuring the I&O of a patient after surgery
    b. Assessing the skin of a newly admitted patient
    c. Providing a bed bath for a patient with hemiparesis
    d. Offering apple juice to a patient on a clear liquid diet

28. Several nurses complain to the Nurse Manager that one of the Patient Care Aides constantly takes extensive lunch breaks. The Nurse Manager should:
    a. Convene a group meeting of all the Patient Care Aides to review their responsibilities related to time management
    b. Talk with the Patient Care Aide to explore the reasons for the behavior and review expectations
    c. Arrange a meeting with the nurses so that they can confront the Patient Care Aide as a group
    d. Document the Patient Care Aide's behavior and place it in the Aide's personnel file

29. To ensure efficiency when organizing the daily workload, the Registered Nurse should:
    a. Provide care to a patient in isolation first
    b. Plan activities to promote nursing convenience
    c. Organize care around legally required activities
    d. Perform routine bed baths between 8 and 10 AM

30. A nurse arrives on the unit during the last 5 minutes of a 20 minute change of shift report for the second time within a week. The nurse in charge should handle this situation by:
    a. Writing an Incident Report concerning the lateness
    b. Ignoring the lateness and intervening if it should happen again
    c. Including the lateness in the nurse's yearly performance evaluation
    d. Discussing the lateness with the nurse in private immediately after the report

31. Which action associated with restraint use can be delegated to an unlicensed nursing team member?
    a. Assessment of a patient's safety needs
    b. Evaluation of a patient's response to restraint use
    c. Provision of movement of the patient after release of a restraint
    d. Selection of the appropriate type restraint to meet a patient's needs

32. When a Supervisor communicates expectations about a task to be completed and then delegates the task, which management function is being implemented by the Supervisor?
    a. Planning
    b. Directing
    c. Controlling
    d. Organizing

33. The leadership style that empowers group members to be creative and independent is:
    a. Directive
    b. Autocratic
    c. Democratic
    d. Laissez-faire

34. Which is most important when the student nurse is given a patient assignment in the clinical area?
    a. Accepting the role of leader of the patient's health team
    b. Completing the care indicated on the patient's plan of care
    c. Assuming accountability for the tasks that are assigned by the instructor
    d. Helping other students to complete their patient care whenever necessary

35. Between 80 and 90% of a manager's day is spent:
    a. Planning
    b. Assessing
    c. Evaluating
    d. Communicating

36. Which statement is most significant in relation to the concept of change theory in the health care environment?
    a. Overcoming barriers to change requires embracing new ideas uncritically
    b. Change generates anxiety by moving away from the comfortable
    c. Behaviors are easy to change when change is supported
    d. Change is most effective when spontaneous

37. A discharge task that can be delegated to a Nursing Assistant is:
    a. Teaching the patient how to measure weight using a standing scale
    b. Obtaining the patient's temperature, pulse, and respiratory rate
    c. Determining if the patient knows how to measure I&O
    d. Demonstrating to the patient how to use a walker

38. Management's major focus is on:
    a. Accomplishing an objective
    b. Empowering others
    c. Problem solving
    d. Planning

39. The most effective resource in helping a staff nurse identify a solution to a complex problem is the?
    a. Organizational Chart of the institution
    b. Nursing Procedure Manual
    c. Unit's Nurse Manager
    d. Nursing Supervisor

40. When delegating a specific procedure to a Patient Care Aide, the Aide refuses to perform the procedure. The nurse should first:
    a. Assign the procedure to another Patient Care Aide
    b. Explain that it is part of the Patient Care Aide's job description
    c. Explore why the Patient Care Aide refused to perform the procedure
    d. Send the Patient Care Aide to the procedure manual to review the procedure

41. A Registered Nurse identifies that a postoperative patient is hemorrhaging. The nurse directs another Registered Nurse to immediately call the surgical resident and sends a Nurse Aide to gather specific equipment from the clean utility room and then proceeds to implement measures to stem the bleeding. Which style of leadership did the nurse use in this situation?
    a. Autocratic
    b. Democratic
    c. Bureaucratic
    d. Laissez-faire

42. The task that should be delegated to a Registered Nurse is:
    a. Taking a patient's vital signs
    b. Evaluating a patient's response to Demerol
    c. Administering a cleansing enema to a patient
    d. Transporting a patient to the operating room for surgery

43. When planning to apply for a new position within an agency, what is the first thing the nurse should do?
    a. Review the job description
    b. Provide at least 3 positive references
    c. Identify the power associated with the position
    d. Locate the position on the agency's Table of Organization

44. The most important reason why a Nurse Aide must fully understand how to implement a delegated procedure is because the Nurse Aide must be able to:
    a. Explain the procedure to the patient
    b Teach a Nurse Aide the procedure
    c. Perform the procedure quickly
    d. Complete the procedure safely

45. The nursing team leader delegates a wound irrigation to a Licensed Practical Nurse (LPN). It has been a long time since the LPN performed this procedure. To ensure patient safety the nursing team leader should:
    a. Verbally describe to the LPN how to perform the procedure
    b. Have the LPN demonstrate how to perform the procedure
    c. Assign another LPN to assist with the procedure
    d. Delegate the procedure to another LPN

1. a. Collaborative is not a classical leadership style. Collaborative refers to the democratic leadership style. Democratic leaders encourage discussion and decision making within the group, which requires collaboration, coordination, and communication among group members.
   b. **This is the most appropriate leadership style in a crisis when urgent decisions are necessary. In a crisis, one person needs to assume the responsibility for decisions. Autocratic leaders give orders and directions and make decisions for the group.**
   c. This leadership style is not appropriate in a crisis when urgent decisions are necessary. Laissez-faire leaders are nondirective and permissive which allows for self-regulation, creativity, and autonomy, but limits fast-acting efficiency.
   d. This leadership style is not appropriate in a crisis when urgent decisions are necessary. Democratic leaders encourage discussion and decision making within the group, which takes time.

2. a. **This is essential to overcome resistance to change. There are many different reasons people resist change. Each reason will respond to different strategies. There are four different types of interventions to overcome resistance: providing information; disproving currently held beliefs; maintaining psychological safety; and by administrative order or command.**
   b. Modifying a goal compromises the integrity of the planned change. All ramifications associated with the change should be explored before beginning and all contingencies planned for so that modifying a goal will be unnecessary.
   c. Although emphasizing the positive consequences of the change might be done, another option is a more important action that can be implemented by the Nurse Manager to overcome resistance to change.
   d. Although it is important to state the purpose of the change clearly and concisely, another option is a more important action that can be implemented by the Nurse Manager to overcome resistance to change.

3. a. **Leaders can inspire others with their vision and gain cooperation through their persuasion and communication skills (influence power), the respect others have for their knowledge and abilities (expert power), and their charisma and prior success (referent power).**
   b. Creating change is the major function of a change agent, not a leader. Change agents are often managers rather than leaders because managers have responsibility for ensuring that the work of the organization is done.
   c. Controlling others is a function of a manager, not a leader.
   d. Producing a product is a function of a manager, not a leader. The manager is responsible for ensuring that the work of the organization is done and this often requires the development of such things as a policy or procedure, management reports, and work schedules.

4. a. Effective leaders and managers have vision.
   b. Effective leaders and managers have charisma.
   c. Effective leaders and managers have confidence.
   d. **Managers, not leaders, have responsibility. Leaders can be formal or informal. Informal leaders are not assigned to direct others. They are viewed as leaders by the members of the group because of their experience, vision, charisma, confidence, expertise, or age.**

5. a. This person has not directly delegated the care to the Nursing Assistant and, therefore, is not the person most responsible for the safe performance of the care.
   b. Although the Nursing Assistant is responsible for his/her own actions, the primary legal responsibility lies with a person listed in another option.
   c. **The Registered Nurse is accountable for tasks delegated to other nursing team members. The nurse must ensure that a delegated task is within each team member's scope of practice and that the person is capable and competent to perform all the critical elements of the task safely.**
   d. This person has not directly delegated the care to the Nursing Assistant and, therefore, is not the person most responsible for the safe performance of the care.

6. a. Taking the vital signs of all the patients on the unit at the same time is called functional nursing and is unrelated to the adage in the question.
   b. **This action is an appropriate example of the adage, "A stitch in time saves nine." It means that if you sew a tear when it is small you need less stitches and time to repair it than when it is large. The same adage can be applied to the collection of equipment before a procedure. If the nurse has all the equipment that is needed before beginning a procedure less time is used than when forgotten equipment is obtained later. Every time the nurse leaves the room for forgotten equipment, the patient is inconvenienced and time is wasted.**
   c. Delegation is related to the efficient use of staff and is unrelated to the adage in the question.
   d. This example is unrelated to the adage in the question. Whether the nurse documents every two hours or at longer intervals will not alter how long the nurse spends documenting by the end of the shift.

7. a. Delegation is unrelated to creating change. Delegation is the transfer of responsibility for the performance of a task to another while remaining accountable for the actions of the person to whom the task was delegated. Creating change is associated with responding to a stressor that is either planned or unplanned, which results in change that is positive or negative.
   b. Delegation is unrelated to networking. Networking occurs when a person makes connections with others for sharing ideas, knowledge, information, and professional support.
   c. **Delegation allows the Registered Nurse to assign tasks to various individuals on the nursing team**

who are best qualified to complete the task. In today's health care environment, nursing team members have different levels of educational preparation. The Registered Nurse must take into account the qualifications and scope of practice of each professional and nonprofessional nursing team member and assign tasks accordingly. When this is done, each person's skills and abilities are used most appropriately and productivity increases.

d. The person who is assigned a task is responsible for the outcome of the assigned task. However, the Registered Nurse delegating the task is not relieved of accountability but is responsible for the actions of the person to whom the task was delegated as well as the outcome of the intervention.

8. a. The Nurse Manager can provide negative feedback in a manner that is firm without being assertive. Not yielding under pressure (firm) is less confrontational than being confident in a persistent way (assertive).

b. When providing negative feedback, the exploration of alternative solutions is performed later in the counseling session.

c. **Feedback is essential to identify the problem. Problem recognition is the first step in the problem-solving process. Once the unacceptable behavior is identified and acknowledged, then the reasons for the problem can be explored, solutions suggested, and expectations reinforced.**

d. Although this should be done, it is not feedback. Feedback is necessary for the nurse to recognize one's offending behavior. In addition, documentation is the last, not the first, step in the counseling process.

9. a. Directive is not one of the four classical leadership styles.

b. The autocratic leadership style is probably the least effective style to use with a professionally mature and motivated staff. Autocratic leaders give orders and directions and make decisions for the group. There is little freedom and a large degree of control by the leader, which frustrates motivated and professionally mature staff members.

c. The democratic leadership style is the second best style to use when the staff is motivated and professionally mature. The democratic style offers fewer opportunities for autonomy for staff members who are mature and motivated than a leadership style in another option.

d. **This is correct. The laissez-faire leadership style is appropriate for a group of individuals who have an internal locus of control and desire autonomy and independence. Individuals who are professionally mature and motivated more often have an internal locus of control.**

10. a. **A task of this complexity requires the knowledge and judgment of a Registered Nurse. This task has great potential for harm if the caregiver misdiagnoses the patient's condition and it has an unpredictable outcome. In addition, it requires problem solving that may call for innovation in the form of an individually designed plan of care to address the presence of a dysrhythmia.**

b. Applying a condom catheter is not a complex task. It requires simple problem-solving skills, involves a predictable outcome, and employs a simple level of interaction with the patient. Although this task has the potential to cause harm if the critical elements of the skill are not implemented, it is within the scope of practice of an unlicensed Nursing Assistant. It does not require the more advanced competencies of a Registered Nurse.

c. Making an occupied bed is not a complex task. It requires simple problem-solving skills, involves a predictable outcome, and employs a simple level of interaction with the patient. Although this task has the potential to cause harm if the critical elements of the skill are not implemented, it is within the scope of practice of an unlicensed Nursing Assistant. It does not require the more advanced competencies of a Registered Nurse.

d. Transferring a patient is not a complex task. It requires simple problem-solving skills, involves a predictable outcome, and employs a simple level of interaction with the patient. Although this task has the potential to cause harm if the critical elements of the skill are not implemented, it is within the scope of practice of an unlicensed Nursing Assistant. It does not require the more advanced competencies of a Registered Nurse.

11. a. Exploring possible alternative solutions occurs before achieving a consensus. A consensus is achieved when all or most agree or have the same opinion.

b. Consensus, not flexibility, is the goal. However, some members of the group may be flexible and change their opinion to ensure the achievement of a consensus.

c. **Cooperation and teamwork is essential for the achievement of any goal. If a consensus is achieved about the value of the expected outcome, people are more likely to work together constructively.**

d. Autocratic decision making does not seek a consensus when making a decision within a group. Autocratic leaders give orders and directions and make decisions for the group. There is little freedom within the group

12. a. Evaluating the performance of a subordinate does not fall under the planning function of management. Planning activities involves assessment, problem identification, establishment of goals, planning interventions based on the priority identified, and how outcomes will be evaluated.

b. Evaluating the performance of a subordinate does not fall under the directing function of management. Directing activities involve getting the work accomplished and includes such activities as assigning and communicating tasks and expectations, guiding and teaching, and decision making.

c. **The controlling function of management includes the evaluation of staff members. This is in addition to ensuring that plans are carried out and the outcomes evaluated.**

d. Evaluating the performance of a subordinate does not fall under the organizing function of management. Organizing activities include sharing expectations, identifying the chain of command, and determining responsibilities. In addition, since the manager is responsible for delegating tasks to subordinates, the manager is responsible for ensuring that policies and procedures clearly describe standards of care and expected outcomes.

13. a. A clear and concise description of the objective and expected outcomes need to be communicated to whom the task is being delegated. This is not related to the Right of Delegation associated with the appropriateness of the task in light of the person's scope of practice.
    b. Feedback is associated with evaluating the implementation and outcome of the delegated task, not ensuring that the intervention can be legally implemented by the assigned person.
    c. The right person does not refer to ensuring that the delegated intervention can legally be implemented by the assigned person. The right person refers to whether or not the person to whom the task is being delegated is qualified to do the job. Although a person's job description and credentials legally permit a person to be delegated a particular task, the person may not have the ability or experience to carry out the task safely.
    d. **This is correct. The right task refers to a task that can be legally delegated because it is within the legal scope of practice of the person to whom the task is being delegated.**

14. a. There is no end to a system. Individual parts of a system are interrelated and the whole system responds in an integrated way to changes within a part.
    b. Systems do not function in a linear (straight-line) format. Systems are complex.
    c. Trial and error is unrelated to Systems Theory. Trial and error is a problem-solving method whereby a number of solutions are tried until one is found that solves the problem.
    d. **Systems Theory is a cyclical process in which a whole is broken down into parts and the parts are studied individually as well as how they work together within the system. Every system consists of matter, energy and communication. Because each part of a system is interconnected, the whole system reacts to changes in one of its parts. The concept of treating a patient holistically is based on an understanding of Systems Theory.**

15. a. **Effective management depends on careful planning. Planning activities involves deciding what is to be done, when to do it, where and how to do it, and who will do it and with what level of assistance. Planning involves assessment, problem identification, establishment of goals, identifying interventions based on priorities, and how outcomes will be evaluated.**
    b. Getting the work accomplished (directing) is associated with only one step in the management process.
    c. Ensuring that plans are carried out and the outcomes evaluated (controlling) is associated with only one step in the management process.

    d. Sharing expectations, identifying the chain of command, and determining responsibilities (organizing) are associated with only one step in the management process.

16. a. Providing fluids based on a physician's order is a dependent, not independent, function of the nurse.
    b. **Delegating tasks within the scope of nursing practice is an independent function of the nurse and does not require a physician's order.**
    c. Wound care is a dependent function of the nurse and requires a physician's order.
    d. Applying heat requires a physician's order and is a dependent function of the nurse.

17. a. **This is an example of the authoritarian leadership style. Authoritarian leaders give orders and directions and make decisions for the group. There is little freedom and a large degree of control by the leader.**
    b. This is not an example of the bureaucratic leadership style. Bureaucratic leaders rely on the policies, procedures, and rules of the agency to direct the work efforts of the group.
    c. This is not an example of the laissez-faire leadership style. Laissez-faire leaders are nondirective and permissive, which allows for self-regulation and autonomy.
    d. This is not an example of the democratic leadership style. Democratic leaders encourage discussion and decision making within the group.

18. a. Although confrontation may be used occasionally, it can be learned as one socializes into the role of Nurse Manager and is not as important as a competency identified in another option.
    b. **Strong communication skills are an essential competency of a Nurse Manager. Research demonstrates that 80 to 90% of a manager's day is spent communicating verbally and in writing. Managers need to express their thoughts clearly, concisely, and accurately.**
    c. Although this is important, it can be learned as one socializes into the role of Nurse Manager and is not as important as a competency identified in another option.
    d. Recognition by peers as a leader is not as important as a competency identified in another option. A person is generally promoted to a management position because upper management recognizes leadership qualities. As a Nurse Manager grows into the role, peers will recognize the leadership ability of the Nurse Manager.

19. a. This is not an example of influence power. Influence power is the use of persuasion and communication skills to exercise power informally without using the power associated with formal authority.
    b. This is not an example of coercive power. The leader bases coercive power on the fear of the punitive withholding of rewards or retribution.
    c. This is not an example of referent power. Referent power is associated with respect for the leader because of the leader's charisma and prior successes.
    d. **This is an example of expert power. Expert power is the respect one receives based on one's ability, skills, knowledge, and experience.**

20. **a.** The right preceptor is not one of the Four Rights of Delegation. A preceptor is an experienced person who functions as a role model and facilitates an orientee's introduction to new responsibilities.
    b. Feedback is one of the Five Rights of Delegation. Feedback is associated with evaluation of the implementation and outcome of the delegated task in a timely manner.
    c. The right route refers to the Five Rights of Medication Administration, not the Four Rights of Delegation.
    d. The right place is not one of the Four Rights of Delegation.

21. **a.** Change that is consistent with current values and beliefs is easier to implement than change that is inconsistent with current values and beliefs. Values and beliefs are difficult to change.
    b. This is not the priority intervention. Although incentives might motivate some individuals, it does not motivate all because some people have an internal rather than an external locus of control.
    c. Although small steps are more effective than large steps because they are easier to achieve and once achieved are motivating, it is not the first thing the nurse should do to overcome resistance to change.
    d. Although one person sharing explanations with another (informational power) is helpful when trying to change behavior, it is not the most effective type of power to use when trying to effect change. Another option identifies an action that the nurse should do first.

22. **a.** The collection of sputum for cytology does not require the use of sterile technique and can be delegated to an unlicensed Nursing Assistant.
    b. The collection of urine for specific gravity does not require the use of sterile technique and can be delegated to an unlicensed Nursing Assistant.
    c. The collection of stool for ova and parasites does not require the use of sterile technique and can be delegated to an unlicensed Nursing Assistant.
    d. Collecting a specimen for culture and sensitivity requires understanding of and the ability to collect a specimen using sterile technique, which is in the scope of practice of a Licensed Practical Nurse.

23. **a.** This is not the best example of role modeling from the options offered.
    b. This is not the best example of role modeling from the options offered.
    c. When the Nurse Manager follows policies and procedures, the manager is demonstrating the behavior that is expected. Role modeling is more effective than telling as a teaching strategy.
    d. This is not the best example of role modeling from the options offered.

24. **a.** The word *directive* refers to the autocratic, not democratic, leadership style.
    b. The word *permissive* refers to the laissez-faire, not democratic, leadership style.
    c. *Oppressive* is the way some people refer to the autocratic, not democratic, leadership style. There is little freedom and a large degree of control by the

autocratic leader, which frustrates motivated and professionally mature staff members.
    d. The word *consultative* is most closely related to the democratic leadership style. Democratic leaders encourage discussion and decision making within the group. The leader facilitates the work of the group by making suggestions, offering constructive criticism, and offering information.

25. **a.** Primary nursing is a case management approach where one nurse is responsible for a number of patients 24 hours a day, 7 days a week. It was instituted as a way of providing comprehensive, individualized and consistent nursing care.
    b. Critical pathways are not a nursing care delivery model based on case management. Critical pathways are tools used in managed care that are sets of concurrent and sequential actions by nurses as well as other health care professionals to achieve a specific outcome. They represent specific practice patterns in relation to specific medical populations.
    c. Diagnostic Related Groups (DRGs) is not a nursing care delivery model based on case management. Diagnostic Related Groups is a prospective reimbursement plan where patients are grouped based on medical diagnoses for the purposes of reimbursing the cost of hospitalization.
    d. Patient classification systems are not a nursing care delivery model based on case management. Patient classification systems are designed to assign an acuity level to patients based on their needs for the purpose of determining the number of nursing care hours needed to provide care.

26. **a.** Risks and benefits must be carefully analyzed before initiating change. Some change is not worth the risk, because the consequences of failure are greater than the benefits.
    b. The stages of change are not always predictable. Although effective change moves through three zones—comfort, discomfort, and new comfort,—what happens in each stage is not always predictable and change is not always successfully achieved. Change is dynamic and the stages are not rigid.
    c. Outcomes of change can be positive or negative. Sometimes well-planned change meets with resistance and the change effort can terminate in a loss of credibility, lack of achieving the goal, and confusion.
    d. Smaller goals are much easer to achieve than a large goal. Smaller goals are generally designed to ensure achievement, which is motivating.

27. **a.** This task is not complex, has little potential for harm, requires simple problem-solving skills, employs a simple level of interaction with the patient, and is within the scope of practice of an unlicensed Nursing Assistant. It does not require the more advanced competencies of a Registered Nurse.
    b. A task of this complexity requires the knowledge and judgment of a Registered Nurse. This task has great potential for harm if the caregiver misdiagnoses the patient's condition and it has an unpredictable outcome. It requires an assessment

of numerous systems and risk factors, a complex level of interaction with the patient, and problem solving abilities. In addition, it requires innovation in the form of an individually designed plan of care that addresses protecting the patient's skin.

c. This task is not complex, requires simple problem-solving skills, involves a predictable outcome, and employs a simple level of interaction with the patient. Although this task has the potential to cause harm if the critical elements of the skill are not implemented, it is within the scope of practice of an unlicensed Nursing Assistant. It does not require the more advanced competencies of a Registered Nurse.

d. This task is not complex, has little potential for harm, requires only simple problem-solving skills, involves a predictable outcome, employs a simple level of interaction with the patient, and is within the scope of practice of an unlicensed Nursing Assistant. It does not require the more advanced competencies of a Registered Nurse.

28. a. It is the Patient Care Aide who is late, takes extensive lunch breaks, and who needs to review the responsibilities related to time, not the Patient Care Aides who follow the rules.

b. **Recognition of a problem is the first step in the problem-solving process. Once the unacceptable behavior is identified and acknowledged, then the reasons for the problem can be explored, solutions suggested, and expectations reinforced.**

c. It is not the responsibility of peers to confront the employee who is late for work and takes extensive lunch breaks. The employee reports to the Nurse Manager who is superior in the chain of command of the organization. The Nurse Manager should meet with the employee. In addition, counseling sessions with employees should be confidential and conducted in private.

d. This is premature. The Nurse Manager first needs to implement an action identified in another option.

29. a. This may not be possible depending upon the needs of patients.

b. Patient needs are the priority, not the convenience of the nurse.

c. **Legally required activities must be accomplished because they are dependent functions that support the medical regimen of care. Although legally required activities should be accomplished first, many independent actions by the nurse must also be implemented to maintain a basic standard of care and patient safety. Some nursing interventions, which are not essential, can be implemented after the required activities.**

d. This may not be possible depending upon the needs of patients.

30. a. An Incident Report is not the appropriate format to document this event. Incident Reports are used to document unusual events associated with the performance of healthcare activities and includes events such as falls, medication or treatment errors or omissions, and any situation that causes an injury to a patient, visitor or staff member.

b. The nurse's lateness should not be ignored because it is the second time it has happened.

c. This is too long a time to wait to address the nurse's lateness.

d. **The nurse's behavior needs to be addressed by the Nurse Manager and the expected behavior reinforced. Counseling sessions with employees should be confidential and conducted in private as soon as possible after the offending event.**

31. a. Assessment of patient needs requires the knowledge and judgment of a licensed nurse. This task has great potential for harm if the caregiver misdiagnoses the patient's condition and involves an unpredictable outcome. In addition, it requires an assessment of numerous systems and risk factors, a complex level of interaction with the patient, problem solving, and innovation in the form of an individually designed plan of care that provides for the patient's safety.

b. The skill of evaluation requires the knowledge and judgment of a licensed nurse. This task has great potential for harm if the caregiver misdiagnoses the patient's response and it involves an unpredictable outcome. In addition, it requires an assessment of numerous systems and risk factors; a complex level of interaction with the patient, problem solving, and innovation in the form of an individually designed nursing plan of care that provides for the patient's safety.

c. **This task is not complex, requires simple problem-solving skills, involves a predictable outcome, and employs a simple level of interaction with the patient. Although this task has the potential to cause harm if the caregiver fails to notice compromised circulation or impaired movement, it is within the scope of practice of an unlicensed Nursing Assistant. It does not require the more advanced competencies of a licensed nurse.**

d. The choice of the type of restraint is based on the physician's order.

32. a. This is not an example of the planning function of management. Planning involves assessment, problem identification, establishment of goals, planning interventions based on the priority identified, and how outcomes will be evaluated.

b. **This is an example of the directing function of management. Directing involves getting the work accomplished and includes such activities as assigning and communicating tasks and expectations, guiding and teaching, and decision making.**

c. This is not an example of the controlling function of management. Controlling activities ensure that plans are carried out and the outcomes and staff are evaluated.

d. This is not an example of the organizing function of management. Organizing activities include sharing expectations, identifying the chain of command, and determining responsibilities. In addition, since the manager is responsible for delegating tasks to subordinates, the manager is responsible for ensuring that policies and procedures clearly describe standards of care and expected outcomes.

33. a. Directive is not a classical leadership style.
    b. This is not an example of the autocratic leadership style. Autocratic leaders give orders and directions and make decisions for the group. There is little freedom and a large degree of control by the leader.
    c. This is not an example of the democratic leadership style. Democratic leaders encourage discussion and decision making within the group.
    d. **This is an appropriate example of the laissez-faire leadership style. Laissez-faire leaders are nondirective and permissive, which allows for self-regulation, creativity, and autonomy.**

34. a. Students are assigned to care for patients for a specific time period and are generally included as members, not leaders, of the nursing team.
    b. Although students are expected to complete all planned care, the patient's condition can change or some unforeseen event may interfere with the plan. The student must keep the instructor or preceptor informed about the patient's condition, and use the instructor or preceptor as a resource person when the unexpected occurs or guidance is needed.
    c. **Students are accountable for the tasks assigned by the instructor or preceptor. As part of accountability, students are obligated to keep the instructor or preceptor informed about the status of the patient, how the assignment is progressing, and whether all interventions are implemented as planned.**
    d. Students should not help other students unless specifically assigned to do so by the instructor or preceptor. An exception occurs when assistance is needed to ensure patient safety in an emergency.

35. a. Planning does not consume 80 to 90% of a manager's day.
    b. Assessing does not consume 80 to 90% of a manager's day.
    c. Evaluating does not consume 80 to 90% of a manager's day.
    d. **Research demonstrates that this is true. Strong communication skills are an essential competency of a Nurse Manager. They communicate verbally and in writing and need to express their thoughts clearly, concisely, and accurately.**

36. a. Before initiating change, barriers need to be anticipated and addressed. All aspects of the new idea are best accomplished when critically analyzed.
    b. **Change causes one to move from the comfortable to the uncomfortable and is known as *unfreezing* in Lewin's Change Model. It involves moving away from that which is known to the unknown, from the routine to the new, and from the expected to the unexpected. The unknown, new, and unexpected can be threatening, which can increase anxiety.**
    c. Behavior is not easy to change even when supported. Most people do not like to function in an unfamiliar environment. In addition, change challenges one's comfort zone in each level of Maslow's Hierarchy of Needs.
    d. Planned, not spontaneous, change is most effective because it is organized, systematic, and purposeful.

37. a. Teaching requires the knowledge and judgment of a Registered Nurse. Teaching requires a complex level of interaction with the patient, problem solving, and innovation in the form of an individually designed teaching plan of care that addresses the specific learning needs of the patient. In addition, the outcome is unpredictable and it has the potential to cause harm if the skill is taught incorrectly.
    b. **Obtaining vital signs can be delegated to a Nursing Assistant because it is not a complex task. It requires simple problem-solving skills and a simple level of interaction with the patient. Although this task has the potential to cause harm if the critical elements of the skill are not implemented appropriately, it is within the scope of practice of an unlicensed Nursing Assistant. It does not require the more advanced competencies of a Registered Nurse.**
    c. Assessing a patient's level of understanding is a complex task that requires knowledge and judgment and is within the scope of practice of a Registered Nurse. This task requires a complex level of interaction with the patient, problem solving, and innovation in the form of an individually designed teaching plan of care that addresses the specific learning needs of the patient.
    d. Teaching requires the knowledge and judgment of a Registered Nurse. Teaching requires a complex level of interaction with the patient, problem solving, and innovation in the form of an individually designed teaching plan of care that addresses the specific learning needs of the patient. In addition, the outcome is unpredictable and it has the potential to cause harm if the skill is taught incorrectly.

38. a. **Although planning, problem solving, and empowering others are goals of a manager, the bottom line is for the manager to accomplish the work of the organization.**
    b. Although empowering others is one of the goals of a manager, the major objective is identified in another option.
    c. Although problem solving is one of the goals of a manager, the major objective is identified in another option.
    d. Although planning is one of the goals of a manager, the major objective is identified in another option.

39. a. The Organizational Chart schematically plots the reporting relationship of every position within the organization. It does not help a staff nurse identify a solution to a complex problem.
    b. The Nursing Procedure Manual is not designed to help a staff nurse identify a solution to a complex problem. The Nursing Procedure Manual contains details of policies relative to nursing practice and nursing procedures along with the purpose and all the steps that one must follow to implement the procedure safely.
    c. **Generally, in the chain of command of an organization the staff nurse works under the direction of and reports to the unit's Nurse Manager. The Nurse Manager is generally an experienced nurse and is the primary resource**

person for the staff nurse. The staff nurse should seek guidance from the Nurse Manager when assistance is needed to solve a complex problem.

d. The Nursing Supervisor is higher up the chain of command in a Table of Organization than another employee who would be the best person for the staff nurse to seek assistance from when needing help to solve a complex problem.

40. a. This action is premature. Another option has priority.
    b. The employee may be fully aware of the requirements of the job description and not need to have them described. Even though a task is within one's job description a person can refuse to perform a procedure because of a reason that is considered acceptable.
    c. This is the issue that the Nurse Manager needs to explore. The employee may have an acceptable reason for refusing to comply. When the reason is identified, then the Nurse Manager can take an informed action.
    d. The reason for refusal may have nothing to do with the lack of understanding of the procedure.

41. a. This is an appropriate example of the autocratic leadership style. Autocratic leaders make the decisions for the group.
    b. This is not an example of the democratic leadership style. Democratic leaders encourage group discussion and decision-making.
    c. This is not an example of the bureaucratic style of leadership. The bureaucratic leader relies on policies, procedures, and rules to direct the decision-making process.
    d. This is not an example of the laissez-faire leadership style. The laissez-faire leader assumes a hands-off permissive approach, which allows for self-regulation.

42. a. Taking routine vital signs is not complex, has little potential for harm, requires only simple problem-solving skills, involves a simple level of interaction with the patient, and is within the scope of practice of an unlicensed Nursing Assistant. It requires the more advanced competencies of a Registered Nurse only when previous vital signs have been abnormal.
    b. Evaluation requires the knowledge and judgment of a Registered Nurse. The skill of evaluation requires reassessing, synthesizing and analyzing data, determining significance of data, and diagnosing and responding to the data. In addition, it involves an unpredictable outcome and requires problem solving that may call for innovation in the form of an individually designed plan of care to address the patient's need for pain relief if pain is still being experienced.
    c. Administering an enema is not a complex task. It requires simple problem-solving skills, involves a predictable outcome, and employs a simple level of interaction with the patient. Although this task has the potential to cause harm if the critical elements of the skill are not implemented, it is within the scope of practice of an unlicensed Nursing Assistant. It

does not require the more advanced competencies of a Registered Nurse.

d. Transporting a patient is not a complex task. It requires simple problem-solving skills, involves a predictable outcome, and a simple level of interaction with the patient. Although this task has the potential to cause harm if the critical elements of the skill are not implemented, it is within the scope of practice of an unlicensed Nursing Assistant. It does not require the more advanced competencies of a Registered Nurse.

43. a. This is one of the most important actions by the nurse seeking a new position. The job description provides an overview of the requirements and responsibilities of the role. Job descriptions include things such as educational and experiential requirements, job responsibilities, subordinates to be supervised, and whom one reports to in the chain of command.
    b. Requesting references protects the hiring agency, not the nurse. This is not the most important thing the nurse should do when applying for a new position within an agency.
    c. Although understanding the power of the position may help a person meet the responsibilities associated with the job description, it is not the priority when applying for a new position.
    d. Although it is important to recognize where the new position fits into the organization's Table of Organization, it is not the priority when applying for a new position. A Table of Organization schematically plots the reporting relationship of every position within the organization.

44. a. Although this is important, it is not the priority.
    b. Nurse Aides are trained and supervised by the nurse, not other Nurse Aides.
    c. Although this may be desirable, it is not the priority.
    d. Safety of the patient is the priority. The Nurse Aide must perform only the skills that are within the legal role of the Nurse Aide, are understood, have been practiced, and have been performed correctly on a return demonstration.

45. a. This is unsafe. This does not ensure that cognitive information can be converted to a psychomotor skill.
    b. Demonstration is the safest way to assess whether a person has the knowledge and skill to safely perform a procedure. A superior delegating care is responsible for ensuring that the person implementing the care is legally qualified and competent.
    c. A peer should not be held responsible for the care assigned to another team member. The Registered Nurse who delegates a procedure to a subordinate is directly responsible for ensuring that the care is safely delivered to patients.
    d. This intervention does not address the original LPN's need to know how to perform the procedure safely. This procedure is within the legal scope of practice of a Licensed Practical Nurse.

Healthcare Delivery

KEYWORDS

The following words include English vocabulary, nursing/medical terminology, concepts, principles, or information relevant to content specifically addressed in the chapter or associated with topics presented in it. English dictionaries, your nursing textbooks, and medical dictionaries such as *Taber's Cyclopedic Medical Dictionary* are resources that can be used to expand your knowledge and understanding of these words and related information.

Access to health care
Acuity
Advocate
Baby boomers
Beliefs
Burnout
Career ladder
Case manager
Comprehensive care
Continuity of care
Cost containment
Counselor
Critical pathways
Demographics
Diagnostic Related Groups (DRGs)
Functional nursing
Healthcare professionals
   Activity Therapist
   Certified Social Worker
   Clinical Nurse Specialist
   Licensed Practical Nurse
   Nurse Anesthetist
   Nurse Assistant
   Nurse Midwife
   Nurse Practitioner
   Occupational Therapist
   Pastoral care provider
   Patient
   Patient's family members
   Physical Therapist
   Physician
   Physician's Assistant
   Registered Dietitian
   Registered Nurse

   Speech Therapist
Healthcare settings
   Acute care – hospitals
   Adult day-care
   Ambulatory care centers
   Assisted-living residence
   Clinics
   Extended care
   Home health services
   Hospice (inpatient, residential, in the home)
   Industrial or occupation settings
   Life-care community
   Long term care – nursing homes
   Neighborhood community health center
   Physician's offices
   Psychiatric facilities
   Rehabilitation centers
   School settings
   Urgent visit centers
Health Maintenance Organization
Hospice
Indigent
Length of stay
Levels of healthcare
   Primary healthcare
   Secondary healthcare
   Tertiary healthcare
Levels of prevention
   Primary prevention
     Health promotion
     Health protection
     Preventive health services

   Secondary prevention
   Tertiary prevention
Managed care
Medicaid
Medicare
Metropolitan
Multidisciplinary
Occupancy rate
Patient classification system
Population
Poverty
Preauthorization
Preferred Provider Organization
Primary nursing
Prospective payment system
Provider
Reengineering
Reimbursement
Resource Utilization Groups
Rural
Socialized healthcare
Suburban
Surrogate
Teacher
Third party payers
Types of agencies
   Official – governmental
   Proprietary – for profit
   Voluntary – not for profit
Under-served population
Undocumented immigrants (aliens)
Urban

1. Which word best describes the role of the nurse when identifying and meeting the needs of the patient?
   a. Teacher
   b. Advocate
   c. Surrogate
   d. Counselor

2. Which is the most under-served population in the receipt of healthcare benefits in the United States?
   a. Children
   b. Older adults
   c. Pregnant women
   d. Middle-aged men

3. Which is the main effect of Diagnostic Related Groups (DRGs) on the healthcare system?
   a. Increased quality of medical care
   b. Increased reliability of research statistics
   c. Decreased acuity of hospitalized patients
   d. Decreased length of an average hospital stay

4. Which level healthcare service is reflected when providing medical and nursing intervention for a person with an infection in a hospital setting?
   a. Emergency
   b. Secondary
   c. Tertiary
   d. Primary

5. The cornerstone of *Nursing's Agenda For Health Care Reform* is:
   a. A standardized package of healthcare services must be provided by the federal government
   b. Advanced practice nurses should play a prominent role in the provision of primary care
   c. Services need to be provided in environments that are accessible, familiar, and friendly
   d. Nursing must provide for the central focus for the healthcare delivery system

6. What is the primary role of the nurse when functioning as a Case Manager? *social worker*
   a. Coordinator
   b. Counselor
   c. Provider
   d. Teacher

   cope w/ problems result y from long term illness injury - prevent

7. Which is the best example of an inpatient care setting?
   a. Ambulatory care center *— outpatient*
   b. Extended-care facility
   c. Day-care center
   d. Hospice

8. In which area would people have the most problems with having their healthcare needs met?
   a. Metropolitan areas
   b. Suburban areas
   c. Urban areas
   d. Rural areas

9. What should the nurse do if a patient is on a special diet and a food that the patient has requested has not appeared on the tray?
   a. Check the diet manual
   b. Schedule a conference with the dietitian
   c. Inform the supervisor of food services about the oversight
   d. Ask the physician to consider modifying the diet order to include the requested food

10. In the future, which change will most affect healthcare delivery in the United States?
    a. Less emphasis will be placed on prolonging life
    b. The proportion of older adults in society will increase
    c. More people will seek health care in an acute care setting
    d. Genetic counseling will decrease dramatically the number of ill infants born

11. Diagnostic Related Groups were mainly instituted by the federal government to reduce the:
    a. Number of professionals working in hospitals
    b. Focus on illness and place it on prevention
    c. Fragmentation of care
    d. Cost of health care

12. What characteristic is unique to the nurse-patient relationship?
    a. Patient's needs are satisfied
    b. There is a social component
    c. The nurse is the leader of the team
    d. Both are working toward a common goal

13. What is the best thing the nurse can do to prevent professional burnout?
    a. Get adequate sleep and exercise each day
    b. Challenge the "how" and "why" of one's role
    c. Clarify expectations, strengths, and limitations
    d. Seek a balance between seriousness and humor

14. In the emerging healthcare delivery system in the United States a professional who can provide independent healthcare with third party reimbursement is a:
    a. Licensed Registered Nurse
    b. Clinical Nurse Specialist
    c. Physician Assistant
    d. Nurse Practitioner

15. Critical pathways in healthcare refer to:
    a. Educational career ladders for healthcare professionals
    b. Multidisciplinary plans with predetermined patient outcomes
    c. Times during life when certain health problems are more likely to occur
    d. Organizations that provide services that progress from acute care to long term care

16. Which setting is the organizational center of the United States healthcare system?
    a. Clinic setting
    b. Acute care setting
    c. Community setting
    d. Long-term care setting

17. The word that is most associated with the nurse when functioning as caregiver is:
    a. Facilitate
    b. Evaluate
    c. Counsel
    d. Teach

18. Which is an example of an official agency?
    a. American Heart Association
    b. National League for Nursing
    c. Non-profit community hospital
    d. Veterans Administration Hospital

19. A major trend in healthcare is that:
    a. Individuals and the family have primary responsibility for making healthcare decisions
    b. Healthcare providers control the direction and development of healthcare services
    c. Striving for longevity will take on greater concern than quality-of-life issues
    d. Social issues are taking a back seat as a result of the advances in technology

20. Mammography screening reflects which Level of Prevention?
    a. Secondary
    b. Tertiary
    c. Primary
    d. Acute

21. Which new trend in healthcare delivery has influenced how healthcare services are provided in the United States?
    a. Agencies experiencing an increase in the numbers of volunteers
    b. Extended care facilities providing a variety of new therapies
    c. Older-adult day-care centers providing support for wellness
    d. Hospitalized patients being discharged before full recovery

22. Rehabilitation begins after the patient is:
    a. Conscious
    b. Diagnosed
    c. Discharged
    d. Ambulatory

23. Nurses should be role models for healthy living because nurses:
    a. Need to be as healthy as possible to fight invasion of pathogens
    b. Know that the immune system can be affected by an unhealthy life style
    c. Recognize that patients often look at what nurses do rather than what they say
    d. Must be able to deal with the physiological demands of the profession of nursing

24. Which most likely pays for the majority of the healthcare costs of people over 65 years of age?
    a. Medicare
    b. Medicaid
    c. Blue Cross
    d. Blue Shield

25. Which result of reengineering in hospital settings has raised the greatest concerns for patient safety?
    a. Decreased hospital occupancy rates
    b. Increased acuity of hospitalized patients
    c. Hospitals merging with larger institutions
    d. Substitution of less skilled workers for nurses

26. The major concern associated with early discharge as a result of Diagnostic Related Groups (DRGs) is:
    a. Providing for continuity of care
    b. Ordering equipment to be used in the home
    c. Accepting discharge by the patient and family
    d Ensuring hospital reimbursement for services rendered

27. Which generates the most anxiety after a goal is set during patient healthcare planning?
    a. Change
    b. Beliefs
    c. Values
    d. Role

28. How does the nurse function when helping a patient negotiate the healthcare system?
    a. Leader
    b. Resource
    c. Surrogate
    d. Counselor

29. What type of relationship has been entered when three hospitals agree to work collectively to provide a full range of healthcare services in their neighborhoods?
    a. Integrated healthcare service network
    b. Third-party reimbursement system
    c. Health Maintenance Organization
    d. Diagnostic Related Groups

30. Which statement is most important to consider when planning actions that address patients' health needs?
    a. Health and illness are clearly separated at the middle of the Health-Illness Continuum
    b. The demographics of the population of the United States are changing drastically
    c. Mainly external factors are the cause of most illnesses
    d. Most people view health as the absence of disease

31. The factor that most affects healthcare delivery to the older-adult population is that older adults:
    a. Require the services of long term care institutions at the end of life
    b. Will have an increase in numbers within the poverty level
    c. Suffer from significant cognitive deficits as they age
    d. Tend to fall requiring expensive hospital services

32. Which activity reflects care on the Primary Level of Healthcare delivery?
    a. Requesting hospice services
    b. Receiving care in a Coronary Care Unit
    c. Seeking emergency care at a local hospital
    d. Attending a Smoke Ender's meeting weekly

33. The activity that best reflects the role of the nurse as counselor would be when the nurse helps the patient:
    a. Understand and use resources in the healthcare system
    b. Integrate emotions and reality into a total experience
    c. Negotiate the healthcare delivery system
    d. Learn how to change a dressing

34. What should the nurse do first when unsure of the steps in a nursing procedure?
    a. Call the staff education department to arrange for an in-service
    b. Refer to a fundamentals of nursing skills textbook
    c. Check the nursing Policy and Procedure Manual
    d. Refuse to do the nursing procedure

35. Which action is common to the majority of Registered Nurse positions in different settings in which nurses work?
    a. Serving in an administrative capacity
    b. Developing patient plans of care
    c. Providing direct physical care
    d. Assisting the physician

36. In the United States predetermined hospital reimbursement based on the medical problem is associated with:
    a. Diagnostic related groups
    b. Managed care organizations
    c. Retrospective payment systems
    d. Socialized health insurance plans

37. Care associated with learning how to live with limitations after an accident is best delivered in which setting?
    a. Assisted-living residence
    b. Adult day-care program
    c. Extended-care facility
    d. Acute care

38. The largest group of healthcare professionals in the United States is:
    a. Social workers
    b. Nurse aides
    c. Physicians
    d. Nurses

39. What is the major factor that prevents an overhaul of the healthcare delivery system of the United States?
    a. Need for elected officials to respond to the pressure of political constituencies
    b. Explosion of technical advances within the profession of medicine
    c. Complexity of the problems associated with healthcare reform
    d. Physician resistance to reform

40. Which mechanism is designed to facilitate tracking a patient's progress as a cost containment strategy in managed care?
    a. Primary nursing
    b. Critical pathways
    c. Functional method
    d. Quality management

41. Which is emphasized in the traditional healthcare delivery system in the United States?
    a. Health promotion
    b. Illness prevention
    c. Diagnosis and treatment
    d. Rehabilitation and long term care

42. A patient classification system is designed to:
    a. Document resource needs for the purpose of establishing reimbursement
    b. Provide data about patient acuity to help assign nursing staff
    c. Establish that quality standards have been met
    d. Identify standardized expected outcomes

43. Which person is best prepared to track a client's progress through the healthcare system?
    a. Home Care Nurse
    b. Primary Nurse
    c. Case Manager
    d. Charge Nurse

44. Which statement reflects a significant change in the thinking of the general public about concepts related to healthcare delivery and its definition as determined in recent surveys?
    a. "Institutional based care will have to be increased as baby boomers age."
    b. "More services need to address the secondary healthcare needs of the community."
    c. "Individuals can influence their own health through behavior and lifestyle changes."
    d. "Healthcare providers have to be charged with the primary responsibility to provide appropriate healthcare services."

45. An increase in the size of which group is the greatest challenge to the financing of health care in the United States?
    a. Undocumented immigrants
    b. Medically uninsured
    c. Preterm infants
    d. Older adults

46. What has been the main cause of the shift of healthcare delivery from the hospital to the home?
    a. Use of Resource Utilization Groups to categorize needs of clients
    b. Need for hospital beds to be available for the acutely ill
    c. Limits on length of stay by reimbursement sources
    d. Shortage of qualified Registered Nurses

47. Which statement best describes the Medicaid program?
    a. Federally funded health insurance program for individuals with low incomes
    b. United States federal health insurance program for individuals aged 65 years or older
    c. A federal program requiring physician's to be providers of care to people living below the designated poverty level
    d. A retrospective healthcare reimbursement program that pays for the costs incurred by healthcare agencies for the care of the indigent

48. What word best describes the role of the nurse when functioning as a patient advocate?
    a. Provider
    b. Nurturer
    c. Protector
    d. Evaluator

49. Preauthorization for surgery means that:
    a. Medicare/third-party payers have approved the surgery and will reimburse the facility for costs
    b. All required preoperative medical and laboratory tests have been completed
    c. The preoperative check list has been completed and verified by the nurse
    d. The patient has signed the legal consent form for the surgery

50. When preparing for a patient's return from the operating room to a semi-private room, the nurse should first ensure that the patient's roommate is:
    a. Emotionally stable
    b. Able to communicate
    c. In the bed by the window
    d. Physiologically compatible

ANSWERS AND RATIONALES

1. a. The role of teacher is only one area of nursing practice and a word in another option has a stronger relationship with the role of the nurse when identifying and meeting the needs of the patient. Teaching is related only to helping patients learn about their health and healthcare practices.
   b. The role of advocate is the most important role of the nurse because in this role the nurse protects and supports patients' rights. Advocacy combines the roles of teacher, counselor, and leader so that the best interests of patients are protected, particularly when patients are most vulnerable.
   c. The surrogate role is not a professional role of the nurse. A surrogate role is assigned to a nurse when a patient believes that the nurse reminds them of another and projects that role and the feelings one has for the other person onto the nurse.
   d. The role of counselor is only one area of nursing practice and a word in another option has a stronger relationship with the role of the nurse when identifying and meeting the needs of the patient. Counseling is related only to helping a patient recognize and cope with emotional stressors, improve relationships, and promote personal growth.

2. a. In the United States the current healthcare system neglects the overall needs of children. One in 5 children lives in poverty and only half of these children receive Medicaid. One in 5 children does not have health insurance. Over 35% of preschool children are not immunized. In addition, children are vulnerable because they cannot be their own advocates.
   b. Although older adults are a vulnerable population, they are not as underserved as a group in another option because of the availability of Medicare.
   c. Although pregnant women are a vulnerable population, they are not as underserved as a group in another option.
   d. Middle-aged men are the least underserved population of the options offered.

3. a. The DRGs were designed to decrease the cost, not increase the quality, of healthcare.
   b. DRGs are unrelated to increasing or decreasing reliability of research statistics. Reliability is the degree of consistency with which a research study measures a hypothesis and depends on how well the measurement tool and the research methods are designed.
   c. DRGs have increased, not decreased, the acuity of the hospitalized population. Patients who in the past were treated in the hospital are now treated in the home, ambulatory care settings, or in less acute care settings such as rehabilitation or extended care centers.
   d. The DRGs, pretreatment diagnoses reimbursement categories, were designed to decrease the average length of a hospital stay, which in turn reduces costs.

4. a. Emergency care is not a level of care in the healthcare system. Emergency care is a description of one type of service provided on the Secondary Care level in the healthcare system.
   b. This is an example of the Secondary Care level of the healthcare system. Secondary level care is associated with intense and elaborate diagnosis and treatment of disease or trauma and includes critical care and emergency treatment. The Levels of Healthcare should not be confused with Levels of Prevention. The healthcare system has three Levels of Healthcare that describe the scope of services and settings where healthcare is provided and includes Primary, Secondary, and Tertiary. The Levels of Prevention identify three levels of prevention that focus on healthcare activities such as Primary Prevention (avoiding disease through health promotion and disease prevention), Secondary Prevention (early detection and treatment), and Tertiary Prevention (reducing complications, rehabilitation, restoration and maintenance of optimal function).
   c. This is not an example of the Tertiary Care level of the healthcare system. Tertiary Care is associated with the provision of specialized services.
   d. This is not an example of the Primary Care level of the healthcare system. Primary Care is associated with early detection and routine care.

5. a. Although this is a component of *Nursing's Agenda for Health Care Reform*, it is not the cornerstone of the document.
   b. Although this is a component of *Nursing's Agenda for Health Care Reform*, it is not the cornerstone of the document.
   c. This is the cornerstone of *Nursing's Agenda For Health Care Reform*. All people have a right to receive health care but this right is useless unless the care is easily reached and used.
   d. Although this is a component of *Nursing's Agenda for Health Care Reform*, it is not the cornerstone of the document.

6. a. The primary role of a Case Manager is to coordinate the activities of all the other members of the healthcare team and ensure that the patient is receiving care in the most appropriate setting.
   b. Counseling is not the primary role of a Case Manager. When counseling, the nurse helps a patient recognize and cope with emotional stressors, improve relationships, and/or promote personal growth.
   c. Providing care is not the primary role of the Case Manager. When providing care, the nurse is in the caregiver role. Care giving involves identifying and meeting the patient's needs by helping the patient regain health through the caring process.
   d. Teaching is not the primary role of the Case Manager. When teaching, the nurse helps the patient learn about health and healthcare practices.

7. a. Ambulatory care centers are not an inpatient care setting. Although some may be located in a hospital, they are more often in convenient locations such as a shopping mall or store front. They provide services

such as emergency walk-in care, ambulatory surgery, and health prevention and health promotion interventions.

b. An extended-care facility is an inpatient setting where a client lives while receiving sub-acute medical, nursing, or custodial care. It includes facilities such as intermediate care and skilled nursing facilities (nursing homes), assisted living centers, rehabilitation centers, and residential facilities for the mentally or developmentally disabled.

c. Day-care centers are not an example of an inpatient care setting. Day-care centers provide care for people who arrive in the morning and go home at the end of the day. They provide care for healthy children or older adults so that significant others can work or they provide specialized services to specific populations such as individuals with cerebral palsy or mental health problems.

d. Although hospice services may be provided in an inpatient hospice or residential hospice setting, the majority of hospice services are provided in the home. Hospice agencies provide multiple specialized services to support the dignity and quality of life of individuals who are dying and their family members who are caring for them at home.

8. a. A metropolitan area is a major city with smaller surrounding communities. The cities in the United States have a high concentration of healthcare organizations, health professionals, and specialty medical services, which provide opportunities for access to healthcare.

b. A suburban area is a residential district on the outskirts of a city. The cities in the United States have a high concentration of healthcare organizations, health professionals, and specialty medical services, which provide opportunities for access to healthcare. Because of the close proximity of a suburb to a city, residents usually have opportunities to access the healthcare available in the city.

c. An urban area is a city or town with the characteristics of a city. Urban areas in the United States have a high concentration of healthcare organizations, professionals, and specialty services, which provide opportunities for access to healthcare.

d. **Rural areas are usually geographically remote areas with few healthcare providers, healthcare organizations that may be hundreds of miles away, and specialty medical services that may be thousands of miles away. In addition, rural areas tend to have a healthcare culture that values self-sufficiency and many people are self-employed and do not have health insurance.**

9. a. **The nurse needs to first check the diet manual to see if the food that the patient requested is permitted on the ordered diet. The next action will depend on whether or not the food is permitted.**

b. This is premature. The first thing the nurse should do is indicated in another option.

c. It may not be an oversight. The first thing the nurse should do is indicated in another option.

d. This is premature. The nurse needs more information.

10. a. Although this remains to be seen, the explosion in knowledge and technology usually results in treatments that prolong life.

b. **This is a statistically supported fact. The percentage of older adults in the United States is expected to increase from the current 12% of the population to 22% by the year 2030. Fourteen percent of the 22% will be people over the age of 85. Because chronic illness is more prevalent among older adults, additional healthcare services will be needed in the future, raising costs.**

c. More people will seek healthcare in the home and community, not the acute care setting. In 1992 the National League for Nursing predicted that home care will become the center of healthcare and that community nursing centers and community health programs will focus on illness prevention and health promotion.

d. This may or may not occur because of a multiplicity of factors such as religious beliefs, unplanned pregnancies, and lack of seeking genetic counseling.

11. a. This is not the reason why DRGs were instituted. In addition, the DRGs have increased the acuity of hospitalized patients requiring a lower ratio of nurses to patients. However, many hospitals have not increased the numbers of nurses because of reengineering and the lack of available qualified nurses.

b. This is not the reason why DRGs were instituted. Although there is a current trend in the United States with more people focusing on health promotion and illness prevention, it is unrelated to DRGs.

c. DRGs were not instituted to solve fragmentation of care. Fragmentation of care is generally caused by overspecialization and caregivers failing to address patients' needs holistically and comprehensively.

d. **The DRGs, pretreatment diagnoses reimbursement categories, were designed to decrease the average length of a hospital stay, reducing costs.**

12. a. Because of circumstances, a nurse's intervention may not always be able to meet a patient's perceived needs.

b. The nurse-patient relationship is a therapeutic, not social, relationship.

c. The patient, not the nurse, is the leader of the health team.

d. **When planning patient care the nurse and patient work together to identify appropriate goals and interventions to facilitate goal achievement.**

13. a. Although it is important to reduce the effects of stress, it does not reduce the contributing factors that cause the stress.

b. How one practices nursing and why one is a nurse are based on enduring values and beliefs. Although it is important to be aware of how one practices nursing and why one is a nurse, confronting, taking exception to, and calling into question one's enduring values is not where the problem lies in burnout. Burnout occurs generally because nurses are unable to practice nursing as they were taught to practice nursing based on principles and standards of practice. Nurses experience stress because of such factors as understaffing, increased patient care assignments, shift work, excessive mandatory overtime, inadequate support, and caring for patients who are more critically ill and dying.

c. When faced with any stressful situation that can lead to feelings of burnout, the nurse must begin with self awareness and identify personal expectations, strengths, and limitations associated with the job. After the assessment is complete and problems are identified, the nurse can explore options to reduce factors contributing to job related stress. The nurse needs to employ strategies to manage stress to prevent the physical and emotional exhaustion associated with burnout and not wait until these responses occur.

d. Although there is an element of truth in this statement, providing nursing care is a serious responsibility and humor is not an effective strategy to cope with the major issues that contribute to burnout.

14. a. Licensed Registered Nurses do not receive third party reimbursement for their services.
b. Clinical Specialists are not healthcare professionals who receive third party reimbursement. Clinical Specialists have been on the scene since the decade of the 60's. They are Masters-prepared nurses with a specialty in areas such as medical-surgical nursing, pediatrics, psychiatry etc. or they may have advanced education and experience in caring for individuals with special needs such as wound care, enterostomal care, or care of the patient with diabetes.
c. Physician Assistants are not healthcare professionals who receive third party reimbursement directly. They work under the supervision of a physician in many different settings and are paid by the physician in private practice or by the organization that hired them. They assist physicians by carrying out common, routine medical treatments and they have prescriptive authority.
d. This is a relatively new trend in healthcare delivery. Nurse Practitioners generally are Masters-prepared individuals who work independently or collaboratively with physicians to provide primary healthcare services. Nurse Practitioners work independently under their own license, are accountable for their own practice, have prescriptive authority, and receive third party reimbursement, depending on the state in which they work. In the states that do not permit this level of healthcare delivery, Nurse Practitioners work under the license of a physician who supervisors their practice.

15. a. Critical pathways are not an educational career ladder for health professionals. A career ladder is the organization of educational experiences so that professional growth progresses in a planned manner.

b. Critical pathways are a case management system that identifies specific protocols and timetables for care and treatment by various disciplines designed to achieve expected patient outcomes within a specific timeframe.
c. This is a definition of critical time, not critical pathways.
d. This is unrelated to critical pathways.

16. a. The clinic setting is not the organizational center of the United States healthcare system.
b. The acute care setting is the organizational center of the United States healthcare system today. Specialized services (tertiary level of care) and emergency, critical care, and intense diagnosis and treatment (secondary level of care) of illness and disease are provided for in hospitals (acute care setting). In 1991 the American Nurses Association published Nursing's Agenda for Health Care Reform which made recommendations for healthcare reform in many areas. The major trend identified as a result of implementation of the recommendations would be a shift of the focus of healthcare from illness and cure to one of wellness and care. If this occurs, the healthcare system of the United States will shift from the acute care setting to the home and community.
c. The community setting is not the organizational center of the United States healthcare system.
d. The long-term care setting is not the organizational center of the United States healthcare system.

17. a. The caregiver role is associated with facilitating the achievement of goals identified in the patient's plan of care.
b. Of the options offered, the word evaluate is not the word most associated with the nurse functioning as a caregiver. Although, evaluation is important in relation to the nursing process and care giving, it is only one aspect of care giving.
c. Of the options offered, the word counsel is not the word most associated with the nurse functioning as a caregiver. When counseling, the nurse helps a patient recognize and cope with emotional stressors, improve relationships, and/or promote personal growth and it is only one aspect of care giving.
d. Of the options offered, the word teach is not the word most associated with the nurse functioning as a caregiver. When teaching, the nurse helps the patient learn about health and healthcare practices and is only one aspect of care giving.

18. a. The American Heart Association is a voluntary not-for-profit organization, not an official organization.
b. The National League for Nursing (NLN) is a not-for-profit organization founded in 1952 to foster the development and improvement of nursing education and services. The NLN is not an official organization.
c. Non-profit community hospitals are voluntary, not official, organizations.
d. The Veterans Administration is an official organization because it comes under the umbrella of government supported and operated healthcare financed by taxation.

19. a. The patient is the center of the health team and has primary responsibility for making healthcare decisions. Consumers are more knowledgeable than ever before, have a greater awareness of health issues, and have a desire to be responsible for healthcare decisions. In addition, more knowledgeable consumers (patients and families) have made a major impact on the delivery of healthcare services in the United States because they have made their opinions and preferences known.

   b. Educated consumers, not healthcare providers, control the direction and development of healthcare services. Citizens are active members of the Boards of Trustees of healthcare agencies in all settings, community organizations have political action committees that lobby government representatives to shape the political agenda, and the consumer movement with its demands and expectations all impact on the direction of healthcare reform.

   c. Although some people strive to sustain life at any cost, most people prefer to seek ways to support and maintain quality, over longevity, of life. The hospice movement, which is increasing, is based on the concept of maintaining quality of life by caring for dying people in their homes surrounded by family and friends and making remaining days as comfortable and meaningful as possible.

   d. Social issues are taking a front, not back, seat as a result of advances in technology. Technological advances and specialized treatments are extremely expensive. The United States spends over 1 billion dollars a day on healthcare and it continues to increase (a 400% increase since 1965). Social issues include who will pay for healthcare costs, who has access to healthcare, and who will care for older adults and the uninsured (both of whom are increasing in numbers). In addition, ethical issues are becoming prominent in response to advances in areas such as transplant and beginning of life technology.

20. a. Screening surveys and procedures are examples of Secondary Prevention. Secondary Prevention is associated with early detection, early and quick intervention, health maintenance, and prevention of complications. The Levels of Prevention identify three levels of prevention that focus on healthcare activities such as Primary Prevention (avoiding disease through health promotion and disease prevention), Secondary Prevention (early detection and treatment), and Tertiary Prevention (reducing complications, rehabilitation, restoration and maintenance of optimal function).

   b. This is not an example of Tertiary Prevention. Tertiary Prevention begins after a situation is stabilized and the focus is on rehabilitation and restoration within the limits of the disability.

   c. This is not an example of Primary Prevention. Primary Prevention is associated with activities that promote health and protect against disease.

   d. Acute is not one of the Levels of Prevention. The word acute refers to the type of care that is provided on the Secondary Care Level of the healthcare delivery system.

21. a. Volunteerism has generally remained the same because of two factors. More women are working to help support their families and people are retiring earlier and engaging in volunteer work.

   b. Extended care facilities are the result of a trend rather than the cause of a trend in how healthcare services are provided in the United States.

   c. Older-Adult Day-Care Centers have always provided for the support of wellness and is not a new trend in healthcare delivery.

   d. The DRGs, pretreatment diagnoses reimbursement categories, were designed to decrease the average length of a hospital stay, reducing costs. As a result, patients are being discharged not fully recovered and still in need of medical and nursing support services. These services are being provided in a variety of extended care facilities such as nursing homes and rehabilitation centers as well as in the home. This trend has dramatically changed the way healthcare services are provided to all but those who are acutely ill.

22. a. Rehabilitation interventions begin whether the patient is conscious or unconscious.

   b. As soon as a patient is diagnosed with a problem, rehabilitation interventions begin.

   c. This is too late to begin rehabilitation interventions.

   d. Rehabilitation interventions begin whether the patient is ambulatory or non-ambulatory.

23. a. Although this is a true statement, it does not explain why nurses need to be role models for healthy living.

   b. Although this is a true statement, it does not explain why nurses need to be role models for healthy living.

   c. This is true. Congruity must exist between what nurses say and what they do. For nurses to be credible and attentive to the health needs of patients, nurses must work at maintaining their own health. By caring for themselves, nurses demonstrate values that they believe in and behaviors that support health and wellness. Actions speak louder than words.

   d. Although this is a true statement, it does not explain why nurses need to be role models for healthy living.

24. a. Virtually everyone in the United States over 65 years of age is protected by hospital, post-hospital extended care, and home health benefit insurance under Part A of Medicare. Patients pay a coinsurance of 20% and the other 80% is paid by the government.

   b. Medicaid is not a program that pays for the majority of healthcare costs of people over 65 years of age. Medicaid is a United States federal program, that is state operated, that provides medical assistance for people with low incomes.

   c. Blue Cross is a not-for-profit medical insurance plan that pays for hospital services for people of all ages, not just people over 65 years of age.

   d. Blue Shield is a not-for-profit medical insurance plan that pays for care provided by healthcare professionals for all age groups, not just for people over 65 years of age.

25. a. Reengineering has not reduced hospital occupancy

rates. Decreased hospital occupancy rates are directly related to Diagnostic Related Groups and the resultant decrease in lengths of stay. The concerns about a decrease in occupancy rates are not related to patient safety, but rather fiscal issues.

b. Reengineering has not increased patient acuity in the hospital setting. Although the increased acuity of hospitalized patients is a real concern when providing for patient safety, if a unit is adequately staffed with the appropriate mix of nurses to ancillary staff, safety should not be an issue.

c. Reengineering does not precipitate hospital mergers. Hospital mergers and the resulting reengineering should not impact on patient safety if professional practice standards are maintained.

d. Reengineering is concerned with training a less well educationally prepared nursing assistant to implement nursing tasks that were formerly associated with the practice of nursing. This trend poses a serious threat to the safety and welfare of patients because tasks requiring the complex skills of a nurse are being delegated to minimally prepared individuals. This is particularly dangerous in the present healthcare environment where hospitalized patients are more acutely ill than ever before.

26. **a. Providing for continuity of care is the major concern with early discharge as a result of DRGs. It requires careful planning to ensure that services, personnel, and equipment are provided in a timely and comprehensive manner and care is not fragmented and disorganized.**

b. Although this is a concern for some individuals, if the discharge planner plans early for the patient's discharge, all interventions should be in place before the patient is discharged.

c. Although this is a concern for some individuals, if patients receive supportive emotional intervention and are prepared for discharge from the first day of admission, patients generally would rather be at home than in the hospital.

d. Hospitals are pleased when they are able to discharge a person earlier than the designated length of stay indicated by the DRGs because the hospital keeps the unused portion of the DRG reimbursement.

27. **a. Change almost always causes anxiety because it requires one to move from that which is comfortable and familiar to that which is uncomfortable, unfamiliar, unpredictable, and threatening.**

b. A belief is an opinion or a conclusion that one accepts as true and may be based on either faith and/or facts and should not generate anxiety. People generally set healthcare goals that do not conflict with their beliefs.

c. A value is an enduring attitude about something that is cherished and held dear to one's heart and should not generate anxiety. People generally set healthcare goals that do not conflict with their values.

d. A role is a set of expectations about how one should behave. Although a healthcare goal may conflict with a role one sets for oneself, another option has greater ability to contribute to anxiety than one's role.

28. a. Although the leadership role is an important role and can be demonstrated on many different levels in the nursing profession, a word in another option has a stronger relationship with the role of the nurse when helping a patient negotiate the healthcare system.

b. The healthcare delivery system in the United States is complex and can be confusing at a time when patients have the least energy to explore and negotiate intervention options. When functioning as a resource person, the nurse identifies resources, provides information, and makes referrals.

c. The surrogate role is not a professional role of the nurse. A surrogate role is assigned to a nurse when a patient believes that the nurse reminds them of another and projects that role and the feelings one has for the other person onto the nurse.

d. The role of counselor is only one area of nursing practice and a word in another option has a stronger relationship with the role of the nurse when helping a patient negotiate the healthcare system. Counseling is related only to helping a patient recognize and cope with emotional stressors, improve relationships, and promote personal growth.

29. **a. This is an example of an integrated healthcare service network. Hospitals are joining networks to decrease costs and increase reimbursement. This is accomplished by expanding the breadth of services while avoiding duplication of services, keeping clients within the network, negotiating the price of supplies and equipment, and centralizing departments which results in fewer personnel (e.g., administration, staff education, and human resource departments, etc.).**

b. This is not an example of a third-party reimbursement system. Third-party reimbursement refers to when someone other than the receiver of healthcare (generally an insurance company) pays for the services provided.

c. This is not an example of a Health Maintenance Organization (HMO). An HMO is an organization that provides primary healthcare for a preset fee.

d. The DRGs are pretreatment diagnoses reimbursement categories designed to decrease the average length of a hospital stay, reducing costs.

30. a. There is no clear separation between health and illness on the health-illness continuum. Each individual's personal perceptions of multiple factors determine where a person places himself or herself on the health-illness continuum.

b. Demographics are changing rapidly in the United States as we become a heterogeneous, multicultural, multiethnic society. Because of the increasing diversity of the population of the United States, nurses need to use transcultural knowledge in a skillful way to provide culturally appropriate, competent care.

c. Internal as well as external factors are the cause of illness.

d. Most people do not view health as the absence of disease. There is no one definition of health because there are so many different factors that impact on one's definition of health. Therefore, a definition of health depends on each individual person's own perspective.

31. a. Only approximately 4% of older adults require long term care at the end of life.
    b. The percentage of older adults below the designated poverty level has been declining with less than 15% falling in this category in the year 2000.
    c. Although older adults may take more time to process and respond to information, only approximately 4 to 5% of older adults experience dementia.
    d. Studies report that one third of older adults 75 years of age and older experience at least 1 fall each year. Half of these older adults experience multiple falls each year. Twenty percent of hospital and 40% of nursing home admissions of older adults are associated with falls or complications experienced as a result of falls.

32. a. This is an example of care associated with the Tertiary Level of the healthcare system. Tertiary Care is associated with long-term, chronic, and hospice care and specialized service.
    b. This is an example of care on the Secondary Level of the healthcare system. Secondary Care (acute care) includes emergency treatment, critical care, and care associated with intensive and elaborate diagnosis and treatment.
    c. This is an example of care on the Secondary Level of the healthcare system. Secondary Care (acute care) includes emergency treatment, critical care, and care associated with intensive and elaborate diagnosis and treatment.
    d. **This is an example of the Primary Level of the healthcare system. It is associated with activities that promote health and protect against disease. The healthcare system has three Levels of Healthcare that describe the scope of services and settings where healthcare and include Primary, Secondary, and Tertiary.**

33. a. The nurse functions as a resource, not counselor, when the nurse helps the patient understand and use services provided by agencies in the healthcare system.
    b. **This is an example of the nurse functioning as a counselor. When counseling, the nurse helps a patient recognize and cope with emotional stressors, improve relationships, and promote personal growth.**
    c. The nurse functions as an advocate, not counselor, when the nurse helps the patient negotiate the healthcare delivery system.
    d. The nurse functions as a teacher, not counselor, when the nurse helps a patient to learn how to change a dressing.

34. a. This would not be the first thing to do when unsure of the steps in a nursing procedure.
    b. Fundamental nursing textbooks are not the best source for a step-by-step review of a nursing skill. Generally, fundamental nursing textbooks do not address every nursing skill in a step-by-step approach nor do they include intermediate or advanced skills.
    c. **This is the first resource the nurse should use when unsure of the steps in a nursing procedure.**

A review of the procedure in the Procedure Manual may refresh the memory or support the confidence of the nurse so that it is safe to proceed.
    d. This is premature. Another action should be implemented first.

35. a. Only nursing management positions contain an administrative component.
    b. **Nurses work in a variety of settings; however, a component that is common to all settings is the use of the nursing process to develop patient plans of care.**
    c. Not all Registered Nurse positions include direct physical care of patients. For example, many positions in home care, clinics, industry, and schools focus on case finding, on-going monitoring of progress, and teaching rather than direct physical care.
    d. The majority of nurses' time is concerned with implementing independent and dependent functions within the scope of nursing practice, not spent assisting the physician. In most settings, the nurse and physician work in a collaborative relationship to help patients cope with human responses to illness and disease.

36. a. **The DRGs, pretreatment diagnoses reimbursement categories, were designed to decrease the average length of a hospital stay, reducing costs.**
    b. Predetermined hospital reimbursement based on a medical problem provides reimbursement for care received in a hospital, whereas, managed care organizations generally are associated with predetermined reimbursement for healthcare costs outside of the hospital. Health Maintenance and Preferred Provider Organizations are examples of managed care. They are designed to provide cost-effective quality care with a focus on health promotion, illness prevention, customer satisfaction, and cost control.
    c. Retrospective (after an event) payment systems reimburse healthcare after it is delivered and is not based on a schedule of reimbursement based on a predetermined medical problem.
    d. The United States does not have a national socialized health insurance plan. Canada has a mandatory socialized plan that provides universal coverage to all citizens. Hospital and physician reimbursement are insured through the plan with no consumer billing and it is paid for through taxation.

37. a. Once stabilized and out of danger, the individual in the scenario needs intensive rehabilitation services that generally cannot be provided in an Assisted-Living Residence. An Assisted-Living Residence (apartment, villa, or condominium) provides limited assistance with activities of daily living, meal preparation, laundry services, transportation, and opportunities for socialization. Residents are relatively independent.
    b. Once stabilized and out of danger, the individual in the scenario needs intensive rehabilitation services that generally cannot be provided in Day-Care

Centers. These centers provide care for people who arrive in the morning and go home at the end of the day. They generally provide care for healthy children or older adults so that significant others can work or they provide specialized services to specific populations such as individuals with cerebral palsy or mental health problems.

c. An extended-care facility is an inpatient setting where people live while receiving sub-acute medical, nursing, and rehabilitative care. Extended-care facilities that would meet the needs of this individual include intermediate-care facilities, nursing homes with sub-acute care or skilled nursing care, or rehabilitation centers.

d. This is generally not the best setting to provide extensive rehabilitation services. The acute care setting provides services that medically and emotionally support the patient during the critical and acute phases right after the traumatic event until the patient is stable and out of danger.

38. a. This is not the largest group of healthcare professionals in the United States.
b. This is not the largest group of healthcare professionals in the United States.
c. This is not the largest group of healthcare professionals in the United States.
d. **Nurses comprise the largest group of healthcare professionals in the United States. There are not enough Registered Nurses to meet the present demand. It is predicted that if the demand for nurses continues at the present rate and even if the present rate of graduating nurses increases slightly each year, by the year 2020 the nation's supply of Registered Nurses will only meet 72% of the demand.**

39. a. This is not a major factor that prevents an overhaul of the healthcare delivery system of the United States. Most elected officials recognize the need for healthcare reform and the need to respond to the desires of their political constituencies if they are to be reelected.
b. This is not a major factor that prevents an overhaul of the healthcare delivery system of the United States.
c. **Healthcare delivery in the United States is an extremely complex service industry consisting of public, voluntary, and proprietary businesses with multiple disciplines of healthcare workers represented. The system is influenced by federal, state, and local social, economic, ethical, and consumer driven issues.**
d. Physician input is only one factor that may prevent an overhaul of the healthcare delivery system of the United States. Although the American Medical Association has a strong political action committee it was unable to prevent the institution of prospective reimbursement systems that in many ways dramatically changed the work world of the physician as well as placing limits on financial compensation for medical services provided.

40. a. Primary nursing is not a cost containment strategy in managed care, but rather a nursing care delivery system that ensures a comprehensive and consistent

approach to identifying and meeting patients' needs. Primary nursing occurs when one nurse is assigned the 24 hour responsibility for the planning and delivery of nursing care to a specific patient for the duration of the patient's hospitalization.

b. **Critical pathways are a case management system that identifies specific protocols and timetables for care and treatment by various disciplines designed to achieve expected patient outcomes within a specific timeframe. The purpose is to discharge patients sooner, thereby reducing the cost of healthcare.**

c. Functional method refers to a model of nursing care delivery that assigns a specific task for a group of patients to one person. Although it is efficient, it is impersonal and contributes to fragmentation of care because it is task oriented rather than patient centered.

d. Quality management (also known as continuous quality improvement, total quality management, or persistent quality improvement) refers to a program designed to improve, not just ensure, the quality of care delivered to patients. It also includes an educational component to support growth and provide for corrective action.

41. a. Health promotion is not emphasized in the traditional healthcare delivery system in the United States. However in 1992 the National League for Nursing predicted that in the future healthcare in the United States will move from the traditional hospital setting to the community with an emphasis on health promotion.
b. Illness prevention is not emphasized in the traditional healthcare delivery system in the United States. In 1992 the National League for Nursing predicted that in the future healthcare in the United States will move from the traditional hospital setting to the community with an emphasis on illness prevention.
c. **Traditional healthcare delivery has always centered on activities associated with diagnosing, treating, and curing illness and disease. In addition, hospitals account for the largest proportion of money spent on healthcare and employs the largest number of healthcare workers.**
d. Rehabilitation and long term care are not emphasized in the traditional healthcare delivery system in the United States.

42. a. This is not the purpose of a patient classification system.
b. **A Patient Classification System or Acuity Reports are designed to rate patients in terms of high or low acuity based on the amount of time and nursing resources that are needed to care for the patient. A patient who is unstable and requires constant monitoring and nursing intervention will be rated a higher acuity score than a patient who is stable and relatively self-sufficient in activities of daily living.**
c. On-going Quality Improvement Programs are designed to establish whether or not standards of care have been met, not a patient classification system.

d. Standardized expected outcomes are established by professional educational and practice organizations, credentialing bodies, and critical pathways, not by a patient classification system.

43. a. A Home Care Nurse provides and coordinates health services in the home.
    b. A Primary Nurse has total responsibility for the planning and delivery of nursing care to a specific patient for the duration of the patient's hospitalization. Primary nursing is a nursing care delivery system that attempts to prevent fragmentation of care and ensure a comprehensive and consistent approach to meeting patients' needs while in the hospital.
    c. **A Case Manager coordinates and links healthcare services to clients and their families at single levels of care (e.g., during hospitalization) and across levels of care (e.g., progression through hospitalization, extended-care facilities, and home care).**
    d. A Charge Nurse is a unit manager within an organization. A manager's job is to ensure that the objectives and goals of the organization are met appropriately, efficiently, and in a cost-effective manner.

44. a. Studies and position papers from all segments of the healthcare industry indicate the need to provide more healthcare services in the community and not the institutional setting. To meet the healthcare needs of older adults in the future, efforts have to begin now to provide more community-based support services so that people can remain in their own homes and not have to move to an institutional setting.
    b. More services need to address the primary, not secondary, healthcare needs of the community. Secondary healthcare services include emergency care, acute care, diagnosis, and complex treatment. The present healthcare system has an infrastructure that supports the delivery of secondary healthcare services. More emphasis must be placed on providing services that meet the primary healthcare needs of society, which includes health promotion, illness prevention, health education, environmental protection, and early detection and treatment.
    c. **Consumers are more aware than ever before that change in their own behavior and life style will have a major influence on their own health status. Public health service announcements, community health education programs, and even television programs and media print materials (newspapers and magazines) have improved consumer awareness.**
    d. Consumers, not healthcare providers, have to be charged with the primary responsibility for providing appropriate healthcare services. As individuals or as groups, consumer demands and expectations will have the greatest impact on the delivery of health care.

45. a. Although undocumented immigrants are increasing in numbers, it is not the group posing the greatest challenge to financing healthcare in the United States.
    b. Although the medically uninsured are increasing in numbers, it is not the group posing the greatest challenge to financing healthcare in the United States.
    c. Although the number of preterm infants has increased from 7.5 to 11.6% because of an increase in multiple-gestations and the failure to receive early prenatal care in singletons, it is not the group posing the greatest challenge to financing healthcare in the United States.
    d. **The percentage of older adults in the United States is expected to increase from the current 12% of the population to 22% by the year 2030. Fourteen percent of the 22% will be people over the age of 85. Because chronic illness is more prevalent among older adults, additional healthcare services will be needed in the future. The need for increased services will increase costs.**

46. a. Resource Utilization Groups (RUGs) is the patient classification system used to determine reimbursement rates to nursing homes and is unrelated to the shift of healthcare delivery from the hospital to the home.
    b. This is not the reason for the shift of healthcare delivery from the hospital to the home. As a result of Diagnostic Related Groups, many hospitals are downsizing to reduce costs and do not need more hospital beds.
    c. **This is the reason for the shift from the hospital to the home because patients are discharged earlier in an effort to reduce the cost of healthcare.**
    d. Although there is a shortage of Registered Nurses, this has not caused a shift of healthcare delivery from the hospital to the home. It is predicted that if the demand for nurses continues at the present rate and even if the present rate of graduating nurses increases slightly each year, by the year 2020 the nation's supply of Registered Nurses will only meet 72% of the demand.

47. a. **Medicaid is a federally funded, but state regulated, health insurance program for individuals with low incomes.**
    b. This describes Medicare, not Medicaid.
    c. Federally funded programs providing care to people living below the designated poverty level are voluntary, not mandatory.
    d. Healthcare reimbursement in the hospital setting in the United States is based on a prospective, not retrospective, reimbursement formula. Diagnostic Related Groups is a predetermined hospital reimbursement rate based on a medical problem.

48. a. When functioning as a provider, the nurse is in the caregiver, not advocate, role. Care giving involves identifying and meeting the patient's needs by helping the patient regain health through the caring process.
    b. When functioning as a nurturer, the nurse is in the caregiver, not advocate, role. Nurture means to encourage, foster, and promote, all of which are components of care giving. Advocate means to plead another's cause.
    c. **Of the options offered, the word protector best**

describes the role of the nurse when functioning as the patient's advocate. In the role of advocate, the nurse protects and supports patients' rights and assists in asserting those rights when patients are unable to defend themselves.

d. Evaluation does not describe patient advocacy. Evaluation is an important function, not role, of the nurse. Evaluation is the last step in the nursing process and is a determination of whether or not the patient's goals are achieved.

49. a. To maintain quality control and cost containment, third party payers have preauthorization criteria for surgery that may include requirements such as second opinions, initial conservative therapies, or certain diagnostic tests.

b. These are not related to the concept of preauthorization. They are obtained to identify actual or potential health problems that may influence or be affected by the surgery.

c. This is unrelated to preauthorization. A checklist summarizes the patient's preoperative preparation to ensure that all significant activities and safety precautions have been completed.

d. This is unrelated to preauthorization. Informed Consent is a legal document giving permission for surgery including the procedure, surgical site, and surgeons.

50. a. Many hospitalized patients may be emotionally fragile because of the stress of the experience. It is only when patients are a threat to themselves or others that they should not be placed with another patient and they should be under constant supervision.

b. This is not a requirement for roommates. A patient does not have to converse with or be responsible for another patient.

c. The location of a bed within a room is insignificant. When two beds are available, the choice may be left to patient preference.

d. One patient's physical condition should not influence another patient's physical condition. For example, a patient with a communicable disease should be in a private room and a patient with an incision or an open wound should not be in a room with a patient with an infection.

Community-Based Nursing

KEYWORDS

The following words include English vocabulary, nursing/medical terminology, concepts, principles, or information relevant to content specifically addressed in the chapter or associated with topics presented in it. English dictionaries, your nursing textbooks, and medical dictionaries such as *Taber's Cyclopedic Medical Dictionary* are resources that can be used to expand your knowledge and understanding of these words and related information.

Case management
Coalition
Collaboration
Collegial
Community
Continuity
Demographics
Discharge planning
Epidemiology
Focus group
Global initiatives
Health care settings
  Acute care – hospitals
  Adult day-care
  Ambulatory care centers
  Assisted-living residence
  Clinics
  Extended care
  Home health services
  Hospice (inpatient, residential, in the home)
  Industrial or occupation settings

Life-care community
Long term care – nursing homes
Neighborhood community health center
Physician's offices
Psychiatric facilities
Rehabilitation centers
School settings
Urgent visit centers
Health care reform
Healthy People 2000
Holistic
Hospice
Initiatives
Levels of healthcare
  Primary healthcare
  Secondary healthcare
  Tertiary healthcare
Levels of prevention
  Primary prevention
    Health promotion
    Health protection

Preventive health services
Secondary prevention
Tertiary prevention
Managed care
Metropolitan
Nursing's Agenda for Health Care Reform
Occupational nurse
Outreach
Population
Primary care
Public health nurse
Public policy
Referral
Respite care
Rural
Self-help group
Suburban
Urban
Vulnerable populations
Wellness

QUESTIONS

1. Which is a need that falls within the category of Tertiary Healthcare service?
   a. Critical care
   b. **Long term care**
   c. Diagnostic care
   d. Preventive care

2. Which support would generally provide the most benefit to a person at home recovering from an illness that has caused functional deficits?
   a. Meals on Wheels program
   b. Church outreach program
   c. **Home care agency**
   d. A hospice

3. The major role of the nurse in the community setting is:
   a. Advisor
   b. Teacher
   c. Counselor
   d. Surrogate

4. Which statement accurately reflects a concept about a healthy community?
   a. Health of a community is based on the sum of the health of its individuals
   b. In community health the focus is primarily on the health of each member of society
   c. The focus of community health is mainly on healing the sick and preventing disease
   d. Promotion of health is one of the most important components of community health practice

5. A feature common to most containers for prescription medications that are used in the home is:
   a. Drip proof tops
   b. Unit dose packages
   c. Sun repellent plastic
   d. Child-resistant covers

6. Which is the most important factor associated with being able to provide nursing services in the home setting?
   a. The patient must be able to perform some self care
   b. The family has the financial resources to pay for the care
   c. Additional family members need to be available for support
   d. Intervention must be ordered by a provider with a license to prescribe

7. When assessing variables from a cultural perspective, it is most important for the nurse to:
   a. Use the patient as the main source of data
   b. Interview the members of the patient's family
   c. Recognize beliefs common to the patient's ethic group
   d. Recall experiences of caring for patients with a similar background

8. In which setting do nurses most often need to *wear many hats*?
   a. Urban centers
   b. Rural communities
   c. Acute care hospitals
   d. Rehabilitation facilities

9. Which factor is essential to promote healthy lifestyles and behaviors within the community setting?
   a. The entire family must be committed to making changes
   b. A practitioner's order is necessary before care can be provided
   c. There must be resources available to support the desired changes
   d. The focus must be on the community as a whole, not on individuals

10. Which has noticeably declined in the United States over the last several years?
    a. Public health services
    b. At risk client groups
    c. Cost of healthcare
    d. Self-help groups

11. Which is an example of an intervention associated with Secondary prevention?
    a. Conducting a cardiac risk assessment for people over 40 years of age
    b. Teaching a low-fat diet to a person with high cholesterol
    c. Immunization of a child during the first year of life
    d. Monthly self-breast examinations by women

12. Which is an example of an agency that provides respite care?
    a. Hospice program
    b. Meals on Wheels
    c. Ambulatory care center
    d. Alcohol treatment center

13. An important role of the nurse that takes on more emphasis in the delivery of healthcare in the home than in the acute care setting is:
    a. Modifying the environment
    b. Providing for healthy meals
    c. Delivering skilled nursing care
    d. Coordinating the efforts of the health team

14. The difference between the acute and home care settings is that in the home care setting the:
    a. Patient is the center of the health team
    b. Nurse functions as an advocate for the patient
    c. Nurse is responsible for coordinating the efforts of the health team
    d. Patient is not discharged until counseling and teaching are completed

15. The action related to advocacy that reflects the nurse's attempt to work with families to explore the nature and consequences of their choices is:
    a. Affirming
    b. Informing
    c. Mediating
    d. Interviewing

16. In an acute care setting, activities related to the concept of community nursing begin:
    a. On first contact with the patient
    b. After the patient is admitted to the institution
    c. When the practitioner writes the discharge orders
    d. At the time referrals to community resources are made

17. When collecting information about a community to identify its needs, the most significant assessment is:
    a. The demographics of the community
    b. What the community thinks is important
    c. How many support services are available
    d. Environmental data as it relates to safety

18. The individual who will have the most difficult time adjusting because of the need for long-term home healthcare is the:
    a. Middle-school-aged child
    b. Pre-school-aged child
    c. Adolescent
    d. Older adult

19. A factor that differentiates nursing care in the home from care in the acute setting is that in the home:
    a. Nurses work more independently
    b. Nurses need excellent communication skills
    c. Patients have needs that require less technical nursing skills
    d. Patients need to be taught about how to care for themselves

20. Which activity is associated with Tertiary prevention of disease?
    a. Seeking pregnancy testing
    b. Providing family planning
    c. Attending an AA meeting
    d. Teaching infant bathing

21. A patient has effective discharge planning and returns home seven days after the surgical creation of a colostomy. While all professional roles of the nurse are important, which role of the Registered Nurse takes priority in the home setting during this patient's initial return to the home?
    a. Practitioner
    b. Surrogate
    c. Specialist
    d. Teacher

22. After arriving at a home location that has a history of domestic violence, the home-care nurse believes that the environment may be unsafe. The nurse should:
    a. Call the police for an escort
    b. Leave the home immediately
    c. Attempt to defuse the situation in the home
    d. Complete the visit quickly while remaining alert

23. To best prevent a child from ingesting prescription medications in a home environment, parents should be taught to keep medications:
    a. On a high shelf
    b. In a locked cupboard
    c. In the medicine cabinet in a bathroom
    d. On a shelf in the back of the refrigerator

24. The most important team member in an assisted-living facility would be the:
    a. Occupational Therapist
    b. Nurse Aide
    c. Patient
    d. Nurse

25. Continuation of services to an individual receiving care from a home-care program depends on:
    a. The presence of a physician's order
    b. Retrospective audits of quality management
    c. Nursing documentation that there is a need for the care
    d. Patient and family satisfaction with the care being provided

26. The underutilization of services in a rural community is often the result of:
    a. The varieties of ethnic origin
    b. The culture of independence
    c. A disinterest in health
    d. A lack of intelligence

27. Which factor is essential to the health of a community?
    a. Availability of medical specialists
    b. Consumers having health insurance
    c. Everyone having access to healthcare
    d. Public Health Nurses working in the community

28. According to the document, *Healthy People 2000*, an activity associated with Health Protection would be:
    a. Administering immunizations to children
    b. Encouraging children to be physically fit
    c. Teaching a program about alcohol abuse
    d. Working as an occupational nurse in a factory

29. After identifying the health needs of members of a community the nurse's most efficient initial approach to meet those needs would be to:
    a. Involve community leaders to work within the political arena to obtain funding for programs
    b. Write research grants to explore the community's health needs in more detail
    c. Design educational programs that address the identified needs
    d. Make residents aware of the resources in the community

30. Which is the most essential assessment that must be made by the nurse in the home setting?
    a. Can the home environment support the safety of the client?
    b. Is the family willing to participate in the client's recovery?
    c. Does the client have the potential for self-care?
    d. Can the patient participate in the plan of care?

31. The statement that is most reflective of hospice care in healthcare delivery is, "Hospice:
    a. Clients must have less than a year to live to receive services."
    b. Care is more expensive than in the acute care setting."
    c. Mainly provides physical care to the dying person."
    d. Is a method of care rather than a location."

32. During the process of performing a community assessment, members of the community are invited to come and share opinions and concerns about a particular issue. This method of data collection is called:
    a. An opinion survey
    b. A community forum
    c. A demographic assessment
    d. An observation of participants

33. The major role of the nurse in the home care setting is:
    a. Case management
    b. Discharge planning
    c. Modifying client values
    d. Enlisting family support

34. Which type of agency is designed primarily to provide for a continuum of comprehensive healthcare after discharge from the hospital?
    a. Home care agencies
    b. Urgent visit centers
    c. Physicians' offices
    d. Respite programs

35. When conducting a community assessment the nurse should first collect data about the:
    a. General health of community members
    b. Physical environment of the community
    c. Characteristics of the community members
    d. Health and social services available in the community

36. Which patient, who has bilateral long leg casts applied for three months, probably will require a setting other than the home to recover?
    a. Adolescent living in a nuclear family
    b. Independently living older adult
    c. Middle-aged married male
    d. Infant with two parents

37. In the United States families:
    a. Are groups of people related by blood, marriage, adoption, or birth
    b. Are made up of fathers, mothers, and their children
    c. Vary based on their structural composition
    d. Live in the same household

38. Which is an example of a Tertiary healthcare service?
    a. Teaching about how to use a wheel chair after a stroke
    b. Administering a measles, mumps and rubella vaccine
    c. Conducting a smoking cessation class
    d. Changing a dressing after surgery

39. The major role of the nurse in the home associated with infection control is the role of:
    a. Counselor
    b. Caregiver
    c. Advocate
    d. Teacher

40. The most important thing the nurse can convey to caregivers who care for family members in the home who have a stable but chronic illness is to:
    a. Have extra equipment and supplies in the home for emergencies
    b. Plan a daily and monthly schedule of care-giving activities
    c. Care for themselves as well as the family member
    d. Keep a daily journal of the client's status

1. a. Critical care lies in the category of Secondary, not Tertiary, Healthcare. The Secondary Level of Healthcare is associated with acute care, complex diagnosis, treatment of disease and illness, and emergency care.
    b. **This is correct. Long term care lies in the category of Tertiary Healthcare. Tertiary Healthcare is associated with rehabilitation, care of the dying, and long term care.**
    c. Diagnostic care lies in the category of Secondary, not Tertiary, Healthcare.
    d. Preventive care lies in the category of Primary, not Tertiary, Healthcare. Primary Healthcare services are concerned with promoting health, preventing disease, early and basic detection and treatment of disease, environmental protection, and health education.

2. a. Meals on Wheels provides for only the nutritional needs of a client.
    b. Although church outreach programs may be able to provide some support services, it is generally not as an effective agency as another option to provide the multiple services needed or to coordinate the continuum of comprehensive services that a person with functional deficits will need. Many church outreach programs generally serve as a source of information about services and programs available in the community and they provide additional support that augments home care services.
    c. **A home healthcare agency is designed to coordinate the comprehensive services that a client may need to recover from an illness that has caused functional deficits. This person may need help in areas such as assistance with activities of daily living, physical and occupational rehabilitation, direct nursing care, counseling, etc.**
    d. A hospice program is designed to assist clients who have less than six months to live and who have chosen to forego additional curative treatment for palliative care and support of quality of life. Hospice programs also provide support services to members of the client's family as well as bereavement care after the death of the client.

3. a. Nurses should not advise or tell patients what to do. Patients need to make their own choices based on information and their own values, beliefs, and goals.
    b. **Of the roles presented in the options, the role of teacher is most important in the home care setting. As a teacher, the nurse helps clients manage, maintain or restore their health, identifies the client's learning needs, readiness, and motivation to learn, formulates a teaching plan in conjunction with the client, employs appropriate teaching strategies, and evaluates outcomes of learning.**
    c. Although nurses function as counselors, a role in another option is more frequently employed in the home care setting.
    d. The surrogate role is not a professional role of the nurse. A surrogate role is assigned to a nurse when a patient believes that the nurse reminds them of another and projects that role and the feelings one has for the other person onto the nurse.

4. a. A healthy community seeks to provide infrastructure, resources, and activities that support a healthy community and is not just reflective of the health of its members.
    b. Community health focuses on families, groups, and the community, not just individuals.
    c. This statement focuses on illness and is too limited in relation to community health.
    d. **Health promotion has taken on new meaning as consumers take more and more responsibility for their health status. Teaching about promoting health is a more positive perspective than teaching about preventing illness, which is a negative perspective.**

5. a. This is not common to all medication containers. Only medications in liquid form need to have drip proof tops.
    b. Most prescriptions filled for home use are in multi-dose containers.
    c. Not all medications need to be protected from the sun.
    d. **All prescriptions filled for home use are dispensed in containers with child-resistant tops as required by law. If a person has a physical limitation such as arthritis that interferes with one's ability to open a medication container, the person can request that a non-safety top be provided. The pharmacy will generally document the request in their computer and may even require that a waiver be signed and witnessed for the record.**

6. a. This is not necessary. In some instances, the family members provide total care with no help from the patient.
    b. A person does not have to be wealthy to receive nursing services in the home. For example, Medicare, Medicaid, or private healthcare insurance plans assume some of the costs of care provided in the home.
    c. The presence of family members is not a requirement for home care services. However, if it is unsafe for the patient to be home alone or unattended for long periods, the home may not be the most appropriate setting. In addition, patients who have no family support may rely on a friend, neighbor or volunteers from a neighborhood outreach group to help in a supportive way.
    d. **Healthcare professionals who have prescriptive licenses (physicians, nurse practitioners, physician's assistants) must order home care nursing services. Providers with prescriptive licenses are required if a home care agency is to receive reimbursement from third party sources (government, medical insurance plans, etc.). Orders written by these professionals direct the medical plan of care. Although the nurse is only one professional on the health team, the nurse is the patient's advocate and generally the Case Manager in the home care setting.**

7. a. **The patient is the center of the health team and is the most important source of information about one's perspective.**

b. Family members provide only their own views which are not the most important when assessing variables that affect a patient from a cultural perspective.

c. Each patient is an individual and generalizations should not be made based on a person's ethnic or cultural group. Generalizations are often based on stereotypes that are preconceived and untested beliefs about people based on their culture, race, and/or ethnic backgrounds.

d. This would deny the individuality of the patient. Generalizations are often based on stereotypes, which are preconceived and untested beliefs about people based on their culture, race, and/or ethnic backgrounds. Stereotyping a patient can lead to inaccurate assessments and result in inappropriate or potentially harmful actions or omission of care.

8. a. Of the options presented, nurses working in urban centers are less likely to wear many hats. Urban centers refer to cities with a population of more than 50,000 individuals. Urban areas tend to have a concentration of specialized services where nurses have specific roles and responsibilities.

b. **Nurses working in rural communities wear many hats. The adage *wear many hats* refers to someone with many different roles and responsibilities. Rural refers to *the country* or *the farm* where communities are less populated and are a great distance from physicians and healthcare services. Because of the uneven distribution of healthcare professionals and services in rural areas versus urban areas, nurses working in a rural area will assume many different roles and perform multiple tasks.**

c. Of the options presented, nurses working in the acute care setting are less likely to wear many hats. Generally, nurses working in acute care settings have specific roles and responsibilities.

d. Of the options presented, nurses working in a rehabilitation setting are less likely to wear many hats. Generally, nurses working in a rehabilitation setting have specific roles and responsibilities.

9. a. Each individual person is responsible for one's own health seeking actions and behavior. It would be ideal if all members of a family were interested and motivated to promote a healthy lifestyle; however, not all members of a family are committed to this value.

b. Educational intervention is an independent function of the nurse and does not require a practitioner's order. Education is the key in relation to recognizing and understanding the importance of behaviors that support a healthy life style.

c. **Resources that support Health Promotion, Health Protection, and Preventive Health Services are essential if one expects members of the community to engage in healthy lifestyles and behaviors. Resources, such things as availability of health professionals, sites for Primary Health Prevention programs for meetings and provision of services, consumables in the form of equipment and medications (immunizations), etc., must be available to promote and support health.**

d. Although programs are designed to meet the needs of groups in a community, each individual must be reached and influenced when promoting healthy lifestyles and behaviors.

10. a. The services of public health agencies established at the federal, state, and local levels to safeguard and improve the physical, mental and social well being of an entire community are on the decline. In an effort to reduce the escalating rise in the budgets of public health agencies, programs and services have been reduced or terminated.

b. Client groups at risk are on the rise; for example, groups such as older adults, the homeless, the uninsured, people living below the poverty level, single parent families, and immigrants.

c. The cost of healthcare is dramatically on the rise. More than 18% of the Gross Domestic Product is spent on healthcare costs and is still rising. In addition, healthcare costs have increased over 400% since 1965. To put this into perspective, healthcare costs are more than the budgets of both educational services and defense in the United States combined and we spend more than 1 billion dollars a day on healthcare costs.

d. Self-help groups are on the rise. More than 500 self-help groups represent almost all the major health problems, life events, or crises. The National Self-Help Clearinghouse provides information about existing groups and guidelines on how to begin a new group. Consumer access to The World Wide Web and the Internet has disseminated information about self-help groups.

11. a. This is Primary, not Secondary prevention. Primary prevention is concerned with generalized health promotion and specific protection against disease. Risk assessments for specific diseases are included in Primary prevention.

b. A low-fat diet is generally part of a medical management program for a person who is overweight or who has high cholesterol. This is Tertiary, not Secondary, prevention. Tertiary prevention is associated with attempts to reduce the extent and severity of a health problem in an effort to limit disability as well as restore and maintain function.

c. This is Primary, not Secondary prevention. Primary prevention includes protecting people from disease.

d. **This is correct. Secondary prevention is associated with early detection of disease and prompt intervention.**

12. a. **A hospice program is an example of an agency that might provide respite care in an inpatient setting or in the home. The care-giving role is physically and emotionally grueling and family members may need relief from the care-giving role or a break to attend a family function or go on vacation.**

b. Meals on Wheels does not provide respite care. It provides nutritious, low-cost meals for homebound people so that they can remain in their own homes.

c. Ambulatory care centers do not provide respite care. Ambulatory care centers provide care for conditions that do not require hospitalization. Services may include diagnosis and treatment of disease and illness as well as simple surgical procedures where the patient returns home the same day.

    d. An alcohol treatment center does not provide respite care. It provides a specialized service in the care and treatment of individuals who abuse alcohol.

13. a. The hospital environment rarely requires modification because it is designed to provide for the safety needs of patients. However, in the home setting, a home hazard assessment needs to be implemented to identify potential problems with walkways and stairways, floors, furniture, bathrooms, kitchens, electrical and fire protection, toxic substances, communication devices and issues associated with medications and asepsis. Although the nurse may not be able to change a client's living space and lifestyle, recommendations can be made that will eliminate or minimize risks.
    b. Ensuring that clients receive healthy meals is an important responsibility of the nurse in all settings in which nurses work.
    c. Delivering skilled nursing care is an important responsibility of the nurse in all settings in which nurses work.
    d. Coordinating the efforts of the health team is an important responsibility of the nurse in all settings in which nurses work.

14. a. The patient is the center of the health team in all settings.
    b. The nurse functions as an advocate for the patient in both the acute and home care settings. The role of advocate is important in all settings because in this role the nurse protects and supports patients' rights.
    c. The nurse is responsible for coordinating the efforts of the members of the health team in both the acute and home care settings.
    d. **Because of shorter length of hospital stays, patients are being discharged before teaching and counseling are completed. However, in the home care setting, patients are provided with appropriate care including counseling and teaching until they are able to care for themselves without needing ongoing home care intervention.**

15. a. Affirm means to state positively, to declare firmly, to ratify, and to assert. Exploring the nature and consequences of choices is not affirming.
    b. **Informing is an important role of the nurse when functioning as a patient advocate. Inform means to give information, to enlighten, and to give knowledge. When working with families to explore the nature and consequences of their choices, the nurse can provide information so that people understand the ramifications of their choices. An informed decision is a decision based on an understanding of the facts and ramifications associated with the choice.**
    c. Mediation means to negotiate or intercede. Exploring the nature and consequences of choices is not mediating.
    d. Interview means to meet and talk for the purpose of collecting information. Exploring the nature and consequences of choices is not interviewing.

However, interviewing skills may be employed when the nurse explores with the patient the nature and consequences of choices.

16. a. **This is correct. As soon as contact with the patient is made, planning and teaching should begin so the patient is prepared for discharge and returned to the community.**
    b. The nurse does not have to wait until the patient is admitted to the hospital to begin preparing for the patient's return to the community.
    c. This is too late to prepare the patient for the return to the community.
    d. This is too late. Referrals can be anticipated before admission in most cases.

17. a. This is not as important as an assessment presented in another option. The demographics of a community are only one component of a community assessment.
    b. **The members in the community are the primary source of data about the community and their needs. Just as the patient is the center of the health team when caring for an individual, the collective membership of a community is the center of the health team when caring for the healthcare needs of a community.**
    c. This does not help to identify the needs of a community. After the needs of the community are identified, then the ability of the healthcare system to deliver the necessary services is assessed.
    d. This is not as important as an assessment presented in another option. Environmental data is only one component of a community assessment.

18. a. A middle-school-aged child has to deal with the developmental task of Industry versus Inferiority. Tasks associated with this age, deriving pleasure from accomplishments and developing a sense of competence, can be facilitated in the home setting. Although a middle-school-aged child will have to adjust to the need for long-term home healthcare, there are fewer crises occurring during the middle-school years that impact on development than the number of crises occurring in a group in another option.
    b. A pre-school-aged child is dependent on a parent to provide for basic human needs and meeting the developmental task of Initiative versus Guilt. Tasks associated with this age, the development of confidence in ability and having direction and purpose, can be facilitated in the home setting. Although a pre-school-aged child will have to adjust to the need for long-term home healthcare, there are fewer crises occurring during the pre-school years that impact on development than the number of crises occurring in a group in another option.
    c. **The adolescent will generally have the hardest time adjusting to the need for long-term home healthcare than any other stage of development. Adolescents experience multiple and complex physiological, psychological, and social developmental milestones. Adolescents want to be attractive to others, similar to their peers, and accepted within a group. It is common for adolescents to experience mood swings, make**

decisions without having all the facts, challenge authority, and assert the self. This is a turbulent time as the adolescent internalizes the dramatic physical changes and the psychological stressors of new social conflicts. Being relatively isolated in the home for an extended period will pose serious stressors associated with adjustment, which can dramatically influence the outcome of the developmental tasks of adolescence.

d. The developmental task of Ego Integrity versus Despair challenges older adults to understand their worth and accept the end of life. Although older adults will have the second hardest time adjusting to the need for long-term home healthcare of the options offered, there are fewer crises occurring during the older adult years that impact on development than the number of crises occurring in a group in another option.

19. a. In the home setting patients tend to have less physicians' orders and therefore nurses work more independently. In addition, the roles of the nurse in community-based practice today are expanding dramatically. In 1991 the American Nurses Association published *Nursing's Agenda for Health Care Reform*, which made recommendations for healthcare reform. The major predictions influencing nurse accountability included: nurses will become community leaders; community-nursing centers will expand and focus on preventing disease and promoting health; and the center of healthcare will shift to the home setting. Nurses already work independently in such programs as community outreach, nursing centers, nurse sponsored wellness and health promotion programs, and independent practice. These roles require the nurse to utilize nursing theory and skills that are in the scope of the legal definition of nursing practice and do not require dependence upon physician's orders.

b. Excellent communication skills are essential in both the acute care and community-based settings.

c. Excellent technical skills are essential in both the acute care and community-based settings. Patients at home receive highly technical therapy such as hemodialysis, intravenous therapy, wound care, and ventilator support.

d. Teaching occurs in both the acute care and community-based settings. In addition, some patients may never be able to care for themselves.

20. a. This action is associated with Secondary, not Tertiary, prevention. Secondary prevention activities are associated with early detection and encouragement of treatment when actions may contribute to the control or elimination of an already present risk factor, illness or disease.

b. This is Primary, not Tertiary, prevention. Primary prevention is associated with health teaching and actions that relate to specific protection and prevention of disease or injuries. Primary prevention activities precede disease or dysfunction and include actions generally applied to a healthy population.

c. This is correct. Alcoholism is a disease. Tertiary

prevention is associated with attempts to reduce the extent and severity of a health problem/disease in an effort to limit disability and restore, maintain, or maximize function or quality of life.

d. This is Primary, not Tertiary, prevention. Primary prevention is associated with health teaching and actions that relate to specific protection and prevention of disease or injuries. Primary prevention activities precede disease or dysfunction; includes actions generally applied to a healthy population.

21. a. The Registered Nurse providing home care does not function as a practitioner. A practitioner is a person with a prescriptive license such as a physician, nurse practitioner, or physician's assistant.

b. The surrogate role is not a professional role of the nurse. A surrogate role is assigned to a nurse when a patient believes that the nurse reminds them of another and projects that role and the feelings one has for the other person onto the nurse.

c. Home care nurses are generalists, not specialists. If the home care nurse believed that this patient would benefit from the services of a nurse specialist in enterostomal care, the home care nurse could make a referral for the provision of this type of service.

d. Functioning as a teacher is critical when caring for a patient at home with a new colostomy. The patient has so much to learn to become self-sufficient and comfortable with the colostomy. New learning will include topics such as skin and stoma care, colostomy appliances, diet, asepsis, bowel irrigation, potential complications, available self-help groups, etc.

22. a. This could inflame the situation and/or take too long.

b. Nurses need to immediately remove themselves from any environment that they believe is unsafe.

c. This could place the nurse at additional risk by making matters worse.

d. This could place the nurse at additional risk.

23. a. This is not a safe place to keep medications. Children have natural curiosity, problem solving abilities, and the agility to climb to a top shelf.

b. A locked area is the safest place to store prescription as well as over-the-counter medications to prevent accidental ingestion by children.

c. This is not a safe place to keep medications. Children have natural curiosity, problem solving abilities, and the agility to climb up to a medicine cabinet.

d. This is not a safe place to keep medications. Children have natural curiosity and problem solving abilities, and could get to the back of a shelf in a refrigerator.

24. a. The Occupational Therapist is not the most important member of the health team. An Occupational Therapist (OT) is generally not a member of the health team in an assisted-living residence. On occasion, a physician may order occupational therapy and the resident will either go to an Occupational Therapist to receive therapy or one will come to the person and provide therapy.

b. Although Nurse Aides are the people who provide

the bulk of the assistance needed by residents in an assisted-living residence, they are not as important as another member of the health team.

c. **The patient is always the center of the health team in every setting and is the most important member.**

d. The nurse is not the most important team member in an assisted-living facility. An assisted-living residence (apartment, villa, or condominium) provides limited assistance with activities of daily living, meal preparation, laundry services, transportation, and opportunities for socialization, not extensive nursing services.

25. a. The physician is generally not the healthcare professional making the decision whether a patient is eligible for continuation of services or is ready for discharge from the home-care program. In the home-care setting a physician's order is necessary to initiate home-care services as well as orders directing the nurse in the dependent functions of the nurse.

b. Quality Management activities are unrelated to whether a patient is to receive a continuation of services or is to be discharged from a home healthcare program. Ongoing Quality Management Programs are designed to monitor the quality of care being delivered and identify problem areas so that efforts can be employed to improve care.

c. **Case management by the nurse in the home-care setting includes determining when the patient is ready for discharge. After the nurse determines that the patient is ready for discharge, it is conveyed to the physician and the physician discharges the patient. Nursing documentation supports the decision. Often the nurse needs to document objectively the status of the patient to convince the healthcare provider and the insurer that the patient needs a continuation of services.**

d. Dissatisfaction with the services of a home-health agency could influence whether or not the family wanted a continuation of services. However, family satisfaction or dissatisfaction would not influence whether the patient still needed the services of the home-healthcare agency.

26. a. Although culture and the inability to speak English may be a factor in underutilization of services in rural communities, it is not the main reason services are underutilized. In addition, there are more ethnic ghettoes in urban and suburban, not rural, areas.

b. **Rural communities are more isolated from services, stores, and resources and therefore people tend to be self-sufficient, independent, and autonomous. Because they are more self-reliant and the need to seek healthcare intervention generally requires travel, they tend to first attempt to deal with healthcare issues with home remedies. In addition, because they fear becoming dependent and losing control over themselves and their decisions, they may be wary about seeking outside help.**

c. Interest is not a factor in underutilization of healthcare services in rural communities. People in rural areas are no less interested in health and healthcare than people who live in other areas of the country.

d. Intelligence is not a factor in underutilization of healthcare services in rural communities. People in rural areas may be somewhat less sophisticated than city dwellers but they are no less intelligent.

27. a. Although it is important to have access to medical specialists, another option has priority. In addition, the availability of primary care practitioners, not specialists, is more essential because Primary healthcare addresses health promotion, illness prevention and entry into Secondary healthcare (diagnosis and treatment of illness and disease).

b. Although individuals with health insurance have better access to healthcare services, it is not essential to have health insurance to receive healthcare. People can pay privately or if indigent, they can apply for various government and non-profit supported programs that provide basic care. In addition, hospital emergency departments, by law, cannot turn patients away who need emergency care.

c. **For a healthy community, all members of the community must have access to healthcare. The health of a community depends on each member of the community having appropriate and comprehensive healthcare.**

d. Public Health Nurses work for only the federal, state, or local governments implementing programs supported by taxes. These programs are only a small percentage of the multitude of programs and services that are designed to support community health.

28. a. According to the document *Healthy People 2000*, this is a Preventive Health Service, not an activity associated with Health Protection.

b. According to the document *Healthy People 2000*, this is a Health Promotion, not Health Protection, activity.

c. According to the document *Healthy People 2000*, this is a Health Promotion, not Health Protection, activity.

d. **This is correct. In 1990, *Healthy People 2000*, a document prepared by the United States Department of Health and Human Services with input from 24 national nursing organizations, outlined 298 health related objectives. This document differentiated the Primary Prevention Level of Healthcare into three areas: Health Promotion, Health Protection, and Preventive Health Services. Health Protection was defined as actions by the government and industry to reduce environmental factors that are a threat to health. It included activities such as controlling factors that maintain occupational safety, preventing accidents and infectious diseases and controlling environmental toxic agents and radiation.**

29. a. This is not the most efficient approach. This may be necessary if present resources are not available to meet the needs of the community.

b. The health needs of the members of the community are identified already. Further study at this time does not appear to be appropriate.

c. This is not the most efficient approach. This may eventually be done after an action in another option is implemented first.

d. This is the most efficient initial approach to meeting the identified needs of the members of the community. The use of presently available resources is more efficient than the other options presented.

30. a. The first and most important assessment made by the home care nurse focuses on determining whether the client's home environment is safe. Safety and security are basic needs identified by Maslow's Hierarchy of Needs.

b. Although it is often helpful when family members participate in a home care client's recovery, it is not necessary.

c. A client's potential for self-care is not a criterion for receiving home care services. Clients who have little or no potential for self-care receive home care services.

d. Clients who are unable to participate in the plan of care because they are mentally, emotionally, or physically disabled are still eligible for home care.

31. a. To be eligible for hospice services, an individual must be diagnosed as having less than 6 months to live, not a year.

b. Although there are inpatient hospice programs, palliative care units in hospitals, and residential hospice settings, most hospice care is delivered in patients' homes. The home is a less expensive setting than other healthcare settings because family members provide most of the care supported by a team of professionals, nonprofessionals, and volunteers.

c. Hospice services include not only palliative care and support of quality of life for the terminally ill patient but supportive care to family members and support persons. In addition, it includes services that assist family members with bereavement and adjustment after the death of the patient.

d. This is true. Hospice is not a setting but a movement. It focuses on providing supportive, palliative services that focuses on managing pain, treatment of symptoms and helping patients maintain their quality of life so they can live the remainder of their lives to the fullest.

32. a. This is not an example of an opinion survey. An opinion survey is designed to collect each individual person's perspective about the problem being studied. Results are tallied to identify the major concerns. Opinion surveys are generally questionnaires.

b. A forum is defined as an opportunity for open discussion. Inviting people from the community to share opinions and concerns about a particular issue for the purpose of collecting data is called a community forum.

c. This is not an example of a demographic assessment. A demographic assessment is the quantitative study of the characteristics of a population. A demographic assessment might include information such as distribution of the population by gender, size, growth, density, and ethnicity.

d. This is not an example of an observation of participants. Direct observation is a method of data collection that might be used to determine whether individuals follow a specific procedure or behave in an expected manner.

33. a. Case management is the major role of the nurse in the home care setting. The nurse engages in activities such as assessing, planning, coordinating nursing care and professional services, making referrals, monitoring medical progress, maintaining documentation, evaluating and monitoring outcomes, determining closure and discharging the client after goal achievement.

b. Although discharge planning is a component of the role of the nurse in the home care setting, it is not the role with the highest priority. Traditionally, discharge planning is focused on moving a person from the hospital to the home. However, in the present healthcare environment, discharge planning is conducted when moving a client from one level of care to another and occurs in many settings.

c. The role of the nurse is to help the client achieve expected outcomes that are within the client's present value and belief systems. Although a client might be healthier if other behaviors are adopted, it is difficult and sometimes impossible to change or modify a person's values and beliefs.

d. Although family support is helpful, it is the patient's interest and motivation in achieving expected outcomes that is the most important contributing factor to success.

34. a. Home care agencies are responsible for coordinating and providing for a continuum of comprehensive healthcare services after a patient is discharged from the hospital. Because of the decreased length of stay in the hospital setting, patients are being discharged sooner than ever before and are in need of home care services.

b. Urgent visit centers are designed to deal with the treatment of non-critical emergencies such as infections, minor injuries, and physical responses to disease or illness as well as primary care services.

c. Physicians' offices are the traditional primary care setting for ambulatory care. Patients go to physicians' offices for routine physicals and the diagnosis and treatment of routine illnesses or diseases.

d. Respite programs provide for short stay, intermittent, inpatient or day-care services to patients who are generally cared for at home. This service provides a rest period for family members who have the responsibility of sustained care giving.

35. a. Although the general health of the members of a community is important, it is not the first data that the nurse should collect when assessing a community.

b. Although a community's physical environment (including information such as whether it is rural, suburban, or urban, physical boundaries, density, size, types of lodgings, incidence of crime, etc.) is important to know, it is not the first data that the nurse should collect when assessing a community.

c. Acquiring core information about the people in the community is the first stage in assessing a community. Core characteristics about the members of a community include information such as vital statistics, values and beliefs, demographics, religious groups, etc.

d. Although it is important to know information such as healthcare facilities, agencies, and services provided, the accessibility to healthcare services, sources of health information, transportation services, routine caseloads etc., it is not the first data that the nurse should collect when assessing a community.

36. a. A nuclear family of siblings and parents should be able to provide an adolescent with the assistance needed to meet basic human needs, and should not need a setting other than the home to recover.
   b. **A person with bilateral long leg casts for three months will have to rely on others to provide for one's basic needs such as food and assistance with activities of daily living. An independently living older adult would not have the daily assistance needed to recover at home and, therefore, would be a candidate for a nursing home.**
   c. A middle-aged married male could rely on the spouse to provide the needed assistance to meet basic human needs and would not require a setting other than the home to recover.
   d. The infant could depend on the parents to provide for basic human needs and therefore would not need a setting other than the home to recover.

37. a. Families are not limited to individuals who are related by blood, marriage, adoption, or birth.
   b. This is an example of a nuclear family and is only one example of a family structure.
   c. **This is correct.** A family is defined as a social group whose members are closely related by blood, marriage, or friendship. Today, family structure is diverse and includes families such as traditional nuclear families, single-parent families, blended families, cohabitating families, gay and lesbian families, families with foster children, and single people living alone but who are part of an extended family.
   d. Family members remain connected by their relationships, not because they all live in the same household.

38. a. **Teaching a patient how to use a wheelchair after a stroke is an example of Tertiary healthcare. Tertiary healthcare is associated with rehabilitation, long-term care, and care of the dying. The Levels of Healthcare, which describe the scope of services and settings where healthcare is provided, includes Primary, Secondary, and Tertiary. The Levels of Healthcare should not be confused with Levels of Prevention.**
   b. Immunizations are an example of Primary, not Tertiary, healthcare. Primary healthcare services are concerned with promoting health, preventing disease, early and basic detection and treatment of disease, environmental protection, and health education.
   c. This is an example of a service provided on the Primary, not Tertiary, Level of Healthcare. The Primary Level of Healthcare services is associated with illness prevention, health promotion, early detection and routine treatment, environmental protection and health education.
   d. Changing a dressing after surgery is care associated with the Secondary, not Tertiary, Level of Healthcare. The Secondary Level of Healthcare

services is associated with acute care, complex diagnosis and treatment of disease and illness, and emergency care.

39. a. Counseling is related to helping a patient recognize and cope with emotional stressors, improve relationships, and promote personal growth, not dealing with infection control issues.
   b. Although the term caregiver is broad and could include many different roles of the nurse, caregiver generally refers to direct *laying on of the hands* when providing direct care. This is not the major role of the nurse when dealing with infection control issues in the home setting.
   c. The role of advocate is not the most appropriate role of the roles presented in the options when dealing with infection control issues in the home setting. In the role of advocate, the nurse protects and supports patients' rights and assists in asserting those rights when patients are unable to defend themselves, not dealing with infection control issues.
   d. **Of the roles presented in the options, the role of teacher is most important in the home care setting when addressing infection control issues. Nurses need to teach patients and their family members how to maintain a clean environment, modifications to the environment that may be necessary to support asepsis, and procedures associated with aseptic and sterile technique to prevent infection. Nurses can also teach patients and their family members about the steps in the Chain of Infection and actions that they can implement to reduce the risk of infection. Because the nurse is only in the home for a limited amount of time at each visit, it is important that the nurse teach the patient and family members how best to reduce the risk of infection on a daily basis.**

40. a. Although this is a good idea, it is not the most important thing a home care nurse can convey to a person caring for a family member in the home.
   b. Although this might contribute to efficiency as well as gaining a feeling of control over the activities that must be accomplished, it is not the most important thing a home care nurse can convey to a person caring for a family member in the home.
   c. **Caregiver role strain experienced by a family member is a serious concern of home care nurses. Caregivers often fail to address their own health needs because of the extraordinary burden of the caregiver role, which can jeopardize their own health and well-being. Caregivers should be encouraged to delegate responsibilities to other family members, to get adequate sleep, rest and nutritional intake, to seek assistance from agencies that provide respite services, to take time for leisure activities and a vacation, and to join a caregiver support group.**
   d. A daily journal of the client's status is unnecessary when a client is in stable condition. If the client experienced an acute episode then a record of the client's daily status could be helpful in monitoring progress or lack of progress.

Psychosociocultural Nursing Care

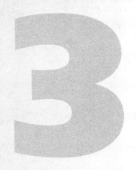

Nursing Care Across The Lifespan

KEYWORDS

The following words include English vocabulary, nursing/medical terminology, concepts, principles, or information relevant to content specifically addressed in the chapter or associated with topics presented in it. English dictionaries, your nursing textbooks, and medical dictionaries such as *Taber's Cyclopedic Medical Dictionary* are resources that can be used to expand your knowledge and understanding of these words and related information.

Accommodation
Adolescent (teenager)
Ageism
Anorexia nervosa
Assimilation
Berry Brazelton
Bonding
Bulimia nervosa
Cephalocaudal
Child abuse
Cognitive Development Theory
Congenital anomalies
Critical Time
Developmental
Developmental milestones
Developmental stressor
Developmental Task Theory of Development
Developmental tasks
Differentiated development
Egocentrism
Embryo
Erikson's Theory of Personality Development
Failure to thrive
Fetal alcohol syndrome
Fetus

First, second, and third trimester of development
Gender-role development
Attention-deficit/hyperactivity disorder (ADHD)
Genetics
Growth
Gynecomastia
Human Needs Theory
Infancy - infant
Intellect – intellectual
Latchkey children
Lawrence Kohlberg
Learning disability
Life-cycle
Life-events
Low-birth weight
Menarche
Menopause
Middle adulthood
Middle-school-aged child
Midlife crisis
Moral Development Theory
Moral reasoning
Newborn
Nocturnal emission
Organogenesis

Older adult
Physique
Polypharmacy
Pre/postmenopausal
Pre-school-aged child
Preschooler
Preterm
Proximodistal
Puberty
Regression
Reminiscence
Retirement
Role reversal
Sandwich generation
Scoliosis
Senescence
Short stature
Sibling
Sibling rivalry
Sigmund Freud
Substance abuse
Sudden infant death syndrome
Teratogenic
Toddler
Young Adulthood

1. Which age group generally demonstrates an inefficiency of adaptation?
   a. 60 plus years
   b. 40 to 60 years
   c. 12 to 19 years
   d. 3 to 11 years

2. Erikson's theory of personality development includes the concept that:
   a. Basic level needs have to be met before higher level needs
   b. Biologic needs must be met before fulfillment of one's unique potential
   c. Once a developmental stage is passed it cannot be revisited and relearned
   d. Cultural and interpersonal tasks have to be accomplished to grow developmentally

3. Which issue is of major concern when providing drug therapy for older adults?
   a. Alcohol is often used by older adults to cope with the multiple problems of aging
   b. Older adults experience an increased difficulty swallowing tablets
   c. Hepatic clearance is reduced in older adults
   d. Older adults are less motivated

4. At which age is death first recognized as irreversible, universal, and natural?
   a. 6
   b. 9
   c. 12
   d. 15

5. Which behavior in an adult indicates an unresolved developmental conflict associated with adolescence?
   a. Being overly concerned about following daily routines
   b. Requiring excessive attention from others
   c. Relying on oneself rather than others
   d. Failing to set goals in life

6. Which concept associated with development factors and quality of sleep must the nurse understand to best plan nursing care?
   a. Pregnant women have a decreased need for sleep
   b. Adolescents need less sleep than the average young adult
   c. Aging is associated with an increased risk of sleep disorders
   d. Healthy older adults have more efficient sleep times than younger people

7. An individual who nurtures, teaches, and gives to others reflects which stage of Erikson's Stages of Development?
   a. Generativity versus Stagnation
   b. Ego Integrity versus Despair
   c. Industry versus Inferiority
   d. Initiative versus Guilt

8. Which comment best demonstrates ageism? "He is 75 years old and:
   a. Has outlived his usefulness."
   b. Reads the newspaper with difficulty."
   c. Reminisces about his World War II experience."
   d. Is most happy when working in his home workshop."

9. When planning nursing care the nurse needs to remember that energy expenditure and nutrient requirements are higher during the:
   a. First year of life
   b. Early adult years
   c. Middle adult years
   d. End of the life cycle

10. One of the most effective nursing actions that can reduce anxiety in a hospitalized child is:
    a. Instructing the parent to bring in the child's favorite cuddly toy
    b. Inviting parents to be involved in the daily care of the child
    c. Engaging in activities that refocus the child's attention
    d. Taking the child to the playroom

11. According to Erikson, establishing relationships based on commitment mainly occurs in which stage of psychosocial development?
    a. Generativity versus Stagnation
    b. Identity versus Role Diffusion
    c. Intimacy versus Isolation
    d. Trust versus Mistrust

12. Which age group is reflected in the statement, "More time is spent in bed but less time is spent asleep?"
    a. Two-year-olds
    b. Forty-year-olds
    c. Seventy-year-olds
    d. Fourteen-year-olds

13. A common stressor associated with the developmental stage of early childhood (1–3 years) would be:
    a. Accepting limited dietary choices
    b. Adjusting to a change in physique
    c. Responding to life-threatening illness
    d. Resolving conflicts associated with independence

14. Many foods are ingested by the adolescent because of:
    a. Taste
    b. Routine
    c. Pressure
    d. Preference

15. Which response to medication occurs most frequently in the older adult?
    a. Toxicity
    b. Side effects
    c. Hypersensitivity
    d. Idiosyncratic effects

16. Which age group has the greatest potential to demonstrate regression when ill?
    a. Infant
    b. Toddler
    c. Adolescent
    d. Young adult

17. Which behavior in an adult may indicate an unresolved developmental task of infancy?
    a. Avoiding assistance from others
    b. Rationalizing unacceptable behaviors
    c. Being overly concerned about cleanliness
    d. Apologizing constantly for small mistakes

18. Successful aging depends on a person's ability to:
    a. Adapt to social isolation
    b. Adjust to the change in social roles
    c. Associate with members of all age groups
    d. Increase the number of meaningful relationships

19. Which age group tends to be more involved with expanding and refining spiritual beliefs?
    a. Adolescents
    b. Older adults
    c. Young adults
    d. Middle-aged adults

20. Which change in skin is the older adult most likely to experience?
    a. Increased tone
    b. Decreased dryness
    c. Increased elasticity
    d. Decreased thickness

21. Which patient is at the greatest risk when taking a drug that has a high teratogenic potential?
    a. Older adult man
    b. Pregnant woman
    c. Four-year-old child
    d. One-month-old baby

22. Which is a common behavioral adaptation in the older adult to sensory overload caused by the hospital environment?
    a. Dementia
    b. Confusion
    c. Drowsiness
    d. Bradycardia

23. According to Erikson, which individual would have the greatest risk of experiencing a negative outcome in relation to a developmental task?
    a. A toddler who cries when left with a baby sitter
    b. A toddler who delays gratification of immediate needs
    c. A school-aged child with a majority of friends of one gender
    d. A teenager who had an arm amputated because of a car accident

24. When assessing the older adult, the nurse may expect to identify an increase in:
    a. Nail growth
    b. Skin elasticity
    c. Urine residual
    d. Nerve conduction

25. Which word is unrelated to principles of growth and development?
    a. Unpredictable
    b. Sequential
    c. Integrated
    d. Complex

26. The people within which age group have the greatest individual differences in appearance and behavior?
    a. Children
    b. Adolescents
    c. Older adults
    d. Middle-aged adults

27. Which concept associated with drug therapy and quality of sleep is important to understand to best plan nursing care?
    a. Sedatives are not well tolerated by older adults
    b. Anti-anxiety drugs are the least helpful in supporting sleep
    c. The effectiveness of hypnotics increases with prolonged use
    d. Melatonin is the drug of choice for long term use in sleep disorders

28. Which concept is reflective of Erikson's Theory of Personality Development?
    a. Defense mechanisms help to deal with anxiety
    b. Moral maturity is a central theme in all stages
    c. Achievement of developmental goals is affected by the social environment
    d. Two continual processes, assimilation and accommodation, stimulate intellectual growth

29. According to Erikson, reminiscence of life events occurs in which stage of psychosocial development?
    a. Autonomy versus Shame and Doubt
    b. Generativity versus Stagnation
    c. Identity versus Role Diffusion
    d. Ego Integrity versus Despair

30. In addition to administering medication to a child experiencing acute pain, the most effective intervention is to:
    a. Use a new toy to distract the child
    b. Support frequent rest periods to reduce fatigue
    c. Encourage a parent to stay with the child for support
    d. Allow the child to engage in any activity that alters pain perception

31. Which physiologic change commonly is seen among older adults?
    a. Increase in sebaceous gland activity
    b. Deterioration of joint cartilage
    c. Loss of social support system
    d. Increased need for sleep

32. When screening for eating disorders, the nurse should expect more problems to become evident during:
    a. Toddlerhood
    b. Adolescence
    c. Senescence
    d. Infancy

33. The group that has the greatest risk for iron deficiency anemia is:
    a. Postmenopausal women
    b. Older adults
    c. Teenagers
    d. Infants

34. Which age group would be at the greatest risk for constipation?
    a. School-aged children
    b. Middle-aged adults
    c. Older-aged adults
    d. Bottle-fed infants

35. A developmental crisis that is more often precipitated during middle adulthood occurs when there is an inability to:
    a. Achieve a concept of success
    b. Develop peer relationships
    c. Delay satisfaction
    d. Face death

36. A 2-year-old child is trying to eat with a spoon and is making a mess. The caregiver should:
    a. Provide finger foods until the child is older
    b. Offer praise and encouragement as the child eats
    c. Feed the child along with the child's attempts at eating
    d. Take the spoon and feed the child until the child is more capable

37. An individual who is preoccupied with reliving life because of dissatisfaction with the past reflects a negative resolution of which stage of Erikson's Stages of Development?
    a. Generativity versus Stagnation
    b. Identity versus Role Diffusion
    c. Ego Integrity versus Despair
    d. Intimacy versus Isolation

38. According to Erikson, antisocial behavior in an adult most commonly would be associated with a negative resolution of which stage of development?
    a. Preschool age
    b. Adolescence
    c. School age
    d. Infancy

39. When planning to meet the needs of patients in pain, the nurse must recognize that the age group that is most sensitive to pain is:
    a. Infants
    b. Adolescents
    c. Older adults
    d. Pregnant women

40. The decline of which system most often influences an older adult's ability to maintain safety?
    a. Sensory
    b. Respiratory
    c. Integumentary
    d. Cardiovascular

41. Which psychodynamic theorist believed that 10-year-old children gain pleasure from accomplishments?
    a. Lawrence Kohlberg
    b. Sigmund Freud
    c. Berry Brazelton
    d. Erik Erikson

42. Which age group generally has the most difficulty adapting to major losses?
    a. Middle-aged adults
    b. Older adults
    c. Young adults
    d. Adolescents

43. According to Erikson, the person who becomes self-absorbed and obsessed with one's own needs is having difficulty resolving which stage of psychosocial development?
    a. Industry versus Inferiority
    b. Ego Integrity versus Despair
    c. Identity versus Role Diffusion
    d. Generativity versus Stagnation

44. One of the participants attending a parenting class asks the teacher, "What is the leading cause of death during the first month of life?" Besides exploring the person's concerns, the nurse should respond:
    a. Sudden infant death syndrome
    b. Congenital abnormalities
    c. Low birth weight
    d. Infection

45. The person at greatest risk for problems with regulating body temperature is the:
    a. Toddler
    b. Teenager
    c. Older adult
    d. School-aged child

46. An individual who is preoccupied with work and the drive to succeed at the expense of emotionally committing to others reflects a negative resolution of which stage of Erikson's Stages of Development?
    a. Autonomy versus Shame and Doubt
    b. Identify versus Role Diffusion
    c. Ego Integrity versus Despair
    d. Intimacy versus Isolation

47. Which age group is at the greatest risk for injury?
    a. 6 to 10
    b. 12 to 16
    c. 26 to 40
    d. 65 and over

48. Which group has the most problems with sleep as a result of multiple, complex developmental factors?
    a. Infants
    b. Toddlers
    c. Adolescents
    d. Preschoolers

49. To what is a person referring when during an interview the person says, "I am a member of the *sandwich generation*?
    a. Cares for children and aging parents at the same time
    b. There is a role reversal between parents and self
    c. Assists own parents and spouse's parents
    d. Has both older and younger siblings

50. When providing drug therapy for older adults, an issue of major concern is that older adults:
    a. Experience an increase in absorption of drugs from the GI tract
    b. Often use alcohol to cope with the multiple stressors of aging
    c. Are less motivated to follow a prescribed drug regimen
    d. Have a decreased risk for adverse reactions to drugs

51. The most important concept related to the stages of growth and development is that:
    a. Individuals experience growth and development at their own pace
    b. Each task must be achieved before moving on to the next task
    c. Family members provide safe and supportive environments
    d. Once a task is achieved regression is minimal

52. Which stage of development is most unstable and challenging with regard to the development of a personal identity?
    a. Toddlerhood
    b. Adolescence
    c. Childhood
    d. Infancy

53. Drug toxicity occurs in the older adult primarily because of a decrease in:
    a. Serum calcium
    b. Glomerular filtration
    c. Red blood cell count
    d. Frequency of voiding

54. Which patient is at the greatest risk for complications during surgery?
    a. Middle-aged adult
    b. Pregnant woman
    c. Adolescent
    d. Infant

55. What is a word that describes the process of growth and development?
    a. Fast
    b. Simple
    c. Limiting
    d. Individual

1. a. When a person reaches sixty years of age and older all physiologic systems are less efficient, which reduces compensatory reserve.
   b. In the 40- to 60-year-old age group a person will begin to see the earliest signs of aging. Changes are gradual and insidious and generally do not impact on function.
   c. In the 12- to 19-year-old age group the adolescent is experiencing rapid growth and a beginning transition to adulthood, not a decline in the ability to adapt.
   d. In the 3- to 11-year-old age group children are growing at a continuous pace in their ability to adapt to the world around them, not declining in their ability to adapt.

2. a. This statement reflects Maslow's Hierarchy of Needs, not Erikson's Stages of Psychosocial Development.
   b. This statement reflects Maslow's Hierarchy of Needs, not Erikson's Stages of Psychosocial Development.
   c. Erikson emphasized that a person might regress to an earlier stage to seek comfort and reduce anxiety when unable to cope with a stressful event, situation, or illness.
   d. Erikson emphasized the importance of environment as being extremely influential in achievement or non-achievement of developmental tasks. Culture and social and family relationships are factors that have tremendous impact on one's environment.

3. a. Older adults often reduce alcohol intake because of concerns with drug interactions and a decline in one's ability to metabolize alcohol.
   b. Dysphagia is not a normal process of aging.
   c. This is a major concern. The risk of potential accumulation of a drug in the body increases because of decreased liver function and excretion that accompanies aging.
   d. Motivation does not generally decline as one ages. While it may take older adults longer to process and respond to information, they generally are motivated to achieve goals.

4. a. A 6-year-old child is developing an understanding of the differences among the concepts of past, present, and future. A 6-year-old child believes that death is temporary, can be caused by bad thoughts, may be a punishment, and that magic can make the dead person alive.
   b. A 9-year-old child has a more realistic understanding of death than a younger child and recognizes that death is universal, irreversible, and natural. A 9-year-old child has a beginning knowledge of his/her own mortality and may fear death.
   c. Recognizing that death is irreversible, universal, and natural occurs at an earlier age than 12 years.
   d. Recognizing that death is irreversible, universal, and natural occurs at an earlier age than 15 years.

5. a. This relates to Freud's Anal Stage of development (1 to 3 years). If a parent is strict, overbearing, and oppressive during toilet training the child may develop traits of an anal retentive personality (obsessive-compulsive tendencies, rigid thought patterns, stinginess, and/or stubbornness).
   b. Seeking excessive attention from others is most likely the result of an unresolved task of the 6- to 12-year-old age group (school-age), Industry versus Inferiority. Seeking attention often is an attempt to increase self-esteem.
   c. People who have difficulty accepting help from others or who would rather do things themselves generally have not completely resolved the developmental task of infancy, Trust versus Mistrust.
   d. The main developmental task of adolescence is forming a sense of personal identity as a foundation for the tasks of young adulthood, making decisions regarding career choices, and selecting a mate. An adult who has difficulty setting goals in life or who is unable to make a commitment to others indicates an unresolved conflict of Identity versus Role Diffusion.

6. a. The need for sleep increases, not decreases, because of the physical demands of pregnancy. In addition, pregnant women often have a decreased quality of sleep because a comfortable position may be difficult to assume as the uterus enlarges.
   b. Adolescents need more, not less, sleep than the average young adult because of accelerated growth and high energy expenditure. Adolescents need 8 to 10 hours of sleep a day.
   c. Half of all older adults have difficulty sleeping. Insomnia is the most common complaint. Frequent awakening, physical discomfort and pain, and shortened REM sleep associated with aging contribute to a decrease in the quality of sleep. Older adults sleep 5 to 7 hours a day and often take a daytime nap.
   d. Older adults have a decrease, not increase, in sleep efficiency. The fact that older adults sleep only 5 to 7 hours a day is a result of a decreased need for sleep, not a more efficient sleep time than younger people.

7. a. The 25- to 65-year-old adult (Generativity versus Stagnation) strives to fulfill life goals associated with family, career, and society as well as being able to give to and care for others. A positive resolution of the conflict associated with this age group is often displayed in teaching, counseling, and community volunteer work.
   b. Adults 65 years of age and older strive to resolve the conflict of Ego Integrity versus Despair. Successful resolution results in accepting one's life, recognizing the good and accepting the mistakes, willing to face death, and having a sense of integrity and wholeness.
   c. The 6- to 12-year-old child (Industry versus Inferiority) strives to gain control over the self, develop feelings of confidence and adequacy, and achieve the ability to carry out a task to completion.
   d. The 3- to 6-year-old child (Initiative versus Guilt) strives to become purposeful and self-directed.

8. a. This statement is a clear example of ageism whereby older adults are systematically stereotyped and discriminated against because they are old. This is a form of prejudice, an

unfavorable opinion without concrete information about the individual. Ageism is based on the misconceptions that older adults are no longer productive, are narrow minded, are unable to learn, are dependent, experience memory loss, live in a nursing home, are ill, boring, etc.

b. This is not a discriminatory statement indicative of ageism.

c. This is not a discriminatory statement indicative of ageism.

d. This is not a discriminatory statement indicative of ageism.

9. a. During the first year of life nutritional needs per unit of body weight are the greatest in comparison to any other time during the life-span. Birth weight generally doubles in 4 to 6 months and triples by the end of the first year.

b. Although young adults tend to be active and require nutrients adequate to meet a high energy expenditure, physical growth slows and the basal metabolic rate begins to stabilize, so they require fewer calories than do other age groups.

c. During the middle-adult years energy expenditure decreases and nutritional needs stabilize. People in other age groups have greater needs for nutrients to meet physiologic demands than do those in the middle-adult years.

d. Older adults experience a decrease in basal metabolic rate, lean body mass, and physical activity, which contribute to a decrease in caloric needs.

10. a. Although a favorite cuddly toy provides for a friendlier environment and, being something familiar to the child, supports comfort and security, it is not as high a priority as one of the other options.

b. **Children tend to feel physically and psychologically safe and secure in the presence of parents. Children generally trust parents to protect, support, accept, and love them unconditionally, which is comforting and reassuring to the child.**

c. Although refocusing may temporarily distract the child, it ignores the child's anxiety and is not the best intervention of the options offered.

d. Therapeutic play therapy, not just going to a playroom, can help alleviate the stress of hospitalization. To be most effective, it should be facilitated by a professional with training in play therapy.

11. a. Middle-aged adults (25 to 65 years—Generativity versus Stagnation) strive to fulfill life goals associated with family, career, and society as well as to give to and care for others.

b. Adolescents (12 to 20 years—Identity versus Role Diffusion) strive to make the transition from childhood to adulthood with a sense of personal self.

c. **Young adults (18 to 25 years—Intimacy versus Isolation) strive to establish mature relationships, commit to suitable partners, and develop social and work roles acceptable to society. Unsuccessful resolution results in self-absorption, egocentricity, and emotional isolation.**

d. Infants (newborn to 18 months—Trust versus Mistrust) strive to have their needs met through interacting with others. When their needs are consistently met they develop a sense of trust in their caregivers.

12. a. Toddlers are active once awake and rarely spend much time in bed when not sleeping. Toddlers sleep 12 to 14 hours a day, including one or two day-time naps.

b. Middle-aged adults sleep about 6 to 8 hours a day. Although middle-aged adults spend more time in bed awake than when they were younger, they spend less time in bed awake than an age group in another option.

c. **Older adults generally spend more time in bed awake because of the decreased need for sleep and more frequent awakening. They often go to bed earlier in an effort to get more sleep and end up spending more time in bed awake. Older adults often misinterpret the decreased need for sleep as insomnia and are concerned about not getting enough sleep.**

d. Adolescents sleep 8 to 10 hours a day. Adolescents generally have high activity levels and stay up late. It may seem as though adolescents are always sleeping because they sleep later in the morning, but generally they go to bed much later at night.

13. a. More often people in the older age group need to adapt to the stress of a declining ability to ingest, digest, and/or absorb particular food. This might be required of an older adult who is learning to adjust to a therapeutic diet.

b. This is a normal developmental task of adolescence, not early childhood. Many bodily changes occur in this transitional period, such as a growth spurt and sexual maturity.

c. This is not a normal developmental stressor of this age group. Only a small percentage of the population of 18-month- to 3-year-old children face the challenge of a life-threatening illness.

d. **During early childhood the child gains independence through learning right from wrong. Independence occurs with guidance from parents as the child learns self-control without feeling shame and doubt. When parents are overly protective or critical, feelings of inferiority will develop.**

14. a. Although taste influences choices of foods ingested by the adolescent, a factor identified in another option generally has more influence over what adolescents eat.

b. Adolescents tend to have few rigid routines because of their busy schedules. A factor identified in another option generally has more influence over what adolescents eat than do routines.

c. **Peers often dictate the dietary choices of adolescents. Fad dieting and demands of socialization that generally involve fast food are commonly seen among adolescents.**

d. Although personal preferences may influence choices of foods ingested by the adolescent, a factor identified in another option generally has more influence over what adolescents eat.

15. a. This is a serious concern because of a decrease in efficiency of hepatic metabolism and renal excretion of drugs in the older adult.
    b. Although side effects are a concern in the older adult, another option is a greater concern.
    c. Although hypersensitivity is a concern in the older adult, another option is a greater concern.
    d. Although idiosyncratic effects are a concern in the older adult, another option is a greater concern.

16. a. Infants already demonstrate behavior on the most basic level.
    b. Toddlers are less able to understand and interpret what is happening to them when ill; therefore, they commonly regress to a previous level of development in an attempt to reduce anxiety.
    c. Adolescents generally want to behave in an adult manner and, therefore, demonstrate a controlled behavioral response to illness.
    d. Although some young adults may regress to an earlier level of development as a coping strategy, regression is not commonly used as a defense mechanism when coping with illness.

17. a. People who avoid help from others and who would rather do things themselves generally have not completely resolved the developmental task of Trust versus Mistrust during infancy.
    b. Rationalizing unacceptable behaviors is a defense mechanism, not an indication of an unresolved developmental task of infancy. Rationalization is used to justify in some socially acceptable way ideas, feelings, or behavior through explanations that appear to be logical.
    c. This behavior relates more to the Anal Stage of Freud's Psychosexual Theory of Development. Freud believed that when toilet training is approached in a rigid and demanding manner, a child develops into an adult who is overly concerned with orderliness and cleanliness.
    d. This would indicate an unresolved conflict of Autonomy versus Shame and Doubt associated with the 18-month- to 3-year-old age group. One of the developmental tasks of this age group is learning right from wrong. When parents are overly critical and controlling, a child may develop an overly critical Superego and become an adult who feels the need to constantly apologize for small mistakes.

18. a. Although social isolation is a risk for some older adults because of declining health, death of family members and friends, fear of crime or injury precipitating a desire not to leave the house, most older adults seek opportunities to maintain and build social contacts via the telephone, Internet, community groups, senior centers, life-care communities, etc.
    b. The older adult needs to adjust to multiple changes in social roles to emerge emotionally integrated with an intact ego and sense of wholeness. Changes in social roles are often dramatic as the result of retirement, death of significant others, changing responsibilities within the extended family structure, moving to different living quarters, and decreasing finances.
    c. Although older adults associate with members of all age groups, they generally establish an explicit affiliation with members of their own age group. This supports a sharing of common interests and concerns as well as meeting belonging and self-esteem needs as older adults seek status among their peers.
    d. Older adults do not always have the energy or stamina needed to invest in increasing the number of new meaningful relationships. In addition, they tend to experience a decrease, not increase, in meaningful relationships because of the death of members of their circle of friends and relatives.

19. a. During adolescence the individual is beginning to question life-guiding values such as spirituality. However, it is not uncommon for the adolescent to turn away from religious practices as part of dealing with role confusion and exploration of self-identity. Faith becomes centered around the peer group and away from the parents. This stage is called Synthetic-Conventional Faith by James Fowler.
    b. Although older adults often refine spiritual beliefs in response to life events, beliefs are generally greatly expanded upon at an earlier stage of development. Some unique adults are able to achieve Universalizing Faith identified by James Fowler, which is a world view stressing living out the vision of justice, love, and compassion.
    c. Young adults are just beginning to think about spirituality more introspectively at this age. Young adults generally enter a reflective period of time as discovery of values in relation to social goals are explored within their own frame of reference rather from the peer group frame of reference as during adolescence. This stage is called Individuative-Reflective Faith by James Fowler.
    d. Middle-aged adults tend to engage in refining and expanding spiritual beliefs through questioning. Middle-aged adults are reported to have greater faith, more reliance on personal spiritual strength, and be less inflexible in spiritual beliefs. Middle-aged adults integrate other viewpoints about faith which introduces tension while working toward resolution of spiritual beliefs. This stage is called Conjunctive Faith by James Fowler.

20. a. As a person's skin ages it decreases, not increases, in tone because of loss of dermal mass. This occurs because of flattening of the dermal-epidermal junction, reduced thickness and vascularity of the dermis, and slowing of epidermal proliferation.
    b. As a person's skin ages it increases, not decreases, in dryness because of a reduction in moisture content, sebaceous gland activity, and circulation to the skin.
    c. As a person's skin ages it decreases, not increases, in elasticity because collagen fibers become coarser and more random, and there is a degeneration of elastic fibers in the dermal connective tissue.
    d. This is true. The skin of the older adult decreases in thickness because of loss of dermal and subcutaneous mass. This occurs in response to a flattening of the dermal-epidermal junction, reduced thickness and vascularity of the dermis, and slowing of epidermal proliferation.

21. a. An older adult man is not at risk when receiving a medication that has a teratogenic effect.
    b. A pregnant woman would be at risk. Teratogenic refers to a substance that can cross the placental barrier and interfere with normal growth and development of the fetus.
    c. A 4-year-old child is not at risk when receiving a medication that has a teratogenic effect.
    d. A newborn baby is not at risk when receiving a medication that has a teratogenic effect.

22. a. Dementia is a progressive irreversible decline in mental function that is not caused by sensory overload.
    b. **Confusion is a common response to sensory overload. Because of excessive sensory stimulation a person is unable to perceive the environment accurately or respond appropriately.**
    c. Sensory overload generally precipitates anxiety, agitation, and restlessness, not drowsiness.
    d. If sensory overload precipitates anxiety and the autonomic nervous system is stimulated by the *fight or flight* mechanism, tachycardia, not bradycardia, will occur.

23. a. During early childhood (18 months to 3 years—Autonomy versus Shame and Doubt) children move from complete dependence to beginning independence. Experience with short periods of separation from parents helps toddlers to develop a reliance on self.
    b. The developmental task of early childhood (18 months to 3 years—Autonomy versus Shame and Doubt) is to learn self-control. Delaying gratification of an immediate need until a more socially acceptable time requires the child to curb impulses and control the expression of self-centered feelings and is normal for this age group.
    c. School-aged children (6 to 12 years—Industry versus Inferiority) generally participate in competitive and cooperative activities primarily with children of the same gender, which is normal for this age group.
    d. **Adolescents (12 to 20 years—Identity versus Role Diffusion) have multiple and complex physiological, psychological, and social developmental milestones. Adolescents want to be attractive to others, similar to their peers, and accepted within a group. An amputation of a limb at this age can alter an evolving body image and impose physical and social limitations.**

24. a. Nails tend to grow thicker and become brittle and yellowed rather than to grow longer in the older adult.
    b. Skin elasticity decreases, not increases, in the older adult. Elasticity declines because collagen fibers become coarser and more random, and there is a degeneration of elastic fibers in the dermal connective tissue.
    c. **Residual urine increases in the older adult because of loss of bladder and urethral muscle tone. In addition, older adults may delay responding to the need to void, which further contributes to a decrease in bladder tone.**
    d. Nerve conduction decreases, not increases, in the older adult. Neurologic changes include a decreased

number of neurons, slower transmission of nerve impulses, reduced production of chemical neurotransmitters, and lower sensory thresholds.

25. a. **Growth and development is an orderly process that follows a predictable, not unpredictable, path. There are three predictable patterns: cephalocaudal—proceeding from head to toe; proximodistal—progressing from gross motor to fine motor movements; and symmetrical—both sides developing equally. Growth is marked by measurable changes in the physical aspects of the life-cycle and development is marked by behavioral changes that occur because of achievement of developmental tasks and their resulting functional abilities and skills.**
    b. Growth and development follow a sequential timetable whereby multiple dynamic changes occur in a systematic and orderly manner.
    c. Individuals grow and develop in the physiologic, cognitive, psychosocial, moral and spiritual realms in an integrated way, with each one influencing the others.
    d. Growth and development is a complex process that involves multiple influencing variables, such as genetics, experience, health, culture, and environment.

26. a. School-aged children (6 to 12 years) tend to have fewer differences in appearance and behavior from their peers. These children begin to be involved with formalized groups where conformity is expected.
    b. Although adolescents may be viewed as different from the norms of their parents, they are similar to their peers. In their search for self-identity, adolescents experience role confusion. To control anxiety with role confusion, they are attracted to and conform with peer groups, which provide a sense of security.
    c. Although there is diversity in this age group, individuals have to adjust to common experiences such as physical decline, retirement, multiple losses, and changes in social roles. Older adults commonly seek out people of the same age to share similar interests and find status among their peers.
    d. **Middle-aged adults (40 to 60 years) are in a time of transition between young adulthood and older adulthood. Therefore, individuals in this group, more so than in any other age group, have the greatest individual differences in appearance and behavior as they span the norms seen in young adulthood, middle adulthood, and older adulthood.**

27. a. **Sedatives are not well tolerated by older adults because a decrease in the absorption, metabolism, and excretion of the drug can result in toxicity. In addition, they may experience idiosyncratic (unexpected or opposite) effects.**
    b. Anti-anxiety drugs depress the central nervous system and therefore are helpful in supporting sleep.
    c. The effectiveness of hypnotics decreases, not increases, with prolonged use. They should be used only as a short-term intervention because tolerance and rebound insomnia occur in approximately 4 weeks.

    d. Although melatonin demonstrates promise as a drug to support sleep, it is not the drug of choice because its safety and efficacy are not yet established.

28. a. Sigmund Freud, not Erikson, identified that defense mechanisms were used to reduce anxiety by preventing conscious awareness of threatening thoughts or feelings.
    b. Lawrence Kohlberg, not Erikson, established a framework for understanding the development of moral maturity, which is the ability to independently recognize what is right and what is wrong.
    c. Erikson expanded on Freud's Theory of Personality Development by giving equal emphasis to the influence of a person's social and cultural environment. Erikson stressed that psychosocial development depends on an interactive process between the physical and emotional variables during a person's life at eight distinct stages. Each stage requires resolution of a developmental conflict that has opposite outcomes and that requires interaction within the self and with others in the environment.
    d. Assimilation and accommodation of new information necessary to stimulate intellectual growth is a concept basic to Jean Piaget's Theory of Cognitive Development, not Erikson's Theory of Personality Development. Assimilation involves the process of organizing new information into one's present body of knowledge, and accommodation involves rearranging and restructuring thought processes to deal with the imbalance caused by new information and thereby increase understanding.

29. a. The 18-month- to 3-year-old child (Autonomy versus Shame and Doubt) strives for independence.
    b. The 25- to 65-year-old adult (Generativity versus Stagnation) strives to fulfill life goals associated with family, career, and society as well as being able to give to and care for others.
    c. The 12- to 20-year-old adolescent (Identity versus Role Diffusion) strives to make the transition from childhood to adulthood with a sense of personal self.
    d. The adult 65 years and older (Ego Integrity versus Despair) conducts a review of life events and seeks to come to terms with and accept responsibility for one's own life, including what it was in light of what one had hoped it would be.

30. a. Although refocusing may temporarily distract the child, it is not the best intervention.
    b. Although reducing fatigue can increase pain tolerance, it is not the best intervention.
    c. Anxiety reduces pain tolerance. Therefore, it is important to employ actions that help to reduce anxiety. Children tend to feel physically and psychologically safe and secure in the presence of parents. Children generally trust parents to protect, support, accept, and love them unconditionally, which is comforting and reassuring to the child.
    d. Not all activities or positions may be permitted based on the needs of the child. This action assumes that there are no limits on the child's activity.

31. a. Sebaceous gland activity decreases, not increases, during the older-adult years.
    b. Older adults generally experience a deterioration of the cartilage surface of joints and often form spurs or projecting points that limit joint motion.
    c. Loss of a social support system is a psychosocial, not physiologic, change commonly experienced by older adults.
    d. Older adults have a decreased, not increased, need for sleep.

32. a. Although toddlers may experience an eating disorder called *failure to thrive* in which they fail to ingest enough nutrients to be adequately nourished, it is not as common as an eating disorder in an age group in another option.
    b. Studies report that 10% to 15% of young women in the United States between 12 to 25 years of age experience one of the following eating disorders: anorexia nervosa (self-imposed dieting leading to starvation); bulimia (destructive episodic binge eating followed by purging/self-induced vomiting to prevent weight gain); and obesity (weight 20% greater than ideal body weight).
    c. Although older adults have many stressors in relation to nutrition such as decline in metabolism, difficulty with procuring, cooking and chewing food, and physiologic changes affecting absorption and utilization of nutrients, they are not at as high a risk for eating disorders as members in another age group.
    d. Although infants may experience an eating disorder called *failure to thrive* in which they fail to ingest enough nutrients to be adequately nourished, it is not as common an eating disorder as in another age group.

33. a. Cessation of estrogen and progesterone production during menopause does not contribute to iron deficiency anemia.
    b. Although older adults are at risk for iron deficiency anemia because of decreased intake and less efficient absorption of nutrients, they are not at as high a risk as an age group in another option
    c. Although teenagers are at risk for iron deficiency anemia because of rapid growth and diets high in fat and low in vitamins, they are not at as high a risk as an age group in another option.
    d. This age group is at the highest risk for iron deficiency anemia because of the increased physiological demand for blood production during growth, inadequate solid food intake after 6 months of age, and formula not fortified with iron. In addition, premature or multiple birth infants are at special risk because of inadequate stores of iron during the end of fetal development.

34. a. Although school-aged children often experience constipation because they are too busy or are uncomfortable with an unfamiliar bathroom to toilet, they are not at as great a risk for constipation as an age group in another option.

b. Although middle-aged adults experience a slower gastrointestinal motility than when they were younger, they are not at as great a risk for constipation as an age group in another option.

c. Older adults are at the greatest risk for constipation because of decreases in activity levels, intake of high-fiber foods, peristalsis, digestive enzymes, and fluid intake.

d. Constipation in infants is uncommon except when they are weaned from formula to cow's milk or when their diet is mismanaged.

35. a. The major task of middle adulthood is successfully fulfilling life-long goals that involve family, career, and society. If these goals are not achieved, a crisis is often precipitated.

b. Developing peer relationships is one of the developmental tasks of the 6- to 12-year-old child, not the middle-aged adult.

c. Delaying satisfaction is one of the developmental tasks of the 18-month- to 3-year-old child, not the middle-aged adult.

d. Facing death is one of the developmental tasks of the 65-year-old and older adult, not the middle-aged adult.

36. a. Although finger foods help to avoid a mess during meal time, the child needs to learn how to use utensils when eating. This intervention interferes with the achievement of the task associated with this age group.

b. From 18 months to 3 years of age (Autonomy versus Shame and Doubt) the child strives for independence. Attempts to feed oneself should be encouraged and enthusiastically praised even though the child may make a mess. It allows the child to practice and perfect new skills, helps to develop fine motor skills, and supports control of the self and the environment.

c. This should be avoided. When children are made to feel that the job they are doing is not good enough, it conveys a sense of shame and doubt and will make them feel inadequate.

d. This is discouraging to the child and may precipitate feelings of inadequacy, shame, and doubt. When caregivers always do what children should be learning, children are not permitted to learn for themselves.

37. a. The 25- to 65-year-old adult who is unable to successfully resolve the conflict of Generativity versus Stagnation becomes egocentric, disinterested in others, and self-absorbed. Successful resolution results in the ability to give to and care for others.

b. The 12- to 20-year-old adolescent strives to resolve the conflict of Identity versus Role Diffusion. Unsuccessful resolution of the conflict of Identity versus Role Diffusion results in self-doubt, dysfunctional relationships, and even antisocial behavior. Successful resolution results in a personal integration of a self-identity.

c. The adult 65 years and older who is preoccupied with reliving life because of dissatisfaction with the past would reflect a negative resolution of the task of Ego Integrity versus Despair.

Conducting a review of life events, seeking to come to terms with and accepting responsibility for one's own life, and accepting what it was in light of what one had hoped it would be reflects successful resolution of the task of Ego Integrity versus Despair.

d. Young adults 18 to 25 years of age who are self-absorbed, egocentric, and emotionally isolated reflect a negative resolution of the conflict of Intimacy versus Isolation. Successful resolution results in the ability to establish mature relationships, commit to a suitable partner, and develop social and work roles acceptable to society.

38. a. Preschoolers (3 to 5 years—Initiative versus Guilt) learn to separate from parents and develop a sense of initiative. Negative resolution will result in guilt, rigidity, and a hesitancy to explore new skills or challenge abilities.

b. Adolescents (12 to 20 years—Identity versus Role Diffusion) strive to develop a personal identity and autonomy. This is a turbulent time as the adolescent internalizes the dramatic physical changes and the psychological stressors of new social conflicts. It is common for adolescents to experience mood swings, make decisions without having all the facts, challenge authority, and assert the self. However, these behaviors are left behind when the developmental tasks of adolescence are positively resolved. Negative resolution results in assertive, rebellious, and antisocial behavior.

c. School-aged children (6 to 12 years—Industry verses Inferiority) learn to compete, compromise, and cooperate, develop relationships with peers, and win recognition through productivity. Negative resolution results in feelings of inadequacy, low self-esteem, and a reluctance to explore the environment.

d. Infants (birth to 18 months—Trust versus Mistrust) learn to depend on others to meet their needs, thereby developing trust and a beginning sense of self. Negative resolution of this task results in mistrust, dependency, lack of self-confidence, and shallow relationships in later stages of development.

39. a. Infants react to pain in an intense way with physical resistance and lack of cooperation. Separation of an infant from the usual comforting contact with parents contributes to separation anxiety which in turn lowers pain tolerance, which intensifies the pain experience. Infants express pain by irritability, rolling of the head, flexing the extremities, overacting to common stimuli, an inability to be comforted by holding and rocking, and physical responses indicating stimulation of the sympathetic nervous system.

b. Adolescents are less sensitive to pain than an age group in another option. Adolescents generally want to behave in an adult manner and, therefore, demonstrate a controlled behavioral response to pain.

c. Older adults have a decreased capacity to sense pain and pressure. Older adults often fail to notice situations that would cause acute pain in younger people.

d. Pregnant women are generally no more sensitive to pain than when not pregnant.

40. a. A decline in vision, hearing, tactile sensation to pain and pressure, and a slower response time have the greatest impact on an older adult's ability to maintain safety over all of the systems offered in the other options.
    b. Although there is a decline in respiratory functioning, it does not pose as great a threat to safety when compared to a decline in another system of the body.
    c. Alterations in the integumentary (skin) system generally do not pose a threat to safety when compared to a decline in another system of the body.
    d. Although a decline in cardiovascular functioning can contribute to decreased physical activity, endurance, balance, and orthostatic hypotension, it does not pose as great a threat to safety as a decline in another system of the body.

41. a. Kohlberg is best known for his Theory of Moral Development. People move through 6 stages of moral reasoning where the concepts about what is right and what is wrong progressively become more complex.
    b. Freud identified the 6- to 12-year-old age group to be a period of latency during which sexual development lies dormant and emotional tension is reduced.
    c. Brazelton is known for his Neonatal Assessment Scale, which is used to assess an infant's integrative behavioral processes in relation to various stimuli.
    d. Erik Erikson believed that 6- to 12-year-old children are in conflict over the developmental task of Industry versus Inferiority. Ten-year-old children strive to work or produce, compete and cooperate, and be competent.

42. a. The developmental tasks of middle-aged adults are not as numerous or complex as tasks associated with the age groups listed in other options.
    b. Older adults often deal with multiple losses in a shorter period of time, and the longer a person lives the more loss one experiences. A multiplicity of stressors increases the difficulty of coping. Older adults may lose their spouse (the most stressful of all life events), home, health, independence, role, self-esteem, and hope for the future.
    c. Young adults have the least difficulty adapting to major losses. Young adults have a mature understanding of loss and have fewer and less complex developmental tasks that could interfere with grieving than the age groups listed in the other options.
    d. The adolescent age group is the second group of all the options offered to have the most difficulty adapting to major losses. Although developmental, physical, and psychosocial milestones are stressful during adolescence, an age group listed in another option has more difficulty adapting to major loss.

43. a. The 6- to 12-year-old child strives to resolve the conflict of Industry versus Inferiority. Unsuccessful resolution results in lack of motivation and feelings of inadequacy, inferiority, and guilt. Successful resolution results in a positive control over the self, feelings of confidence and adequacy, and the ability to carry a task to completion.
    b. Adults 65 years of age and older strive to resolve the conflict of Ego Integrity versus Despair. Unsuccessful resolution results in a fear of death and dissatisfaction with one's life. Successful resolution results in accepting one's life (recognizing the good and accepting the mistakes), having a sense of integrity and wholeness, and being willing to face death.
    c. The 12- to 20-year-old adolescent strives to resolve the conflict of Identity versus Role Diffusion. Unsuccessful resolution results in self-doubt, dysfunctional relationships, and even antisocial behavior. Successful resolution results in personal integration of a self identity.
    d. The 25- to 65-year-old adult who is unable to successfully resolve the conflict of Generativity versus Stagnation becomes egocentric, disinterested in others, and self-absorbed. Successful resolution results in the ability to give to and care for others.

44. a. The highest incidence of SIDS (109 infants per 100,000 live births) occurs during the third and fourth months of life, not during the first month.
    b. One hundred and twenty nine infants per 100,000 live births die of congenital anomalies, the leading cause of death during the first month of life. Congenital anomalies also cause 49 infant deaths per 100,000 live births after the first month of life to 1 year of age.
    c. This is not the leading cause of death during the first month of life. One hundred and five infants per 100,000 live births die of disorders related to short gestation and low birth weight during the first month of life.
    d. Infection is not one of the four leading causes of death of infants under 1 month of age. Pneumonia and influenza cause 10 infant deaths per 100,000 live births after the first month to 1 year of age.

45. a. Toddlers generally are able to regulate body temperature as long as they are basically healthy.
    b. Adolescents generally are able to regulate body temperature as long as there are no coexisting health problems.
    c. Regulation of body temperature depends on the ability to dilate or constrict blood vessels and control the activity of sweat glands. In the older adult: the production of sweat glands decreases, reducing a person's ability to perspire and resulting in risk for heat exhaustion; there are decreased amounts of muscle mass and subcutaneous fat, which lead to increased susceptibility to cold; there is inefficient vasoconstriction in response to cold and inefficient vasodilation in response to heat; and there is a diminished ability to shiver, which increases body temperature.
    d. School-aged children generally are able to regulate temperature as long as there are no other underlying medical conditions.

46. a. The 18-month- to 3-year-old child who has feelings of self-doubt, low self-control and self-esteem reflects difficulty in resolving the conflict of Autonomy versus Shame and Doubt. Successful resolution results in independence, displays of emerging willpower, and a sense of control.

    b. The 12- to 20-year-old adolescent who has self-doubt, dysfunctional relationships, and even antisocial behavior reflects a negative resolution of the conflict of Identity versus Role Diffusion. Successful resolution results in a personal integration of a personal self.

    c. The adult 65 years and older who is preoccupied with reliving life because of dissatisfaction with the past reflects a negative resolution of the task of Ego Integrity versus Despair. Conducting a review of life events, seeking to come to terms with and accepting responsibility for one's own life, and accepting what it was in light of what one had hoped it would be reflects successful resolution of the conflict of Ego Integrity versus Despair.

    d. **Young adults 18 to 25 years of age who are self-absorbed, egocentric, and emotionally isolated reflect a negative resolution of the conflict of Intimacy versus Isolation. Successful resolution results in the ability to establish mature relationships, commit to a suitable partner, and develop social and work roles acceptable to society.**

47. a. Although children 6 to 10 years of age are at risk for injury because of such things as automobile accidents, cognitive immaturity, and risky play (skate boards, bicycles, skates), they are not at as great a risk for injury as an age group in another option.

    b. Although adolescents are at risk for injury because of impulsive behavior, a sense of invulnerability, rebellion, and testing of limits, they are not at as great a risk for injury as an age group in another option.

    c. Although young and middle-aged adults are at the greatest risk for occupational health hazards and automobile accidents (particularly because of alcohol use), they are not at as great a risk for injury as an age group in another option.

    d. **The older adult is at the greatest risk for injury because of a decline in vision, hearing, and sensory ability; decreased muscle strength, mass, and flexibility; delayed reaction time and reflexes; increased incidence of orthostatic hypotension; and decreased bone density, a cause of fractures and falls. In addition, older adults experience more acute and chronic illnesses, which further contribute to physical decline and risk for accidents.**

48. a. Infants initially sleep 17 to 20 hours a day and by the end of the first year are sleeping 12 to 16 hours a day. Frequent awakening for feeding is normal and not a sleep problem for the infant.

    b. Toddlers (18 months to 3 years) generally sleep 12 to 15 hours a day with one or two naps. Toddlers will occasionally awaken during the night because of teething pains, illness, separation anxiety, and loneliness; this is considered normal. If caregivers establish regular bedtime routines and provide emotional comfort, sleep problems are minimal during this age group.

    c. Adolescents (12 to 20 years) have more multiple and complex physiological (e.g., puberty), psychological (e.g., self identity and independence issues), and social (e.g., peer pressure, altered roles, and maturing relationships) milestones than any other stage of development. Anxiety associated with all of these stressors contributes to altered sleep patterns and sleep deprivation. Adolescents generally need 8 to 10 hours of sleep a day; however, adolescents' sleep needs vary widely.

    d. Preschoolers (3 to 5 years) have well established sleep-wake cycles, they sleep 10 to 12 hours a day, and daytime napping decreases. Dreams and nightmares, which can awaken the child, are common but are not considered abnormal. Establishing consistent rituals that include quiet time helps to minimize nighttime awakening.

49. a. **When middle-aged adults are caring for their children and their aging, dependent parents at the same time, they are referred to as the** *sandwich generation.* **Their parents and children represent the bread and they are the meat in between.**

    b. Role reversal is not a definition of *sandwich generation.*

    c. Assisting both sets of parents is not a definition of *sandwich generation.*

    d. Being a middle child between older and younger siblings is not the definition of *sandwich generation.*

50. a. Older adults experience a decreased, not increased, absorption of drugs from the GI tract.

    b. Although approximately 10% of older adults have some problem with alcohol use late in life, the literature supports the fact that there is a decrease, not increase, in the incidence of alcoholism with the aged.

    c. **The literature documents that 75% of older adults are to some degree intentionally non-compliant with drug therapy because of inconvenience, side effects, and/or perceived ineffectiveness of the drugs.**

    d. Older adults have an increased, not decreased, risk for adverse reactions to drugs. Adverse effects are any effects that are not therapeutic. Side effects are minor adverse effects that in most cases can be tolerated.

51. a. **Although there is a predictable sequence to growth and development, there are individual differences in the rate and pace in which developmental milestones are achieved. Therefore, achievement of milestones is measured in ranges of time to allow for individual differences.**

    b. Task achievement refers to Erikson's Theory of Personality Development, which is only one aspect of growth and development. Erikson believed that each stage of personality development is characterized by the need to achieve a specific developmental task, and that achievement of each task is affected by the social environment and influence of significant others.

c. Unfortunately, not all families provide safe and supportive environments for the growing child. In addition, the family is only one of many factors that influence the stages of growth and development.

d. This is untrue. Regression is possible at any stage when one attempts to cope with a threat to the Ego.

52. a. Although toddlers (18 months to 3 years; early childhood—Autonomy versus Shame and Doubt) experience a number of developmental milestones, it is not as unstable or complex as another stage of development. Toddlers explore and test the environment, develop independence, and have a beginning ability to control the self.

    b. **Adolescents (12 to 20 years—Identity versus Role Diffusion) have multiple and complex physiological (e.g., puberty), psychological (e.g., self identity and independence), and social (e.g., peer pressure, altered roles, and maturing relationships) milestones than any other stage of development. The multiplicity of these stressors can have a major impact on the development of the adolescent's personal identity and sense of self.**

    c. Although children in early childhood or toddlerhood (18 months to 3 years—Autonomy versus Shame and Doubt) and late childhood (3 to 6 years—Initiative versus Guilt) experience a number of developmental milestones, they are not as unstable or complex as another age group. The main tasks of childhood are achievement of self-control, initiation of one's own activities, and development of purpose and competence.

    d. Although infants (birth to 18 months—Trust versus Mistrust) experience a number of developmental milestones, it is not as unstable or complex as another age group. The main tasks of infancy are to adjust to living in and responding to the environment and the development of trust.

53. a. Calcium is essential for normal functioning, but it is unrelated to the risk for drug toxicity in the older adult. Calcium is essential for cell membrane structure, wound healing, synaptic transmission in nervous tissue, membrane excitability, muscle contraction, tooth and bone structure, blood clotting, and glycolysis.

    b. **The glomerular filtration rate is reduced by as much as 46% at 90 years of age. In addition, decreased cardiac output can reduce the amount of blood flow to the kidneys by as much as 50%. When the glomerular filtration rate declines, the time necessary for half of a drug to be excreted increases by as much as 40%, which places the older adult at risk for drug toxicity.**

    c. Red blood cells are responsible for delivering oxygen to cells, and are unrelated to the risk for drug toxicity in the older adult.

    d. Frequency of voiding is unrelated to the risk for drug toxicity in the older adult.

54. a. Middle-aged adults usually are safe candidates for surgery.

    b. Although a pregnant woman has unique needs during surgery, as long as the mother's cardiovascular and fluid and electrolyte status are maintained the fetus is supported and safe.

    c. Although the adolescent has needs related to body image and separation from friends, the physiologic risk of surgery is not increased.

    d. **Infants are at risk for volume depletion because of a small blood volume and limited fluid reserves. In addition, immature liver and kidneys affect the ability to metabolize and eliminate drugs, an undeveloped immune system increases the risk of infection, and immature temperature regulating mechanisms increase the risk of hyperthermia and hypothermia.**

55. a. Some stages are faster and some are slower depending on the person and the developmental level.

    b. The growth and development process is very complex and influenced by many different factors.

    c. Just the opposite; the growth and development process helps people to extend themselves to be the most that they can be.

    d. **Although people follow a general pattern, they do not grow and develop at exactly the same rate or extent.**

Communication

The following words include English vocabulary, nursing/ medical terminology, concepts, principles, or information relevant to content specifically addressed in the chapter or associated with topics presented in it. English dictionaries, your nursing textbooks, and medical dictionaries such as *Taber's Cyclopedic Medical Dictionary* are resources that can be used to expand your knowledge and understanding of these words and related information.

Active listening
Assertive skills
Barriers to communication
   Advising
   Direct questions
   Disapproving
   False reassurance
   Moralizing
   Patronizing
   Probing
Body language
Cliché
Communication process
   Encoding by sender
   Message
   Channel of communication
      Auditory
      Kinesthetic
      Visual
   Decoding by receiver
   Feedback
Confidential
Confidentiality
Confrontation

Congruence
Content themes
Conversation
Empathy
Exploring
Focus
Formal interview
Gossip
Group dynamics
Inference
Informal interview
Interaction
Interpersonal communication
Intrapersonal communication
Listening skills
Nonverbal
Organizational communication
Rapport
Response
Space
   Intimate
   Personal
   Social
   Public

Sympathy
Territoriality
Therapeutic communication skills
   Clarifying
   Focusing
   General leads
   Indirect question
   Open-ended question
   Paraphrasing
   Reflection
   Responding
   Silence
   Summarizing
   Touching
   Validating
Therapeutic relationship, phases
   Orientation
   Working
   Termination
Verbal
Verbalization
Visual cues

QUESTIONS

1. A patient states, "Do you think I could have cancer?" The nurse responds, "What did the doctor tell you?" What interviewing approach did the nurse use?
   a. Paraphrasing
   b. Confrontation
   c. Reflective technique
   d. Open-ended question

2. The main purpose of the working phase of a therapeutic relationship is to:
   a. Establish a formal or informal contract that addresses the patient's problems
   b. Implement nursing interventions that are designed to achieve expected patient outcomes
   c. Develop rapport and trust so the patient feels protected and an initial plan can be identified
   d. Clearly identify the role of the nurse and establish the parameters of the professional relationship

3. Reflective technique focuses on:
   a. Feelings
   b. Content themes
   c. Clarification of information
   d. Summarization of the topics discussed

4. A patient says, "I don't know if I'll make it through this surgery." Which response by the nurse would block further communication by the patient?
   a. "You sound scared."
   b. "You think you will die."
   c. "Surgery can be frightening."
   d. "Everything will be all right."

5. The patient states, "My wife is going to be very upset that my prostate surgery probably is going to leave me impotent." What is the best response by the nurse?
   a. "I'm sure your wife will be willing to make this sacrifice in exchange for your well being."
   b. "The doctors are getting great results with nerve sparing surgery today."
   c. "Your wife may not put as much emphasis on sex as you think."
   d. "Let's talk about how you feel about this surgery."

6. The patient states, "I think that I am dying." The nurse responds, "You feel as though you are dying?" What interviewing approach did the nurse use?
   a. Focusing
   b. Reflecting
   c. Validating
   d. Paraphrasing

7. Which is the best intervention for a patient who is having a problem with speaking?
   a. Limit the number of visitors at one time
   b. Use visual cues when communicating
   c. Correct errors as they occur gently
   d. Allow adequate time to respond

8. The most important thing the nurse can do to foster a therapeutic relationship with a patient is to:
   a. Work on establishing a friendship with the patient
   b. Use humor to defuse emotionally charged topics of discussion
   c. Demonstrate respect that is not based on the patient's behavior
   d. Sympathize with the patient when the patient shares sad feelings

9. A patient who is NPO in preparation for a bronchoscopy says, "I'm worried about the test and I can't even have a drink of water." What is the best response by the nurse?
   a. "Let's talk about your concerns regarding the test."
   b. "I'll see if the doctor will let you have some ice chips."
   c. "The doctor will review the results of the test as soon as possible."
   d. "As soon as the test is over I'll get you whatever you would like to drink."

10. What is the first thing the nurse should do to confirm the meaning of a patient's nonverbal behavior?
    a. Look for similarity in meaning between the patient's verbal and nonverbal behavior
    b. Ask family members to help you interpret the patient's behavior
    c. Validate your inferences by asking the patient direct questions
    d. Recognize that what a patient says is most important

11. The patient appears tearful and is quiet and withdrawn. The nurse says, "You seem very sad today." What interviewing approach did the nurse use?
    a. Examining
    b. Reflecting
    c. Clarifying
    d. Orienting

12. Which action best reflects the concept of therapeutic communication?
    a. Using interviewing skills to discuss the patient's concerns
    b. Letting the patient control the focus of conversation
    c. Setting time aside to interact with the patient
    d. Agreeing with a patient's statements

13. A factor that is unique to a helping relationship is that it is:
    a. Characterized by the patient's assuming the dominant role
    b. Distinguished by an equal sharing of information
    c. Specific to a person and guided by a purpose
    d. Based on the needs of both participants

14. The patient appears agitated and states, "I'm not sure that I want to go through with this surgery." Which response by the nurse uses the technique of paraphrasing?
    a. "Are you saying that you want to postpone the surgery?"
    b. "You are undecided about having this surgery?"
    c. "You seem upset about this surgery."
    d. "Tell me more about your concerns."

15. The most important purpose of the orientation phase of the assessment interview is to:
    a. Collect data
    b. Build rapport
    c. Identify problems
    d. Establish priorities

16. When collecting data for an admission nursing history, which would be best to open the discussion?
    a. "What brought you to the hospital?"
    b. "Would it help to discuss your feelings?"
    c. "We don't need to talk unless you want to."
    d. "Perhaps you would like to talk about why you are here?"

17. Which interviewing technique is used primarily in a focused interview?
    a. Probing
    b. Clarification
    c. Direct questions
    d. Paraphrasing statements

18. An agitated 80-year-old patient states, "I'm having trouble with my bowels." Which response by the nurse would be the interviewing skill of reflection?
    a. "You seem distressed about your bowels."
    b. "You're having trouble with your bowels?"
    c. "It's common to have problems with the bowels at your age."
    d. "When did you first notice having trouble with your bowels?"

19. What is the best response when a patient says, "I have something important to tell you but you have to promise me that you will not tell anyone."
    a. "Anything you tell me I will share with the health team because we are here to help you."
    b. "Something is clearly upsetting you for you to place such a restriction on our interaction."
    c. "Whatever you tell me is between us because your personal information is confidential."
    d. "You will have to trust me that I will maintain your confidentiality as long as it will not cause harm to you or others."

20. The statement that is most accurate about communication is:
    a. Communication is inevitable
    b. Behavior clearly reflects feelings
    c. The hands are the most expressive part of the body
    d. Verbal communication is essential for human relationships

21. The patient is upset and crying and mentions something about her job that the nurse cannot understand. The nurse's best response would be:
    a. "It's natural to be worried about your job."
    b. "Your job must be very important to you."
    c. "Calm down so that I can understand what you are saying."
    d. "I'm not quite sure I heard what you were saying about your work."

22. When providing nursing care, humor should be used to:
    a. Diminish feelings of anger
    b. Refocus the patient's attention
    c. Maintain a balanced perspective
    d. Delay dealing with the inevitable

23. Therapeutic communication is evaluated as being effective when:
    a. Verbal and nonverbal communication is congruent
    b. Interaction is conducted in a professional manner
    c. Common understanding is achieved
    d. Thoughts can be put into words

24. A patient comes to the Emergency Department with multiple trauma from a suspected assault by a boyfriend. When the patient seems reluctant to talk with the nurse, an appropriate leading statement would be:
    a. "Did your boyfriend do this to you?"
    b. "You really got beat up pretty badly this time."
    c. "Would you like to talk about how this happened to you?"
    d. "Sometimes people are embarrassed to share information about their situation."

25. A patient is admitted to the hospital with cirrhosis of the liver caused by long term alcohol abuse. What is the best response by the nurse when the patient says, "I really don't believe that my drinking a couple of beers a day has anything to do with my liver problem?"
    a. "You find it hard to believe that beer can damage the liver?"
    b. "How long have you been drinking a couple of beers a day?"
    c. "You may believe that beer is not harmful but research shows that it is just as bad for you as hard liquor."
    d. "Are you aware that each beer is equivalent to one shot of liquor so it's just as damaging to the liver as hard liquor?"

26. The patient states, "I can't believe that I couldn't even eat half my breakfast." Which statement by the nurse uses the interviewing skill of reflection?
    a. "Would it help to talk about your inability to eat?"
    b. "What part of your breakfast were you able to eat?"
    c. "How long have you been unable to eat most of your breakfast?"
    d. "You seem surprised that you were unable to eat all your breakfast."

27. Which is the most important action when communicating with a person who is hearing-impaired?
    a. Raise the volume of your voice and speak directly towards the patient's good ear
    b. Lower the pitch of your voice when speaking with the patient
    c. Exaggerate lip movements when speaking with the patient
    d. Stand directly in front of the patient when speaking

28. What is the best response by the nurse when the patient's husband says, "I just don't know what to say to my wife if she asks how I feel about her breast cancer."
    a. "How do you feel about your wife's diagnosis?"
    b. "This is a difficult topic. Would you like to talk about it?"
    c. "She needs you to be as caring and supportive as you can possibly be."
    d. "Men don't always understand what women are going through. Ask her about how she feels."

29. What is being communicated when the nurse leans forward during a patient interview?
    a. Interest
    b. Anxiety
    c. Aggression
    d. Positive self-esteem

30. What best describes the proverb, *What you do speaks so loudly I cannot hear what you say?*
    a. Nonverbal messages are often more meaningful than words
    b. Hearing ability is an important factor in the communication process
    c. Listening to what people say requires attention to what is being said
    d. When people talk too loudly it is hard to understand what is being said

31. A mother whose young daughter has died of leukemia is crying, and is unable to talk about her feelings. What is the best response by the nurse?
    a. "Everyone will remember her because she was so cute. She was one of our favorites."
    b. "As hard as this is, it is probably for the best because she was in a lot of pain."
    c. "She put up the good fight but now she is out of pain and in heaven."
    d. "I feel so sad. It must be hard to deal with such a precious loss."

32. The most important concept that nurses must recognize to make accurate assessments is that nonverbal behavior:
    a. Is controlled by the conscious mind
    b. Carries less weight than what the patient says
    c. Does not have the same meaning for everyone
    d. Is a generally a poor reflection of what the patient is feeling

33. The goals of communication mainly should depend on the:
    a. Environment in which communication takes place
    b. Role of the nurse in the particular clinical setting
    c. Concerns of the patient and family members
    d. Skill level of the nurse in the situation

34. A male adolescent who had a leg amputated because of trauma says, "No one will ever choose to love a person with one leg." What is the best response by the nurse?
    a. "You are a good looking young man and you will have no trouble meeting someone who cares."
    b. "You may feel that way now, but you will feel differently as time passes."
    c. "Do you feel that no one will marry you because you have one leg?"
    d. "How do you see your situation at this point?"

35. A confused patient becomes upset. What is the best action by the nurse?
    a. Speak louder with a lower pitch to the voice
    b. Use touch to communicate caring and concern
    c. Talk to the patient in a way that is simple and direct
    d. Administer medication to minimize the patient's anxiety

36. Which level of space around a patient is being entered when changing a patient's dressing over a wound?
    a. Personal
    b. Intimate
    c. Social
    d. Public

37. The stage of an interview that establishes the relationship between the nurse and the patient is the:
    a. Opening stage
    b. Working stage
    c. Surrogate stage
    d. Examining stage

38. The patient is exhibiting anxious behavior and states, "I just found out that I have cancer everywhere and I don't have very long to live. My life is over." What is the best response by the nurse?
    a. "Shall I call your wife? It might be good if she was here right now."
    b. "What might be the best way to approach this terrible news?"
    c. "That is so sad. You must feel like crying."
    d. "It sounds like you feel hopeless."

39. Which interviewing skill is being used when the nurse says, "You mentioned before that you are having a problem with your colostomy?"
    a. Focusing
    b. Clarifying
    c. Paraphrasing
    d. Acknowledging

40. What would be the best question to ask when obtaining an admission history from a patient being admitted to the hospital with a medical diagnosis of diverticulitis?
    a. "Have you ever had any previous episodes of diverticulitis?"
    b. "What did you eat the day before you were admitted?"
    c. "What led up to your coming to the hospital today?"
    d. "When were you diagnosed with diverticulitis?"

41. The patient says, "I am really nervous about having a spinal tap tomorrow." The best response by the nurse would be:
    a. "I'll ask the doctor for a little medication to help you relax."
    b. "It's OK to be nervous. I don't ever remember anyone who wasn't."
    c. "Patients who have had a spinal tap say it is not that uncomfortable."
    d. "The doctor is excellent and is very careful when spinal taps are done."

42. A patient is being admitted to the Emergency Department with chest pain. When asked about next of kin the patient states, "Don't bother calling my daughter, she is always too busy." What is the best response by the nurse?
    a. "She might be upset if you don't call her."
    b. "What does your daughter do that makes her so busy?"
    c. "Is there someone else that you would like me to call for you?"
    d. "I can't imagine that your daughter wouldn't want to know that you are sick."

43. Effective therapeutic communication mainly depends on the nurse's ability to:
    a. Send a verbal message
    b. Use interviewing skills
    c. Be assertive when collecting data
    d. Display sympathy when communicating

44. *Active listening* means:
    a. Identifying the patient's concerns by exploring with "why" questions
    b. Determining the content and feeling of the patient's message
    c. Employing silence to encourage the patient to talk
    d. Using nonverbal skills to display interest

45. The patient appears agitated and states, "I'm not sure that I want to go through with this surgery." Which is the best response by the nurse to focus on feelings?
    a. "You don't want to have surgery?"
    b. "You seem upset about this surgery."
    c. "I'll call the doctor to come talk with you."
    d. "Are you saying that you want to postpone the surgery?"

46. An older adult in a nursing home was talking about her early life as a young woman and said, "I had no choice in life. It was expected that I was to get married and be a stay-at-home wife and mother." What is the best response by the nurse?
    a. "Why didn't you explain to your parents how you felt? Maybe they would have understood."
    b. "You feel that there were things you would have liked to have had the opportunity to do?"
    c. "Times are different. Thank goodness women have so many more choices today."
    d. "I could understand how frustrating that could be. I would have just rebelled."

47. A patient who has had a number of postoperative complications appears upset and agitated, yet withdrawn. The most appropriate statement by the nurse would be:
    a. "You seem agitated. Tell me why you are upset."
    b. "You've been having a pretty rough time of it since surgery."
    c. "It's not uncommon to have complications after the kind of surgery that you had."
    d. "I'm not sure that I know everything that has been happening to you since surgery."

48. Which is most important when facilitating communication between the nurse and the patient?
    a. Using interviewing techniques to control the direction of the communication
    b. Minimizing energy spent by the patient on negative feelings and concerns
    c. Ensuring that the patient has an effective way to communicate with staff
    d. Refocusing to the positive aspects of the patient's situation and progress

49. When directing a very confused patient with Alzheimer's disease to eat, what should the nurse say?
    a. "Please eat your meat."
    b. "It's important that you eat."
    c. "What would you like to eat?"
    d. "If you don't eat, you can't have dessert."

50. A patient with terminal cancer says to the nurse, "I've been fairly religious, but sometimes I wonder if the things I did were acceptable to God." The nurse's best response would be:
   a. "Not knowing what the future brings can be scary."
   b. "God will appreciate that you went to church."
   c. "If you were good, you have nothing to fear."
   d. "In life, all we have to do is try to be good."

1. a. The nurse's response is not an example of paraphrasing, which is restating the patient's basic message in similar words.
   b. This is not an example of confrontation. A confronting or challenging statement fails to consider feelings, puts the patient on the defensive, and is a barrier to communication.
   c. The nurse's response is not an example of reflective technique, which is referring back the basic feelings underlying the patient's statement.
   d. **This open-ended statement invites the patient to elaborate on the expressed thoughts with more than a one or two word response.**

2. a. Formal or informal contracts are established during the introductory (orientation), not working, phase of a therapeutic relationship.
   b. **During the working phase of the therapeutic relationship, nursing interventions have a twofold purpose: assisting patients to explore and understand their thoughts and feelings, and facilitating and supporting patient decisions and actions.**
   c. The development of trust is the primary goal of the introductory (orientation), not working, phase of a therapeutic relationship. Trust is achieved through respect, concern, credibility, and reliability.
   d. These tasks are achieved during the introductory (orientation), not working, phase of a therapeutic relationship.

3. a. **Reflective technique requires active listening to identify the underlying emotional concerns or feelings contained in patients' messages. These feelings are then referred back to patients to promote a clearer understanding of what they have said.**
   b. Content themes are referred back to patients through paraphrasing, which is a restatement of what was said in similar words.
   c. When seeking clarification the nurse can confess confusion, restate the message or ask the patient to elaborate in attempt to make the patient's message more understood.
   d. Summarization reviews the significant points of discussion to reiterate or clarify information.

4. a. This example of reflective technique identifies feelings, which promotes communication.
   b. This example of paraphrasing restates the content of the patient's message, which promotes communication.
   c. This example of reflective technique focuses on feelings, which promotes communication.
   d. **This response is false reassurance. It denies the patient's concerns about survival and does not invite the patient to elaborate.**

5. a. This response is false reassurance. Only the wife can make this statement.
   b. Although a true statement, this response negates the patient's concerns and cuts off communication.
   c. This may or may not be a true statement. Only the wife can make this statement.
   d. **The patient may be using projection to cope with**

the potential for impotence. This response reflects that it is acceptable to talk about sexuality and invites the patient to verbalize concerns.

6. a. This is not an example of focusing, which centers on the key elements of the patient's message in an attempt to eliminate vagueness. It keeps a rambling conversation on target to explore the major concern.
   b. This is not an example of reflecting, which focuses on feelings. The use of the word "feel" does not make the nurse's statement an example of reflection.
   c. This is not an example of validating. Consensual validation, a form of clarification, verifies the meaning of specific words rather than the overall meaning of the message. This ensures that both patient and nurse agree on the meaning of the words used.
   d. **The nurse's response is an example of paraphrasing because it uses similar words to restate the patient's message.**

7. a. This is not necessarily helpful for a patient who is having difficulty communicating a message. This is advisable when a patient is having difficulty receiving a message, not sending a message.
   b. This will not improve a patient's ability to speak. This is advisable when a patient is having difficulty receiving, not sending, a message.
   c. This is demeaning, and may promote a low self-esteem.
   d. **This intervention demonstrates respect and supports the patient's self-esteem. Patients who have difficulty formulating and communicating a message should be afforded ample time to complete the task without being rushed.**

8. a. The nurse should maintain a professional relationship with the patient. Nurses may be "friendly" toward but should not establish a "friendship" with a patient.
   b. Humor with emotionally charged issues may be viewed as minimizing concerns or frivolous, and could be a barrier to communication.
   c. **Emotionally charged topics should be approached with respectful, sincere interactions that are accepting and nonjudgmental, which will promote further verbalizations.**
   d. Sympathy denotes pity, which should be avoided. The nurse should empathize, not sympathize, with the patient.

9. a. **This response encourages the patient to explore concerns. Verbalization of concerns, validation of feelings, and patient teaching may help reduce anxiety.**
   b. This intervention bypasses data collection. In addition, ice chips are composed of water, which is contraindicated before and after a bronchoscopy because of the risk for aspiration.
   c. This response ignores both of the patient's concerns and addresses a completely different issue.
   d. Fluid and food are not permitted after a bronchoscopy until the gag reflex returns.

10. a. The patient is the primary source of information. When nonverbal communication reinforces the verbal message, the message reflects the true feelings of the patient because nonverbal behavior is under less conscious control than verbal statements.
    b. This abdicates the nurse's responsibility to others and obtains a response that is influenced by emotion and subjectivity.
    c. Direct questions are too specific. Open-ended questions or pointing out the incongruence between actions and words are more effective techniques than direct questions in this situation.
    d. Nonverbal behaviors, rather than verbal statements, better reflect true feelings. Actions speak louder than words!

11. a. Examining is not an interviewing technique.
    b. Reflective technique refers to feelings implied in the content of verbal communication or in exhibited nonverbal behaviors. Patients who are crying, quiet, and withdrawn often are sad.
    c. This is not an example of clarifying, which is a use of a statement to better understand a message when communication is rambling or garbled.
    d. This is not an example of orienting. Reality orientation is a nursing technique used to assist patients in restoring an awareness of what is actual, authentic, or real.

12. a. Therapeutic communication is patient-centered and goal-directed. It facilitates the exploration of the patient's thoughts and feelings and helps to establish a constructive relationship between the nurse and patient.
    b. Although this often is done, there are many times when the patient may ramble and need to be refocused by the nurse.
    c. Although this often is done, therapeutic communication can occur at any time, such as when providing physical hygiene or performing a procedure.
    d. Although this often is done, there are many times when this response would be inappropriate.

13. a. There are times that the nurse must assume a dominant role; examples include when the patient is unconscious, out of touch with reality, in a crisis, or experiencing panic.
    b. In a therapeutic relationship, the focus is on the patient, not the nurse.
    c. The helping relationship (interpersonal relationship, therapeutic relationship) is a personal, client-focused, goal-oriented process whereby the nurse assists a person to problem solve and meet needs.
    d. The purpose of a therapeutic relationship is to focus on and meet the needs of the patient, not the nurse.

14. a. This is an inference based on inadequate data.
    b. This is an example of paraphrasing, which restates the content of the patient's message in similar words.
    c. This is an example of reflective technique, which focuses on feelings.
    d. This is an example of an open-ended statement, which invites the patient to elaborate on the stated concern.

15. a. The majority of the collection and analysis of data is conducted during the working, not orientation, phase of a therapeutic relationship.
    b. The orientation phase (also called the introductory or prehelping phase) of a therapeutic relationship sets the tone for the rest of the relationship. A rapport develops when the patient recognizes that the nurse is willing and able to help and can be trusted.
    c. Problems are identified, explored, and dealt with during the working, not orientation, phase of a therapeutic relationship.
    d. Prioritiy needs are identified and interventions planned and implemented during the working, not orientation, phase of a therapeutic relationship.

16. a. This open-ended statement invites the patient to communicate while focusing on the reason for seeking health care.
    b. This direct question can be answered with a yes or no response.
    c. This statement may discourage communication. Emphasis should be placed on promoting communication to collect important data.
    d. The desire to talk and the need to talk are different issues. It is helpful if health care providers collect as much significant data as possible.

17. a. Probing questions violate the patient's privacy, may cut off communication, and are inappropriate even in a focused interview. Probing interviewing occurs when the nurse persistently attempts to obtain information even after the patient indicates an unwillingness to discuss the topic or pursues information out of curiosity, rather than because the information is significant.
    b. Although clarification may be used during a focused interview to understand what the patient is saying, it is not the primary technique utilized for seeking specific information.
    c. A focused interview explores a particular topic or obtains specific information. Direct questions meet these objectives and avoid extraneous information.
    d. Paraphrasing may be used during a focused interview to redirect ideas back to the patient so that the patient can verify that the nurse received the message accurately or to allow the patient to hear what was said. However, it is not a technique that obtains specific information quickly.

18. a. This response recognizes and reflects back the underlying feeling in the patient's message (reflective technique). When people are in trouble they usually feel threatened or stressed.
    b. This restates the patient's comment in similar words and is an example of paraphrasing, not reflection.
    c. This negates the patient's concerns and shuts off communication.
    d. This is not an example of reflection; it is a direct question that collects specific information.

19. a This statement is a barrier to communication. Most

information communicated by the patient can remain confidential.

b. This effective open-ended statement invites the patient to continue talking; however, it does not set up the parameters of the therapeutic relationship.

c. Personal information remains confidential even if significant other members of the health team are aware of the information. This is known as the circle of confidentiality.

d. **This statement is an open, honest response and sets up the parameters of the therapeutic relationship. The nurse must be credible, that is trustworthy, reliable, caring, supportive, and honest.**

20. a. **Watzlawick's theory indicates that all behavior has meaning, people are always behaving, and we cannot stop behaving or communicating; therefore, communication is inevitable.**

b. Behavior may imply, not clearly reflect, feelings. The nurse should obtain verbal feedback from the patient regarding assumptions about behavior.

c. The face, not the hands, is the most expressive part of the body.

d. All communication, not just verbal communication, is essential for human relationships.

21. a. This may or may not be an accurate assumption.

b. This makes an assumption that may be erroneous.

c. This patronizing response treats the patient in a condescending manner. The patient cannot calm down.

d. **This response requests additional information in an attempt to clarify an unclear communication.**

22. a. Humor used inappropriately can cause anger to be increased, suppressed or repressed. Anger should be expressed safely.

b. The focus should be on the patient's concerns.

c. **Humor is an interpersonal tool and a healing strategy. It releases physical and psychic energy, enhances well being, reduces anxiety, increases pain tolerance, and places experiences within the context of life.**

d. Coping strategies should not be delayed because delay increases stress and anxiety and prolongs the process.

23. a. This just ensures that the message probably reflects the true feelings of the patient.

b. Interactions, even if conducted in a professional manner, may or may not be effective.

c. **Understanding is the foundation of therapeutic communication. When the nurse comprehends, appreciates, and empathizes with the patient, therapeutic communication is effective. The working phase of the helping relationship can then move forward and is productive.**

d. This just ensures that ideas or feelings are communicated.

24. a. This probing question attempts to seek information about a topic the patient is unwilling to explore. This direct question may put the patient on the defensive and further shut off communication.

b. This judgmental statement may cut off further communication.

c. This direct question will probably elicit a response of "No" because the patient appears reluctant to talk.

d. **This statement identifies a common reaction to an emotionally charged situation. It is an accepting open-ended remark that provides an opportunity for the patient to talk with the nurse.**

25. a. **This is an example of paraphrasing. It repeats the content in the patient's message in similar words to provide feedback to let the patient know whether the message was understood and to prompt further communication.**

b. This response does not address the content or emotional theme of the patient's statement. In addition, this probing question may be a barrier to further communication.

c. This assertive, confronting, judgmental response will put the patient on the defensive and cut off communication.

d. This response is condescending, judgmental, and confrontational, which will put the patient on the defensive and inhibit further communication.

26. a. This direct question can be answered with a yes or no response.

b. This direct question elicits a minimal amount of information about only one aspect of eating.

c. This direct question focuses on just one aspect of the problem, duration.

d. **This question is an example of reflective technique because it focuses on the feeling of surprise.**

27. a. This is demeaning and may be viewed by the patient as aggressive behavior.

b. This may or may not be effective. Although this may be helpful with the older adult whose hearing loss typically involves high-pitched sounds first, there is no reference to this patient's age or type of hearing loss.

c. This may be demeaning and ineffective because the patient may not be able to read lips.

d. **This focuses the patient's attention on the nurse. A hearing-impaired receiver must be aware that a message is being sent before the message can be received and decoded.**

28. a. This question is too direct. The husband may not be in touch with his feelings and will be unable to answer the question.

b. **This response acknowledges that the patient is in a dilemma and it offers an opportunity to explore the situation. Validation and an invitation to talk provide emotional support.**

c. This response focuses on the patient's needs and ignores the husband's concerns.

d. This response is condescending and focuses on the patient's, not the husband's, needs.

29. a. **Leaning forward is a nonverbal behavior that conveys involvement. It is a form of physical attending, which is being present to another.**

b. A closed posture, avoidance of eye contact, increased muscle tension, and increased motor activity convey anxiety.

c. Piercing eye contact, increased voice volume,

challenging or confrontational conversation, invasion of personal space, and inappropriate touching convey aggression, which is a hostile, injurious, or destructive action or outlook.

   d. Self-esteem is not reflected by leaning forward during an interview. Self-esteem is one's judgment of one's own worth, including how the person's standards and performances compare to others and to one's ideal self. A person has a positive self-esteem when one's self-concept matches the ideal self.

30. a. **Nonverbal communication (body language) conveys messages without words and is under less conscious control than verbal statements. When a person's words and behavior are incongruent, nonverbal behavior most likely reflects the person's true feelings.**
   b. Although hearing, one aspect of decoding a message, is an important factor in the communication process, it is unrelated to the stated proverb.
   c. Although this true statement reflects *active listening*, it is unrelated to the stated proverb.
   d. This statement is unrelated to the stated proverb. The volume of a message may or may not influence understanding of the message. The volume of a message occurs on the physiologic level, while understanding a message occurs on the cognitive level.

31. a. This response is not therapeutic because it focuses on the nurses rather than on the patient.
   b. The first part of this response minimizes the loss. The second part of the response focuses on the pain experienced by the child, which may increase the mother's grief.
   c. This response minimizes the loss and focuses on the pain experienced by the child, which may increase the mother's grief.
   d. **The first sentence communicates empathy. The second sentence focuses on the feelings surrounding loss and provides an opportunity for the patient to verbalize. Both of these are therapeutic responses to the situation.**

32. a. Nonverbal behavior is controlled more by the unconscious than by the conscious mind.
   b. Nonverbal behavior carries more, not less, weight than verbal interactions because nonverbal behavior is influenced by the unconscious.
   c. **Transculturally, nonverbal communication varies widely. For example, gestures, facial expressions, eye contact, and touch may reflect opposite messages among cultures and among individuals within a culture.**
   d. The opposite is true. Nonverbal behaviors often directly reflect feelings.

33. a. Although the environment may enhance or be a barrier to communication, it does not determine the goals of communication.
   b. The role of a nurse in a particular setting does not dictate the goals of communication.
   c. **The patient and significant others and their needs are always the focus of nursing interventions, including the goals of communication.**

   d. Although the interviewing skills of the nurse may determine the effectiveness of communication, it does not set the goals of communication.

34. a. This negates the patient's concerns. The patient needs to focus on the "negative" before focusing on the "positive." In addition, only the future will tell if the patient meets someone who cares.
   b. This is false reassurance. There is no way the nurse can ensure that his belief will change.
   c. **This is an example of paraphrasing, which restates the patient's message in similar words. It promotes communication.**
   d. This statement is unnecessary. The patient has already stated his point of view.

35. a. A confused patient does not necessarily have hearing problems. This approach is appropriate for some people with a hearing impairment.
   b. A confused person might interpret touch as an aggressive act and respond by being frightened or agitated.
   c. **Simple direct statements are messages that require minimal effort and time to decode, resulting in better understanding by the confused patient.**
   d. Medication is used as a last resort. Nursing interventions often can calm an upset confused patient.

36. a. "Laying on of the hands" does not occur with personal distance. Personal space ($1\frac{1}{2}$ to 4 feet) is effective for communicating with another. It is close enough to imply caring and is not extended to the distance that implies lack of involvement.
   b. **Physically caring for a patient involves inspection and touch that invades the instinctual, protective distance immediately surrounding an individual. Intimate space (physical contact to $1\frac{1}{2}$ feet) is characterized by body contact, visual exposure, and low-volume interactions.**
   c. Invasive touching does not occur with social distance. Social space (4 to 12 feet) is effective for more formal interactions or group conversations.
   d. Touching is not used with public distance. Public space (12 feet and beyond) is effective for communicating with groups or the community. Individuality is lost.

37. a. **The purposes of the opening stage of an interview are to establish rapport and orient the interviewee. A relationship is established through a process of creating goodwill and trust. The orientation focuses on explaining the purpose and nature of the interview and what is expected of the patient.**
   b. This is not the purpose of the working stage. In the working stage, also called the body stage, of an interview patients communicate how they think, feel, know, and perceive in response to questions by the nurse.
   c. There is no stage called the surrogate stage in an interview. Hildegard Peplau identified six roles that nurses assume during therapeutic relationships, and one of these is the surrogate role. The nurse may be assigned a surrogate role by a patient to help resolve

problems that need to be worked out in a supportive environment.

d. There is no stage called the examining stage in an interview. Examining takes place during a physical assessment, when specific skills are used to collect data systematically to detect health problems.

38. a. This response abdicates the nurse's responsibility to explore the patient's concerns immediately. In addition, it could be an erroneous assumption.

b. The patient is in the shock and disbelief mode of coping and would not be able to explore approaches to coping. In addition, using the words "terrible news" may increase anxiety and hopelessness.

c. This response ignores the patient's feelings and imposes the nurse's feelings into the situation.

d. **This is an example of reflective technique. When no solutions to a problem are evident, a person becomes hopeless (despair, despondent).**

39. a. **This example of focusing helps the patient explore a topic of importance. The nurse selects one topic for further discussion from among several topics presented by the patient.**

b. This is not an example of clarifying, which lets the patient know that a message was unclear and seeks specific information to make the message clearer.

c. This is not an example of paraphrasing, which is restating the patient's message in similar words.

d. This is not an example of acknowledging, which is providing nonjudgmental recognition for a contribution to the conversation, a change in behavior, or an effort by the patient.

40. a. Although this historical information eventually may be obtained, it is not the immediate priority.

b. This question is too focused and should include dietary intake for the previous 24 hours, not the day before.

c. **This invites the patient to expand on and develop a topic of importance that relates to the current problem.**

d. Although this historical information eventually may be obtained, it is not the immediate priority.

41. a. This statement avoids the patient's feelings and fails to respond to the patient's need to talk about concerns. It cuts off communication.

b. **This statement is therapeutic. It recognizes the patient's feelings, gives the patient permission to feel nervous, and reassures the patient that one's behavior is not unusual. This statement sets the groundwork for the next question, such as, "Let's talk a little bit about the spinal tap and the concerns you may have."**

c. This is a generalization that minimizes the patient's concern and should be avoided.

d. This is false reassurance, which discourages discussion of feelings and should be avoided.

42. a. This response will put the patient on the defensive and jeopardize the nurse-patient relationship.

b. This response will require the patient to rationalize the daughter's behavior and focuses on information that is not significant at this time.

c. **This response lets the patient know that the message has been heard and moves forward to**

meet the need to notify a significant other of the patient's situation.

d. This provides false reassurance. Only the daughter can convey this message.

43. a. Communication involves both verbal and nonverbal messages.

b. **Communication is facilitated by interviewing techniques that include attitudes, behaviors, and verbal messages. Interviewing skills promote therapeutic communication because they are patient-centered and goal-directed.**

c. Assertiveness when collecting data may be perceived by the patient as aggression, which is a barrier to communication.

d. A therapeutic relationship should avoid sympathy because it implies pity. The nurse should empathize, not sympathize, with patients.

44. a. "Why" statements are direct questions that tend to put the patient on the defensive and cut off communication.

b. **Active listening is the use of all the senses to comprehend and appreciate the patient's verbal and nonverbal thoughts and feelings.**

c. Silence is passive, not active. Silence allows the patient time for quiet contemplation of what has been discussed.

d. When talking with patients, verbal and nonverbal cues are used to indicate care and concern, which promote communication.

45. a. This is an example of paraphrasing. It may be perceived as a challenging statement that may put the patient on the defensive.

b. **This open-ended question reflects the patient's feelings and invites the patient to talk about concerns in more detail.**

c. This statement abdicates responsibility, delays a discussion about the patient's feelings, and is inappropriate

d. This is not the best response of the options offered. Although it may at first appear appropriate because it seeks clarification, it puts words into the patient's mouth and unnecessarily escalates the situation by challenging the patient.

46. a. This is a judgmental or disapproving statement and is not constructive. The patient cannot change the past. In addition, *why* questions should be avoided because they can be interpreted as accusations, which can cause resentment and mistrust.

b. **This therapeutic open-ended statement gently seeks clarification. It gives the lead to the patient to share whatever thoughts and feelings that the patient may wish to express.**

c. This focuses attention away from the patient's needs and is not therapeutic.

d. The first half of the statement reflects the patient's feelings of frustration, which is appropriate. However, the second half of the statement is judgmental and imposes the nurse's standards on the patient, which is not therapeutic.

47. a. The first part of this statement uses the therapeutic interviewing technique of reflection, which identifies the underlying feelings of the patient and is

appropriate. However, the second half of the statement is asking for an explanation, which is inappropriate. Patients often interpret *why* questions as accusations which can cause resentment and mistrust and should be avoided.

b. This is an example of the therapeutic interviewing skill of an open-ended statement. It demonstrates that the nurse recognizes what the patient is going through and the broad opening encourages free verbalization by the patient. At the very least, it demonstrates caring and concern.

c. This statement minimizes the patient's feelings and is not supportive.

d. This statement would not inspire confidence in the nurse. Nurses should know what is happening if care is to be comprehensive and patient-centered.

48. a. The patient, not the nurse, should direct the flow of communication.

b. Negative feelings or concerns must be addressed. Both physical and psychic energy are used when coping with stress.

c. Communication between the patient and healthcare providers is essential, particularly for obtaining subjective data and feedback. Speech, pantomime, writing, touch, and picture boards are examples of channels of transmission (mediums used to convey a message).

d. The focus must be on the patient's present concerns before refocusing to other issues because anxiety increases if immediate concerns are not addressed.

49. a. Confused patients more easily understand simple words and sentences.

b. This may not be understood by the confused patient.

c. A confused patient may not be able to make a decision.

d. This is a threat and should be avoided when talking with patients.

50. a. This recognizes the patient's feelings.

b. This denies the patient's feelings and gives false reassurance.

c. This denies the patient's feelings.

d. This denies the patient's feelings and gives false reassurance.

Psychological Support

KEYWORDS

The following words include English vocabulary, nursing/medical terminology, concepts, principles, or information relevant to content specifically addressed in the chapter or associated with topics presented in it. English dictionaries, your nursing textbooks, and medical dictionaries such as *Taber's Cyclopedic Medical Dictionary* are resources that can be used to expand your knowledge and understanding of these words and related information.

Acceptance
Agitation
Alzheimer's disease
Anticipatory grieving
Anxiety: mild, moderate, severe, panic
Autonomy
Behavior modification
Beliefs
Bereavement
Body image
Confrontational
Confusion
Conscious, unconscious, subconscious
Coping
Crisis
Crisis intervention
Defense mechanisms
    Compensation
    Conversion
    Denial
    Depersonalization
    Dissociation
    Identification
    Intellectualization
    Introjection
    Minimization
    Projection
    Rationalization
    Reaction formation
    Regression
    Repression
    Sublimation

Substitution
Suppression
Transference
Delirium
Delusions
Dementia
Dependence
Depression
Desensitization
Dysfunctional grieving
Ego
Ego integrity
Egocentric (self-absorbed)
Empathy
Endorphin
Fantasy
Frustration
Gratification
Grief
Grief cycle
Grieving
Guided imagery
Hallucinations
Hopelessness
Id
Identity
Loss
Meditation
Memory
Mid-life crisis
Mourning
Orientation

Panic attack
Perception
Personal identify
Positive mental attitude
Powerlessness
Progressive relaxation
Psyche
Psychodynamic
Psychosocial development
Psychotherapy
Relocation stress syndrome
Resilience
Respect
Role
Role ambiguity
Role conflict
Role strain
Sandwich generation
Self-concept
Self-esteem
Situational crisis
Social isolation
Somatic responses
Spiritual distress
Spirituality
Suicidal
Superego
Sympathy
Trust
Values
Withdrawn

QUESTIONS

1. After being hospitalized for a surgical procedure a man who was impressed with the care he received from the nurses decides to change careers and become a nurse. This is an example of:
   a. Fantasy
   b. Projection
   c. Identification
   d. Intellectualization

2. Anxiety always occurs in response to:
   a. Identifiable fears
   b. Unexpected events
   c. Threats to ego integrity
   d. Anticipated dependence

3. To best deal with a patient who is being demanding, the nurse should:
   a. Set limits verbally
   b. Alternate care with another nurse
   c. Point out the behavior to the patient
   d. Attempt to see the situation from the patient's perspective

4. Which situation reflects the defense mechanisms of displacement?
   a. A woman is very nice to her mother-in-law whom she secretly dislikes
   b. A man says that he is not so bad, so don't believe what they say about him
   c. An adolescent puts a poor grade on a test out of his mind when at his after-school job
   d. An older man gets angry with friends after family members attempt to talk with him about his illness

5. Which is the best way to support patients' self-esteem needs across the life span?
   a. Employing a positive mental attitude
   b. Providing a non-judgmental environment
   c. Supporting the use of defense mechanisms
   d. Encouraging social interaction with others

6. An adaptation that demonstrates mild anxiety is:
   a. Alertness
   b. Fearfulness
   c. Preoccupation
   d. Forgetfulness

7. The underlying basis of all the defense mechanisms is:
   a. Rationalization
   b. Suppression
   c. Regression
   d. Repression

8. Fear is most commonly experienced when the precipitating cause is:
   a. Life-threatening
   b. Unexpected
   c. Recurrent
   d. Unknown

9. Which nursing diagnosis becomes a priority when a patient expresses a sense of hopelessness?
   a. Ineffective Individual Coping
   b. Risk for Self-Directed Violence
   c. Powerlessness
   d. Fatigue

10. When assessing the patient for anxiety, the nurse recognizes that anxiety is a:
    a. Reaction triggered by a known stressor
    b. Response that is avoidable
    c. Universal experience
    d. Threat to the Id

11. A woman with diabetes does not follow her prescribed diet and states, "Everyone with diabetes cheats on their diet." This is an example of:
    a. Rationalization
    b. Sublimation
    c. Undoing
    d. Denial

12. Which is a defining characteristic of the nursing diagnosis Powerlessness?
    a. Inability to communicate
    b. Experiencing multiple losses
    c. Inability to control prognosis
    d. Progressive debilitating disease

13. Which word reflects a concept that is nonessential for the nurse to establish a therapeutic relationship?
   a. Trust
   b. Caring
   c. Control
   d. Empathy

14. The most important thing that the nurse can do to reduce anxiety associated with hospitalization is to:
   a. Teach relaxation techniques
   b. Validate the anxious feelings
   c. Minimize environmental stimuli
   d. Explain procedures to the patient

15. A man with a heart condition continues to perform strenuous sports against medical advice. This is an example of:
   a. Denial
   b. Repression
   c. Introjection
   d. Dissociation

16. Which question would be most helpful when assessing the effectiveness of a patient's coping ability?
   a. "What has been the most stressful event that has happened during this hospitalization?"
   b. "Have you received treatment for any stress-related problems in the past?"
   c. "How have you coped with similar stressors before?"
   d. "How do you feel when you are stressed?"

17. Which is the best intervention by the nurse that supports a patient with a comprehension deficit?
   a. Ask that unclear words be repeated
   b. Speak directly in front of the patient
   c. Make a referral for a hearing evaluation
   d. Establish a structured environment and routine

18. An important concept to understand about anxiety in order to provide appropriate nursing care is that:
   a. Panic attacks generally have a slow onset that can be prevented if identified early
   b. One can conceptualize anxiety as being similar to the health-illness continuum
   c. People who lead healthy lifestyles rarely experience anxiety
   d. Anxiety is an abnormal reaction to realistic danger

19. Which situation reflects the defense mechanism of sublimation?
   a. A child always makes excuses for not attaining goals
   b. A short man acts aggressively to compensate for his size
   c. An adolescent who is focused on sexuality becomes active in sports
   d. An older woman becomes more dependent on the nurse than is necessary

20. Which word reflects the ability of a person to perceive another person's emotions accurately?
   a. Trust
   b. Empathy
   c. Sympathy
   d. Autonomy

21. Which nursing diagnosis is unrelated to older adults who are clinically depressed?
   a. Fatigue
   b. Stress Incontinence
   c. Activity Intolerance
   d. Disturbed Sleep Pattern

22. When considering the concepts regarding the defense mechanism of projection, the person who fears being taken advantage of is usually:
   a. In denial
   b. An opportunist
   c. Depersonalizing
   d. Eager to please others

23. Denying a patient the use of a defense mechanism will:
    a. Damage the Id
    b. Cause more anxiety
    c. Facilitate effective coping
    d. Encourage emotional growth

24. Which nursing intervention would best support a patient's sense of self?
    a. Maintaining a respectful relationship
    b. Verbalizing realistic expectations
    c. Exploring maladaptive responses
    d. Referring to counseling services

25. What defense mechanism is being used when a patient who has just been diagnosed with terminal cancer calmly says, "I'll have to get on the Internet to assess my options?"
    a. Intellectualization
    b. Introjection
    c. Depression
    d. Denial

26. When helping family members deal with conflicts that arise from developmental differences, what should the nurse do first?
    a. Identify one's own values
    b. Demonstrate an attitude of acceptance
    c. Foster an environment that is non-judgmental
    d. Encourage open communication among family members

27. Which defense mechanism does an alcoholic person use when making the statement, "I just drink a little to help me relax after a hard day at work?"
    a. Substitution
    b. Suppression
    c. Rationalization
    d. Intellectualization

28. In what stage of anxiety would a person most likely exhibit the presence of noticeable elevations in pulse, respirations, and blood pressure?
    a. Mild
    b. Moderate
    c. Severe
    d. Panic

29. Which defense mechanism is being used when an adolescent who is a poor student excels in sports?
    a. Projection
    b. Sublimation
    c. Displacement
    d. Compensation

30. Which action best demonstrates support of human dignity in the practice of nursing?
    a. Maintaining confidentiality of information about clients
    b. Supporting the rights of others to refuse treatment
    c. Obtaining sufficient data to make sound inferences
    d. Staying at the scene of an accident

31. The patient who is diabetic and continues to eat candy and foods high in sugar is using the defense mechanism of:
    a. Intellectualization
    b. Introjection
    c. Regression
    d. Denial

32. Which is the most important action when a patient is experiencing a panic attack?
    a. Demonstrate the use of progressive muscle relaxation for the patient
    b. Explore positive and negative stressors in the patient's life
    c. Stay with the patient throughout the event
    d. Assess the patient's vital signs

33. To provide the most effective psychosocial support, which data would be the most helpful to the nurse?
    a. Progress notes
    b. Medical history
    c. Patient's concerns
    d. Family contributions

34. Which defense mechanism is being used when an adolescent who has poor self-esteem states, "Nobody likes me at school?"
    a. Rationalization
    b. Displacement
    c. Introjection
    d. Projection

35. Which is the best way to help a patient reduce anxiety?
    a. Involve significant others
    b. Use distraction techniques
    c. Foster verbalization of feelings
    d. Use progressive desensitization strategies

36. A bathrobe is draped over the chair of a confused patient. What is the best response when the patient says, "Tell that scary man to get out of my chair"?
    a. "Tell me more about the scary man that you see sitting in the chair."
    b. "The medication is making you confused. There is nobody sitting in the chair."
    c. "I understand you are afraid, but there is no one there. Your bathrobe on the chair may look like a person."
    d. "It's not uncommon for people in an unfamiliar environment to think that they see things that are not there."

37. The woman who remembers only the good times after the death of her husband is using the defense mechanism of:
    a. Compensation
    b. Minimization
    c. Repression
    d. Regression

38. A patient strongly states the desire to go to the hospital coffee shop for lunch regardless of hospital policy. This behavior most likely reflects:
    a. The need to regain some measure of control
    b. Anger with the policies of the hospital
    c. Disappointment with hospital food
    d. A desire for a change of scenery

39. Physical exercise reduces anxiety by:
    a. Reducing metabolism of adrenaline
    b. Stimulating endorphin production
    c. Interfering with concentration
    d. Decreasing acidity of blood

40. Which defense mechanism is used by a woman who decides to forgo motherhood and chooses to place energy into nurturing a rose garden?
    a. Sublimation
    b. Suppression
    c. Identification
    d. Rationalization

41. Which additional nursing diagnosis in the psychosocial area might the nurse assess for when the patient's assessment data supports the nursing diagnosis, Self-Care Deficit Syndrome Related to Partial Paralysis?
    a. Risk for Self-Harm
    b. Risk for infection
    c. Risk for Constipation
    d. Risk for Powerlessness

42. Which situation stimulates the greatest anxiety for most people?
    a. Accepting assistance from non-family members
    b. Arranging for home care upon discharge
    c. Carrying out self-care activities when ill
    d. Managing uncertainty about an illness

43. Which statement by the patient would best support the nursing diagnosis, Ineffective Denial?
    a. "I'll take care of the tumor after I get back from vacation."
    b. "I just don't think that I can ask for help."
    c. "I really don't care what you do to me."
    d. "I feel like I'm losing it."

44. Which statement best reflects the dimensions of self-esteem?
    a. "I really like the me that I see."
    b. "What do I want to achieve?"
    c. "How do I appear to others?"
    d. "I like to do things my way."

45. The patient is scheduled for life-threatening surgery. Which defense mechanism is being used when the patient says to the daughter, "Be brave?"
    a. Rationalization
    b. Minimization
    c. Substitution
    d. Projection

46. Which is the most appropriate nursing diagnosis for a patient who says, "I'm the same age as my father when he died. Am I going to die of my cancer?"
    a. Powerlessness related to feelings of loss of control
    b. Fear related to perceived threat to biological integrity
    c. Anticipatory Grieving related to perceived impending death
    d. Ineffective Individual Coping related to inadequate psychological resources

47. Which unconscious psychologic response reduces anxiety?
    a. The Local Adaptation Syndrome
    b. One's value system
    c. Suppression
    d. Denial

48. A patient who has been withdrawn says, "When I have the opportunity, I am going to commit suicide." The best response would be:
    a. "You have a lovely family. They need you."
    b. "Let's explore the reasons you have for living."
    c. "You must feel overwhelmed to want to kill yourself."
    d. "Suicide does not solve problems. Tell me what is wrong."

49. A dying patient is withdrawn and depressed. The action that would be most therapeutic would be:
    a. Assisting the patient in focusing on positive thoughts
    b. Explaining that the patient still can accomplish goals
    c. Accepting the patient's behavioral adaptation
    d. Offering the patient advice when appropriate

50. A male patient has been told by his physician that he has metastatic lung cancer and he is seriously ill. After a severe episode of coughing and shortness of breath he says, "This is just a cold, I'll be fine once I get over it." The best response would be:
    a. "Didn't the doctor talk to you about your illness?"
    b. "The doctor had some bad news for you today."
    c. "Tell me more about your illness."
    d. "It's not a cold, it's lung cancer."

1. a. This scenario is not an example of fantasy. Fantasy is an imagined situation that provides for wish-fulfillment.
   b. This scenario is not an example of projection. Projection is attributing to others unacceptable thoughts, emotions, motives, or characteristics that are within oneself.
   c. **This scenario is an example of identification. Identification helps a person avoid self-deprecation. The person reduces anxiety by emulating the behavior of someone respected.**
   d. This scenario is not an example of intellectualization. Intellectualization is the use of reasoning to avoid facing unacceptable stimuli in an effort to protect the Ego from anxiety.

2. a. Anxiety is triggered by an unknown stressor, whereas identifiable fears contribute to a fear response to a known stressor.
   b. An unexpected event may, or may not, contribute to anxiety.
   c. **Anxiety is a psychological adaptation to a threat to the self or self-esteem. The Ego is the *self*. Therefore, whenever the Ego is threatened a person will become anxious.**
   d. When a person feels a disruption to an identifiable source that is perceived as dangerous, as with an anticipated dependence, the individual will experience fear, not anxiety.

3. a. Setting limits will make the patient more anxious and demanding. Demanding behavior generally is an attempt to gain control over events in an effort to protect the Ego.
   b. **Alternating care with another nurse can be confusing to the patient and increase anxiety. Maintaining continuity in the nurse assignment will support the development of a trusting relationship, enable the nurse to explore the patient's feelings, as well as plan and implement interventions that encourage choices, all of which support feeling in control.**
   c. Pointing out demanding behavior is too confrontational at this time. Demanding behavior generally is a defense mechanism that reduces the anxiety generated by powerlessness. To confront the behavior and take away the patient's coping mechanism will cause the patient to become more anxious.
   d. **This is an example of empathy, which is understanding a patient's emotional point of view. An empathic response communicates that the nurse is listening and cares.**

4. a. This is an example of reaction formation, not displacement. Reaction formation is when a person develops conscious attitudes, behaviors, interests, and feelings that are the exact opposite to unconscious attitudes, interests, and feelings.
   b. This is an example of minimization. Minimization allows a person to decrease responsibility for one's own behavior.
   c. This is an example of suppression, not displacement. Suppression is a conscious attempt to put unpleasant thoughts out of the conscious mind to be dealt with at a later time.
   d. **This is an example of displacement. Displacement is the transfer of emotion from one person or object to another person or object that is more acceptable and less threatening.**

5. a. The nurse's personal attitudes should not be imposed on the patient. An attitude is a mental position or feeling toward a person, object, or idea.
   b. **When the nurse establishes a non-judgmental environment and functions without biases, preconceptions, or stereotypes and avoids challenging a patient's values and beliefs, a patient's self-esteem is supported.**
   c. This should be avoided because support of defense mechanisms results in reality distortion. The nurse just should recognize when defense mechanisms are being used because all behavior has meaning.
   d. This may or may not support self-esteem needs. The benefit of this intervention depends on the relationships that develop and whether or not they promote self-worth.

6. a. **This response occurs when one is mildly anxious. Alertness and vigilance are the result of an increase in one's perceptual field and state of arousal in response to the stimulation of the autonomic nervous system when one feels threatened.**
   b. Fearfulness is not a response to anxiety. Fearfulness is an adaptation to an identifiable source, while anxiety is caused by an unidentifiable source.
   c. This response reflects moderate, not mild, anxiety.
   d. This response reflects moderate, not mild, anxiety. With mild anxiety the person increases arousal and perceptual fields and is motivated to learn. With moderate anxiety the person has a narrowed focus of attention and may forget because of an inability to focus attention.

7. a. Rationalization is not the underlying basis of all defense mechanisms. Rationalization is used to justify in some socially acceptable way ideas, feelings or behavior through explanations that appear to be logical.
   b. Suppression is not the underlying basis of all defense mechanisms. Suppression is a conscious attempt to put unpleasant thoughts out of the conscious mind to be dealt with at a later time.
   c. Regression is not the underlying basis of all defense mechanisms. Regression is resorting to an earlier, more comfortable pattern of behavior that was successful in earlier years and is now inappropriate.
   d. **Repression is the basis of all defense mechanisms. All defense mechanisms contain an element of the need to unconsciously exclude upsetting or painful emotions, thoughts or experiences.**

8. a. **Life-threatening events that intimidate one's safety and security generally precipitate fear in most people.**
   b. An unexpected event may or may not cause fear. A surprise party may be unexpected, yet be pleasant and fun, posing no threat.
   c. A recurrent event may or may not cause fear. A

recurrent event could be a pleasant event, posting no threat.

d. The unknown usually precipitates anxiety, not fear.

9. a. Although a person who expresses hopelessness may also demonstrate an inability to manage stressors because of inadequate physical, psychologic, behavioral, or cognitive resources, another option identifies a nursing diagnosis that has a higher priority.

   b. Risk for Self-Directed Violence takes priority over the other three nursing diagnoses because of the potential for suicide.

   c. Although a person who expresses hopelessness may also perceive a lack of personal control over events or situations, another option identifies a nursing diagnosis that has a higher priority.

   d. Although a person who expresss hopelessness may also experience an overwhelming sense of exhaustion unrelieved by rest, another option identifies a nursing diagnosis that has a higher priority.

10. a. Anxiety is triggered by an unknown stressor, whereas, fear is a response to a known stressor.

    b. Anxiety cannot be avoided. It is a normal aspect of everyday living. Every time someone experiences something new it is a threat to the identity or self-esteem; therefore, people feel anxious.

    c. Anxiety is a common and universal response to a threat. Every time people experience something new that is a threat to the identity or self-esteem they will feel anxious. Anxiety is a psychosocial response to stress that is a vague sense of impending doom or apprehension precipitated by the unknown.

    d. Anxiety is a response to a threat to the Ego, not the Id.

11. **a. This is an example of rationalization. Rationalization is used to justify in some socially acceptable way ideas, feelings, or behavior through explanations that appear to be logical.**

    b. This is not an example of sublimation. Sublimation is the channeling of primitive sexual or aggressive drives into activities or behaviors that are more socially acceptable, such as sports or creative work.

    c. This is not an example of undoing. Undoing is use of actions or words as an attempt to cancel unacceptable thoughts, impulses, or acts. This reduces feelings of guilt through reparation (atonement, retribution).

    d. This is not an example of denial. Denial is an unconscious protective response that involves a person's ignoring or refusing to acknowledge something unacceptable or unpleasant to reduce anxiety.

12. a. This is a *related to* factor, not a defining characteristic.

    b. This is a *related to* factor, not a defining characteristic.

    c. A *defining characteristic* of the nursing diagnosis Powerlessness is an expression of dissatisfaction about an inability to control a situation that is negatively affecting outlook, goals, and lifestyle.

    d. This is a *related to* factor, not a defining characteristic.

13. a. Trust is essential to the therapeutic relationship. A reliance on someone without doubt helps make the patient feel comfortable, rather than anxious.

    b. Caring is essential to the therapeutic relationship. Caring conveys emotional closeness and is demonstrated through compassion, interest, and concern.

    c. Control is nonessential to a therapeutic relationship. The purpose is not to have control over the patient, but to identify and meet the needs of the patient.

    d. Empathy is essential to the therapeutic relationship. It is important for the nurse to understand the patient's emotional state and point of view, which can be accomplished through empathetic listening and responding.

14. a. Relaxation techniques are effective ways to reduce the autonomic nervous system response to a threat. However, they do not reduce the stressor contributing to this response.

    b. Validating a patient's feelings will help the patient feel accepted, understood, and credible. However, it is not as helpful as another option.

    c. Minimizing environmental stimuli may support rest and sleep, which is an essential aspect of stress management in any setting. However, it is not as helpful as another option.

    d. Anxiety is a response to an unknown threat to the self or self-esteem. Therefore, explaining what, how, why, when, and where of every procedure to the patient will reduce anxiety by minimizing the unknown.

15. **a. This scenario is an example of denial. Denial is being used when a person ignores or refuses to acknowledge something unacceptable or unpleasant.**

    b. This scenario is not an example of repression. Repression is an unconscious mechanism whereby painful or unpleasant ideas are kept from conscious awareness.

    c. This scenario is not an example of introjection. Introjection is the taking into one's personality the norms and values of another as a means of reducing anxiety.

    d. This scenario is not an example of dissociation. Dissociation occurs when a person segregates a group of thoughts from normal consciousness or when an object or idea is segregated from its emotional significance in an effort to avoid emotional distress.

16. a. This question assesses the presence of a stressor, not the patient's coping abilities.

    b. Although this information may be helpful to include in the health history, it does not address the patient's present ability to cope with stress.

    c. This question identifies how a patient coped in the past, whether the patient's strategy was problem-focused (taking action to improve a situation) or emotion-focused (thoughts and actions to relieve emotional distress), and whether the strategy was effective or ineffective. This information helps the nurse because the

patient may respond to the present situation in a similar manner.

d. This question explores the patient's feelings, rather than coping abilities, when stressed.

17. a. It is the patient who is having difficulty with comprehension who may need words repeated, not the nurse.

b. This action does not facilitate comprehension. It helps a patient with a hearing deficit recognize that someone is speaking and it facilitates lip reading if the patient has the ability to lip read.

c. The patient's problem is a decreased ability to process and understand information, not a hearing loss.

d. **New experiences require a person to process information and problem solve, which is difficult to do for the person with a comprehension deficit. Lack of understanding is threatening to feelings of safety and security. Structure and routines provide predictability, which limits confusion, disorientation, and anxiety.**

18. a. Panic attacks cannot be prevented if identified early, and they do not have a slow onset. Panic attacks usually occur suddenly and spontaneously, build to a peak in ten minutes or less, and last from several minutes to as long as an hour.

b. **People can experience anxiety along a continuum from no anxiety to mild, moderate, severe, or panic just as health is viewed along a continuum from illness to health.**

c. Healthy people experience anxiety when the Ego is threatened. Anxiety is a universal response to a threat. People will feel anxious when exposed to something new that is a threat to self-identity or self-esteem.

d. A realistic danger triggers a fear response, which is a normal, not abnormal, reaction.

19. a. This is an example of rationalization, not sublimation. Rationalization is used to justify in some socially acceptable way ideas, feelings, or behavior through explanations that appear to be logical.

b. This is an example of compensation, not sublimation. Compensation is observed when an attempt is made to achieve respect in one area as a substitute for a weakness in another area.

c. **This is an example of sublimation. Sublimation is the channeling of primitive sexual or aggressive drives into activities or behaviors that are more socially acceptable, such as sports or creative work.**

d. This is an example of regression, not sublimation. Regression is resorting to an earlier, more comfortable pattern of behavior that was successful in previous years but is now inappropriate.

20. a. Trust is not the nurse's perceiving the patient's emotions accurately. Trust is established when a patient has confidence in the nurse because the nurse demonstrates competence, respect for the patient, and behaves in a predictable way.

b. **Empathy is the nurse's ability to have insight into the feelings, emotions, and behavior of the patient.**

c. Sympathy is more than expressing concern and sorrow for a patient but also contains an element of pity. When sympathetic, the nurse may let one's own feelings interfere with the therapeutic relationship, which can impair judgment and limit the ability to identify realistic solutions to problems. Although sympathy is a caring response, it is not therapeutic, as is empathy.

d. Autonomy is being self-directed, not being able to perceive another person's emotions.

21. a. Fatigue is often associated with depression. A depressed person may become inactive and sedentary, which may cause deconditioning that contributes to fatigue.

b. **Stress incontinence is unrelated to depression. Stress incontinence is a physiological, not psychological, problem caused by an involuntary loss of small amounts of urine in response to a rise in intraabdominal pressure.**

c. Activity intolerance is often associated with depression. A depressed person may become inactive and sedentary, which can cause deconditioning that contributes to activity intolerance.

d. A disturbed sleep pattern is often a response to depression. Anxiety and depression can elevate epinephrine blood levels, which can result in less REM and Stage IV NREM sleep, as well as contribute to frequent awakening.

22. a. The person who fears being taken advantage of is not in denial. When in denial, a person ignores or refuses to acknowledge something unacceptable or unpleasant.

b. **Projection is attributing unacceptable thoughts, emotions, motives, or characteristics within oneself to others. In projection, a person who fears being taken advantage of is usually a person who is an opportunist.**

c. The person who fears being taken advantage of is not depersonalizing. Depersonalization is treating a person as an object instead of as a person.

d. A person who fears being taken advantage of is usually *not* eager, rather than eager, to please others.

23. a. Denying the use of defense mechanisms will stress the Ego, not the Id. Id impulses are physiologic, body processes that are dominated by the pleasure principle, not by psychologic or social processes as seen in the Ego.

b. **Defense mechanisms are used to reduce anxiety and achieve or maintain emotional balance. If a nurse identifies reality and does not recognize the patient's need to use defense mechanisms, the patient will become more anxious, even to the point of panic.**

c. Denying a patient the use of a defense mechanism will contribute to ineffective coping, not facilitate effective coping.

d. Denying the use of defense mechanisms will not encourage emotional growth. Emotional growth develops as a result of gaining insight into behavior, recognizing reality, and addressing problems constructively.

24. a. **Respectful interaction demonstrates to patients**

that they are valuable and important and lays the foundation on which trust can be built between the nurse and patient.

b. Verbalizing realistic expectations may challenge a patient who is not ready to face reality, which may increase anxiety and result in a decrease in a sense of self.

c. Defense mechanisms are the most common maladaptive response to stress in an attempt to reduce anxiety. Confronting maladaptive responses before the patient is capable of dealing with reality will cause anxiety to increase and self-esteem to decrease.

d. Although counseling services are an excellent way for a patient to support the Ego and to increase self-esteem, another option offers a better strategy to support a patient's sense of self.

25. a. **This is an example of intellectualization. Intellectualization is the use of reasoning to avoid facing unacceptable stimuli in an effort to protect the Ego from anxiety.**

b. This is not an example of depression. Depression is not a defense mechanism, it is an altered mood indicated by feelings of sadness, discouragement, and loss of interest in usual pleasurable activities.

c. This is not an example of introjection. Introjection is the taking into one's personality the norms and values of another as a means of reducing anxiety.

d. This is not an example of denial. Denial is ignoring or refusing to acknowledge something unacceptable or unpleasant.

26. a. **It is important for the nurse to examine one's own values because values influence beliefs, attitudes, behaviors, and decisions. This should be done in all situations, not just in situations where there are developmental differences.**

b. Although demonstrating an accepting attitude is an important intervention, the nursing action that takes priority is offered in one of the other options.

c. Although it is important to foster an environment that is nonjudgmental, the nursing action that takes priority is offered in one of the other options.

d. Although encouraging open communication among family members is important, the nursing action that takes priority is offered in one of the other options.

27. a. This scenario is not an example of substitution. Substitution is the replacement of an unattainable, unavailable, or unacceptable goal, emotion, or motive with one that is attainable, available, or acceptable in an effort to reduce anxiety, frustration or disappointment.

b. This scenario is not an example of suppression. Suppression is a conscious attempt to put unpleasant thoughts out of the conscious mind to be dealt with at a later time.

c. **This scenario is an example of rationalization. Rationalization is used to justify in some socially acceptable way ideas, feelings, or behavior through explanations that appear to be logical.**

d. This scenario is not an example of intellectualization. Intellectualization is the use of reasoning to avoid facing unacceptable stimuli in an effort to protect the Ego from anxiety.

28. a. During mild anxiety the pulse, respirations, and blood pressure remain at the resting rate.

b. **During moderate anxiety the pulse, respirations, and blood pressure are noticeably elevated in response to the stimulation of the autonomic nervous system.**

c. During severe anxiety the pulse, respirations, and blood pressure are more than just noticeably elevated. The pulse and respirations are rapid and may be irregular, and the blood pressure is high, not just noticeably elevated.

d. During a panic attack the pulse and respirations are very rapid and may be irregular, the blood pressure will be high, and the patient may hyperventilate. If a panic attack is extreme, the blood pressure may suddenly drop and cause fainting.

29. a. This scenario is not an example of projection. Projection is attributing unacceptable thoughts, emotions, motives, or characteristics within oneself to others.

b. This scenario is not an example of sublimation. Sublimation is diversion of unacceptable instinctive urges or the libido to socially acceptable and personally approved outlets.

c. This scenario is not an example of displacement. Displacement is when emotion is transferred from one person or object to another person or object that is more acceptable and safe.

d. **This scenario is an example of compensation. Compensation is an attempt to achieve respect in one area as a substitute for a weakness in another area.**

30. a. **Confidentiality respects the patient's right to privacy, which is a component of human dignity.**

b. This supports the right of a patient to self-determination, which is based on the concept of freedom, not human dignity.

c. This reflects the nurse's attempt to seek the truth, not support human dignity.

d. This reflects a nurse's attempt to be responsible and accountable, not support human dignity.

31. a. This scenario is not an example of intellectualization. Intellectualization is the use of reasoning to avoid facing unacceptable stimuli in an effort to protect the Ego from anxiety.

b. This scenario is not an example of introjection. Introjection is the taking into one's personality the norms and values of another as a means of reducing anxiety.

c. This scenario is not an example of regression. Regression is resorting to an earlier, more comfortable pattern of behavior that was successful in earlier years but is now inappropriate.

d. **This scenario is an example of denial. Denial is the ignoring of or refusal to acknowledge something unacceptable or unpleasant.**

32. a. The patient who is having a panic attack is incapable of higher-order thinking, immobilized, and experiencing a major distortion of perception. A person in the panic state of anxiety is incapable of learning or following directions as complex as learning progressive muscle relaxation.

b. The patient who is experiencing a panic attack is not capable of rational thought or logical thinking, and does not have the ability to problem solve.

c. Staying with the patient and providing for safety is the main purpose of nursing interventions when caring for a patient during a panic attack. Because of the patient's distorted perceptions, poor motor coordination, unpredictable behavior, increased motor activity, agitation, difficulty focusing, and even inability to communicate clearly, the patient is at high risk for injury and should not be left alone.

d. The patient is in a severe state of *fight-or-flight* and it is expected that the patient will be experiencing significant elevations in pulse, respirations, and blood pressure rates as the sympathetic nervous system prepares the body to protect it from the perceived threat. Although vital signs are important, they are not as important as providing for the patient's safety.

33. a. Progress notes, while helpful, are history and may not reflect the current needs of the patient.

b. A medical history, while helpful, is history and may not reflect the current needs of the patient.

c. The patient is the center of the health team and is the primary source of data. The patient generally can provide subjective data about feelings and concerns regarding her/his illness and its impact that no one else can provide.

d. Family members' contributions generally supplement, clarify, and validate data collected from the patient. Only patients can give first-hand descriptions of how they feel and what concerns them. If a patient is confused, mentally or emotional disabled, unconscious, unable to communicate due to pain or critical illness, or are too young, the family can be a helpful secondary source of data.

34. a. This scenario is not an example of rationalization. Rationalization is used to justify in some socially acceptable way ideas, feelings, or behavior through explanations that appear to be logical.

b. This scenario is not an example of displacement. Displacement is transfer of emotion from one person or object to another person or object that is more acceptable and safe.

c. This scenario is not an example of introjection. Introjection is the taking into one's personality the norms and values of another as a means of reducing anxiety.

d. This scenario is an example of projection. Projection is attribution of unacceptable thoughts, emotions, motives, or characteristics within oneself to others.

35. a. Significant others are generally as anxious as the patient because anxiety is contagious. Anxious significant others bring to the discussion their own emotional problems that can misdirect the focus from the patient as well as compound the problem.

b. Although distraction techniques, such as guided imagery, can help manage stress, another option offers a more effective intervention to reduce anxiety.

c. Using interviewing techniques encourages the patient to verbalize feelings and explore

concerns, which reduce anxiety. Verbalization uses energy, makes concerns recognizable, and promotes problem solving. Talking about one's feelings was called *catharsis* by Freud.

d. Anxiety is not something one can desensitize oneself to by increasing exposure to the stressor. Increasing exposure to the stressor will increase anxiety.

36. a. The patient is experiencing an illusion or hallucination. The nurse needs to orient the patient to reality and not add credibility to the misinterpretation of the environment.

b. A person who is confused may not be able to recognize cause and effect. In addition, to point out to the patient that one is confused because of medication may frighten a patient and contribute to an increase in the patient's anxiety.

c. This statement is therapeutic. The nurse first recognizes that the patient is afraid and addresses the fear. In the second half of the statement the nurse explains what might be contributing to a misinterpretation of environmental stimuli.

d. This minimizes concerns and dismisses the patient's fear response. It is a sweeping statement that demonstrates lack of real interest in the needs of the patient.

37. a. This scenario is not an example of compensation. Compensation is making an attempt to achieve respect in one area as a substitute for a weakness in another area.

b. This scenario not an example of minimization. Minimization is not admitting to the significance of one's own behavior, thereby reducing one's responsibility.

c. This is an example of repression. Repression is an unconscious mechanism whereby painful or unpleasant ideas are kept from conscious awareness.

d. This scenario is not an example of regression. Regression is resorting to an earlier, more comfortable pattern of behavior that was successful in earlier years but is now inappropriate.

38. a. Acting-out behaviors that reflect attempts to control events are often covert expressions of feeling powerless.

b. Patients generally follow hospital policies because they recognize that they are designed to keep patients safe.

c. Patients have an opportunity to choose foods they like from the menu, request alternative meals if they are unhappy with the food that arrives, and to ask family members to bring in food as long as the food is permitted on the ordered diet. Wanting to go to the hospital coffee shop against hospital policy is an inappropriate strategy to deal with the disappointment with hospital food.

d. Most hospital units have a lounge that supports patients' needs to have a change of scenery from their rooms.

39. a. Exercise promotes, not reduces, metabolism of adrenaline and thyroxine thereby minimizing

autonomic arousal and decreasing vigilance associated with the anxious response.

b. Exercise stimulates endorphin production, which promotes a sense of well-being and euphoria. Also, endorphins act as opiates and produce analgesia by modulating the transmission of pain perception.

c. Endorphins improve one's ability to concentrate and problem solve by increasing circulation, which facilitates oxygenation of brain cells.

d. Endorphins increase, not decrease, the acidity of blood. This improves digestion and metabolism and thereby increase one's energy level.

40. a. **This scenario is an example of sublimation. Sublimation is diversion of unacceptable instinctive urges of the libido to socially acceptable and personally approved outlets.**

b. This scenario is not an example of suppression. Suppression is a conscious attempt to put unpleasant thoughts out of the mind, to be dealt with at a later time.

c. This scenario is not an example of identification. Identification helps a person avoid self-deprecation and anxiety by emulating the behavior of someone respected.

d. This scenario is not an example of rationalization. Rationalization is used to justify in some socially acceptable way ideas, feelings, or behavior through explanations that appear to be logical.

41. a. Data that support the nursing diagnosis Self-Care Deficit Syndrome Related to Partial Paralysis do not support the nursing diagnosis Risk for Self-Harm. The major defining characteristics of the nursing diagnosis Risk for Self-Harm is an expression of a desire to harm oneself, commit suicide, or die.

b. Risk for Infection is a nursing diagnosis in the physiologic realm, not the psychosocial realm.

c. Risk for Constipation is a nursing diagnosis in the physiologic realm, not the psychosocial realm.

d. **Self-Care Deficit Syndrome is found in the patient who has a decreased ability to perform activities of daily living in all five categories of self care (feeding, hygiene, dressing, toileting, and instrumental deficits). People who have disabilities in all five areas often perceive a lack of control over events, and the nurse should be alert to the presence of data that supports the nursing diagnosis Risk for Powerlessness.**

42. a. Generally attendance by educated healthcare professionals provides a patient with a sense of security and safety; this reduces, not increases, anxiety.

b. Home care commonly empowers a person, which in turn reduces, not increases, anxiety. The patient is reassured that daily needs will be addressed in the home environment, where patients are generally most comfortable

c. Carrying out one's own activities of daily living supports one's self-esteem and self-identity and most commonly reduces, not increases, anxiety.

d. Uncertainty about an illness or the unknown is a threat to one's life, self-identify, self-esteem,

and/or significant relationships. Uncertainty causes the greatest anxiety for most people.

43. a. When a person puts off treatment for whatever reason, the nurse needs to gather more data in an effort to determine if the delay is logical or if the delay is denial of the seriousness of the situation.

b. This statement is not denying the presence of a problem. The inability to ask for help is a major defining characteristic of the nursing diagnosis Ineffective Individual Coping.

c. This statement reflects apathy, a minor defining characteristic of the nursing diagnosis Powerlessness, not Ineffective Denial.

d. This statement is not denying the presence of a problem. Verbalizing an inability to cope is a major defining characteristic of the nursing diagnosis Ineffective Individual Coping.

44. a. **This statement best reflects the dimensions of self-esteem. Self-esteem is a person's self evaluation of one's own worth or value. A person whose self-concept comes close to one's ideal self will generally have a high self-esteem.**

b. This statement reflects one's self-expectations, not self-esteem. Establishing expectations contributes to the composition of the ideal self.

c. This statement reflects self-concept, not self-esteem. Self-concept is an individual's knowledge about oneself. Self-concept is derived from all the collective beliefs and images about oneself as a result of interaction with the environment, society, and feedback from others.

d. This statement is a reflection of a patient's need to be autonomous and self-reliant. Having confidence in one's ability to complete a task is only one component of self-concept.

45. a. This is not an example of rationalization. Rationalization is used to justify in some socially acceptable way ideas, feelings, or behavior through explanations that appear to be logical.

b. This is not an example of minimization. Minimization is not admitting to the significance of one's own behavior, thereby reducing one's responsibility.

c. This is not an example of substitution. Substitution is replacement of an unattainable, unavailable, or unacceptable goal, emotion, or motive with one that is attainable, available, or acceptable in an effort to reduce anxiety, frustration or disappointment.

d. **This is an example of projection. Projection is attributing unacceptable thoughts, emotions, motives, or characteristics within oneself to others.**

46. a. This statement does not reflect powerlessness. People who are powerless usually do not ask questions.

b. **This statement supports the nursing diagnosis of Fear. A major defining characteristic of the nursing diagnosis Fear is the verbalization of feelings of apprehension and alarm related to an identifiable source.**

c. This statement does not indicate that the patient perceives that his death is imminent. The defining characteristics of the nursing diagnosis Anticipatory Grieving is that the person must express distress regarding a potential loss. This patient is asking questions, not displaying distress related to a perceived impending death.

d. This statement does not indicate that the patient is ineffectively coping or that he has inadequate psychological resources. He is gathering data by appropriately asking questions, which is an effective, task-oriented action in the coping process.

47. a. The Local Adaptation Syndrome is a physiologic, not psychologic, response. The Local Adaptation Syndrome is a nonspecific defensive response of tissue to injury.

b. Values are not responses. One's values influence attitudes and behavioral responses. When one's values are contrary to behavioral expectations anxiety increases.

c. Suppression is a conscious, not unconscious, response.

d. **Denial is an unconscious protective response where a person ignores or refuses to acknowledge something unacceptable or unpleasant, thus reducing anxiety.**

48. a. This statement is inappropriate; the patient is unable to cope, is selecting the ultimate escape, and is not capable of meeting the needs of others; this response may also precipitate feelings such as guilt.

b. This denies the patient's feelings; the patient must focus on the negatives before exploring the positives.

c. **This statement identifies feelings and invites further communication.**

d. This is a judgmental response that may cut off communication. This response is too direct, and the patient may not consciously know what is wrong.

49. a. Focusing on positive thoughts is inappropriate because it denies the patient's feelings; the patient needs to focus on the future loss.

b. Focusing on positive thoughts is inappropriate because it denies the patient's feelings; the patient needs to focus on the future loss.

c. **Depression is the fourth stage of dying according to Kübler-Ross; patients become withdrawn and non-communicative when feeling a loss of control and recognizing future losses. The nurse should accept the behavior and be available if the patient wants to verbalize feelings.**

d. It is never appropriate to offer advice; people must explore their alternatives and come to their own conclusions.

50. a. This is a challenging statement and is inappropriate. It could take away the patient's coping mechanism, is demeaning, and could cut off communication; the patient is using denial to cope with the diagnosis.

b. This response would take away the patient's coping mechanism, is demeaning, and could cut off communication; the patient is using denial to cope with the diagnosis.

c. **This provides an opportunity to discuss the illness; eventually a developing awareness will occur, and the patient will move on to other coping mechanisms.**

d. This response would take away the patient's coping mechanism, is demeaning, and could cut off communication; the patient is using denial to cope with the diagnosis.

Teaching and Learning

The following words include English vocabulary, nursing/medical terminology, concepts, principles, or information relevant to content specifically addressed in the chapter or associated with topics presented in it. English dictionaries, your nursing textbooks, and medical dictionaries such as *Taber's Cyclopedic Medical Dictionary* are resources that can be used to expand your knowledge and understanding of these words and related information.

Accredited
Active participation
Assumption
Behavior modification
Certified
Compliance
Comprehension
Continuing education program
Culturally competent
Expectation
Experiential
Explain
Focus group
Formal teaching
Identify
Illiteracy
Informal teaching
Inservice education program
Intelligence
Interpret
Knowledge
Knowledge deficit
Learning domains
   Affective
      Receiving
      Responding

Valuing
Organizing
Characterizing
Cognitive
   Acquisition
   Comprehension
   Application
   Analysis
   Synthesis
   Evaluation
Psychomotor
   Set
   Guided response
Mechanism
Complex overt response
Adaptation
Origination
Learning styles
Literacy
Locus of control
   External
   Internal
Maturity
Motivation
Orientation program
Pedagogy

Positive feedback
Post-test
Predict
Pre-test
Readiness
Reading level
Reinforcement
Relevant
Repetition
Reward
Self-actualized
Survey
Teaching/learning contract
Teaching methods
   Active learning
   Audiovisual aids
   Case study
   Computer-assisted instruction
   Demonstration
   Discussion
   Lecture
   Programmed instruction
   Return demonstration
   Role-playing
   Simulation
   Written material

QUESTIONS

1. What must the nurse do first before implementing a teaching plan?
   a. Identify the patient's level of recognition of the need for learning
   b. Frame the goal within the patient's value and belief systems
   c. Determine how the patient prefers to learn best
   d. Assess the patient's personal support system

2. A teaching-learning concept basic to all teaching plans is to present content from the:
   a. Cognitive to the Affective Domains
   b. Formal to the informal
   c. Simple to the complex
   d. Broad to the specific

3. Which common factor among older adult patients must be kept in mind when planning a teaching program?
   a. Learning may require more energy
   b. Intelligence decreases as people age
   c. Older adults rely more on visual rather than auditory learning
   d. Older adult patients are more resistant to change and new learning

4. Teaching is determined to be most effective when:
   a. Many questions are asked by the learner
   b. Rewards are used to stimulate motivation
   c. Positive behavioral changes can be documented
   d. The learner can verbally repeat the information being taught

5. When assessing a patient's knowledge about a medication that will have to be continued after discharge, the best question the nurse should ask the patient is:
   a. "What do you know about this medication?"
   b. "Did you read the medication's package insert?"
   c. "Did you ever take this medication before today?"
   d. "What has your physician told you about this medication?"

6. Which method would be most effective when teaching a patient colostomy care in the Affective Domain?
   a. Discussing a pamphlet about colostomy care from the American Cancer Society
   b. Exploring how the patient feels about having a colostomy
   c. Providing a demonstration on how to do colostomy care
   d. Showing a videotape demonstrating colostomy care

7. Role playing is a more effective and creative learning activity than other methods of learning because it:
   a. Is more fun that other methods
   b. Eliminates the need for a teacher
   c. Requires active participation by the learner
   d. Provides the learner the opportunity to be another person

8. To be culturally competent when implementing a teaching plan, the nurse first should assess the patient's:
   a. Religious affiliation
   b. Support system
   c. National origin
   d. Health beliefs

9. Which best describes a patient with an external locus of control? A patient who:
   a. Is self-motivated when implementing health promotion behaviors
   b. Wants to please family members with efforts to get well
   c. Understands the expected outcome of therapy
   d. Is a self-actualized adult

10. When assessing a patient to determine educational needs, which statement is most important to consider?
    a. Make no assumptions about the patient
    b. Teaching may be informal or formal in nature
    c. The teaching plan should be documented on appropriate records
    d. A copy of the teaching/learning contract should be given to the patient

11. Learning in the Psychomotor Domain is demonstrated when a patient:
    a. Accepts the need to have a colostomy
    b. Understands why certain foods should be avoided
    c. Verbalizes the rationale for daily colostomy irrigations
    d. Changes a colostomy bag without contaminating the hands

12. The primary goal of the nurse when functioning as a teacher is to:
    a. Provide
    b. Comfort
    c. Empower
    d. Collaborate

13. What is an essential role of the nurse when the physician orders a low-calorie diet for a patient?
    a. Ensuring that the patient's family understands the dietary modifications
    b. Obtaining the patient's weight before beginning the diet
    c. Assessing the patient's motivation to follow the diet
    d. Monitoring the patient's intake and output

14. What is the best response by the nurse when a patient who is learning to use a syringe to self-administer insulin says, "This is so complicated. I'm never going to learn this."
    a. "Let's take one step at a time and master each step before we go on to the next."
    b. "Most people learn how to do this well. It just takes a little time."
    c. "Would you rather have a family member give you your insulin?"
    d. "A lot of people feel that way in the beginning."

15. When evaluating a patient's learning regarding nutrition, which behavior reflects the highest level of learning in the *Cognitive Domain*?
    a. Modifies favorite recipes by eliminating foods that have to be avoided
    b. Evaluates the benefits associated with avoidance of certain foods
    c. States why a mother's diet may affect breast feeding
    d. Identifies a list of foods to be avoided

16. What is the main purpose of continuing education programs?
    a. Updating professional knowledge
    b. Networking within the nursing profession
    c. Fulfilling requirements for an advanced degree
    d. Graduating from an accredited nursing program

17. When designing a teaching-learning program what should the nurse do first?
    a. Identify the patient's locus of control
    b. Use a variety of teaching methods appropriate for the patient
    c. Formulate an achievable, measurable, and realistic patient goal
    d. Assess the patient's current understanding of the content to be taught

18. The nurse wants to influence a patient's beliefs so that new behaviors can be incorporated into the patient's lifestyle. Within which learning Domain does the nurse need to direct teaching?
    a. Psychomotor
    b. Physiologic
    c. Cognitive
    d. Affective

19. When teaching the older adult, what should the nurse do first?
    a. Plan educational sessions in the late afternoon
    b. Speak louder when talking
    c. Provide large-print books
    d. Assess for readiness

20. When evaluating learning about diabetes in the Psychomotor Domain, the nurse should:
    a. Ask the patient to draw up 3 units of regular insulin in an insulin syringe
    b. Question whether the patient knows what to do when not feeling well
    c. See if the patient can identify the adaptations to excessive insulin
    d. Explore the patient's feelings about adjusting to having diabetes

21. When teaching the older adult, which action is necessary to address a developmental stress of aging?
    a. Speak louder when talking to the patient
    b. Use terminology understandable to the patient
    c. Have the patient provide a return demonstration
    d. Allow more time for the patient to process information

22. What is the first thing the nurse should do before beginning a teaching program for a patient with anxiety?
    a. Begin with simple information first
    b. Determine the patient's level of anxiety
    c. Identify the cause of the patient's anxiety
    d. Encourage the use of progressive relaxation techniques

23. When evaluating a nurse's abilities, the highest level of learning in the *Cognitive Domain* would be demonstrated when the nurse:
    a. Identifies the normal properties of urine
    b. Explains the importance of producing urine
    c. Recognizes when something is contaminated
    d. Interprets laboratory results of diagnostic urine testing

24. What is the best response by the nurse when the patient states, "What does 96 indicate when my blood pressure is 140 over 96?"
    a. "The 96 is the pressure within an artery when the heart is resting between beats."
    b. "The 96 reflects the lowest pressure within a vein when blood moves through it."
    c. "Everyone is different so it's really relative to each individual what it means."
    d. "Let's talk about the concerns you may have about your blood pressure."

25. An important component that can determine the success or failure of a weight loss plan is:
    a. Rewarding compliant behavior with favorite foods
    b. Using an 800-kilocalories-per-day dietary regimen
    c. Encouraging at least one hour of exercise daily
    d. Setting realistic goals

26. In which learning domain has learning occurred when a patient explains the therapeutic action of a medication?
    a. Affective
    b. Cognitive
    c. Sociocultural
    d. Psychomotor

27. Which is the best intervention by the nurse that supports a patient with a comprehension deficit?
    a. Establishing a structured environment
    b. Asking that unclear words be repeated
    c. Speaking directly in front of the patient
    d. Making a referral for a hearing evaluation

28. In which domain is the nurse working when exploring with a patient acceptance of changes in life style associated with an above-the-knee amputation?
    a. Psychomotor
    b. Cognitive
    c. Affective
    d. Personal

29. Every person who attended a smoking cessation educational program completed a questionnaire. This type of evaluation is called a:
    a. Survey
    b. Post-test
    c. Case study
    d. Focus group

30. Which is the most important to assess before developing a teaching plan in the Affective Domain?
    a. Intelligence
    b. Strengths
    c. Maturity
    d. Values

31. What should the nurse do first to support health care compliance?
    a. Encourage healthy behaviors
    b. Develop a trusting relationship
    c. Use educational aids to reinforce teaching
    d. Establish why the client is not following the regimen

32. When teaching people with a hearing impairment, the nurse should:
    a. Limit educational sessions to 10 minutes
    b. Provide information in written format
    c. Use multiple teaching methods
    d. Teach in group settings

33. Which is the best action to effectively support a learner who has an internal locus of control?
    a. Provide feedback to the patient in the form of a special privilege or treat
    b. Praise the patient verbally when positive behaviors are demonstrated
    c. Associate the learning with growth that is important to the patient
    d. Award gold stars when goals are achieved

34. When assessing the results of dietary teaching the nurse would identify that learning occurred in the Affective Domain when the patient:
    a. Discusses which foods are on a diabetic diet and which must be avoided
    b. Adheres to the 1200-calorie diabetic diet ordered by the physician
    c. Compiles a list of foods that are permitted on a diabetic diet
    d. Asks about which foods can be eaten on a diabetic diet

35. Which group would benefit the most from role playing?
    a. Older adults who are preparing to retire from the workforce
    b. Middle-aged adults preparing for total knee replacement surgery
    c. Men who are unwilling to admit that they have a drinking problem
    d. Adolescents who are learning to abstain from recreational drug use

36. Educational medical material should be developed at what grade reading level to be most effective?
    a. Fourth-grade
    b. Sixth-grade
    c. Eighth-grade
    d. Tenth-grade

37. What is the greatest advantage of using computer-assisted instruction as a teaching strategy when teaching patients?
    a. Learners can progress at their own rate
    b. It is the least expensive teaching strategy
    c. There are opportunities for pre- and post-testing
    d. Information is presented in a well-organized format

38. Which behavior would indicate the highest level of learning in the *Psychomotor Domain*?
    a. Demonstrating a well-balanced stance with crutches
    b. Identifying the correct equipment that is needed for a colostomy irrigation
    c. Performing a dry sterile dressing change without contaminating the equipment
    d. Recognizing the difference between systolic and diastolic blood pressure sounds

39. The most important factor that determines that a teaching program is needed is the patient's:
    a. Previous experience
    b. Perceived need
    c. Expectations
    d. Flexibility

40. When teaching a preschool-aged child, the teaching method most appropriate would be:
    a. Demonstrations
    b. Coloring books
    c. Small groups
    d. Videos

41. Which type of program is the nurse attending when participating in a mandatory program about medical asepsis provided by a hospital staff education department?
    a. Continuing education program
    b. Inservice education program
    c. Certification program
    d. Orientation program

42. When arriving at a teaching session the nurse assesses the patient and identifies that the patient is experiencing acute pain of "4" on a scale of 1 to 10. What should the nurse do first?
    a. Offer a back rub and reposition the patient for comfort
    b. Postpone the patient's educational session for another time
    c. Continue with the patient's teaching session as a means of distraction
    d. Medicate the patient for pain and then continue with the teaching session

43. Before implementing a teaching a plan, the nurse first should assess the patient's:
    a. Intelligence
    b. Experience
    c. Motivation
    d. Strengths

44. Which is most relevant when predicting success of a teaching program regarding the learning of a skill?
    a. The learner's cognitive ability
    b. The amount of reinforcement
    c. The extent of family support
    d. The interest of the learner

45. Which psychosocial adaptation to an illness has the greatest impact on a patient's future success when planning to engage the patient in a program to learn about the illness?
    a. Fear
    b. Denial
    c. Fatigue
    b. Anxiety

ANSWERS AND RATIONALES

1. a. **The learner must recognize that the need exists and that the material to be learned is valuable. Motivation is the most important factor influencing learning.**
   b. Although this is important, it is not the first thing the nurse should do before implementing a teaching plan.
   c. Although the teacher should identify a patient's learning style, a variety of teaching methods, not just the patient's preference, should be used. This ensures that as many senses as possible are stimulated when learning, thereby increasing the probability of a successful outcome to the learning.
   d. Although supportive individuals (family members, friends, neighbors, etc.) can assist in helping the patient maintain a positive mental attitude and reinforce learning, another option has a higher priority.

2. a. Teaching and learning involve one or all domains of learning and do not move from one to the other in progressive order. Cognitive learning involves the intellect and requires thinking. Cognitive learning increases in complexity from knowledge to comprehension, application, analysis, synthesis, and evaluation of information. Affective learning involves the expression of feelings and the changing of beliefs, attitudes, or values. Affective learning increases in complexity from receiving to responding, valuing, organizing, and characterizing. In addition, there is the Psychomotor Domain, which is related to mastering a skill and requires motor activity. Learning in this Domain increases in complexity from readiness to take action to a guided response, mechanism, complex-overt response, adaptation, and origination.
   b. Teaching methods that are formal or informal are equally effective. The key is to select the approach that is most likely to be effective for the individual learner. This depends on a variety of factors such as intelligence, content to be taught, learning style preferences, available resources, reading level, etc.
   c. **Understanding complex material is best learned when easily understood aspects of the topic are presented first as a foundation to the more complex aspects. When moving from the simple to the complex a person works at integrating and incorporating the less complex new learning into one's body of knowledge and understanding before moving on to more complex information.**
   d. There is no documented principle that supports the need to present content in the direction of broad to specific rather than specific to broad. Each individual patient and the information to be taught will influence the direction in which content is taught.

3. a. **Various physiological changes of aging impact on the rate of learning (declines in sensory perception and speed of mental processing, and more time needed for recall) requiring the use of multisensory teaching strategies and a slower approach. In addition, older adults may have less physical and emotional stamina because of more chronic illnesses, so they may require shorter and more frequent learning sessions.**
   b. Although some older adults may experience a decline in short-term memory, they are not less intelligent. When older adults experience a decline in sensory function (vision, hearing) they may feel ashamed or frustrated, causing withdrawal. Behaviors reflective of withdrawal may be misperceived as a decline in intelligence.
   c. This is not necessarily true. Individuals usually have learning preferences that persist throughout life.
   d. Older adults are not generally resistant to change. Some older adults may be less motivated to learn if they believe that death is near. However, in this situation when older adults are shown how learning will improve quality of life and independence, they are motivated to learn.

4. a. Asking many questions indicates a readiness to learn, not goal achievement.
   b. Rewards stimulate motivation in the person with an external locus of control; they do not evaluate whether goals are achieved.
   c. **When a person incorporates learning into one's behavior and lifestyle, the learner recognizes the value of the content learned.**
   d. Although knowing content on the cognitive level indicates learning has taken place, another option reflects behavior that demonstrates recognition of the importance of knowing the content.

5. a. **This question asks the patient what is known about the medication from the patient's perspective and level of understanding. This question enables the nurse to identify what the patient still needs to know about the medication and to provide an opportunity to clarify misconceptions and answer questions.**
   b. Just because a patient has read the package insert does not mean that the patient understands what was read.
   c. This is the least helpful question to elicit information about a patient's understanding about the medication.
   d. This is the second best question of the options offered. However, this reports only the patient's understanding of what the physician said about the medication. Information, misinformation, past experiences, etc. may all affect the patient's understanding and concerns about the medication.

6. a. This option reflects learning in the Cognitive Domain. Cognitive learning involves the intellect and requires thinking.
   b. **This option reflects learning in the Affective Domain. Affective learning is concerned with feelings, emotions, values, beliefs, and attitudes about the colostomy.**
   c. Providing a demonstration on colostomy care is an example of a teaching strategy in the Psychomotor Domain. The Psychomotor Domain is related to mastering a skill and requires the use of physical and motor activity.
   d. Showing a video tape demonstrating colostomy care is an example of a teaching strategy in the Psychomotor Domain. This is an example of learning on the Perception Level in the Psychomotor Domain. It reflects a beginning awareness of the

objects needed for and steps to be implemented in a skill.

7. a. Role-playing is no more or less fun than many other active and creative learning strategies.
    b. A teacher is always needed to facilitate learning. With role-playing the teacher offers guidance and feedback while providing a safe, supportive environment.
    c. **Learning activities that actively engage the learner have been shown to be more effective as well as more fun than methods that do not actively engage the learner. When learners are actively involved, they assume more responsibility for their own learning and develop more self-interest in learning the content.**
    d. Role-playing is designed to support rehearsing a desired behavior in a safe environment. In addition, it offers the learner the opportunity to play another person, which allows one to view a situation from another vantage point. Although both of these are advantages, they are not the most important reasons why role-playing is effective.

8. a. Although religious affiliation may be important to know, it is only one part of a patient's sociocultural makeup. Another option has a higher priority.
    b. Although the level of support is important to know, it is only one part of a patient's sociocultural makeup. Another option has a higher priority.
    c. Although national origin is important to know, it is only one part of a patient's sociocultural makeup. In addition, nurses have to be careful not to make generalizations and stereotype an individual because of national origin, because each person is an individual.
    d. **Individuals have their own beliefs associated with cultural health practices, faith beliefs, diet, illness, death and dying, and lifestyle, which all have a major impact on health beliefs.**

9. a. A self-actualized adult is motivated by an internal locus of control. According to Maslow, the self-actualized person is an individual who has a need to develop to one's maximum potential and personally realize one's qualities and abilities.
    b. **The person with an external locus of control is motivated by rewards that center on privileges, incentives, or praise received from pleasing significant others or members of the health team.**
    c. Understanding the expected outcome of therapy is associated with recognizing the goal one is working to achieve; it does not describe an external locus of control.
    d. This behavior indicates an internal, not external, locus of control. People with an internal locus of control are motivated by personal internal rewards such as achieving a personal goal, pleasing oneself, returning to a normal lifestyle, and avoiding complications.

10. a. **Many variables influence an individual's willingness and ability to learn (readiness, motivation, physical and emotional abilities, education, age, cultural and health beliefs, cognitive abilities, etc.). Since everyone is a**

unique individual with individual needs, the nurse must avoid making assumptions and generalizations.
    b. The patient's needs must be identified before teaching formats and strategies are designed.
    c. The patient's needs must be identified before the teaching plan is designed and documented.
    d. The patient's needs must be identified before a plan is designed and a contract is written.

11. a. Accepting the need to have a colostomy indicates learning on the Valuing Level in the Affective, not Psychomotor, Domain. Valuing is demonstrated when learning is incorporated into the learner's behavior because it is perceived as important.
    b. Understanding why certain foods have to be avoided indicates learning on the Comprehension Level in the Cognitive, not Psychomotor, Domain. Learning on the Comprehension Level is reflected in the ability to understand the meaning of learned content.
    c. Understanding the rationale for daily colostomy irrigation indicates learning on the Comprehension Level in the Cognitive, not Psychomotor, Domain. Learning on the Comprehension Level is reflected in the ability to understand the meaning of learned content.
    d. **Changing a colostomy bag without contaminating the hands is an example of learning in the Psychomotor Domain. Learning in the Psychomotor Domain is related to mastering a skill and requires motor activity.**

12. a. Although a teacher may *provide* opportunities for learning, it is not the best word to describe the goal of the nurse when functioning as a teacher.
    b. Although a teacher may *comfort* the patient when teaching, it is not the best word to describe the goal of the nurse when functioning as a teacher.
    c. **The purpose of teaching patients is to ensure that they have the knowledge and authority (empower) to respond most effectively to their own situation.**
    d. Although a teacher may *collaborate* with other health team members to provide the best learning opportunities for the patient, it does not describe the relationship with a patient in a teaching/learning relationship and is not the primary goal of the nurse.

13. a. Although it is important to engage family members and significant others in the care of loved ones to reinforce learning and help maintain lifestyle changes, it is not the option with the highest priority.
    b. Although it is important for the nurse to assess the patient's weight to establish a baseline, another option has a higher priority.
    c. **Motivation is the most important factor influencing learning. The learner must recognize that the need exists and that the need will be addressed through the learning.**
    d. The physician's order for a low-calorie diet does not indicate a need for monitoring the patient's fluid intake and output.

14. a. **This addresses the patient's immediate concern, breaks the task into manageable steps, and ensures mastery of each step so that the patient**

does not feel overwhelmed. In addition, it communicates to the learner that the teacher is there for the patient and that they will tackle the problem together.

b. This is false reassurance, minimizes the patient's concerns and feelings, and cuts off communication.

c. This statement is an inappropriate response. This statement puts thoughts into the patient's mind and does not focus on the patient's concerns and feelings.

d. This minimizes the patient's feelings, concerns, and cuts off communication.

15. a. This reflects learning on the Characterizing Level and is the highest level out of 5 levels of learning in the Affective, not Cognitive, Domain.

b. **This is an appropriate example of learning on the Evaluation Level and is the highest level of learning out of the 6 levels of learning in the Cognitive Domain.**

c. This reflects learning on the Comprehension Level, which is the second out of 6 levels of learning in the Cognitive Domain.

d. Identifying a list of foods to avoid reflects learning on the Knowledge Level, which is the first of 6 levels of complexity in the Cognitive Domain of learning.

16. a. **Continuing education programs are formal learning experiences designed to update and enhance professional knowledge or skills. This is necessary because of the explosion in information and technology within health care. Some states require evidence of continuing education units (CEUs) for license renewal.**

b. Although nurses who attend continuing education programs have the opportunity to professionally network with other nurses, it is not the main purpose of attending a continuing education program.

c. Continuing education programs do not fulfill requirements for an advanced degree. Master's and Doctoral programs grant advanced degrees in specialty areas (parent-child health, psychiatry, medical-surgical nursing, gerontology, etc.) and practice roles (nurse practitioner, education, administration, etc.).

d. Continuing education programs do not prepare a person to graduate from an accredited nursing degree program. Associate Degree programs, Baccalaureate Degree programs, and Diploma Schools of Nursing prepare graduates to take the NCLEX examination.

17. a. Although this may be done to determine if the patient has an internal locus of control (those who do are more likely to take responsibility for their own learning), it is not the first thing the nurse should do of the options offered.

b. Although a variety of teaching methods should be used so that all the senses are engaged in learning, it is not the first thing the nurse should do of the options offered.

c. Goal setting is accomplished after the nurse gathers essential information that will influence the goal, particularly in relation to the achievable and realistic factors of a goal.

d. **Learners bring their own lifetimes of learning to the learning situation. The nurse needs to**

customize each teaching plan, capitalize on the patient's previous experience and knowledge, and identify what the patient still needs to know before teaching can begin.

18. a. This is not an example of learning in the Psychomotor Domain. Learning in the Psychomotor Domain includes using motor and physical abilities to master a skill. It requires the learner to practice to improve coordination and dexterity manipulating the equipment associated with the skill.

b. There is no learning domain known as Physiologic.

c. This is not an example of learning in the Cognitive Domain. In the Cognitive Domain, learning is concerned with intellectual understanding and includes thinking on many levels, with progressively increasing complexity.

d. **This is an example of learning in the Affective Domain. In the Affective Domain, learning is concerned with feelings, emotions, values, beliefs, and attitudes.**

19. a. Late in the afternoon is not the best time to schedule teaching sessions for older adults. They may tire from the energy and effort required to perform daily activities, and therefore they may be too tired to concentrate.

b. Speaking in a lower-pitch tone rather than speaking louder is more effective. Older adults often experience a decline in the ability to hear high-pitch tones.

c. Not all older adults have vision problems. This should be done for the patient who has visual problems.

d. **If the patient does not recognize the need to learn or value the information to be learned, the patient will not be ready to learn.**

20. a. This is an example of evaluating learning associated with the Psychomotor Domain. Learning in the Psychomotor Domain is related to mastering a skill and requires motor activity. When the learner is able to perform a motor skill involving a complex movement pattern, learning has taken place on the Complex-Overt Response Level of learning in the Psychomotor Domain.

b. This is an example of evaluating learning associated with the Cognitive Domain. Learning in the Cognitive Domain is concerned with intellectual understanding and includes thinking on many levels, with progressively increasing complexity. When the learner is able to use newly-learned ideas in a life-like situation, learning has occurred on the Application Level in the Cognitive Domain.

c. This is an example of evaluating learning associated with the Cognitive Domain. Learning in the Cognitive Domain is concerned with intellectual understanding, and includes thinking on many levels with progressively increasing complexity. Being able to recall new information reflects learning on the Knowledge Level in the Cognitive Domain.

d. This is an example of the nurse assessing learning in the Affective Domain. Affective learning involves the expression of feelings and the changing of beliefs, attitudes, or values. Affective learning increases in complexity from receiving to responding, valuing, organizing, and characterizing. Since the outcome is still unknown, it is impossible to determine what level in the Affective Domain the patient has achieved.

21. a. This is not only unnecessary but also contraindicated in some older adults who have hearing loss with recruitment. Recruitment occurs when a slight increase in sound intensity causes discomfort or pain. In addition, although hearing acuity declines in older adults, they often wear hearing aids that correct hearing to a functional level. High-pitch hearing loss is the most common hearing loss in the older adult and can be addressed by the teacher lowering the pitch of the voice, not by speaking louder.
    b. This teaching principle is common to all age groups, not just older adults.
    c. This teaching principle is common to all age groups, not just older adults. This ensures that the learner has learned all the critical elements associated with the skill.
    d. **Reaction time will slow with aging; therefore, older adults need more time to process and respond to information or perform a skill. In addition, some older adults may have less energy, experience more fatigue, and may need shorter, frequent learning sessions.**

22. a. Although this should be done in every teaching situation, an action in another option has priority.
    b. **This is the first thing the nurse should do because the patient's level of anxiety will affect the teaching/learning process. Mild anxiety is generally motivating. Moderate, severe, and panic stages of anxiety, exhibited by progressive worsening of one's ability to retain rational thought processes, to remain focused, and to be calm, interfere with learning. If the nurse identifies that the patient has a moderate or more severe level of anxiety, the learning session should be rescheduled and actions taken to reduce the patient's anxiety.**
    c. Although the nurse may want to address the cause of a patient's anxiety before teaching (the patient will not be able to focus on learning), an action in another option has priority.
    d. Although this might eventually be done if the learner has a moderate or severe level of anxiety, an action in another option has priority.

23. a. Identifying the normal properties of urine reflects learning on the Knowledge Level, which is the first of 6 levels of complexity in the Cognitive Domain.
    b. Explaining the importance of producing urine reflects learning on the Comprehension Level, which is the second of 6 levels of complexity in the Cognitive Domain.
    c. Recognizing when something is contaminated reflects learning on the Comprehension Level, which is the second level of 6 levels of complexity within the Cognitive Domain.
    d. **This is the highest level of learning in the Cognitive Domain of the choices offered. Interpretation of laboratory results of urine**

testing reflects learning on the Analysis Level, which is the fourth of 6 levels of learning in the Cognitive Domain.

24. a. **This is the correct response to this patient's question. The nurse's response is simple, direct, and uses language that is easily understood.**
    b. This is incorrect. This is the pressure in the artery, not the vein.
    c. This does not answer the question, which can be frustrating to the patient. When a question receives a meaningless response, the patient may perceive that the nurse is not interested in taking the time to explain the concept.
    d. The patient is requesting simple information. The question has to be answered first and then any concerns can be addressed.

25. a. Learning is encouraged when positive behaviors are reinforced with a reward. However, food in this scenario should be avoided as a reward because it may foster old habits that contributed to the original weight gain. For people with an internal locus of control, rewards should center on recognition of personal achievement such as pleasing oneself, returning to a normal lifestyle, avoiding complications, and in this scenario losing weight. For the person with an external locus of control, rewards might center on privileges or praise received from pleasing significant others or members of the health team.
    b. This is a dependent function of the nurse and requires a physician's order. In addition, an 800-calorie diet is too few calories to acquire basic nutrients to maintain adequate health. Weight loss diets should be between 1200 and 1500 calories for women and between 1500 and 1800 for men.
    c. Although exercise is an important component of any weight loss program, exercise alone will not determine the success or failure of a weight loss program.
    d. **Setting realistic goals is important to the success of a weight loss plan. Since achieving success is largely dependent upon motivation, the teacher should design goals that demonstrate immediate progress or growth. One strategy is to design numerous realistic short-term intermediary goals that are more easily achieved than one long-term goal.**

26. a. In the Affective Domain, learning is concerned with feelings, emotions, values, beliefs, and attitudes, not facts about a medication, which is in another domain.
    b. **Learning the therapeutic action of a medication reflects the acquiring of knowledge in the Cognitive Domain. In the Cognitive Domain learning is concerned with intellectual understanding, and includes thinking on many levels with progressively increasing complexity.**
    c. There is no domain known as Sociocultural.
    d. Learning in the Psychomotor Domain includes using motor and physical abilities to master a skill. Learning in this domain requires practice to improve coordination and dexterity manipulating the equipment associated with the skill.

27. a. For people who have difficulty with comprehension, participating in a learning program often makes them feel overwhelmed and threatened. The teacher needs to provide a structured environment where variables are controlled to reduce anxiety and support comprehension. The nurse should minimize ambiguity, provide a familiar environment, teach at the same time each day, limit environmental distractions, and provide simple learning materials.
    b. This action helps the nurse understand what the patient is saying; it does not help the patient with a comprehension deficit to understand.
    c. This helps the patient who is hearing-impaired, not the patient who has a comprehension deficit.
    d. The patient does not need a hearing evaluation. The patient's problem is a diminished capacity to understand, not a hearing loss.

28. a. Learning in the Psychomotor Domain would be associated with learning how to safely put on, or ambulate with, a prosthetic extremity.
    b. Learning in the Cognitive Domain would be associated with learning what foods would be important to eat to facilitate wound healing after having surgery to amputate a leg.
    c. Learning to accept changes in life style associated with an above-the-knee amputation is associated with the Affective Domain. Learning in the Affective Domain involves the expression of feelings and the changing of beliefs, attitudes, or values. Affective learning increases in complexity from receiving to responding, valuing, organizing, and characterizing. A learner who assumes a normal lifestyle after having an above-the-knee amputation and who has positive self-esteem has achieved learning on the Charactering Level (the highest level) in the Affective Domain.
    d. There is no teaching-learning domain known as Personal.

29. a. The terms *questionnaire* and *survey* are used interchangeably to describe a type of evaluation tool designed to gather data about a topic.
    b. A post-test is not a questionnaire. A post-test is an examination given to assess cognitive learning after an educational program is completed.
    c. A case study is not a questionnaire. A case study is a teaching tool that presents a scenario and a sequence of data to which the learner is required to analyze and respond.
    d. A focus group is not a questionnaire. A focus group is designed to gather opinions and suggestions from a group of people about a particular topic using a discussion, not survey, format.

30. a. A general assessment of intelligence is common to all learning domains. It is important to design learning content and strategies based on the learner's level of intellectual ability to avoid teaching below or above the learner's intellectual capabilities.
    b. An assessment of a patient's strengths is common to all learning domains. Prior knowledge needs to be determined so the nurse knows where to begin teaching new content. Learning is most effective when built upon prior learning.
    c. A general assessment of a learner's level of maturity is common to all learning domains. Teaching and learning is fundamentally different during various phases of the lifespan. The level and amount of information needs to be geared to the learner's developmental stage and cognitive level.
    d. In the Affective Domain, learning is concerned with values, feelings, emotions, beliefs, and attitudes.

31. a. Several other important factors that support health care compliance come before encouraging healthy behaviors.
    b. A trusting relationship between the patient and the nurse is an essential. The patient has to be confident that the nurse will maintain confidentiality, has credibility, and is genuinely interested in their success.
    c. Although using education aids to reinforce teaching supports health care compliance, an action in another option has priority.
    d. This is not the first thing the nurse should do to facilitate health care compliance. After it is determined that the patient is not following the healthcare regimen, then the nurse can assess the factors contributing to noncompliance.

32. a. This is unnecessary. Hearing is the problem, not fatigue.
    b. It is not necessary to limit teaching methods to print material for the hearing impaired. Print material lends itself mainly to learning in the Cognitive Domain. Print material is not as effective in facilitating learning in the Affective and Psychomotor Domains, which require different learning strategies.
    c. Varieties of teaching methods facilitate learning because a variety of senses are stimulated. When we see, hear, and touch, learning is more effective than when we see or hear alone. In addition, research demonstrates that we remember only 10% of what we read, 20% of what we hear, 30% of what we see, 50% of what we see and hear, and 80% of what we say and do.
    d. A group setting would be the least desirable teaching format for hearing-impaired individuals. One-on-one learning sessions limit background noise and distractions that hinder learning. In addition, a one-on-one session allows for individual feedback that ensures that the message is received as intended.

33. a. Physical rewards or incentives support an external, not internal, locus of control. People who are motivated by an external locus of control need to receive some form of praise or reward from an outside source.
    b. Praise supports an external, not internal, locus of control. People who are motivated by an external locus of control need to receive some form of praise or reward from an outside source.
    c. This reflects an action that supports an internal locus of control. A patient who is motivated by the desire for personal growth or self-

satisfaction rather than the approval of others or some external reward has an internal locus of control.

d. Gold stars support an external, not internal, locus of control. People who are motivated by an external locus of control need to receive some form of praise or reward from an outside source.

34. a. This is an example of learning on the Knowledge Level in the Cognitive, not Affective, Domain. Cognitive learning involves the intellect and requires thinking. It increases in complexity from knowledge to comprehension, application, analysis, synthesis, and evaluation of information.

b. **This is an example of learning on the Valuing Level in the Affective Domain.** Valuing is demonstrated when learning is incorporated into the learner's behavior because it is perceived as important. Affective learning involves the expression of feelings and the changing of beliefs, attitudes, or values. Affective learning increases in complexity from receiving to responding, valuing, organizing, and characterizing.

c. This is an example of learning on the Knowledge Level in the Cognitive, not Affective, Domain. Cognitive learning involves the intellect and requires thinking. It increases in complexity from knowledge to comprehension, application, analysis, synthesis, and evaluation of information.

d. This is not an outcome demonstrating learning. This is an example of a question a learner might ask when learning content on the Knowledge Level in the Cognitive Domain. Cognitive learning involves the intellect and requires thinking. It increases in complexity from knowledge to comprehension, application, analysis, synthesis, and evaluation of information.

35. a. This technique is least likely to be used by adults preparing to retire. Role-playing is most often used when learning parenting and other interpersonal skills such as interviewing.

b. This technique is least likely to be used by adults preparing for knee replacement surgery. Role-playing is most often used when learning parenting and other interpersonal skills such as interviewing.

c. Men who are unwilling to admit that they have a drinking problem are not demonstrating readiness to learn. In addition, role-playing requires a person to assume a role for the purpose of learning a new behavior. These men are demonstrating an unwillingness to learn new behavior.

d. **This group would benefit most from role-playing.** Role-playing provides a safe environment in which to practice interpersonal skills. It enables the adolescent to rehearse what should be said, learn to respond to the emotional environment, and experience the pressures of the person playing the peer using drugs.

36. a. Twenty percent of Americans read at or below the fifth-grade reading level and are considered functionally illiterate. Studies demonstrate that people generally read 3 to 5 grades below their highest grade of education.

b. Randomized studies demonstrate that the average reading level of individuals who need health teaching is 6.8 grades of schooling.

c. The eighth-grade reading level is too high a reading level for educational medical material. Randomized studies demonstrate that only 22% of individuals needing health teaching are able to profit from written health materials on the eighth-grade reading level.

d. **The tenth-grade reading level is too high a reading level for educational medical material.** Twenty percent of Americans read at or below the fifth-grade reading level and are considered functionally illiterate.

37. a. **Learners progress through a program at their own pace viewing informational material, answering questions, and receiving immediate feedback. Some programs feature simulated situations that require critical thinking and a response. Correct responses are rationalized, praise is offered, and incorrect responses trigger an explanation of why the wrong answer is wrong and offer encouragement to try again. This is a superior teaching strategy for the learner who may find that group lessons are paced either too fast or too slow for effective learning.**

b. Computer assisted instruction (CAI) is not the least inexpensive teaching strategy. CAI requires a computer, keyboard and station, software, technical support to install, maintain, and repair equipment, and a computer-literate teaching staff to preview, select, and implement CAI programs.

c. Although individual computer assisted programs (CAI) often include pre- and post-testing components, it is not the greatest advantage of CAI as a teaching strategy.

d. Although computer assisted programs (CAI) generally are well organized in a programmed instruction (step-by-step) format, it is not the greatest advantage of using CAI as a teaching strategy.

38. a. When a person achieves the ability to perform a behavior with confidence (demonstrates a well-balanced stance with crutches), learning has been achieved on the Mechanism Level.

b. When the patient is able to identify the correct equipment for a colostomy irrigation, a readiness for action has been demonstrated. This example indicates learning on the Set Level of the Psychomotor Domain.

c. **This option reflects the highest level of learning of the options offered. When a person achieves the ability to perform a behavior that requires a complex movement pattern with confidence, learning has been achieved on the Complex-Overt Response Level of learning in the Psychomotor Domain.**

d. When a person achieves the ability to perform a behavior with confidence (recognize the difference between systolic and diastolic blood pressure sounds), learning has been achieved on the Mechanism Level.

39. a. Although previous experience is important to know

when designing a teaching program, it is not as important as another option when determining whether a teaching program is needed.

b. **Readiness to learn and motivation, which are closely tied together, are the two most important factors contributing to the success of any learning program. The learner must recognize that the learning need exists and that the material to be learned is valuable.**

c. Although expectations are important to know so the teacher can incorporate them into the teaching plan, particularly when goal-setting, it is not as important as another option when determining whether a teaching program is needed.

d. Although it is important to know how flexible a patient is when designing a teaching plan, particularly when goal-setting, it is not as important as another option when determining whether a teaching program is needed.

40. a. Demonstrations are generally used for teaching a skill. Skills involve learning about equipment, rationales and sequencing multiple steps and are too cognitively complex for the developmental abilities of a preschooler. A teaching method in another option is more age-appropriate for a preschooler.

b. **This is the best approach because it requires preschoolers to be active participants in their own learning. In addition, the child has a product to take home and be proud of, it reduces anxiety associated with learning because coloring is an activity most preschoolers are familiar with, and it is within a preschooler's cognitive level.**

c. Preschoolers are just beginning to interact with peers, have a short attention span, and get distracted easily, and therefore need a one-on-one relationship with the teacher. The teacher facilitates the learning specifically for the individual, keeps the learner focused, and permits reinforcement on the learner's cognitive level. Other age-specific strategies include games, storybooks, the use of dolls, puppets or toys, and role-playing.

d. A video requires concentration and an attention span that may be beyond the developmental abilities of a preschooler.

41. a. This is not an example of a continuing education program. Continuing education (CE) refers to formal professional development experiences designed to enhance the knowledge or skills of practitioners.

b. **Mandated programs are an example of an inservice education program. Inservice programs generally are provided by healthcare agencies to reinforce current knowledge and skills or provide new information about such things as policies, theory, skills, practice or equipment.**

c. This is not an example of a certification program. The American Nurses Association has a certification program where nurses can demonstrate minimum competence in specialty areas. Achievement of certification demonstrates advanced expertise and a commitment to ensuring competence.

d. This is not an example of an orientation program. An orientation program is provided by a healthcare agency to introduce new employees to the policies, procedures, departments, services, table of organization, expectations, equipment, etc. within the agency.

42. a. This is not the first thing the nurse should do. In addition, many in the pain management field believe that pain on a level of "4" should receive pharmacologic intervention.

b. **This is the first thing the nurse should do. Pain on a level of "4" depletes energy, interferes with concentration and comprehension, and requires immediate pain relief measures.**

c. Distraction is used to reduce the perception of pain when pain is mild. A pain level of "4" is considered moderate pain, and distraction is less effective on this level. In addition, distraction techniques include watching television, listening to the radio, rocking, slow rhythmic breathing, not learning new content that requires concentration and attention.

d. Although medicating the patient is appropriate, continuing with the teaching session is inappropriate. Generally when people are medicated to relieve pain, time is necessary to have the medication take effect and provide rest to recover from the painful experience.

43. a. Intelligence may actually increase, not decrease, as one ages. However, declining functional abilities may alter learning, and debilitating diseases may impair the intellectual functioning of some individuals and thus weaken their ability to learn.

b. Although it is important to assess a patient's experience before implementing a teaching plan, it is not the first thing the nurse should do of the options offered.

c. **If the patient does not recognize the need to learn or value the information to be learned, the patient will not be ready to learn.**

d. Although it is important to assess a patient's strengths before implementing a teaching plan, it is not the first thing the nurse should do of the options offered.

44. a. Although a teaching program must be designed within the patient's developmental and cognitive abilities, it is not the most relevant factor when predicting success of the options presented.

b. Although this is important, it is not the most relevant factor when predicting success of the options presented.

c. Although family support is important, it is not the most relevant factor when predicting success of the options presented. Not all patients have a family support system.

d. **The motivation of the learner to acquire new attitudes, information, or skills is the most important component for successful learning; motivation exists when the learner recognizes the future benefits of learning.**

45. a. Although fear will affect the success of a teaching program and will need to be assessed and modifications employed, it is not the factor that will have the greatest impact on the future success of a teaching program. Fear that causes mild anxiety is motivating. Fear that causes moderate anxiety will motivate a patient to learn but may require the nurse

to keep concepts and approaches simple. The person with moderate anxiety may need to be focused and distractions minimized to facilitate learning. If fear causes severe anxiety or panic, the teaching program will have to be postponed until the patient is less anxious.

b. **Of all the options presented, the patient in denial is the person least ready and motivated to learn. The patient in denial is unable to recognize the need for the learning.**

c. Fatigue is a physiologic, not psychosocial, adaptation to an illness. When teaching, the nurse needs to assess the patient's stamina and modify the teaching program so as not to unduly stress the patient, and yet meet the objectives.

d. Although anxiety is important, it is not the factor that has the greatest impact on the future success of a teaching program. Mild anxiety is motivating. Moderate anxiety will motivate a patient to learn but may require the nurse to keep concepts and approaches simple. The person with moderate anxiety may need to be focused, and distractions minimized to facilitate learning. If fear causes severe anxiety or panic, the teaching program will have to be postponed until the patient is less anxious.

Essential Components of Nursing Care

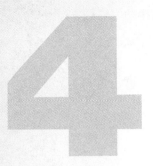

Nursing Process

KEYWORDS

The following words include English vocabulary-, nursing/ medical terminology, concepts, principles, or information relevant to content specifically addressed in the chapter or associated with topics presented in it. English dictionaries, your nursing textbooks, and medical dictionaries such as *Taber's Cyclopedic Medical Dictionary* are resources that can be used to expand your knowledge and understanding of these words and related information.

Achievement
Actual outcome
Analyze
Assessment
Care plan conferences
Care plan types
   Individualized
   Standardized
   Computerized
   Case management
   Clinical pathway
Cluster of data
Collaborative problem
Conclusion
Contributing factor
Corrective action
Database
Data collection methods
   Interview
   Inspection
   Observation
   Palpation
   Percussion
   Examination
   Auscultation
Decision-making process
Deductive reasoning
Defining characteristic
Dependent functions of the nurse
Diagnostic label
Diagnostic reasoning process
Discharge planning
Documentation of care

Dynamic
Effective
Etiology
Evaluation
Expected outcome
Formulate
Goal
Goal—components
   Achievable
   Measurable
   Realistic
   Time frame
   Parameters
Gordon's Functional Health Patterns
Holistic Identity
Implementation
Independent functions of the nurse
Inductive reasoning
Inference
Information-processing theory
Interdependent functions of the nurse
Interpret
Intervention skills
   Teaching
   Collaborating
   Managing
   Coordinating
   Monitoring
   Assisting
   Supporting
   Protecting
   Sustaining
Medical diagnosis

Medical record, parts of
   History and Physical
   Admission Sheet
   Progress notes
   Flow sheets
   Doctor's orders
   Consents
   Laboratory results
   Medication administration record
Nursing care plan
Nursing Diagnosis
Nursing Process
Objective data
Organize
Policy
Primary source
Priority
Problem statement
Procedure
Protocols
Rationale
Risk factors
Secondary source
Secondary to factor
Significance
Signs
Standards of practice
Subjective data
Symptoms
Taxonomy
Variance

1. When two nursing diagnoses appear closely related what should the nurse do first to determine which diagnosis most accurately reflects the needs of the patient?
   a. Reassess the patient
   b. Examine the *related to* factors
   c. Analyze the *secondary to* factors
   d. Review the defining characteristics

2. The nurse completes an admission assessment primarily to:
   a. Diagnose if the patient is at risk for falls
   b. Ensure that the patient's skin is intact
   c. Establish a therapeutic relationship
   d. Identify clusters of data

3. Which statement by the patient is an example of subjective data?
   a. "I'm not sure that I am going to be able to manage at home by myself."
   b. "I can call Home Care Services if I feel I need help at home."
   c. "What should I do if I have uncontrollable pain at home?"
   d. "A home health aide will help me with my care at home."

4. Evaluation relates most directly to which aspect of the Nursing Process?
   a. Goal
   b. Problem
   c. Etiology
   d. Implementation

5. What step of the Nursing Process is being used when the nurse comes to the conclusion that a patient's elevated temperature, pulse, and respirations may be interrelated?
   a. Implementation
   b. Assessment
   c. Evaluation
   d. Diagnosis

6. The most appropriate goal associated with medications is: "The patient will:
   a. Be taught the common side effects of medications."
   b. Have a good understanding of the drugs ordered."
   c. Self-administer medications correctly in 1 week."
   d. Be administered medications as ordered."

7. When considering the Nursing Process "identify" is to "recognize" as "do" is to:
   a. Plan
   b. Evaluate
   c. Diagnose
   d. Implement

8. Which data collection method is best when assessing for subjective data associated with a patient's anxiety?
   a. Observing
   b. Inspecting
   c. Auscultation
   d. Interviewing

9. Which action reflects an activity associated with the diagnosing step of the Nursing Process?
   a. Formulating a plan of care
   b. Identifying the patient's potential risks
   c. Designing ways to minimize a patient's stressors
   d. Making decisions about the effectiveness of patient care

10. What step of the Nursing Process is being used when the nurse says to a newly admitted patient, "You look tired"?
    a. Diagnosis
    b. Evaluation
    c. Assessment
    d. Implementation

11. Which would be an example of objective data? The patient:
    a. Is anorexic
    b. Feels warm
    c. Ate half of lunch
    d. Has the urge to void

12. Which is an example of subjective data? The patient states:
    a. "I just went in the urinal and it needs to be emptied."
    b. "My pain feels like a "5" on a scale of 1 to 5."
    c. "The doctor said I can go home today."
    d. "I only ate half my breakfast."

13. During which of the five steps in the Nursing Process are outcomes of care determined to be achieved?
    a. Implementation
    b. Evaluation
    c. Diagnosis
    d. Planning

14. When considering the Nursing Process "observe" is to "assess" as "determine" is to:
    a. Plan
    b. Analyze
    c. Diagnose
    d. Implement

15. An essential concept related to understanding the Nursing Process is that it:
    a. Is dynamic rather than static
    b. Focuses on the role of the nurse
    c. Moves from the simple to the complex
    d. Is based on the patient's medical problem

16. Which is the most accurately stated goal? "The patient will:
    a. Be taught how to use a urinal when on bed rest."
    b. Experience fewer incontinence episodes at night."
    c. Be assisted to the toilet every two hours and whenever necessary."
    d. Transfer independently and safely to a commode before discharge."

17. Which word best describes the role of the nurse when identifying and meeting the needs of the patient holistically?
    a. Teacher
    b. Advocate
    c. Counselor
    d. Surrogate

18. The word most closely associated with scientific principles is:
    a. Data
    b. Problem
    c. Rationale
    d. Evaluation

19. Which part of the nursing diagnosis is most directly related to the concept of a pebble dropped into a pond causing ripples on the surface of the water?
    a. Defining characteristics
    b. Outcome criteria
    c. Etiology
    d. Goal

20. Which would be an example of subjective data?
    a. Jaundice
    b. Dizziness
    c. Diaphoresis
    d. Hypotension

21. The patient comes to the Emergency Department complaining of chest pain and dyspnea. When taking the patient's vital signs the nurse is:
    a. **Assessing**
    b. Evaluating
    c. Diagnosing
    d. Implementing

22. Which statement by the nurse is an inference? The patient is:
    a. Hypotensive
    b. **Withdrawn**
    c. Jaundiced
    d. Oliguric

23. What step of the Nursing Process is being used when the nurse teaches a patient the use of visualization to cope with chronic pain?
    a. Planning
    b. Diagnosis
    c. Evaluation
    d. **Implementation**

24. Where in the patient's chart would the nurse find documentation of the current medical diagnosis?
    a. Physician's History and Physical
    b. Social Service Record
    c. Admission Sheet
    d. **Progress Notes**

25. During which of the five steps in the Nursing Process are data analyzed critically?
    a. **Diagnosis**
    b. Clustering
    c. Collection
    d. Assessment

26. Which is a well-designed goal? The patient will:
    a. Have a lower temperature
    b. Be given aspirin Gr. X q8hrs prn
    c. Be taught how to take an accurate temperature
    d. **Maintain fluid intake sufficient to prevent dehydration**

27. During the evaluation step of the Nursing Process the nurse must:
    a. Establish outcomes
    b. Determine priorities
    c. **Take corrective action**
    d. Set the time frames for goals

28. Determining what nursing actions will be employed occurs in which step of the Nursing Process?
    a. Implementation
    b. Assessment
    c. Diagnosis
    d. **Planning**

29. When considering the Nursing Process the words "present" is to "future" as "plan" is to:
    a. Diagnosis
    b. **Implement**
    c. Evaluation
    d. Assessment

30. The appropriateness of a Nursing Diagnosis is supported by its:
    a. **Defining characteristics**
    b. Planned interventions
    c. Diagnostic statement
    d. Related risk factors

31. The primary goal of the assessment phase of the Nursing Process is to:
    a. Build trust and rapport with the patient
    b. Identify goals and outcomes with the patient
    c. Collect and organize information about the patient
    d. Identify and validate the patient's medical diagnosis

32. Which would be an example of objective data?
    a. Pain of "5" on a 1-to-10 pain scale
    b. Irregular radial pulse
    c. Shortness of breath
    d. Dizziness

33. What step in the Nursing Process is being used when the nurse who is assisting a postoperative patient to ambulate says, "You look tired?"
    a. Diagnosis
    b. Evaluation
    c. Assessment
    d. Implementation

34. The Planning step of the Nursing Process is most directly influenced by the:
    a. Related factors
    b. Diagnostic label
    c. Medical diagnosis
    d. Secondary factors

35. Once data is collected, the nurse then:
    a. Writes a patient-centered goal
    b. Formulates a nursing diagnosis
    c. Designs a plan of nursing interventions
    d. Determines the significance of the information

1.
   a. If a thorough assessment is completed initially, a reassessment should not be necessary.
   b. To establish which of two nursing diagnoses is most appropriate is not dependent upon identifying the factors that *contributed to* (also known as *related to* or *etiology of*) the nursing problem. These factors are identified after the problem statement is identified.
   c. To establish which of two nursing diagnoses is more appropriate is not dependent upon analyzing the *secondary to* factors. *Secondary to* factors are generally medical conditions that precipitate the *related to* factors. The *secondary to* factors are identified after the *related to* factors of the problem are identified.
   d. **The first thing the nurse should do to differentiate between two closely associated nursing diagnoses is to compare the data collected to the major and minor defining characteristics of each of the nursing diagnoses being considered.**

2.
   a. Data must be collected and significance determined before a nursing diagnosis can be made.
   b. Although completing a nursing admission assessment includes an assessment of the skin, it is only one component of the assessment.
   c. Although completing a nursing admission assessment helps to initiate the nurse-patient relationship, it is not the primary purpose of completing a nursing admission assessment.
   d. **This is the primary purpose of a nursing admission assessment. Data must be collected, analyzed to determine significance, and grouped in meaningful clusters before a nursing diagnosis can be made.**

3.
   a. **This is subjective information because it is the patient's perception and can be verified only by the patient. Subjective data are those adaptations, feelings, beliefs, preferences, and information that only the patient can confirm.**
   b. This is neither subjective nor objective. It is a statement indicating an understanding of how to seek home care services after discharge.
   c. This is neither subjective nor objective. It is a question indicating that the patient wants more information about how to control pain when at home.
   d. This is neither subjective nor objective. It is a patient statement indicating an understanding of who will provide assistance with care once the patient goes home.

4.
   a. **To evaluate the effectiveness of a nursing action, the nurse needs to compare the *actual* patient outcome with the *expected* patient outcome. The expected outcomes are the measurable data that reflect goal achievement, and the actual outcomes are what really happened.**
   b. The problem is associated with the first half (problem statement) of the Nursing Diagnosis, not the Evaluation, step of the Nursing Process.
   c. Etiology is a term used to identify the factors that *relate to* the problem statement of the Nursing Diagnosis, not the Evaluation, step of the Nursing Process.
   d. Implementation is a step separate from Evaluation in the Nursing Process. Nursing care must be implemented before it can be evaluated.

5.
   a. This is not an example of the Implementation step of the Nursing Process. During the Implementation step, nursing care that is planned is delivered.
   b. This is not an example of the Assessment step of the Nursing Process. Although data may be gathered during the Assessment step, the manipulation of the data is conducted in a different step of the Nursing Process.
   c. This is not an example of the Evaluation step of the Nursing Process. Evaluation occurs when actual outcomes are compared with expected outcomes, which reflect attainment of the goal.
   d. **During the Diagnosis step of the Nursing Process, data are critically analyzed and interpreted; significance of data is determined; inferences are made and validated; cues and clusters of cues are compared with the defining characteristics of nursing diagnoses; contributing factors are identified; and nursing diagnoses are identified and organized in order of priority.**

6.
   a. This is an action the nurse plans to implement; it does not identify a patient goal or expected outcome.
   b. This goal is inappropriate because the word *good* is not specific, measurable, or objective.
   c. **This is a well written goal. Goals must be patient-centered, measurable, realistic, and indicate the time frame in which the expected outcome is to be accomplished. The word *correctly* implies that critical elements are used as standards to measure the patient's actions when self-administering medications.**
   d. This is an action the nurse plans to implement; it does not identify a patient goal or expected outcome.

7.
   a. The words *identify* and *recognize* have the same definition. They both mean the same as that which is known. The word *plan* does not fit the analogy because the definitions of *plan* and *do* are different. The word *plan* means a method of proceeding. The word *do* means to carry into effect or to accomplish.
   b. The words *identify* and *recognize* have the same definition. They both mean the same as that which is known. The word *evaluate* does not fit the analogy because the definitions of *evaluate* and *do* are different. The word *evaluate* means to determine the worth of something, whereas the word *do* means to carry into effect or to accomplish.
   c. The words *identify* and *recognize* have the same definition. They both mean the same as that which is known. The word *diagnose* does not fit the analogy because the definitions of *diagnose* and *do* are different. The word *diagnose* means to identify the patient's human response to an actual or potential health problem. The word *do* means to carry into effect or to accomplish.
   d. **This is the correct analogy. The words *identify***

and *recognize* have the same definition. They both mean the same as that which is known. The words *do* and *implement* both have the same definition. They both mean to carry out some action.

8. a. Observation is the deliberate use of all the senses, and involves more than just inspection and examination. It includes surveying, looking, scanning, scrutinizing, and appraising. Although the nurse makes inferences based on data collected by observation, this is not as effective as another data collection method to identify subjective data associated with a patient's anxiety

   b. Inspection involves the act of making observations of physical features and behavior. Although the nurse observes behaviors and makes inferences based on their perceived meaning, another data collection method is more effective in identifying subjective data associated with a patient's anxiety.

   c. Auscultation is listening for sounds within the body. This collects objective, not subjective, data, which are measurable.

   d. **Interviewing a patient is the most effective data collection method when collecting subjective data associated with a patient's anxiety. The patient is the primary source for subjective data about beliefs, values, feelings, perceptions, and fears and concerns.**

9. a. This occurs during the Planning, not Diagnosis, step of the Nursing Process.

   b. **Potential risk factors are identified during the Diagnosis step of the Nursing Process. Risk diagnoses are designed to address situations where patients have a particular vulnerability to health problems.**

   c. This occurs during the Planning, not Diagnosis, step of the Nursing Process.

   d. This occurs during the Evaluation, not Diagnosis, step of the Nursing Process.

10. a. This is not a Nursing Diagnosis. Fatigue, Activity Intolerance, Disturbed Sleep Pattern, and Sleep Deprivation are just a few examples of Nursing Diagnoses associated with a patient's looking tired.

    b. This is not Evaluation. Evaluation occurs when the nurse assesses a patient's response to an intervention. This patient is newly admitted, and nursing care has not yet been planned or implemented.

    c. **This statement is an example of the use of the interviewing skill of clarification to obtain baseline information about the patient during the Assessment step of the Nursing Process.**

    d. This is not Implementation. Implementation occurs when the nurse provides nursing care identified in the patient's nursing plan of care.

11. a. Loss of appetite (anorexia) is an example of subjective, not objective, data. Subjective data are those adaptations, feelings, beliefs, preferences, and information that only the patient can confirm.

    b. Feeling warm is an example of subjective, not objective, data. Subjective data are those adaptations, feelings, beliefs, preferences, and information that only the patient can confirm.

    c. The amount of food eaten by a patient can be objectively verified. The nurse measures and documents the percentage of a meal ingested by a patient to quantify the amount of food consumed.

    d. Having the urge to void is an example of subjective, not objective, data. Subjective data are those adaptations, feelings, beliefs, preferences, and information that only the patient can confirm.

12. a. This is an objective, not subjective, statement indicating something that is checkable and measurable. Objective data can be verified.

    b. **A patient's perception about a pain level is subjective information. Subjective data are those adaptations, feelings, beliefs, preferences, and information that only the patient can confirm.**

    c. This is an objective, not subjective, statement indicating something that is checkable and measurable. Objective data can be verified.

    d. This is an objective, not subjective, statement indicating something that is checkable and measurable. Objective data can be verified.

13. a. During the Implementation step of the Nursing Process, outcomes are not determined, but rather nursing care that has been planned is delivered.

    b. **Evaluation occurs when actual outcomes are compared with expected outcomes that reflect goal achievement. If the goal is achieved, the patient's needs are met.**

    c. During the Diagnosis step of the Nursing Process, outcomes are not determined; rather, the nurse diagnoses human responses to actual or potential health problems.

    d. During the Planning step of the Nursing Process, expected outcomes are determined, but their achievement is measured in another step of the Nursing Process.

14. a. The definitions of the words *observe* and *assess* are similar. Observe means to examine something scientifically, and assess means to determine the significance of something. The word *plan* does not fit the analogy because the definitions of the words *plan* and *determine* are not similar. *Determine* means to reach a decision. *Plan* means to carry into effect or to accomplish.

    b. The definitions of the words *observe* and *assess* are similar. *Observe* means to examine something scientifically, and *assess* means to determine the significance of something. The word *analyze* does not fit the analogy because *analyze* is not a step in the Nursing Process. The steps in the Nursing Process are Assessment, Diagnosis, Planning, Implementation, and Evaluation.

    c. **The definitions of the words *observe* and *assess* are similar. *Observe* means to examine something scientifically, and *assess* means to determine the significance of something. The word *diagnose* appropriately completes the analogy because the definitions of *determine* and *diagnose* are similar. *Determine* means to reach a decision about something and *diagnose* means to make a decision based on the assessment and analysis of a human response.**

d. The definitions of the words *observe* and *assess* are similar. *Observe* means to examine something scientifically, and *assess* means to determine the significance of something. The word *implement* does not fit the analogy because the definitions of *determine* and *implement* are not similar. *Determine* means to reach a decision about something and *implement* means to carry out some action.

15. a. **The Nursing Process is a dynamic five-step problem-solving process (Assessment, Diagnosis, Planning, Implementation, and Evaluation) designed to diagnose and treat human responses to health problems. It is constantly changing in response to the changing needs of the patient.**
    b. The Nursing Process focuses on the needs of the patient, not the role of the nurse.
    c. Moving from the simple to the complex is a principle of teaching, not the Nursing Process. The Nursing Process is a complex interactive five step problem-solving process designed to meet a patient's needs. It requires an understanding of systems and information-processing theory, and the critical-thinking, problem-solving, decision-making, and diagnostic-reasoning processes.
    d. The Nursing Process is concerned with a person's human responses to actual or potential health problems, not the patient's medical problem.

16. a. This is not a goal. This is an action the nurse plans to implement to help a patient achieve a goal.
    b. This goal is inappropriate because the word *fewer* is not specific, measurable, or objective.
    c. This is not a goal. This is an action the nurse plans to implement to help a patient achieve a goal.
    d. **This is a correctly worded goal. Goals must be patient-centered, measurable, realistic, and include the time frame in which the expected goal is to be achieved. The word *independently* indicates that no help is needed, and the word *safely* indicates that no injury will occur.**

17. a. Although functioning as a teacher is an important role of the nurse, it is a limited role compared to another option. As a teacher the nurse helps the patient gain new knowledge about health and health care to maintain or restore health.
    b. **When the nurse supports, protects, and defends a patient from a holistic perspective, the nurse functions as an advocate. Advocacy includes exploring, informing, mediating, and affirming in all areas to help a patient navigate the health care system, maintain autonomy, and achieve the best possible health outcomes.**
    c. Although functioning as a counselor is an important role of the nurse, it is a limited role compared to another option. As counselor the nurse helps the patient improve interpersonal relationships, recognize and deal with stressful psychosocial problems, and promote achievement of self-actualization.
    d. The word surrogate is not the word that best describes this scenario. The nurse is placed in the surrogate role when a patient projects onto the nurse the image of another and then responds to the nurse with the feelings for the image.

18. a. The word *data* (evidence or information) is not associated with the term *scientific principles* (established rules of action).
    b. The word *problem* (difficulty or crisis) is not associated with the term *scientific principles* (established rules of action).
    c. **The word *rationale* (justification based on reasoning) is closely associated with the term *scientific principles* (established rules of action). Scientific principles are based on rationales.**
    d. The word *evaluation* (determining the value or worth of something) is not associated with the term *scientific principles* (established rules of action).

19. a. Defining characteristics do not contribute to the problem statement but support or indicate the presence of the nursing diagnosis. Defining characteristics are the major and minor clinical cues that support the presence of a nursing diagnosis.
    b. Outcome criteria are not a part of the nursing diagnosis. Outcome criteria (goals) are part of the Planning step of the Nursing Process.
    c. **The etiology (also known as related or contributing factors) are the conditions, situations, or circumstances that add to the development of the human response identified in the problem statement of the nursing diagnosis. The etiology precipitates the problem just as a pebble dropped in a pond causes ripples on the surface of water.**
    d. Goals are not part of the nursing diagnosis. Goals are the expected outcomes or what is hoped that the patient will achieve in response to nursing intervention.

20. a. A yellow color of the skin, whites of the eyes, and mucous membranes (jaundice) because of deposition of bile pigments from excess bilirubin in the blood is objective, not subjective, information. Objective data are measurable and checkable.
    b. **This is subjective information because it is the patient's perception and can be verified only by the patient. Subjective data are those adaptations, feelings, beliefs, preferences, and information that only the patient can confirm.**
    c. Excessive sweating (diaphoresis) is objective, not subjective, information. Objective data are measurable and checkable.
    d. Abnormally low systolic and diastolic blood pressure levels (hypotension) can be measured and verified and are therefore objective data.

21. a. **This is correct. During the Assessment step of the Nursing Process data are collected from different sources using various methods such as physical examination, interviewing, and observation. As data are collected, they are clustered into groups that have a relationship.**
    b. Evaluation occurs during the Nursing Process when the nurse assesses a patient's response to an intervention, not when collecting baseline data about a patient's status.
    c. Taking a patient's vital signs is not an example of diagnosing. During the Diagnosis step of the Nursing Process, data are critically analyzed, interpreted, and significance determined; inferences

are made and validated; cues and clusters of cues are compared with the defining characteristics of nursing diagnoses; contributing factors are identified; and nursing diagnoses are identified and organized in order of priority.

    d. This scenario is not an example of the Implementation step of the Nursing Process. Implementation occurs when the plan of care is put into action and nursing care is actually delivered.

22. a. A low blood pressure is an adaptation that can be measured objectively and is not an inference.
    b. The nurse makes an inference when making the statement, "The patient is withdrawn." This inference is based on a pattern of behavior such as lack of eye contact, somnolence (sleepiness), emotional lack of interest, apathy, and the patient's verbalization of defeat.
    c. A yellow color to the skin, mucous membranes, and whites of the eyes as a result of deposition of bile pigment resulting from excess bilirubin in the blood is called jaundice. The presence of bilirubin can be measured objectively by a blood test (serum bilirubin) and is not an inference.
    d. A patient's experiencing urine output of less than 500 cc per 24 hours (oliguria) is measurable and therefore not an inference.

23. a. This is not an example of the Planning step of the Nursing Process. During the Planning step, the nurse identifies and plans the nursing interventions that seem most likely to be effective.
    b. This is not an example of the Diagnosis step of the Nursing Process. During the Diagnosis step of the Nursing Process, data are critically analyzed and interpreted; significance of data are determined; inferences are made and validated; cues and clusters of cues are compared with the defining characteristics of nursing diagnoses; contributing factors are identified; and nursing diagnoses are identified and organized in order of priority.
    c. This is not an example of the Evaluation step of the Nursing Process. Evaluation occurs when actual outcomes are compared with expected outcomes that reflect goal achievement.
    d. This is an example of the Implementation step of the Nursing Process. During the Implementation step, nursing care that is planned is delivered.

24. a. The Physician's History and Physical contains a history of the patient, a physical, and the medical problems on the day of admission to the hospital. The admission medical diagnosis may be different after diagnostic tests are completed.
    b. Although the patient's medical diagnosis might be documented on the patient's Social Service Record, it is not the major source for this information.
    c. This is the best source for identifying the patient's admitting medical diagnosis, but it will not contain the current medical diagnosis if the diagnosis changed after completion of diagnostic tests.
    d. Generally the Progress Notes contain documentation by all members of the health team. After a patient is admitted and diagnostic tests completed, the patient's medical diagnosis

may change. The on-going changes and current status of the patient are documented in the Progress Notes.

25. a. During the Diagnosis step of the Nursing Process, data are critically analyzed and interpreted; significance of data is determined; inferences are made and validated; cues and clusters of cues are compared with the defining characteristics of nursing diagnoses; contributing factors are identified; and nursing diagnoses are identified and organized in order of priority.
    b. Clustering is not a step in the Nursing Process. Clustering occurs during the Assessment step and is a precursor to critical analysis, which occurs in the next step of the Nursing Process.
    c. Collection is not a step in the Nursing Process. During the Assessment step data is collected from different sources using various methods and then it is generally clustered into groups that have a relationship.
    d. During the Assessment step of the Nursing Process data are collected from different sources using various methods. As data are collected they are generally clustered into groups that have a relationship. Although clustering requires interpretation of data, critical analysis of data occurs in the next step of the Nursing Process.

26. a. This goal is inappropriate because the word *lower* is not specific, measurable, or objective.
    b. This is not a goal. This is an action the nurse plans to implement to help a patient achieve a goal.
    c. This is not a goal. This is an action the nurse plans to implement to help a patient achieve a goal.
    d. This is a well written goal. Goals must be patient-centered, specific, measurable, realistic, and have a time frame in which the expected outcome is to be achieved. The words *sufficient* and *dehydration* are based on generally accepted criteria against which to measure the patient's actual outcome. The word *maintain* connotes continuously, which is a time frame.

27. a. Establishing outcomes is part of the Planning, not Evaluation, step of the Nursing Process.
    b. Determining priorities is part of the Diagnosis, not Evaluation, step of the Nursing Process. Priority setting is a decision-making process that ranks a patient's nursing diagnoses in order of importance.
    c. Corrective action takes place in the Evaluation step of the Nursing Process. If during evaluation it is determined that the goal was not met, the reasons for failure have to be identified and the plan modified.
    d. Setting time frames for goals to be achieved is part of the Planning, not Evaluation, step of the Nursing Process.

28. a. This does not occur during the Implementation step of the Nursing Process. During the Implementation step the nurse puts the plan of care into action. Nursing interventions include actions that are dependent (requiring a physician's order), independent (autonomous actions within the nurse's scope of practice), and interdependent (interventions

that require a physician's order but that permit the nurse to use clinical judgment in their implementation).

b. This does not occur during the Assessment step of the Nursing Process. During the Assessment step the nurse uses various skills such as observation, interviewing, and physical examination to collect data from various sources.

c. This does not occur during the Nursing Diagnosis step of the Nursing Process. A nursing Diagnosis is made when the nurse identifies the patient's human responses to actual or potential health problems.

d. **Nursing actions designed to help a patient achieve a goal occur during the Planning step of the Nursing Process.**

29. a. In the first half of the analogy, the *present* happens before the *future*. In the second part of the analogy, *Diagnosis* does not fit because *Planning* in the Nursing Process happens after, not before, the *Nursing Diagnosis*.

b. **The word *implement* appropriately completes the analogy. In the first half of the analogy, the *present* happens before the *future*. In the second part of the analogy, *Planning* happens immediately before *Implementation* in the Nursing Process.**

c. In the first half of the analogy, the *present* happens before the *future*. In the second part of the analogy, *Evaluation* does not fit as well as another option. Although *Planning* happens before *Evaluation*, *Evaluation* is not the immediate step after the planning.

d. In the first half of the analogy, the *present* happens before the *future*. In the second part of the analogy, *Assessment* does not fit because *Planning* in the Nursing Process happens after, not before, the *Assessment*.

30. a. **The defining characteristics are the major and minor cues that form a cluster that support or validate the presence of a Nursing Diagnosis. At least one major defining characteristic must be present for a nursing diagnosis to be considered appropriate for the patient.**

b. Planned interventions do not support Nursing Diagnosis. They are the nursing actions designed to help resolve the *related to* factors and achieve expected patient outcomes that reflect goal achievement.

c. The diagnostic statement cannot support the Nursing Diagnosis because it is the first part of the Nursing Diagnosis. A Nursing Diagnosis is made up of two parts, the *diagnostic statement* (also known as *the problem statement)* and the *related to* factors (also known as factors that *contribute to* the problem or *the etiology*).

d. Related risk factors cannot support the Nursing Diagnosis because they are the second part of the nursing diagnosis. A nursing diagnosis is made up of two parts, the diagnostic statement (also known as *the problem statement)* and the *related to* factors (also known as factors that *contribute to* the problem or *the etiology*).

31. a. Although this is true, it is not the primary purpose.

b. When a five-step Nursing Process is followed, identifying goals and outcomes occur during the Planning, not Assessment, step of the Process.

c. **The primary purpose of the Assessment step of the Nursing Process is to collect data from various sources using a variety of approaches. After data are collected, they are clustered into meaningful categories in preparation for the analysis and interpretation that takes place during the Diagnosis step of the Nursing Process.**

d. Identifying and validating the medical diagnosis are not within a Registered Nurse's legal scope of nursing practice.

32. a. A patient's perception about a pain level is an example of subjective, not objective, data. Subjective data are those adaptations, feelings, beliefs, preferences and information that only the patient can confirm.

b. **An irregular radial pulse is objective, not subjective, information. Objective data are measurable and checkable.**

c. A patient's complaint about shortness of breath is an example of subjective, not objective, data. Subjective data are those adaptations, feelings, beliefs, preferences, and information that only the patient can confirm.

d. A patient's complaint about dizziness is an example of subjective, not objective, data. Subjective data are those adaptations, feelings, beliefs, preferences, and information that only the patient can confirm.

33. a. This is not a Nursing Diagnosis. Fatigue and Activity Intolerance are two nursing diagnoses associated with this scenario.

b. **This statement is an attempt to obtain information about a patient's response to an intervention, ambulation. Assessing a patient's tolerance to ambulation is conducted in the Evaluation step of the Nursing Process.**

c. A step other than Assessment is best reflected in this scenario. Assessment occurs in the first step of the Nursing Process before Diagnosis, Planning, Implementation, and Evaluation.

d. When the nurse assists a patient with ambulation, the nurse is implementing, not evaluating, the nursing plan of care.

34. a. **Related factors contribute to the problem statement of the Nursing Diagnosis and directly impact on the Planning step of the Nursing Process. Nursing interventions are selected to minimize or relieve the effects of the related factors. If nursing interventions are appropriate and effective, the human response identified in the problem statement part of the Nursing Diagnosis will be resolved.**

b. The Planning step of the Nursing Process includes setting a goal, identifying the outcomes that will reflect goal achievement, and planning nursing interventions. Although the wording of the goal is directly influenced by the diagnostic label (problem statement of the Nursing Diagnosis), the selection of nursing interventions is not.

c. The medical diagnosis does not influence the

Planning step of the Nursing Process. The nurse is concerned with *human responses* to actual or potential health problems, not the medical diagnosis.

d. Secondary factors generally have only a minor influence on the Planning step of the Nursing Process.

35. a. Goals are designed after a Nursing Diagnosis is identified, not after data are collected.

b. Once data are collected, the nurse must first organize and cluster the data to determine significance and make inferences. After all this is accomplished, then the nurse can formulate a Nursing Diagnosis.

c. Nursing care is planned after Nursing Diagnoses and goals are identified, not after data are collected.

d. This is correct. After data are collected they are clustered to determine their significance.

Physical Assessment

KEYWORDS

The following words include English vocabulary, nursing/medical terminology, concepts, principles, or information relevant to content specifically addressed in the chapter or associated with topics presented in it. English dictionaries, your nursing textbooks, and medical dictionaries such as *Taber's Cyclopedic Medical Dictionary* are resources that can be used to expand your knowledge and understanding of these words and related information.

Afebrile
Affect
Aneroid manometer
Anterior
Apnea
Arteriosclerosis
Asymptomatic
Attention span
Auscultation
Auscultatory gap
Autonomic nervous system
Balance
Barrel chest
Blood pressure
Blood viscosity
Body weight
Borborygmi
Bowel sounds
Bradycardia
Bradypnea
Breast examination
Breath sounds
  Normal
    Bronchial
    Bronchovesicular
    Vesicular
  Adventitious
    Crackles (rales)
    Gurgles (rhonchi)
    Pleural friction rub
    Stridor
    Wheeze
Capillary refill
Cardiac output
Cheyne-Stokes respirations
Chills
Circadian rhythms
Clubbing
Comatose
Core temperature
Costal breathing (thoracic)

Defervescence
Deformities
Delirium
Dental caries
Dependent edema
Diaphragmatic breathing (abdominal)
Diastolic
Diplopia
Diurnal variations
Doppler
Drowsiness
Ecchymosis
Edema – 1+, 2+, 3+, 4+
Erythema
Erythrocytes
Eupnea
Exacerbation
Examination
Exhalation
External respiration
Febrile
Fever
Functional health patterns
Gait
General Adaptation Syndrome
Health history
Hirsutism
Hyperemia
Hyper/hypotension
Hypovolemic shock
Inhalation
Inspection
Internal respiration
Jaundice
Korotkoff's sounds
Kussmaul respirations
Lateral
Lesion
Lethargy
Leukocytes
Level of consciousness

Local Adaptation Syndrome
Malaise
Memory
Mental status
Mobility
Mood
Neuro-checks
Neutrophils
Night blindness
Objective data
Observation
Orientation
Orthostatic hypotension
Pain assessment scale
Palpation
Pap smear
Papillae on the tongue
Parasympathetic nervous system
Partial thromboplastin time
Percussion
Peripheral vascular resistance
Physical
Plaque
Platelets
Posterior
Posture
Primary source of data
Prostate specific antigens (PSA)
Pruritus
Pulse deficit
Pulse pressure
Pulse sites
  Apical
  Brachial
  Carotid
  Femoral
  Pedal
  Popliteal
  Posterior tibial
  Temporal
  Tibial

Pyrexia
Rash
Red blood cell count
Reflexes
Remission
Sagittal plane
Secondary source of data
Sensation
Shivering
Sigmoidoscopy
Sordes
Sphygmomanometer
Spinal tap
Stance

Stethoscope
Strength
Subjective data
Superior
Symmetry (contour, shape)
Sympathetic nervous system
Systolic
Tachycardia
Tachypnea
Tartar
Texture
Thermometers
　Disposable
　Electronic

Glass
Intravenous catheter
Temperature-sensitive strips
Tympanic
Thrombocytes
Transverse plane
Tremor
Temperature sites
　Axillary
　Oral
　Rectal
Turgor
Urticaria
Variance

QUESTIONS

1. Which adaptation would be most indicative of shock?
   a. Hyperemia
   b. Hypotension
   c. Irregular pulse
   d. Slow respirations

2. When the patient has an irregular pulse the nurse should first monitor the pulse:
   a. At the carotid
   b. With a Doppler
   c. For a full minute
   d. At two different sites

3. The nurse can anticipate a patient's temperature to be at its highest at:
   a. 12–2 AM
   b. 6–8 AM
   c. 4–6 PM
   d. 8–10 PM

4. When assessing for borborygmi, which physical examination method does the nurse use?
   a. Auscultation
   b. Percussion
   c. Inspection
   d. Palpation

5. A patient has a temperature of 102° F and complains of feeling cold. Which additional adaptation would the nurse expect during this onset stage of fever?
   a. Flushed skin
   b. Dehydration
   c. Diaphoresis
   d. Shivering

6. Which method of examination is used when the nurse takes a patient's radial pulse?
   a. Palpation
   b. Inspection
   c. Percussion
   d. Auscultation

7. Which nursing action is common to all instruments when taking a temperature?
   a. Identify that the reading is below 96° F before insertion
   b. Wash with cool soap and water after use
   c. Place a disposable sheath over the probe
   d. Ensure that the instrument is clean

8. It would be most important to assess vital signs when a patient:
   a. Sits on the side of the bed after surgery for the first time
   b. Complains of pressure in the chest
   c. Finishes ambulating in the hallway
   d. Is coughing and sneezing

9. What is a defining characteristic associated with the nursing diagnosis of Hyperthermia?
   a. Mental confusion
   b. Increased appetite
   c. Decreased heart rate
   d. Rectal temperature of 101° F

10. Which assessment takes priority when engaging in an emergency assessment of a patient?
    a. Blood pressure
    b. Airway clearance
    c. Breathing pattern
    d. Circulatory status

11. What should the nurse do before obtaining a urine specimen from a patient with a urinary retention (Foley) catheter?
    a. Cleanse the exit tube at the bottom of the drainage bag with an alcohol swab
    b. Clamp the tubing immediately distal to the collection port
    c. Position the patient in a semi-Fowler's position
    d. Don a pair of clean gloves

12. The information that would be most important to document when taking a blood pressure would be:
    a. Staff member who took the blood pressure
    b. Patient's tolerance to having the blood pressure taken
    c. Position of the patient if the patient is not in a sitting position
    d. Difference between the palpated and auscultated systolic readings

13. Which is a recommended cancer screening guideline for asymptomatic non-risk people?
    a. Prostate-specific antigens yearly for men 30 years of age and older
    b. Mammograms annually for women 30 years of age and older
    c. Pap smears annually for females 13 years of age and older
    d. Sigmoidoscopies every 5 years for patients 50 years of age and older

14. Which would increase heat production?
    a. Vasodilation
    b. Evaporation
    c. Shivering
    d. Radiation

15. Which series of vital signs is most reflective of hypovolemic shock?
    a. P 100, R 24, BP 140/70
    b. P 80, R 22, BP 110/80
    c. P 60, R 20, BP 100/70
    d. P 110, R 26, BP 80/60

16. Which pulse site should not be assessed on both sides of the body at the same time?
    a. Radial
    b. Carotid
    c. Femoral
    d. Brachial

17. Who would most likely have the highest temperature?
    a. A newborn infant
    b. A person with a blood infection
    c. An adolescent who has been doing aerobic exercises
    d. An older adult who just spent 10 minutes in a warm shower

18. Which term best describes a recurrence of symptoms associated with a chronic disease?
    a. Variance
    b. Remission
    c. Adaptation
    d. Exacerbation

19. A temperature would have to be taken via the rectal route for a patient:
    a. Who is a mouth breather
    b. With a history of vomiting
    c. With an intelligence of a 7-year-old child
    d. Who cannot tolerate a semi-Fowler's position

20. When assessing for cyanosis in a dark-skinned person, the nurse should assess the:
    a. Sclera of the eyes
    b. Nail beds of the toes
    c. Lining of the eye lids
    d. Color of the lower legs

21. What action could result in a blood pressure error?
    a. Placing the diaphragm of the stethoscope over the brachial artery
    b. Applying the center of the bladder of the cuff directly over an artery
    c. Ensuring that the bladder of the cuff encircles less than 25% of the arm
    d. Inserting the ear pieces of the stethoscope so that they tilt slightly forwards

22. Which adaptation is associated with a serious Vitamin K deficiency?
    a. Skin lesions
    b. Bleeding gums
    c. Night blindness
    d. Muscle weakness

23. An additional adaptation that would confirm the defervescence (flush) phase of a fever besides skin that feels warm is:
    a. Sweating
    b. Shivering
    c. Cyanotic nail beds
    d. *Goosebumps* on the skin

24. The nurse can anticipate a patient's temperature to be at its lowest at:
    a. 4–6 AM
    b. 8–10 AM
    c. 4–6 PM
    d. 8–10 PM

25. Which method of examination is being used when the nurse's hands are used to assess the temperature of a patient's skin?
    a. Palpation
    b. Inspection
    c. Percussion
    d. Observation

26. To ensure accuracy when assessing for the presence of bowel sounds, the nurse should auscultate the abdomen:
    a. Using a warmed stethoscope
    b. Prior to palpation and percussion
    c. Starting at the left lower quadrant
    d. For at least three minutes in each quadrant

27. Which assessment result would require the nurse to assess the patient further?
    a. A teenager with a pulse rate of 140 after riding 2 miles on an exercise bike
    b. A 50-year-old man with a BP of 112/60 upon awakening in the morning
    c. A 65-year old-man with a respiratory rate of 10
    d. A 40-year-old woman with a pulse of 88

28. The pulse pressure for a patient with a blood pressure of 140/90 is:
   a. 50
   b. 90
   c. 140
   d. 230

29. Which patient statement indicates the onset of a fever? "I feel:
   a. Cold."
   b. Warm."
   c. Sweaty."
   d. Thirsty."

30. The vital sign that would change first indicating that a postoperative patient had internal bleeding would be the:
   a. Body temperature
   b. Blood pressure
   c. Pulse pressure
   d. Heart rate

31. When assessing a patient's strength in preparation for getting out of bed the nurse should:
   a. Ask if the patient is dizzy
   b. Determine if the patient has dependent edema
   c. Instruct the patient to push against leg resistance
   d. Inquire if the patient feels strong enough to get out of bed

32. How often should a patient's temperature be taken who has had a temperature of 101° F for the last 24 hours?
   a. Every 2 hours
   b. Every 4 hours
   c. Every 6 hours
   d. Every 8 hours

33. When a brachial pulse is unable to be palpated, which pulse would indicate adequate brachial blood flow?
   a. Radial
   b. Carotid
   c. Femoral
   d. Popliteal

34. Which is the first action implemented by the nurse when obtaining a 24-hour urine specimen?
   a. Ensure that a basin with ice is ready to hold the collection container
   b. Have the patient empty the bladder before beginning the test
   c. Teach the patient to cleanse the meatus before each voiding
   d. Prepare an I&O sheet to be used to document each voiding

35. Which can cause urine to appear red?
   a. Beets
   b. Strawberries
   c. Cherry Jell-O
   d. Red food dye

36. What is the most important thing the nurse should do when assessing a carotid artery?
   a. Monitor for a full minute
   b. Palpate just below the ear
   c. Press gently when palpating the site
   d. Massage the site before assessing for rate

37. Which would result in an accurate blood pressure for an average size adult male?
   a. Wrapping the lower edge of the cuff over the antecubital space
   b. Positioning the sphygmomanometer above the level of the heart
   c. Pumping the cuff about 60 mmHg above the point where the brachial pulse is lost
   d. Releasing the valve on the cuff so that the pressure decreases at the rate of 2–3 mmHg per second

38. In an adult, what blood pressure result would cause a concern about hypertension?
    a. 120/85
    b. 130/60
    c. 140/92
    d. 135/90

39. When planning to care for a patient who has an intolerance to activity, what is the first assessment that should be made by the nurse?
    a. Influence on the other family members
    b. Impact on functional health patterns
    c. Pattern of vital signs
    d. Range of motion

40. Which is an adaptation to inadequate nutrition?
    a. Presence of surface papillae on the tongue
    b. Reddish-pink mucous membranes
    c. Cachectic appearance
    d. Shiny eyes

41. When taking a rectal temperature the nurse should:
    a. Take the temperature for 5 minutes
    b. Wear gloves throughout the procedure
    c. Place the patient in the right lateral position
    d. Insert the thermometer 2 inches into the rectum

42. Which is usually unrelated to a nursing physical assessment?
    a. Posture and gait
    b. Balance and strength
    c. Hygiene and grooming
    d. Blood and urine values

43. The patient has a temperature of 102° F and complains of feeling thirsty. Which additional adaptation should the nurse expect during this febrile stage of a fever?
    a. Restlessness with confusion
    b. Decreased respiratory rate
    c. Profuse perspiration
    d. Pale, cold skin

44. Which is the most common site for assessing the heart rate?
    a. Radial
    b. Apical
    c. Carotid
    d. Temporal

45. Which characteristic of a blood pressure would indicate shock?
    a. Rising diastolic
    b. Decreasing systolic
    c. Korotkoff's sounds
    d. Widening pulse pressure

46. Which assessment is a subtle indicator of depression?
    a. Unkempt appearance
    b. Anxious behavior
    c. Tense posture
    d. Crying

47. Which would place a person at risk for hypothermia?
    a. Heat stroke
    b. Inability to sweat
    c. Excessive exercise
    d. High alcohol intake

48. Which adaptation would be expected in a patient who has lost 2 units of blood?
    a. Rapid, shallow breathing
    b. Increased urinary output
    c. Hypertension
    d. Bradypnea

49. A concern that is common to the collection of specimens, regardless of their source, for culture and sensitivity tests is:
    a. The specimen should be suspended in a preservative media
    b. The specimen should be collected in the morning
    c. Surgical asepsis must be maintained
    d. Two specimens should be obtained

50. A patient's vital signs are: oral temperature 99° F, pulse 84 beats per minute with a regular rhythm, respirations 16 breaths per minute and deep, and blood pressure 180/110 mmHg. The sign that should cause the most concern would be the:
    a. Pulse
    b. Respirations
    c. Temperature
    d. Blood pressure

1. a. During the compensatory stage of shock, blood is shunted away from, not toward, the periphery. Hyperemia is an increase in blood flow to an area where the overlying skin becomes reddened and warm.
   b. **The circulating blood volume is reduced by 25 to 35% during the compensatory stage of shock and 35 to 50% during the progressive stage of shock as the peripheral vessels constrict to increase blood flow to vital organs. This shunting of blood causes hypotension.**
   c. With shock, the heart rate increases (tachycardia); it is not irregular. The heart rate increases during the compensatory stage of shock to maintain adequate blood flow to body tissues.
   d. During the compensatory stage of shock the respiratory rate increases, not decreases, to maintain adequate oxygenation of body cells.

2. a. The apical, not the carotid, pulse should be obtained when the pulse is irregular.
   b. This is unnecessary because a stethoscope is adequate.
   c. This is necessary to obtain an accurate count. Taking the pulse for 15 seconds and multiplying by 4 or taking the pulse for 30 seconds and multiplying by 2 will result in inaccurate readings and is unsafe.
   d. Initially the response should be to obtain an apical rate. Ultimately, the apical and radial rates are compared to determine if there is a pulse deficit.

3. a. The body temperature is on the decline during this time.
   b. The body temperature is just beginning to rise from its lowest level, which occurs between 4 and 6 AM.
   c. Although the body temperature is rising, it has not reached its peak at this time.
   d. Diurnal variations (circadian rhythms) vary throughout the day with the highest body temperature usually occurring between 8 PM and midnight.

4. a. Auscultation is the process of listening to sounds produced in the body. It is performed directly by just listening with the ears or indirectly by using a stethoscope that amplifies the sounds and conveys them to the nurse's ears. Active intestinal peristalsis causes rumbling, gurgling, and tinkling abdominal sounds known as bowel sounds (borborygmi).
   b. Percussion may stimulate intestinal motility, which increases bowel sounds, but it is not the assessment method used to hear bowel sounds. Percussion is the act of striking the body's surface to elicit sounds that provide information about the size and shape of internal organs or whether tissue is air-filled, fluid-filled, or solid.
   c. Inspection cannot assess bowel sounds. Inspection uses the naked eye to perform a visual assessment of the body.
   d. Palpation may stimulate intestinal motility, which increases bowel sounds, but it is not the assessment method used to hear bowel sounds. Palpation is the examination of the body using the sense of touch.

5. a. The patient will have warm, flushed skin during the defervescence (flush) stage of a fever. During this stage, the fever abates and body temperature returns to normal.
   b. Dehydration can occur during both the febrile (course, plateau) and defervescence (flush) stages of a fever.
   c. Profuse diaphoresis (sweating) occurs during the defervescence (flush) stage of a fever. During this stage, the fever abates and body temperature returns to normal.
   d. Feeling cold, chills, and shivering are adaptations associated with the onset (chill, initiation) stage of a fever. During this stage, the body responds to pyrogens by conserving heat to raise body temperature and reset the body's thermostat.

6. a. Palpation, the examination of the body using the sense of touch, is used to obtain the heart rate at a pulse site. When measuring a pulse an artery is compressed slightly by the fingers so that the pulsating artery is held between the fingers and a bone or firm structure.
   b. A pulse is not measured by using the sense of sight. Inspection uses the naked eye to perform a visual assessment of the body.
   c. Percussion cannot measure a pulse. Percussion is the act of striking the body's surface to elicit sounds that provide information about the size and shape of internal organs or whether tissue is air-filled, fluid-filled, or solid.
   d. Auscultation is used to obtain an apical, not radial, pulse. Auscultation is the process of listening to sounds produced in the body. It is performed directly by just listening with the ears or indirectly by using a stethoscope that amplifies the sounds and conveys them to the nurse's ears.

7. a. This is not true for all thermometers, such as chemical disposable thermometers, temperature-sensitive tape, and electronic thermometers. This is true for glass/plastic thermometers.
   b. This is true only for glass/plastic thermometers.
   c. This is true only for electronic thermometers and sometimes used for glass/plastic thermometers.
   d. This is an acceptable medical asepsis practice. All instruments, regardless of their type, must be clean before use with a patient.

8. a. Vital signs may be monitored before and after, not during, activity to evaluate the patient's response to activity.
   b. Pressure in the chest is one of the classic signs of angina or a myocardial infarction (heart attack). The patient's vital signs should be obtained immediately.
   c. This is useless without having monitored the patient's status before activity. In addition, the response to activity should be monitored whether the activity is inside or outside the patient's room.
   d. Although this should be done, it is not as important as assessing a patient as described in another option.

9. a. Mental confusion is a defining characteristic for the nursing diagnosis Hypothermia, not Hyperthermia.

b. Loss of appetite (anorexia), not an increased appetite, is a defining characteristic of the nursing diagnosis Hyperthermia.

c. An increased heart rate (tachycardia), not a decreased heart rate (bradycardia), is a defining characteristic of the nursing diagnosis Hyperthermia.

d. A rectal temperature of 101° F (38.8° C) or oral temperature of 100° F (37.8° C) is a defining characteristic of the nursing diagnosis Hyperthermia.

10. a. Though important, blood pressure is related to circulation, which is not the first priority.

b. Patient assessment must always be conducted in order of priority of needs. In an emergency, the ABCs of assessment are airway, breathing, and circulation. A clear airway is essential for life and, therefore, has top priority.

c. Though important, breathing is not the first priority.

d. Though important, circulation is not the first priority.

11. a. This is unnecessary. When obtaining a specimen from a retention catheter, the aspiration port of the catheter (not the exit tube) is wiped with a disinfectant before inserting the syringe. Urine specimens from a retention catheter should come from the port, not the bag, because this urine is the most recently excreted.

b. This should not be done until a step mentioned in another option is performed first. The drainage tubing should be clamped approximately 1 to 2 inches below the aspiration port for 15 to 20 minutes to allow urine to accumulate.

c. This is unnecessary to obtain a urine specimen because only 10 to 30 cc are needed. This position is used to move urine toward the trigone (the triangular area at the base of the bladder where the ureters and urethra enter the bladder) where it is accessible to the catheter, which promotes the flow of urine through the urinary catheter to the drainage bag.

d. Wearing personal protective equipment, such as clean gloves, is a medical asepsis practice that protects the nurse from the patient's body fluids.

12. a. Although this should be done, it is not the most important information that should be documented.

b. This would be necessary only if the patient did not tolerate the procedure.

c. The patient's position when the blood pressure is measured may influence results. Generally, systolic and diastolic readings are lower in the horizontal than in the sitting position. There will be a lower reading in the uppermost arm when a person is in a lateral recumbent position. A change from the horizontal to an upright position may result in a temporary decrease (5 to 10 mmHg) in blood pressure; when it exceeds 25 mmHg systolic or 10 mmHg diastolic, it is called orthostatic hypotension.

d. This is unnecessary because they are approximately the same.

13. a. Prostate-specific antigen (PSA) should be performed at age 50 and yearly thereafter.

b. The American Cancer Society recommends a mammography every 12 to 18 months when a woman is between 40 and 49 years of age and annually when 50 years of age or older.

c. A Pap smear should be performed at age 18 and yearly thereafter. If the person is sexually active, has a sexually transmitted disease, has a mother who took diethylstilbestrol during pregnancy, or has a family history of cervical or uterine cancer, a Pap smear should be performed before age 18 and then every subsequent year.

d. A sigmoidoscopy should be performed at age 50 and every 5 years thereafter.

14. a. Vasodilation brings warm blood to the peripheral circulation where it is lost through the skin via radiation.

b. Evaporation (vaporization) is the conversion of a liquid into a vapor. When perspiration on the skin evaporates, it promotes heat loss.

c. Shivering generates heat by causing muscle contraction, which increases the metabolic rate by 100 to 200%.

d. Radiation is the transfer of heat from the surface of one object to the surface of another without direct contact.

15. a. Although the respiratory rate is elevated slightly, the heart rate and blood pressure are within normal limits.

b. Although the respiratory rate is elevated slightly, the heart rate and blood pressure are within normal limits.

c. These vital signs are all within normal limits.

d. The heart and respiratory rates increase to help maintain oxygen to body cells and the blood pressure decreases because of a decreased circulating blood volume. Vital signs within normal limits in an adult are pulse, 60 to 100 beats per minute; respirations, 12 to 20 breaths per minute; and blood pressure, systolic 100 to 140 mmHg and diastolic 60 to 90 mmHg.

16. a. There are no contraindications for palpating both radial arteries at the same time.

b. It is unsafe to palpate both carotid arteries at the same time. Slight compression of both carotid arteries can interfere with blood flow to the brain. In addition, compression of the carotid arteries can stimulate the carotid sinuses, which causes a reflex drop in the heart rate.

c. There are no contraindications for palpating both femoral arteries at the same time.

d. There are no contraindications for palpating both brachial arteries at the same time.

17. a. The normal temperature in a newborn is 98° F (axillary), which is not as high as would occur in another option.

b. A systemic infection in which pathogens are present in the circulating bloodstream (septicemia) causes extremely high fevers and may result in septic shock.

c. Although exercise can cause the body temperature to increase, it would not be as high as would occur in another option.

d. Although a warm shower causes vasodilation, which

may reflect a slight increase in body temperature, it would not be as high as would occur in another option in this question.

18. a. Variance occurs when there is a variation or deviation from a critical pathway, which occurs when goals are not met or interventions are not performed according to the stipulated time period.
    b. A remission is a period during a chronic illness of lessened severity or cessation of symptoms.
    c. An adaptation is a physical or emotional response to an internal or external stimulus.
    d. **An exacerbation is the period during a chronic illness when symptoms reappear after a remission or absence of symptoms.**

19. a. **Mouth breathing allows environmental air to enter the mouth, which results in an inaccurately low reading. To take an oral temperature the instrument must remain under the tongue of a closed mouth until the reading is obtained. This can take as little as several seconds (electronic thermometers) or as long as 3 to 4 minutes (glass/plastic thermometers).**
    b. A history of vomiting does not negate the use of an oral thermometer. If the patient should begin to vomit, the nurse can remove the thermometer.
    c. A 7-year-old child understands cause and effect and can follow directions regarding the use of an oral thermometer.
    d. An oral thermometer can be used with a patient maintained in any position.

20. a. The sclera of the eyes is an excellent location to assess for the presence of jaundice, not cyanosis. Jaundice is a yellow discoloration resulting from an increase in bilirubin.
    b. Although the nail beds are areas of lighter pigmentation in darker-skinned people, the feet are not a reliable body part to assess central cyanosis because they are a distal site that may already be discolored because of diseases of peripheral arteries and veins (peripheral vascular disease).
    c. **Cyanosis, a bluish discoloration of the skin caused by a decreased amount of oxygen in the blood, is best identified in the mucous membranes of the eyes and oral cavity. The mucous membranes usually are pink regardless of the person's skin color, which facilitates an accurate assessment of cyanosis.**
    d. The color of the lower legs is not as reliable a site to assess for cyanosis as is an area listed in another option. The legs are distal sites that may already be discolored because of diseases of peripheral arteries and veins (peripheral vascular disease).

21. a. This is a correct action when obtaining a blood pressure reading. The brachial artery is close to the skin's surface and the diaphragm of the stethoscope is used for low-pitched sounds of a blood pressure reading.
    b. This ensures an accurate reading because it provides uniform and complete compression of the brachial artery.
    c. **The bladder should be of sufficient length to cover at least two-thirds of the limb's**

circumference. **The width of a blood pressure cuff should be 40 percent of the circumference of the arm. When the width of the cuff is too narrow it results in false high readings and when it is too wide it results in false low readings.**
    d. This ensures that the openings in the earpieces of the stethoscope are facing toward the ear canal for uninterrupted transmission of sounds.

22. a. Vitamin K deficiency is not associated with skin lesions. Vitamin C causes small skin hemorrhages and delays wound healing. Riboflavin deficiency causes lip lesions, seborrheic dermatitis, and scrotal and vulval skin changes.
    b. **A disruption in the clotting mechanism of the body can result in bleeding. Vitamin K plays an essential role in the production of the clotting factors II (prothrombin), VII, IX, and X.**
    c. A deficiency in Vitamin A, not K, results in night blindness.
    d. A deficiency in thiamin, not Vitamin K, causes muscle weakness.

23. a. **Profuse diaphoresis (sweating) occurs during the defervescence (flush) stage of a fever. During this stage, the fever abates and body temperature returns to normal.**
    b. Shivering is an adaptation associated with the onset (chill) stage of a fever. During this stage, the body responds to pyrogens by conserving heat to raise body temperature and reset the body's thermostat.
    c. Cyanosis of the nail beds occurs during the onset (chill) stage of a fever. Vasoconstriction and shivering are the body's attempt to conserve heat.
    d. Contraction of the arrector pili muscles (goosebumps), an attempt by the body to trap air around body hairs, is associated with the onset (chill, initiation) stage of a fever. During this stage, the body responds to pyrogens by conserving heat to raise body temperature and reset the body's thermostat.

24. a. **Diurnal variations (circadian rhythms) vary throughout the day with the lowest body temperature usually occurring between 4 and 6 AM. The metabolic rate is at its lowest while the person is sleeping.**
    b. The body temperature is rising during this time.
    c. The body temperature is rising during this time.
    d. The body temperature is at its highest during this time.

25. a. **Gross temperature measurements (cold, cool, warm, hot) can be obtained by palpation. Palpation is the examination of the body using the sense of touch. Sensory nerves in the fingers transmit messages through the spinal cord to the cerebral cortex, where they are interpreted.**
    b. Inspection cannot measure skin temperature. Inspection uses the naked eye to perform a visual assessment of the body.
    c. Percussion cannot measure skin temperature. Percussion is the act of striking the body's surface to elicit sounds that provide information about the size and shape of internal organs or whether tissue is air-filled, fluid-filled, or solid.

d. Observation cannot measure skin temperature. Observation uses the naked eye to perform a visual assessment of the body.

26. a. This is done for patient comfort, not to influence the accuracy of the assessment.
   b. Bowel sounds are auscultated before palpation and percussion because these techniques stimulate the intestines and thus cause an increase in peristalsis and a false increase in bowel sounds.
   c. This is not necessary. Many people begin the systematic 4-quadrant assessment in the lower right quadrant over the ileocecal valve where the digestive contents from the small intestine empty through a valve into the large intestine.
   d. This is unnecessary. Bowel sounds may be hyperactive (1 every 3 seconds) or hypoactive (1 every minute). After a sound is heard, the stethoscope is moved to the next site. For sounds to be considered absent there must be no sounds over 3 to 5 minutes.

27. a. This is an acceptable increase in heart rate with strenuous aerobic exercise.
   b. This is an acceptable blood pressure with the body at rest. The normal blood pressure in an adult is a systolic of 100 to 140 mmHg and a diastolic of 60 to 90 mmHg.
   c. A respiratory rate of 10 is below the expected respiratory rate for an adult and should be assessed further. The normal respiratory rate for an adult is 12 to 20 breaths per minute.
   d. This is within the within normal range of 60 to 100 beats per minute.

28. **a. Performing the following calculation: 140 minus 90 equals 50, which is the pulse pressure for the blood pressure reading 140/90. Pulse pressure is the difference between the systolic and diastolic pressures.**
   b. This number is the product of an incorrect calculation for the pulse pressure for the blood pressure reading of 140/90.
   c. This number is the product of an incorrect calculation for the pulse pressure for the blood pressure reading of 140/90.
   d. This number is the product of an incorrect calculation for the pulse pressure for the blood pressure reading of 140/90.

29. **a. Feeling cold occurs during the onset (chill) stage of a fever because of vasoconstriction, cool skin, and shivering.**
   b. Feeing warm is associated with the defervescence (flush) stage of a fever because of sudden vasodilation.
   c. Feeling sweaty occurs during the defervescence (flush) stage of a fever because of the body's heat loss response. As perspiration collects on the skin and evaporates, it cools the body and results in the person feeling cold.
   d. Feeling thirsty is associated with the febrile (fever) stage of a fever because of mild to severe dehydration.

30. a. Although the body temperature decreases as shock progresses because of a decreased metabolic rate, it is not one of the first signs of shock.
   b. Two other vital signs will alter before blood pressure as the heart attempts to compensate for a decreased circulating blood volume.
   c. Although during shock the pulse pressure will narrow, other vital signs will reflect compensation first. Pulse pressure is the difference between the systolic and diastolic pressures.
   d. The initial stage of shock begins when baroreceptors in the aortic arch and the carotid sinus detect a drop in the mean arterial pressure. The sympathetic nervous system responds by constricting peripheral vessels and increasing the heart and respiratory rates. During the compensatory stage of shock the effects of epinephrine and norepinephrine continue with stimulation of alpha-adrenergic fibers causing vasoconstriction of vessels supplying the skin and abdominal viscera and beta-adrenergic fibers causing vasodilation of vessels supplying the heart, skeletal muscles, and respiratory system.

31. a. This question relates to orthostatic hypotension and balance, not strength.
   b. Dependent edema may make the work of walking more difficult but it relates more to endurance than strength.
   c. A patient's pushing the soles of the feet against the palms of the hands of the nurse provides information regarding the strength of leg muscles. Standing and walking requires the use of the quadriceps, gluteal, and abdominal muscles.
   d. Although this might be asked, the response may not be honest or accurate.

32. a. This is too frequent for routine monitoring of body temperature. Although the set point for body temperature changes rapidly, it takes several hours for the core body temperature to change.
   b. This is an appropriate interval of time for routine monitoring of body temperature. It is frequent enough to identify trends in changes in body temperature while limiting unnecessary assessments.
   c. This is unsafe. This is too long an interval for monitoring a patient with a fever.
   d. This is unsafe. This is too long an interval for monitoring a patient with a fever.

33. **a. The brachial artery splits (bifurcates) into the radial and ulnar arteries. When there is an adequate radial pulse, the brachial artery must be patent.**
   b. This information would be useless. The carotid artery is in the neck while the brachial artery is in the arms. The carotid pulse site is located on the neck at the side of the larynx, between the trachea and the sternomastoid muscle.
   c. This information would be useless. The femoral artery is in the legs while the brachial artery is in the arms. The femoral pulse site is in the groin in the femoral triangle. It is in the anterior, medial aspect of

the thigh, just below the inguinal ligament, halfway between the anterior superior iliac spine and the symphysis pubis.

d. This information would be useless. The popliteal artery is in the legs while the brachial artery is in the arms. The popliteal pulse site is in the lateral aspect of the hollow area at the back of the knee (popliteal fossa).

34. a. This is not done first and may or may not be necessary. The specimen is kept cool or a preservative may be added to the container to prevent the breakdown of certain urinary constituents.

   b. **A 24-hour urine specimen begins and ends with an empty bladder. At the beginning of the 24-hour test, the patient is asked to void and the specimen is discarded. At the end of the 24-hour test, the patient is asked to void and the specimen is added to the collection container, and the entire specimen then is sent to the laboratory.**

   c. This is unnecessary.

   d. This is unnecessary. However, each voiding during the 24 hours of the test must be added to the collection container.

35. a. **Betacyanin, a pigment that gives beets their purplish-red color, is excreted in the urine and feces of some people when it is nonmetabolizd (a genetically determined trait). This bright red pigment turns the urine and feces red for several days after eating beets.**

   b. Strawberries will not turn the urine red. However, they can cause an allergic reaction (reason is unknown), producing the cellular release of histamine and hives.

   c. Many gelatin desserts contain red dye number 3 but it does not turn the urine red. Red dye number 3, found in foods such as maraschino cherries, pistachio nuts, and gelatin desserts, is a suspected carcinogen.

   d. Red food dye does not turn the urine red. Red dye number 3, found in foods such as maraschino cherries, pistachio nuts, and gelatin desserts, is a suspected carcinogen.

36. a. This is unnecessarily long, and even slight compression can interfere with blood flow to the brain.

   b. This is not the site to access the carotid artery. The carotid pulse site is located on the neck at the side of the larynx, between the trachea and the sternomastoid muscle.

   c. **The carotid artery should be palpated with a light touch to prevent an interference in blood flow to the brain and stimulation of the carotid sinus that can cause a reflex drop in the heart rate.**

   d. This is contraindicated. Massage can stimulate the carotid sinus located at the level of the bifurcation of the carotid artery, which results in a reflex drop in the heart rate.

37. a. This will cover the brachial artery and may interfere with the accurate assessment of blood pressure. The

lower edge of the cuff should be approximately 1 inch (2.5 cm) above the antecubital space.

   b. This will result in a false low blood pressure reading.

   c. The sphygmomanometer should be pumped up 30 mmHg, not 60 mmHg, above the palpatory blood pressure reading. This ensures an accurate systolic reading without exerting undue pressure on the tissues of the arm.

   d. **Releasing the valve slowly ensures that all 5 Korotkoff sounds are heard accurately. Deflating the cuff too rapidly can result in a false low systolic reading and deflating the cuff too slowly can result in a false high diastolic reading.**

38. a. This blood pressure reading is within the normal range for an adult.

   b. This blood pressure reading is within the normal range for an adult.

   c. **The systolic reading is on the extreme high side of normal and the diastolic reading is beyond the acceptable normal range. The normal range for blood pressure is a systolic between 100 to 140 mmHg and a diastolic between 60 and 90 mmHg.**

   d. This blood pressure reading is within the normal range for an adult.

39. a. Although this might eventually be assessed, it is not the priority.

   b. Although this might eventually be assessed, it is not the priority.

   c. **Activity intolerance is related to the inability to maintain adequate oxygenation to body cells, which is associated with respiratory and cardiovascular problems. Obtaining the vital signs (temperature, pulse, respirations, and blood pressure) will provide valuable information about these systems.**

   d. Activity intolerance is related to the cardiovascular and respiratory systems, not the nervous and musculoskeletal systems.

40. a. The tongue is normally pink, moist, and smooth, with papillae and fissures present. A beefy red or magenta color, smooth appearance, and an increase or decrease in size indicates nutritional problems.

   b. This is the color of normal mucous membranes because of their rich vascular supply. Pale mucous membranes or the presence of lesions indicates nutritional problems.

   c. **Cachexia is general ill health and malnutrition marked by weakness and excessive leanness (emaciation).**

   d. The eyes are always moist and shiny because lacrimal fluid continually washes the eyes. Pale or red conjunctivae, dryness, and soft or dull corneas are signs of nutritional problems.

41. a. A rectal thermometer must remain in place 2 to 4, not 5, minutes to obtain an accurate reading.

   b. **Gloves, a personal protective piece of equipment, are the best way the nurse is protected from contracting or transmitting a pathogen.**

   c. The left, not right, lateral position is the best position to place a patient when obtaining a rectal temperature because it utilizes the anatomical position of the anus and rectum for easy insertion of the thermometer

   d. This would be too far and could cause damage to the mucous membranes. A lubricated thermometer should be inserted 1.5 inches into the rectum to ensure an accurate reading.

42. a. Assessing posture and gait is within the scope of nursing practice because they reflect human responses.
   b. Assessing balance and strength is within the scope of nursing practice because they reflect human responses.
   c. Assessing hygiene and grooming is within the scope of nursing practice because they reflect human responses.
   d. Ordering and assessing urine and blood values are not in the independent practice of nursing. These assessments are dependent or interdependent functions of the nurse and are covered by specific orders or standing orders respectively.

43. **a. Restlessness with confusion may indicate the beginning of delirium associated with high fevers that alter cerebral functioning. Delirium is associated with the febrile (fever) stage of a fever.**
   b. During the febrile (fever) stage of a fever the pulse and respiratory rates will increase, because of an increase in the basal metabolic rate, in an attempt to pump oxygenated blood to the tissues.
   c. Profuse diaphoresis (sweating) occurs during the defervescence (flush), not the febrile, stage of a fever.
   d. Pale, cold skin occurs during the onset stage of a fever because of vasoconstriction, which is an attempt to conserve body heat.

44. **a. The radial pulse is the most easily found and accessible site for routine monitoring of the pulse, and it provides accurate information when the heart rate is regular. The radial pulse site is where the radial artery runs along the radial bone, on the thumb side of the inner aspect of the wrist.**
   b. The apical pulse requires a stethoscope and partially undressing a patient, which makes this site less convenient than other sites. However, it does provide information that is more accurate when the heart rate is irregular. The apical pulse site is over the apex of the heart in the fourth or fifth intercostal space at the midclavicular line.
   c. This site is used in emergences when the stroke volume is too low for a peripheral pulse to be felt. The carotid pulse site is located on the neck at the side of the larynx, between the trachea and the sternomastoid muscle.
   d. This site is used for infants and young children. The temporal pulse site is located between the eye and the hairline just above the cheekbone (zygomatic bone).

45. a. The diastolic blood pressure decreases, not increases, during shock.
   b. The initial stage of shock begins when baroreceptors in the aortic arch and the carotid sinus detect a drop in the mean arterial pressure. The systolic pressure is the pressure in the arteries during ventricular contraction.
   c. Korotkoff's sounds are the 5 distinct sounds that are heard when auscultating a blood pressure (I—faint, clear tapping; II—swishing sound; III—intense, clear tapping; IV—muffled, blowing sounds; V—absence of sounds).
   d. During shock, there will be a narrowing, not widening, of pulse pressure. Pulse pressure is the difference between the systolic and diastolic pressures.

46. **a. When people are depressed they frequently do not have the physical or psychic energy to perform the activities of daily living, and often exhibit an unkempt appearance. A disheveled, untidy appearance is a covert, subtle indication of depression.**
   b. Anxious behavior is overt and obvious, not covert and subtle.
   c. Tense posture is overt and obvious, not covert and subtle.
   d. Crying is overt and obvious, not covert and subtle.

47. a. Hyperthermia, not hypothermia, is associated with this condition. Heat stroke (heat hyperpyrexia) is failure of the heat regulating capacity of the body, resulting in extremely high body temperatures (105° F).
   b. Hyperthermia, not hypothermia, can result from the lack of sweat. The inability to perspire does not allow the body to cool by the evaporation of sweat (vaporization).
   c. Hyperthermia, not hypothermia, can result from excessive exercise. Exercise increases heat production as carbohydrates and fats break down to provide energy. Body temperature temporarily can raise as high as 104° F.
   d. Excessive alcohol intake interferes with thermoregulation by providing a false sense of warmth, inhibiting shivering, and causing vasodilation, which promotes heat loss. In addition, it impairs judgment, which increases the risk of making inappropriate self-care decisions.

48. **a. With a decrease in circulating red blood cells, the respiratory rate will increase to meet oxygen needs.**
   b. With a reduction in blood volume, there will be less blood circulating through the kidneys, resulting in a decreased (not increased) urinary output.
   c. With a reduction in blood volume, the blood pressure will be decreased, not elevated.
   d. Bradypnea is not associated with blood loss.

49. a. This is not necessary for all specimens.
   b. This is not necessary.
   c. The results of a culture and sensitivity are faulty and erroneous if the collection container or inappropriate collection technique introduces extraneous microorganisms that falsify and misrepresent results. Surgical asepsis (sterile technique) must be maintained.

d. Generally, if a specimen is collected using proper technique, one specimen is sufficient for testing for culture and sensitivity.

50. a. Although this is slightly outside the normal pulse rate of 60 to 80 beats per minute, the rhythm is regular; the patient should be assessed further and the information compared to the patient's baseline data.

b. This is within the normal respiratory rate of 14 to 20 breaths per minute.

c. This is within the normal temperature range of 97.6°F. to 99.6°F. for an oral temperature.

d. The blood pressure is above the normal range of 100/140 mmHg for the systolic reading and 60 to 90 mmHg for the diastolic reading and should cause the most concern of the options presented.

Infection Control

KEYWORDS

The following words include English vocabulary, nursing/ medical terminology, concepts, principles, or information relevant to content specifically addressed in the chapter or associated with topics presented in it. English dictionaries, your nursing textbooks, and medical dictionaries such as *Taber's Cyclopedic Medical Dictionary* are resources that can be used to expand your knowledge and understanding of these words and related information.

Abrasion
Afebrile
Anaerobes
Antibiotics
Antibody
Antigen
Antimicrobial
Antipyretic
Aseptic technique
Bacteria
Biohazardous
Chain of infection
   Characteristics of pathogen
   Portal of entry
   Reservoir
   Portal of exit
   Mode of transmission
   Characteristics of the host
Colonization
Communicable disease
Contamination
Culture and sensitivity
Debridement
Discharge
Endogenous
Erythema
Erythrocyte sedimentation rate (ESR)
Excoriated
Exogenous
Exudate
Febrile

Fever
Fungi
General Adaptation Syndrome
Granulocytes
Harbor
Host
Hyperthermia
Hypothalamus
Hypothermia blanket
Iatrogenic
Immune response
Immune system
Immunity
Immunization
Immunocompromised
Immunosuppression
Incubation
Inflammatory response
Interferon
Invasion
Leukocyte migration
Leukocytosis
Local Adaptation Syndrome
Neutropenia
Normal flora
Nosocomial
Opportunistic
Ova and parasites
Pathogen
Pediculosis
Phagocytosis

Pneumonia
Pressure ulcer
Primary intention
Primary line of defense
Purulent
Pus
Pyrogens
Resistance
Risk
Sanguineous drainage
Scabies
Secondary intention
Secondary line of defense
Septicemia
Serous drainage
Serosanguineous drainage
Specimen
Standard precautions
Subclinical
Surgical asepsis
Susceptible
Systemic
Transmission
Transmission-based precautions
   Airborne precautions
   Contact precautions
   Droplet precautions
Virulence
Virus
Wet to damp dressing
White blood cell count

QUESTIONS

1. What should the nurse do first to prevent infection in hospitalized patients?
   a. Provide small bedside bags to dispose of used tissues
   b. Encourage staff to avoid coughing near patients
   c. Administer antibiotics as ordered
   d. Identify patients at risk

2. The nurse would recognize that a patient was attempting to resist an infection when diagnostic laboratory values reveal an elevated:
   a. Red blood cell count
   b. White blood cell count
   c. Partial thromboplastin time
   d. Leukocyte alkaline phosphatase test

3. Which is a local adaptation to the inflammatory response?
   a. Fever
   b. Erythema
   c. Bradypnea
   d. Tachycardia

4. To best support healing of a wound by secondary intention, the nurse should expect the practitioner's order to be, "Clean wound with:
   a. Normal saline and cover with one 4×4."
   b. Betadine and apply a dry sterile dressing."
   c. Normal saline and apply a wet to damp dressing."
   d. Half peroxide and half normal saline and apply a wet to dry dressing."

5. Which situation would place the patient at the greatest risk for wound infection?
   a. Surgical creation of a colostomy
   b. First-degree burn on the back
   c. Puncture of the foot by a nail
   d. Paper cut on the finger

6. The skin protects the body from infections because the:
   a. Cells of the skin are constantly being replaced, thereby eliminating external pathogens
   b. Epithelial cells are loosely compacted on skin, providing a barrier against pathogens
   c. Moisture on the skin surface prevents colonization of pathogens
   d. Alkalinity of the skin limits the growth of pathogens

7. When collecting the following specimens, which would not require the use of surgical aseptic technique?
   a. Urine from a Foley catheter
   b. Stool for ova and parasites
   c. Specimen for a throat culture
   d. Exudate from a wound for a C&S

8. Which individual is at the greatest risk for developing a nosocomial infection? One who:
   a. Lives in a nursing home
   b. Ingests an inadequate amount of calories
   c. Touches her nose repeatedly with unwashed hands
   d. Wipes his rectum from back to front after a bowel movement

9. Which is a systemic adaptation to a wound infection?
   a. Hyperthermia
   b. Exudate
   c. Edema
   d. Pain

10. Which nursing action will interrupt the transmission link in the chain of infection?
    a. Handwashing before and after providing care to a patient
    b. Positioning a commode next to a patient's bed
    c. Educating a patient about a balanced diet
    d. Changing a dressing when it is soiled

11. The nurse recognizes the need for an increase in caloric intake above average requirements for the patient who has:
    a. Nausea
    b. Dysphagia
    c. Pneumonia
    d. Depression

12. The person with the greatest risk for developing an infection is a:
    a. 2-month-old who is breastfeeding
    b. 20-year-old who works in a movie theater
    c. 40-year-old who is receiving cancer chemotherapy
    d. 60-year-old who is taking antibiotics while having dental surgery

13. Healing by primary intention is most likely to occur with:
    a. Cuts in the skin from a kitchen knife
    b. Excoriated perianal areas
    c. Abrasions of the skin
    d. Pressure ulcers

14. The primary reason why the nurse should avoid glued-on artificial nails is because they:
    a. Interfere with dexterity of the fingers
    b. Could fall off in a patient's bed
    c. Harbor microorganisms
    d. Can scratch a patient

15. Subclinical infections most commonly occur in:
    a. Infants
    b. Adolescents
    c. Older adults
    d. School-aged children

16. Which factor places a patient at the greatest risk for developing an infection?
    a. Burns over 20% of the body
    b. Implantation of a prosthetic device
    c. Presence of an indwelling urinary catheter
    d. Multiple puncture sites from laparoscopic surgery

17. Which is a secondary line of defense against infection?
    a. Mucous membranes of the respiratory tract
    b. Urinary tract environment
    c. Integumentary system
    d. Immune response

18. When performing a physical assessment before surgery, the nurse identifies that a patient has *pediculosis capitis* (head lice). What should the nurse do first?
    a. Move the patient to a private room
    b. Call the physician for a treatment order
    c. Wash the patient's hair with a germicidal shampoo
    d. Inform the operating room and postpone the surgery for 24 hours

19. Which is most directly related to the word "nosocomial?"
    a. Disease-producing
    b. Hospital-acquired
    c. Endogenous
    d. Iatrogenic

20. A common systemic adaptation to infection is:
    a. Pain
    b. Edema
    c. Tachycardia
    d. Hypothermia

21. Which statement indicates that further teaching is necessary regarding how to ensure protection from food contamination?
    a. "I love juicy rare hamburgers with onion and tomato."
    b. "I prefer chicken salad sandwiches with mayonnaise."
    c. "I know to spit out food that doesn't taste good."
    d. "I should defrost frozen food in the refrigerator."

22. Which nursing action protects the patient as a susceptible host in the chain of infection?
    a. Wearing personal protective equipment
    b. Administering childhood immunizations
    c. Recapping a used needle before discarding
    d. Disposing of soiled gloves in a waste container

23. Which is an objective adaptation to an ear infection?
    a. Throbbing pain
    b. Purulent drainage
    c. Dizziness when moving
    d. Hearing a buzzing sound

24. What blood component should the nurse monitor when assessing an individual's ability to withstand exposure to pathogens?
    a. Platelets
    b. Neutrophils
    c. Erythrocytes
    d. Hemoglobin

25. Which patient is at the greatest risk for a urinary tract infection?
    a. Male with nocturia
    b. Uncircumcised male
    c. Premenopausal female
    d. Female with a purulent vaginal discharge

26. Which is a primary (nonspecific) defense that protects the body from infection?
    a. Tears in the eyes
    b. Alkalinity of gastric secretions
    c. Bile in the gastrointestinal system
    d. Moist environment of the epidermis

27. When brushing a patient's hair, the nurse notes white oval particles attached to the hair behind the ears. The nurse should assess the patient further for signs of:
    a. Scabies
    b. Dandruff
    c. Hirsutism
    d. Pediculosis

28. A rise in body temperature is associated with the presence of infection because:
    a. Pain activates the sympathetic nervous system
    b. Erythema increases the flow of blood throughout the body
    c. Leukocyte migration precipitates the inflammatory response
    d. Phagocytic cells release pyrogens that stimulate the hypothalamus

29. An example of an iatrogenic infection would be a:
    a. Vaginal infection in a postmenopausal woman
    b. Respiratory infection contracted from a grandchild
    c. Urinary tract infection in a patient who is sedentary
    d. Wound infection caused by unwashed hands of a caregiver

30. A wound is packed with a wet to damp gauze dressing primarily to:
    a. Prevent infection of the wound
    b. Promote uptake of Vitamin C
    c. Facilitate the healing process
    d. Promote uptake of nutrients

31. A primary (nonspecific) defense that protects the body from infection is:
    a. Antibiotic therapy
    b. The high pH of the skin
    c. Cilia in the respiratory tract
    d. The alkaline environment of the vagina

32. Which is a local adaptation to a wound infection?
    a. Hyperthermia
    b. Neutropenia
    c. Malaise
    d. Edema

33. A patient with septicemia is placed on a cooling blanket to achieve heat loss via:
    a. Radiation
    b. Convection
    c. Conduction
    d. Evaporation

34. Which is unrelated to infection?
    a. Catabolism
    b. Hyperglycemia
    c. Ketones in the urine
    d. Decreased metabolic activity

35. Which nursing action protects the patient from infection at the portal of entry?
    a. Positioning a Foley collection bag below the level of the patient's pelvis
    b. Enclosing a urine specimen in a biohazardous transport bag
    c. Wearing clean gloves when handling a patient's excretions
    d. Handwashing after removal of soiled protective gloves

1. a. Although this is something the nurse may provide to contain soiled tissues, it is not the first action the nurse should implement to prevent infection.
   b. Although this is something the nurse may do to limit airborne or droplet transmission of microorganisms, it is not the first action the nurse should implement to prevent infection.
   c. Antibiotics are generally ordered by a practitioner for patients who have infections. Antibiotics rarely are ordered prophylactically to prevent the development of resistant strains of microorganisms.
   d. **This is the most important first step in the prevention of infection. A patient who is at high risk may need to receive special protective precautions.**

2. a. Red blood cells (erythrocytes) are responsible for delivering oxygen to the cells of the body. An elevation in red blood cells (erythrocytosis) does not indicate that a patient is attempting to resist an infection.
   b. **The main function of white blood cells (leukocytes) is to protect the body when exposed to pathogenic microorganisms. When the white blood cell count is elevated (leukocytosis) above the normal 5,000 to 10,000 cells/mm^3, it indicates that the individual has mounted a defense against pathogens that cause infection.**
   c. A partial thromboplastin time (PTT) measures the normalcy of blood coagulation. An increased value (greater than 25–38 seconds) would indicate a deficiency in blood clotting factors that would increase an individual's risk for hemorrhage, not infection.
   d. This test measures an enzyme present in neutrophilic granules from metamyelocyte to the segmented stage and represents intracellular metabolism. Elevations indicate polycythemia vera, myelofibrosis, and essential thrombocytopenia, not the body's resisting infection.

3. a. A fever is a systemic, not local, response to inflammation.
   b. **Local trauma or infection stimulates the release of kinins, which increase capillary permeability and blood flow to the local area. The increase of blood flow to the area causes erythema.**
   c. Bradypnea is a regular but abnormally slow rate of breathing (less than 12 breaths per minute) and is not an adaptation to the local or general inflammatory syndromes.
   d. Tachycardia is an abnormally elevated heart rate higher than 100 beats per minute and is unrelated to the Local Adaptation Syndrome.

4. a. Although normal saline is appropriate for cleansing a wound, a moist, not dry, environment facilitates epithelialization and minimizes scar formation.
   b. Betadine is cytotoxic and should not be used on clean granulating wounds.
   c. **Cleaning with normal saline will not damage fibroblasts. Wet to damp dressings allow epidermal cells to migrate more rapidly across the wound surface than dry dressings, thereby facilitating wound healing.**

d. Hydrogen peroxide is cytotoxic and should not be used on clean granulating wounds.

5. a. Surgery is conducted using sterile technique. In addition, preoperative preparation of the bowel helps to reduce the presence of organisms that have the potential to cause infection.
   b. There is no break in the skin in a first degree burn; therefore, there is less of a risk for a wound infection than an example in another option.
   c. **Puncture of the foot by a nail has the greatest risk for a wound infection of all the options. A nail is a soiled object that has the potential of introducing pathogens into a deep wound that can trap them under the surface of the skin, a favorable environment for multiplication.**
   d. Paper is generally not heavily soiled and the wound edges are approximated. This is less of a risk than an example in another option.

6. a. **This is true. Epithelial cells of the skin are regularly shed along with potentially dangerous microorganisms that adhere to the skin's outer layers, thereby reducing the risk of infection.**
   b. Epithelial cells on the skin are closely, not loosely, compacted providing a barrier against pathogens.
   c. Moisture on the skin surface facilitates, not prevents, colonization of pathogens.
   d. Acidity, not alkalinity, of the skin limits the growth of pathogens.

7. a. The bladder is a sterile cavity and the nurse must use sterile technique to collect urine from the port of a retention catheter (Foley) so as not to introduce any pathogens. In addition, it is important not to introduce exogenous organisms that may contaminate the specimen and alter the accuracy of test results.
   b. **Stool for ova and parasites does not have to be sterile because test results for the presence of parasitic eggs and parasites are not altered if the specimen is contaminated with exogenous organisms.**
   c. Sterile technique is used to collect a throat culture, to avoid contaminating the specimen with exogenous organisms that may alter the accuracy of test results.
   d. Sterile technique is used to collect exudate from a wound to avoid contaminating the specimen with exogenous organisms that may alter the accuracy of test results.

8. a. **A person living in a nursing home would be at risk for a nosocomial infection. Nosocomial infections are health-care acquired (formerly called hospital-acquired) infections.**
   b. This could compromise a person's ability to fight an infection, but would not by itself place a person at risk for a nosocomial infection.
   c. This would not place a person at risk for a nosocomial infection.
   d. This would not place a person at risk for a nosocomial infection.

9. a. Hyperthermia is a common systemic adaptation to infection. With hyperthermia microorganisms or endotoxins stimulate phagocytic cells that

release pyrogens, which stimulate the hypothalamic thermoregulatory center and cause fever.

b. Exudate is a local, not systemic, response to an injury or inflammation. Exudate is cleared away through lymphatic drainage or exits from the body via a wound.

c. Edema is a local, not systemic, adaptation to infection. Chemical mediators increase the permeability of small blood vessels, thereby causing fluid to enter the interstitial compartment and resulting in local edema.

d. Pain is a local, not systemic, adaptation to inflammation because swelling of inflamed tissue exerts pressure on nerve endings.

10. a. **This is an example of controlling the mode of transmission. Direct transmission of microorganisms from one person to another is interrupted when microorganisms are removed from the skin surface by handwashing. Handwashing is part of hand hygiene, which also includes nail care, skin lubrication, and wearing of minimal jewelry.**

b. This is an example of controlling the reservoir and the portal of exit from the reservoir, not the mode of transmission, link in the chain of infection.

c. This is an example of reducing the susceptibility of the host, not the mode of transmission, link in the chain of infection.

d. This is an example of controlling the reservoir (source) and portal of exit from the reservoir, not the mode of transmission, link in the chain of infection.

11. a. Nausea does not precipitate a need for an increase in caloric intake above average requirements.

b. Dysphagia, difficulty swallowing, does not precipitate a need for an increase in caloric intake above average requirements.

c. **The individual with pneumonia requires an increase in caloric requirements because of an increased resting energy expenditure and hypermetabolic state. With an infection, more energy is needed to regulate an elevated body temperature and extra protein is needed to produce antibodies and white blood cells.**

d. Depression does not precipitate a need for an increase in caloric intake above average requirements. If a depressed patient becomes withdrawn and sedentary, caloric requirements may decrease.

12. a. Young infants who breastfeed receive passive immunity from the mother for protection against childhood diseases such as chickenpox, mumps, measles, and polio.

b. Individuals who are in late adolescence or young adulthood generally have intact immune systems and are able to defend against infection. Although exposure to large groups of people might put a person at risk for infection, it is not as high a risk as an example in another option.

c. **Most chemotherapeutic drugs for cancer are not only cytotoxic to cancer cells but also contribute to bone marrow depression, which interferes with the ability to produce adequate numbers of white blood cells. In addition, chemotherapeutic**

drugs alter the ability of normal cells to defend against infection.

d. Although a person 60 years old may have a depressed immune response as a result of a decline in body function because of the aging process, the older adult is not at as high a risk for infection as an example in another option.

13. a. **A cut in the skin caused by a sharp instrument with minimal tissue loss can heal by primary intention when the wound edges are lightly pulled together (approximated).**

b. Excoriation heals by secondary intention, not primary intention. Excoriation is an injury to the surface of the skin. It can be caused by friction, scratching, and chemical or thermal burns.

c. An abrasion heals by secondary intention, not by primary intention. In an abrasion, friction scrapes away the epithelial layer exposing the underlying tissue.

d. A pressure ulcer heals by secondary intention, not primary intention. Secondary intention healing occurs when wound edges are not approximated because of full thickness tissue loss and the wound is left open until it fills with new tissue.

14. a. Artificial nails do not interfere with finger dexterity if kept at a reasonable length (not longer than $1/4$ inch beyond the end of the finger).

b. Although this is a concern, it is not the main reason they should be avoided.

c. **Studies have demonstrated that artificial nails, especially when cracked, broken, or split, provide crevices in which microorganisms can grow and multiply, and therefore should be avoided by direct care providers.**

d. When artificial nails are cared for so that they remain intact and free of cracks or breaks, they should not scratch the skin.

15. a. Infants generally respond to infections with acute symptoms that are identified easier and earlier than in an age group in another option.

b. Adolescents generally respond to infections with acute symptoms that are identified easier and earlier than in an age group in another option.

c. **Infections are more difficult to identify in the older adult because the symptoms are not as acute and obvious as in other age groups because of the decline in all body systems related to aging.**

d. School-aged children generally respond to infections with acute symptoms that are identified easier and earlier than in an age group in another option.

16. a. **Burns over 20% of a person's total body surface are generally considered major burn injuries. When the skin is damaged by a burn the underlying tissue is left unprotected and the individual is at risk for infection. The greater the extent and the deeper the depth of the burn, the higher the risk for infection. In addition, invasive therapies such as nasogastric tube, indwelling urinary catheter, intravenous line, and wound care all increase the risk for infection.**

b. Although wound infections can occur when

prosthetic devices are implanted, they are surgically implanted under sterile conditions to minimize this risk.

c. Although urinary tract infections can occur with an indwelling urinary catheter even though it is generally a closed system, an example in another option places a person at a greater risk for infection.

d. Laparoscopic surgery is done using sterile technique to minimize the risk of infection. An example in another option places a person at a greater risk for infection.

17. a. Protective mechanisms in the respiratory tract provide a primary, not secondary, line of defense against pathogenic microorganisms. Primary defenses are nonspecific immune defenses that are anatomical, mechanical, or chemical barriers. In the respiratory tract they include intact mucous membranes, mucus, bactericidal enzymes, cilia, sneezing, and coughing.

b. Protective mechanisms in the urinary tract environment provide a primary, not secondary, line of defense against pathogenic microorganisms. These defenses include intact mucous membranes, urine flowing out of the body, and urine acidity.

c. Skin provides a primary, not secondary, line of defense against pathogenic microorganisms. These defenses include intact skin, surface acidity, and the normal flora that is found on the skin.

d. **The immune response is a specific, secondary line of defense against pathogenic microorganisms. The production of antibodies to neutralize and eliminate pathogens and their toxins (immune response) is activated when phagocytes fail to completely destroy invading microorganism. The primary, nonspecific defenses (anatomical, mechanical, chemical, and inflammatory) work in harmony with the secondary defense (immune response) to defend the body from pathogenic microorganisms.**

18. a. A private room is unnecessary. However, the roommate should not use any personal belongings of the infested individual.

b. **The patient's hair should be washed as soon as possible with a medicated shampoo (gamma benzene hexachloride [Lindane], malathion, or pyrethrin) and then combed with a fine toothed comb to remove the nits (eggs). Pediculocidal shampoo requires a practitioner's order.**

c. A pediculocide, not germicide, shampoo is required to medically manage pediculosis.

d. Another option has a higher priority. However, the operating room should be notified because the surgery will have to be canceled and rescheduled.

19. a. Pathogen refers to an organism that is disease-producing, not nosocomial.

b. **Nosocomial refers to hospital-acquired infections but it also includes infections that are acquired in a variety of health care settings. It is also known as health-care acquired infection.**

c. Endogenous refers to an infection that is caused by an organism from within an individual and is unrelated to the word nosocomial.

d. Iatrogenic refers to a disease or adaptation caused by the effects of some medical treatment. It is not as

directly related to the word nosocomial as another option.

20. a. Pain is a local, not systemic, adaptation to inflammation because swelling of inflamed tissue exerts pressure on nerve endings.

b. Edema is a local, not systemic, adaptation to infection. Chemical mediators increase the permeability of small blood vessels, thereby causing fluid to enter the interstitial compartment, resulting in local edema.

c. **Infection causes the hormonal response of an increase in the secretion of epinephrine and norepinephrine, which then causes an increase in the heart rate (tachycardia).**

d. Hyperthermia, not hypothermia, is a common systemic adaptation to infection. With hyperthermia microorganisms or endotoxins stimulate phagocytic cells that release pyrogens, which stimulate the hypothalamic thermoregulatory center causing fever.

21. a. **Hamburger meat should be thoroughly cooked so that disease producing microorganisms within the meat are destroyed.**

b. This statement does not indicate a lack of knowledge about the use or storage of mayonnaise.

c. This statement does not indicate a lack of knowledge about what to do when it is determined that something does not taste right.

d. This is the correct way to defrost frozen food. Food should not be defrosted in an environment between 45 to 140 degrees because bacteria will rapidly grow in this temperature range.

22. a. This is an example of controlling the mode of transmission, not the susceptible host, link in the chain of infection.

b. **This is a good example of an action designed to interrupt the susceptible host link in the chain of infection by increasing the resistance of the host to an infectious agent.**

c. Discarding uncapped, not capped, used syringes in a sharps' container disrupts the chain of infection at the reservoir link in the chain of infection. The nurse should never recap a used needle because of the risk of a needle-stick injury.

d. This is an example of controlling the mode of transmission, not the susceptible host, link in the chain of infection

23. a. Throbbing pain is subjective, not objective, information because pain cannot be observed; it is felt and described only by the patient.

b. **Purulent drainage from the ear is objective information because it can be observed and measured.**

c. Dizziness is subjective, not objective, information because it cannot be measured; dizziness is experienced and described only by the patient.

d. Hearing a buzzing sound (tinnitus) is subjective, not objective, information because it cannot be observed; a buzzing sound is perceived and described only by the patient.

24. a. Platelets are essential for blood clotting and are unrelated to an individual's ability to withstand exposure to pathogens.

b. Neutrophils, the most numerous leukocytes (white blood cells), are a primary defense against infection because they ingest and destroy microorganisms (phagocytosis). When the leukocyte count is low it indicates a compromised ability to fight infection.

c. Red blood cells (erythrocytes) do not reflect an individual's ability to withstand exposure to pathogens. Erythrocytes transport oxygen via hemoglobin molecules.

d. Hemoglobin is the part of the red blood cell that carries oxygen from the lungs to the tissues and is unrelated to the assessment of an individual's ability to withstand exposure to pathogens..

25. a. Voiding prevents urinary stasis and the flow of urine over the neck of the bladder and through the urethra washes away ascending microorganisms; both of these consequences of voiding reduce the risk of infection. In addition, a male is at a lower risk for a bladder infection because of the length of the urethra (approximately 8 inches).

b. If the foreskin is retracted and the glans penis washed daily there should be no more risk for a urinary tract infection in an uncircumcised than a circumcised male.

c. Although a premenopausal female has to provide more frequent perianal hygiene (when menstruating) than a postmenopausal female, if done from the pubis toward the rectum, there should be no increased risk for a urinary tract infection.

d. **This individual is at the highest risk for a urinary tract infection of all the examples presented. The perianal area that is dark, warm, and moist is an environment that facilitates growth of microorganisms increasing the risk of a urinary tract infection. In addition, the short length of the urethra of the female ($1\frac{1}{2}$ to $2\frac{1}{2}$ inches long) increases the risk of urinary tract infection.**

26. a. **Tears flush the eyes of microorganisms and debris and are a primary (nonspecific) defense that protects the body from infection.**

b. Acidity, not alkalinity, of gastric secretions is a primary (nonspecific) defense mechanism that protects the body from infection.

c. Bile helps emulsify fats; it does not protect the body from infection.

d. A dry, not moist, epidermis is a primary (nonspecific) defense mechanism that protects the body from infection.

27. a. This adaptation is not indicative of scabies. Scabies is a communicable skin disease caused by an itch mite (*Sarcoptes scabiei*) and is characterized by skin lesions (small papules, pustules, excoriations, and burrows ending in a vesicle) with intense itching.

b. This adaptation is not indicative of dandruff. Dandruff is the excessive shedding of dry white scales as a result of the normal exfoliation of the epidermis of the scalp. Dandruff scales do not attach to the hair and can be easily brushed away from the hair shaft.

c. This adaptation is not indicative of hirsutism. Hirsutism is the excessive growth of hair or hair growth in unusual places, particularly in females. In females, it is usually caused by excessive androgen production or metabolic abnormalities.

d. **Pediculosis (*Pediculus humanus capitis*) is characterized by white oval particles attached to the hair. When identified, the nurse needs to assess the patient further for the presence of scratch marks on the scalp and by asking the patient if the head feels itchy. In addition, the nurse must assess the extent of infestation and if any other areas of the body are infested with other types of lice (*P. humanus corporis*—body, and *Phthirus pubis*—pubic and axillary hair).**

28. a. Pain does not cause a rise in body temperature directly.

b. Erythema does not increase the flow of blood throughout the body. Increased blood flow causes erythema.

c. Leukocyte migration does not precipitate the inflammatory response but is a phase of the inflammatory response. White blood cells reach a wound within a few hours to ingest bacteria and clean a wound of debris through the process of phagocytosis.

d. **This is true. Microorganisms or endotoxins stimulate phagocytic cells, which release pyrogens that stimulate the hypothalamic thermoregulatory center causing fever.**

29. a. This is not an example of an iatrogenic infection.

b. This is not an example of an iatrogenic infection.

c. This infection is caused by a decrease in bladder tone and urinary residual as a result of inactivity and is unrelated to an iatrogenic infection.

d. **Iatrogenic refers to a disease or adaptation caused by the effects of some medical treatment. When a caregiver does not wash the hands, thereby transmitting a pathogen that causes a wound infection, the result is an iatrogenic infection.**

30. a. Although packing a wound with wet to damp dressings will wick exudate up and away from the base of the wound and therefore help to minimize wound infection, it is not the primary reason for its use.

b. Dressings are not used to promote the uptake of Vitamin C.

c. **Packing a wound with wet to damp dressings allows epidermal cells to migrate more rapidly across the bed of the wound surface than dry dressings, thereby facilitating wound healing. In addition, loosely packing a wound with wet to damp gauze helps to wick drainage upward and away from the base of the wound and thereby facilitates healing.**

d. Wet to damp packing of a wound is not done to promote the uptake of nutrients from a wound. Adequate ingestion of foods high in Vitamin C and protein promote wound healing.

31. a. Antibiotic therapy is the use of chemotherapeutic agents to control or eliminate bacterial infections. It is not a primary (nonspecific) defense that protects

the body from infection. The inappropriate use of antibiotics destroys the normal flora of the body and can predispose an individual to additional infections.

b. The low, not high, pH of the skin protects the body from infection.

c. **Cilia in the respiratory tract are a primary (nonspecific) defense mechanism that protects the body from infection. Mucus, produced by the respiratory tract, traps microorganisms, which are then propelled away from the lungs by cilia.**

d. The acidic, not alkaline, environment of the vagina protects it from the growth of pathogens.

32. a. Hyperthermia is a systemic, not local, adaptation to a wound infection. Microorganisms or endotoxins stimulate phagocytic cells that release pyrogens, which stimulate the hypothalamic thermoregulatory center to produce fever.

b. An increase in white blood cells (leukocytosis), not a decrease in white blood cells (neutropenia), occurs in response to both local and systemic infections.

c. Discomfort, uneasiness, or indisposition (malaise) is a systemic, not local, response to infection.

d. **Chemical mediators increase the permeability of small blood vessels, thereby causing fluid to move into the interstitial compartment, resulting in local edema.**

33. a. Radiation is not related to heat loss via a cooling (hypothermia) blanket. Radiation is heat loss from one surface to another without direct contact.

b. Convection is not related to heat loss via a cooling (hypothermia) blanket. Convention is the loss of heat as a result of the motion of cool air flowing over a warm body. The heat is carried away by air currents that are cooler than the warm body.

c. **Conduction is the transfer of heat from a warm**

object (skin) to a cooler object (cooling blanket) during direct contact.

d. Evaporation is unrelated to heat loss via a cooling (hypothermia) blanket. Evaporation is the conversion of a liquid to a vapor, which occurs when perspiration on the skin is vaporized. For each gram of water that evaporates from the skin, approximately 0.6 of a calorie of heat is lost.

34. a. Catabolism, the destructive phase of metabolism with its resultant release of energy, is related to infection.

b. Serum glucose is elevated (hyperglycemia) in the presence of an infection because of the release of glucocorticoids in the General Adaptation Syndrome.

c. The presence of ketones in the urine, a sign that the body is using fat as a source of energy, is related to infection because of the associated increased need for calories for fighting the infection.

d. **Metabolic activity increases, not decreases, with an infection as the body increases its activity and mounts a defense to fight invading pathogenic microorganisms.**

35. a. **This is an action designed to interrupt the portal of entry link in the chain of infection. By keeping the Foley collection bag below the level of the patient's pelvis back flow is prevented, which reduces the risk of introducing pathogens into the bladder.**

b. This is an example of controlling the reservoir, not the portal of entry, link in the chain of infection.

c. This is an example of controlling the mode of transmission, not the portal of entry, link in the chain of infection.

d. This is an example of controlling the mode of transmission, not the portal of entry, link in the chain of infection.

Safety

The following words include English vocabulary, nursing/medical terminology, concepts, principles, or information relevant to content specifically addressed in the chapter or associated with topics presented in it. English dictionaries, your nursing textbooks, and medical dictionaries such as *Taber's Cyclopedic Medical Dictionary* are resources that can be used to expand your knowledge and understanding of these words and related information.

Asphyxiation
Aspiration
Burns
Call bell
Cardiopulmonary resuscitation
Child-proof devices
Disaster plan
Drowning
Dysphagia
Electrical grounding
Electrical hazards
Electrical surge
Falls
Fire evacuation protocol
Fire extinguishers—A, B, C

Fire safety
Functional alignment
Heimlich maneuver
Incident Report
Injury
Knots
   Clove hitch
   Half bow
   Slip
Latex allergy
Physical hazards
Poisoning
Pollution
RACE—response to a fire
Restraints

Belt
Elbow
Jacket
Mitt
Mummy
Poncho
Vest
Side rails
Smother
Strangulation
Suffocation
Supervision
Three-pronged plug
Trauma

QUESTIONS

1. Which common nursing action takes priority when feeding a patient who has dysphagia?
   a. Ensuring that dentures are in place
   b. Medicating for pain or nausea before meals
   c. Providing verbal cueing to swallow each bite
   d. **Checking the mouth for emptying between every bite**

2. The best way to maintain the safety of a preschool-aged child in the acute-care setting is by:
   a. Teaching the child how to use the call bell
   b. Placing the child in a crib with high side rails
   c. **Keeping the child under constant supervision**
   d. Having the child stay in the playroom most of the day

3. Which is the most important intervention to help prevent falls from physical hazards in a hospital?
   a. Using an over-bed table
   b. **Ensuring adequate lighting**
   c. Storing belongings in a safe place
   d. Positioning the telephone within easy reach

4. After patients are protected from danger and the fire is reported, the nurse should immediately:
   a. Fight the fire
   b. Close doors and windows
   c. Provide emotional support to agitated patients
   d. Determine what type fire extinguisher to use on the fire

5. Which time of day is of most concern when trying to protect a patient with dementia from injury?
   a. Afternoon
   b. Morning
   c. Evening
   d. Night

6. Which is the best type of restraint to use for a patient who is trying to pull out a urinary retention catheter?
   a. Mummy restraint
   b. Elbow restraint
   c. Jacket restraint
   d. Mitt restraint

7. What is the most common intervention that supports patient safety when feeding a patient?
   a. Elevating the head of the bed
   b. Avoiding talking to the patient while eating
   c. Opening and preparing foods before starting
   d. Keeping the upper side rails in the raised position

8. When orienting a patient to the hospital, it is most important to emphasize to the patient how to:
   a. Notify the nurse when help is needed
   b. Get out of the bed to use the bathroom
   c. Raise and lower the head and foot of the bed
   d. Use the telephone system to call family members

9. Which is the single most common intervention to help prevent falls in a hospital?
   a. Placing the bed in the lowest position to the floor
   b. Using a commode for toileting the patient
   c. Transferring patients with two caregivers
   d. Locking the wheels of a wheelchair

10. Profuse smoke is coming out of the heating unit in a patient's room. The nurse should first:
    a. Open the window
    b. Activate the fire alarm
    c. Move the patient out of the room
    d. Close the door to the patient's room

11. To apply a hospital gown appropriately to a patient receiving an intravenous infusion, the nurse should:
    a. Insert the IV bag and tubing through the sleeve from inside of the gown first
    b. Disconnect the IV at the insertion site, apply the gown, and then reconnect the IV
    c. Close the clamp on the IV tubing no more than 15 seconds while putting on the gown
    d. Don the gown on the unaffected arm, drape the gown over the other shoulder, and adjust the closure behind the neck

12. How often should a restraint be removed, the area massaged, and the joints moved through normal range?
    a. Every shift
    b. Every hour
    c. Every two hours
    d. Every four hours

13. The nurse should encourage the patient with difficulty swallowing to:
    a. Tilt the head backward when swallowing
    b. Drink fluids along with bites of solid food
    c. Keep food in the front of the mouth when chewing
    d. Keep environmental stimuli to a minimum when eating

14. Which is the first action the nurse should employ to prevent falls in an older adult?
    a. Conduct a comprehensive risk assessment
    b. Suggest removing all throw and area rugs in the home
    c. Encourage installation of adequate lighting throughout the home
    d. Discuss with the patient the normal changes of aging that place one at risk

15. Which action is most important when preparing a bed to receive a newly admitted patient?
    a. Place the patient's name on the end of the bed
    b. Ensure that the bed wheels are locked
    c. Position the call bell in reach
    d. Make an open bed

16. An appropriately worded goal associated with the nursing diagnosis Risk for Injury is, "The patient will be:
    a. Taught how to call for help to ambulate."
    b. Kept on bed rest when dizzy."
    c. Safe and free from trauma."
    d. Restrained when agitated."

17. In the hospital setting an electrical appliance should have a three-pronged plug because it:
    a. Controls stray electrical currents
    b. Promotes efficient use of electricity
    c. Shuts off the appliance if there is an electrical surge
    d. Divides the electricity among the appliances in the room

18. Which action is most important when using a stretcher?
    a. Guiding a stretcher around a turn leading with the end with the patient's head
    b. Positioning the patient's head at the end with the swivel wheels
    c. Pulling the stretcher on the elevator with the patient's feet first
    d. Pushing the stretcher from the end with the patient's head

19. The most serious risk associated with dysphagia is:
    a. Anorexia
    b. Aspiration
    c. Self-care deficit
    d. Inadequate intake

20. The physician writes the order "Patient may shower." When preparing the patient for the shower the nurse assesses that the patient lacks the strength to tolerate standing for this procedure. The nurse should:
    a. Give the patient a bed bath
    b. Assist the patient into a bathtub
    c. Use a commode chair in the shower
    d. Place the patient in a chair at the sink

21. Which is the most important action by the nurse to prevent falls in patients who are confused?
    a. Encourage use of the corridor handrails
    b. Place in a room near the nurses' station
    c. Reinforce how to use the call bell
    d. Maintain close supervision

22. When teaching children about fire safety procedures, they should be taught that if their clothes catch on fire they should:
    a. Yell for help
    b. Roll on the ground
    c. Take their clothes off
    d. Pour water on their clothes

23. What should the nurse do first when applying a vest restraint?
    a. Ensure that the back of the vest is positioned on the patient's back
    b. Permit 4 fingers to slide between the patient and the restraint
    c. Inspect the patient's skin where the restraint is to be placed
    d. Secure the restraint to the bed frame using a slip knot

24. Which position would be best for an unconscious patient who is vomiting?
    a. Supine
    b. Side-lying
    c. Orthopneic
    d. Low-Fowler's

25. What is most important when assisting a patient with a bedpan?
    a. Dusting powder on the rim before placing the bedpan under the patient
    b. Positioning the rounded rim of the bedpan toward the front of the patient
    c. Ensuring that the bedside rails are raised once the patient is on the bedpan
    d. Encouraging the patient to help as much as possible when using the bedpan

26. A toaster is on fire in the pantry of a hospital unit. The nurse should first:
    a. Unplug the toaster
    b. Activate the fire alarm
    c. Put out the fire with an extinguisher
    d. Evacuate patients from the room next to the kitchen

27. Which would be the most common factor that contributes to falls in the hospital setting?
    a. Wet floors
    b. Frequent seizures
    c. Advanced age of patients
    d. Misuse of equipment by nurses

28. The action that would help prevent the most serious complication associated with a vest restraint is:
    a. Ensuring that the V opening is positioned in the front
    b. Removing the vest every 2 hours for range of motion
    c. Checking the circulation every 30 minutes
    d. Inspecting the skin every 2 hours

29. An adaptation that most indicates that further assessment is necessary to determine if the patient has difficulty swallowing would be:
    a. Abdominal cramping
    b. Epigastric pain
    c. Constipation
    d. Drooling

30. A patient who secretly has been smoking in bed falls asleep and the cigarette ignites the patient's gown. When entering the room the nurse should first:
    a. Close the door
    b. Activate the fire alarm
    c. Roll the patient from side to side
    d. Smother the flames with a blanket

31. Which would be the most important data collected on admission to the hospital that would indicate that the patient was at risk for physical injury?
    a. Weakness experienced during a prior admission
    b. Medication that increases intestinal motility
    c. Two recent falls that occurred at home
    d. The need for corrective eye glasses

32. When turning and positioning a patient who has a urinary retention catheter, an IV, and is receiving oxygen via nasal cannula, what should the nurse do first?
    a. Ensure that the tubes are safely positioned
    b. Enlist the assistance of the patient, if possible
    c. Obtain the assistance of an additional caregiver
    d. Document the need for turning and positioning

33. To best prevent a patient from falling, the nurse should:
    a. Provide a cane
    b. Keep walkways clear of obstacles
    c. Assist the patient with ambulation
    d. Encourage that the patient use the hand rails in the hall

34. The use of mitt restraints would be most therapeutic when they are used to:
    a. Keep a patient from falling out of bed
    b. Prevent a patient from pulling out a feeding tube
    c. Maintain the upper extremities in functional alignment
    d. Remind a patient to call for assistance when getting out of bed

35. Which is the last step in making an occupied bed?
    a. Raise both side rails on the bed
    b. Lower the height of the bed toward the floor
    c. Ensure that the patient is in a comfortable position
    d. Raise the head of the bed to a semi-Fowler's position

36. When caring for a patient with a nasogastric tube for gastric decompression, which nursing action takes priority?
    a. Positioning the patient in the low-Fowler's position
    b. Providing care to the nares at least every 8 hours
    c. Discontinuing wall suction when providing care
    d. Instilling the tube with 30 cc of air every 2 hrs

37. A patient states that when turning on an electric radio a strong electrical shock was felt. What should the nurse do first?
    a. Call maintenance to come and examine the radio
    b. Disconnect the radio from the source of energy
    c. Check the skin for electrical burns
    d. Take the patient's apical pulse

38. The hospitalized patient at the highest risk for injury is a:
    a. Young child
    b. Comatose teenager
    c. Postmenopausal woman
    d. Confused middle-aged man

39. Which information is important to understand when planning nursing care associated with restraint use?
    a. Restraints adequately prevent falls or injury
    b. Restraints cannot be applied without a physician's order
    c. Reasons for physical restraints must be clearly documented
    d. Most patients recognize that restraints contribute to their safety

40. Injuries in hospitalized patients are caused most commonly by:
    a. Malfunctioning equipment
    b. Failure to use restraints
    c. Visitors
    d. Falls

41. Which is the first thing the nurse should do to prevent problems associated with latex allergies for all patients?
    a. Use non-latex gloves
    b. Identify persons at risk
    c. Keep a latex-safe supply cart available
    d. Administer antihistamine prophylactically

42. Which nursing intervention would enhance an older adult's sensory perception and thereby help prevent injury when walking from the bed to the bathroom?
    a. Providing adequate lighting
    b. Raising the pitch of the voice
    c. Holding onto the patient's arm
    d. Removing environmental hazards

43. Health teaching regarding fires in the home should include information about what to do if grease in a frying pan catches on fire. People should be taught to call 911 and then attempt to contain the fire by:
    a. Pouring water in the pan
    b. Putting the lid on the pan
    c. Closing the door to the kitchen
    d. Using a Class A fire extinguisher

44. Which human response to illness would place the patient at greatest risk for aspiration during meals?
    a. Bulimia
    b. Lethargy
    c. Anorexia
    d. Stomatitis

45. Which is most important when preparing a patient for a physical examination?
    a. Determining if there are any positions that are contraindicated for the patient
    b. Exploring the patient's attitude toward health care providers
    c. Inquiring about the other professionals caring for the patient
    d. Asking when the patient last had a physical examination

1. a. Although this should be done if a patient has dentures, it is not the priority.
   b. Although these medications may be administered, antiemetics and analgesics both cause drowsiness that may increase the potential for aspiration in a patient with dysphagia.
   c. Although this should be done, the patient may be physically incapable of following this direction.
   d. **This is the safest way to ensure that a bolus of food is not left in the mouth where it can be aspirated and cause an airway obstruction.**

2. a. A preschool-aged child does not have the cognitive and emotional maturity to use a call bell.
   b. A preschool-aged child might attempt to climb over the side rails. A crib with high side rails is more appropriate for an infant.
   c. **Constant supervision ensures that an adult can monitor the preschool-aged child's activity and environment so that safety needs are met. Preschool-aged children are active, curious, and fearless and have immature musculoskeletal and neurological systems, narrow life experiences, and a limited ability to understand cause and effect. All of these factors place preschool-aged children at risk for injury unless supervised.**
   d. This is inappropriate because most preschoolers still take 1 or 2 daily naps, the patient may be on bed rest, and periods of activity and rest should be alternated to conserve the child's energy.

3. a. This is unsafe. An over-bed table has wheels and therefore cannot provide a firm base of support. Over-bed tables are physical hazards that often contribute to falls if used inappropriately.
   b. **This provides for the safety of patients, staff, and visitors within a hospital. Inadequate lighting causes shadows, a dark environment, and the potential for misinterpreting stimuli (illusions), and is a major cause of accidents in the hospital setting.**
   c. Although this should be done, this is not a physical hazard.
   d. Although this should be done, and reaching for a phone can result in a loss of balance and a fall, it is not the most important intervention to prevent injury in a hospital.

4. a. Attempting to extinguish the fire is the last responsibility of the nurse during a fire after all other responsibilities are accomplished.
   b. **This helps to limit the oxygen source and contain it in one room. During a fire, a nurse's responsibilities follow the sequence of protecting and evacuating patients, reporting the fire, containing the fire, and finally attempting to extinguish the fire.**
   c. In a crisis, the first priority is the physical, not emotional, safety of patients.
   d. Attempting to extinguish the fire is the last responsibility of the nurse during a fire after all other responsibilities are accomplished.

5. a. The sunlight and normal afternoon activities generally help keep patients with dementia more oriented and safe.
   b. The sunlight and the routine morning activities of hygiene, grooming, dressing, and eating generally help keep patients with dementia more oriented and safe.
   c. As the day progresses the concern for safety increases. However, in the evening there are activities of daily living and available caregivers to distract the patient and provide for safety.
   d. **At the end of the day patients with dementia often experience confusion and agitation (sundown syndrome). At night there is less light, less activity, and fewer caregivers, so there are fewer orienting stimuli. Patients who are confused or agitated are at an increased risk for injury because they may not comprehend cause and effect and, therefore, lack the ability to make safe judgments.**

6. a. A mummy restraint usually is used to immobilize an infant or very young child during a procedure.
   b. An elbow restraint usually is used to prevent flexion of the elbow in an infant or young child to prevent the pulling out of tubes.
   c. A jacket restraint usually is used to keep a person from falling out of bed while not immobilizing the extremities.
   d. **A mitt restraint covers the hand to prevent the fingers from grasping and pulling out tubes.**

7. a. **Elevating the head of the bed facilitates swallowing by permitting food and fluid to flow toward the esophagus, and limits regurgitation based on the principle of gravity.**
   b. The patient, not the nurse, should not talk when the patient is eating. Talking opens the glottis, which raises the risk for aspiration when food or fluid is in the mouth.
   c. This is unrelated to safety.
   d. This is unnecessary if the nurse is at the bedside feeding the patient.

8. a. **Explaining how to use a call bell meets safety and security needs. It reinforces that help is immediately available at a time when the patient may feel physically or emotionally vulnerable in an unfamiliar environment.**
   b. Patients generally do not need teaching about how to get out of bed to go to the bathroom. This instruction depends on the individual needs of a patient.
   c. Although this is part of orienting a patient to the hospital environment, it is not the most important point to emphasize with a patient.
   d. Although this is part of orienting a patient to the hospital environment, it is not the most important point to emphasize with a patient.

9. a. **A greater risk for injury to a patient occurs when the mattress of the bed is further from the floor. It is safer if the bed is in the lowest position and the patient's feet are flat on the floor when getting out of bed.**

b. A commode should be used only when a patient does not have the strength to ambulate to the bathroom but is permitted out of bed.

c. This is unnecessary and impractical in most situations.

d. Although this is done, most patients do not need a wheelchair.

10. a. This is contraindicated because environmental air will feed the fire, causing it to increase in severity.

b. Although this will be done, it is not the priority at this point in time.

c. The patient's physical safety is the priority. The patient must be removed from direct danger before the alarm is activated and the fire contained.

d. Although this will be done eventually, it is not the priority at this point in time.

11. a. This ensures that the IV bag and tubing are safely passed through the armhole of the gown before the patient puts the arm with the insertion site through the gown. This prevents tension on the tubing and insertion site, which limits the possibility of the catheter dislodging from the vein.

b. Disconnecting the IV tubing at the catheter insertion site is unsafe. This opens a closed system unnecessarily, increasing the potential for infection.

c. This is unsafe. This stops the flow of the IV solution, which can result in blood coagulating at the end of the catheter in the vein and compromising the patency of the IV tubing.

d. This leaves the patient exposed unnecessarily. It interferes with privacy, and the patient may feel cold.

12. a. This is unsafe because it promotes the development of contractures.

b. This generally is too often.

c. Restraints should be removed every 2 hours. The extremities must be moved through their full range of motion to prevent muscle shortening and contractures. The area must be massaged to promote circulation and prevent pressure injuries.

d. This is too long a period between activity, and promotes the development of contractures.

13. a. This increases the risk of aspiration because it straightens the trachea and anatomically makes it easier for food and fluid to enter the trachea rather than the esophagus.

b. Food and fluid should be consumed separately in the presence of dysphagia. Fluid is more difficult to control with dysphagia and it may flush the solid food toward the trachea where it can cause choking or a partial or total airway obstruction.

c. This will increase the risk for aspiration. Food should be placed in the posterior, not anterior, part of the mouth toward the side. The molars in the back of the mouth are designed for chewing. Placing food to the side keeps it close to the molars for chewing and out of direct line with the trachea. Placing food in the posterior of the mouth limits the need for the tongue to manipulate the bolus of food toward the back of

the mouth in preparation for swallowing (deglutition).

d. A patient with dysphagia should concentrate on the acts of chewing and swallowing. Environmental stimuli can be distracting and can result in inadequate chewing or premature swallowing, which in turn can result in choking and aspiration.

14. a. The best way to prevent falls is by instituting extra fall precautions for those patients at the highest risk. Most hospitals have policies and procedures designed to identify, monitor, and support patients at risk.

b. Although this is advisable, it is not the priority at this time.

c. Although this is advisable, it is not the priority at this time.

d. Although this is advisable, it is not the priority at this time.

15. a. This violates the patient's right to privacy. An identification wristband must be worn for patient identification.

b. Locked bed wheels are an important safety precaution. The bed must be an immovable object because the patient may touch the bed for support, lean against it when getting in or out of bed, or move around when in bed. If the bed wheels are unlocked during these maneuvers, the bed may move and the patient can fall.

c. Although this is done, it is not the most important action to ensure patient safety.

d. Although this is done, it meets comfort, not safety, needs.

16. a. This is a planned intervention, not a goal.

b. This is a planned intervention, not a goal.

c. This is an appropriate goal. It is realistic, specific, measurable, and has a time frame. It is realistic to expect that all patients be safe. It is specific and measurable because safety from trauma can be compared to standards of care within the profession of nursing. It has a time frame because the words *free from* reflect the time frames of *always, constantly, and continuously*.

d. This is a planned intervention, not a goal. In addition, it is inappropriate to restrain a person automatically for agitation. A restraint should be used as a last resort to prevent the patient from self-injury or injuring others.

17. a. A three-pronged plug functions as a ground to dissipate stray electrical currents.

b. This is not the purpose of a three-pronged plug.

c. A surge protector performs this function.

d. A multiple outlet plug performs this function.

18. a. It is too difficult and unsafe to maneuver a stretcher with the non-swivel wheels on the leading end of the stretcher. The end of the stretcher with the patient's head does not have swivel wheels.

b. The swivel-wheeled end of the stretcher should be the leading end of the stretcher, and it is unsafe to lead with the patient's head. In addition, the end of the stretcher with the swivel wheels moves through greater arcs; this can cause dizziness. The swivel wheels of a stretcher should be at the end under the patient's feet, not the head.

   c. This is unsafe and places the patient in physical jeopardy. The elevator doors could inadvertently close by the patient's head while the nurse is pulling the feet end of the stretcher into the elevator. The patient should be moved into an elevator head, not feet, first.

   d. The swivel wheels must be under the patient's feet on the leading end of the stretcher for safe maneuverability. A stretcher is always pushed, not pulled, so that the transporter stays at the patient's head for protection.

19. a. Although lack of an appetite (anorexia) can occur with dysphagia, it is not the most serious associated risk.

   b. When a person has difficulty with swallowing (dysphagia), food or fluid can pass into the trachea and be inhaled into the lungs (aspiration) rather than swallowed down the esophagus. This can result in choking, partial or total airway obstruction, or aspiration pneumonia.

   c. Dysphagia is unrelated to self-care deficit. Feeding self-care deficit occurs when a person is unable to cut food, open food packages, or bring food to the mouth.

   d. Inadequate intake of food and fluid can result with dysphagia because of fear of choking. However, it is not the most serious associated risk.

20. a. This is unnecessary and is not as effective as a shower.

   b. This will require a practitioner's order, and few facilities have bathtubs.

   c. A commode chair or tub/shower chair is a water-resistant chair that allows the patient to sit safely during a shower. It permits a thorough cleansing and minimizes the physical demands on the patient, conserving the patient's energy.

   d. This is unnecessary and is not as effective as a shower.

21. a. A confused patient may not be able to follow directions or understand cause and effect.

   b. This may be impossible and impractical.

   c. A confused patient may not be able to follow directions or understand cause and effect.

   d. Maintaining safety of the confused patient is best accomplished through close or direct supervision. Confused patients cannot be left on their own because they may not have the cognitive ability to understand cause and effect, and therefore their actions can result in harm.

22. a. This may eventually be done, but the child must do something immediately without waiting for help to arrive.

   b. Rolling on the ground will smother the flames and put the fire out.

   c. This may be impossible. In addition, it will take time and the clothing and skin will continue to burn.

   d. Finding and obtaining water will take too much time

and the clothing and skin will continue to burn. Something must be done immediately.

23. a. Although this is done, it is not the first intervention.

   b. This would result in the jacket being too loose. The jacket should be applied so that 2, not 4, fingers can slide between the patient and the restraint.

   c. Even when applied correctly, restraints can cause pressure and friction. A baseline assessment of the skin under the restraint should be made. In addition, the presence of a dressing, pacemaker, or subclavian catheter may influence the use of a jacket restraint.

   d. Although this is done, it is the last, not the first, intervention.

24. a. This position will promote aspiration and should be avoided in this situation.

   b. This position prevents the tongue from falling to the back of the oropharynx, thus blocking vomitus and promoting aspiration. In addition, it allows the vomitus to flow out of the mouth by gravity, preventing aspiration.

   c. This is an unsafe, impossible position in which to maintain an unconscious patient.

   d. This position will promote aspiration and should be avoided in this situation.

25. a. Although this might be done to limit friction and shearing force when placing a patient on and off a bedpan, it is not the most important safety precaution related to the use of a bedpan.

   b. The rounded rim of a bedpan should be placed under the patient's buttocks, not toward the front of the patient.

   c. Patient safety is a priority. A bedpan is not a stable base of support and the effort of elimination may require movements that alter balance. Side rails provide a solid object to hold while balancing on the bedpan as well as supply a barrier to prevent falling out of bed.

   d. Although this is done to promote independence and limit strain on the nurse, it is not the most important factor to consider when assisting a patient with a bedpan.

26. a. This is unsafe because it places the nurse in jeopardy. The nurse could be exposed to an electrical charge or become burned.

   b. Because no patient is in jeopardy, the nurse's initial action should be to activate the alarm. The sooner the alarm is set the sooner professional firefighters will reach the scene of the fire.

   c. The nurse may not be capable of containing or fighting the fire. Not calling for professional firefighting help places the nurse, staff, and patients in jeopardy.

   d. This is premature at this time, but it may become necessary eventually.

27. a. Although wet floors can contribute to falls, it is not the most common factor that contributes to falls in the hospital setting.

   b. Although seizures can contribute to falls, most patients do not experience seizures.

c. Extreme older adults who are hospitalized frequently have multiple health problems, are frail, and lack stamina. All of these contribute to the inability to maintain balance and ambulate safely.

d. Although this occasionally happens and is negligence, it is not the most common factor that contributes to falls in the hospital setting.

28. a. The V opening of a jacket restraint should be in the front of the patient to prevent pressure against the neck, particularly the trachea. The rounded side of the restraint goes across the patient's back.

b. Although a jacket restraint is removed every 2 hours to permit range-of-motion exercises, contractures are not life-threatening and therefore are not the most serious complication associated with a vest restraint.

c. This is too often and unnecessary.

d. Although a jacket restraint is removed every 2 hours to permit inspection of the skin, excoriation and skin compression are not the most serious complications associated with a vest restraint.

29. a. Abdominal cramping is related to problems such as flatus, malabsorption, and increased intestinal motility, not difficulty swallowing.

b. Epigastric pain is related to problems such as gastritis, esophageal reflux disease, cholecystitis, and angina, not difficulty swallowing.

c. Although constipation may result from not eating foods high in fiber because of difficulty with chewing and swallowing, this adaptation is not as directly related to difficulty swallowing as another option.

d. The body continuously secretes saliva (approximately 1000 cc a day) that is usually swallowed. When saliva accumulates and is not swallowed, it dribbles out of the mouth (drooling). This would indicate the need to assess swallowing.

30. a. This will impede the evacuation of the room if it becomes necessary.

b. This is premature at this time, but it may become necessary eventually.

c. This is unsafe. Rolling the patient from side to side fans the flames, which will increase the intensity of the fire.

d. Smothering the flames with a blanket deprives the fire of oxygen. Without oxygen to support combustion, the fire will go out.

31. a. Although this is important information, it is not the most important factor of the options offered in this question. In addition, the prior admission may have been too long ago to have any current relevance.

b. A patient with increased intestinal motility may experience diarrhea, which may place the patient at risk for a fluid and electrolyte imbalance, not a physical injury. Although a person with diarrhea may need to toilet more frequently, a bedside commode or bedpan can be used to reduce the risk of falls.

c. This is significant information that must be considered because if falls occurred before, they are likely to occur again. When a risk is identified, additional injury prevention precautions can be implemented.

d. Although this is important information, it is not the most important factor of the options offered in this question.

32. a. This is essential to prevent their accidental dislodgment or removal.

b. Although at times a patient may assist with tubes, it is not the patient's responsibility to ensure safety of tubes.

c. This may or may not be necessary.

d. This is done last, not first.

33. a. The patient may or may not need a cane. An unnecessary cane actually may increase the risk of a fall.

b. Although this should be done, it is not the best intervention in the options presented.

c. This widens the patient's base of support, which improves balance and decreases the risk of a fall.

d. Although this should be done, it is not the best intervention in the options presented.

34. a. This is the purpose of a jacket restraint.

b. Mitt restraints cover the hands, which prevent the fingers from grasping and pulling out catheters.

c. Pillows, rolls, and wedges, not restraints, are used to maintain the body in functional alignment.

d. This is not the purpose of a mitt restraint.

35. a. This may or may not be necessary. This action should be based on the individual needs of the patient.

b. It is safer if the bed is in the lowest position and the patient's feet are flat on the floor when getting in or out of bed. A greater risk for injury to a patient occurs when the mattress of the bed is further from the floor.

c. This should be done while the bed is at a comfortable working height for the nurse.

d. This may or may not be necessary. This action should be based on the individual needs of the patient.

36. a. A nasogastric (NG) tube for gastric decompression passes down the esophagus, through the cardiac sphincter, and into the stomach. The cardiac sphincter remains slightly open because of the presence of the NG tube. The low-Fowler's position keeps gastric secretions in the stomach via gravity (preventing reflux and aspiration) and allows the gastric contents to be suctioned out by the NG tube.

b. This should be done more frequently to prevent irritation and pressure.

c. This is unnecessary and can result in vomiting and aspiration.

d. Patency of an NG tube should be assessed every 2 hours. After determining placement of the tube, 30 cc of normal saline, not air, can be used as an instillation or irrigation to reestablish patency.

37. a. Although this may be done eventually, it is not the priority at this time.
   b. This action is contraindicated because it could place the nurse in jeopardy.
   c. This is not the priority and electrical burns may or may not be evident.
   d. **An electric shock can interfere with the electrical conduction system within the heart and result in dysrhythmias. An electric shock can be transmitted through the body because body fluids (consisting of sodium chloride) are an excellent conductor of electricity.**

38. a. Although a young child is at risk for injury in a hospital setting, age-related precautions are always instituted. More nurses are generally assigned to pediatric units and frequently family members are at the bedside.
   b. This patient is not at as high a risk for injury as a patient in another option. A comatose patient demonstrates no response to maximum painful stimuli, has an absence of muscle tone and reflexes in the extremities, and appears to be in a deep sleep.
   c. A postmenopausal woman is not at a high risk for injury.
   d. **A confused patient is at an increased risk for injury because of the inability to comprehend cause and effect and, therefore, lacks the ability to make safe decisions.**

39. a. This is not true. Injuries and falls can occur if restraints are not applied appropriately. In addition, research indicates that patients incur less severe injuries if left unrestrained.
   b. Restraints are applied in emergencies to protect patients from harming themselves or others. A physician's order must be obtained for the original restraint within 24 hours. Agencies have protocols concerning how often restraints need to be reordered by the physician (many require reorders every 24 hours).
   c. **All patient care, including the use of restraints, should adhere to standards of care. The reason for the use of restraints must adhere to standards of care and be documented on the patient's hospital record to create a legal record that protects the patient as well as the health care providers.**
   d. The opposite is true. Patients resist the use of restraints and usually are mentally or emotionally incompetent to understand their necessity or benefits.

40. a. This is not true.
   b. This is not true. The use of restraints has declined dramatically and now is used only when patients may harm themselves or others.
   c. This is not true.
   d. **Research demonstrates that most injuries experienced by hospitalized patients occur from falls. Failing to call for assistance, inadequate lighting, and the physical condition of the patient all contribute to falls.**

41. a. This may or may not be necessary depending on the patient.
   b. **Patient allergies must be identified (e.g., latex, food, medication, etc.) before any care is provided, documented in the patient's hospital record, and appear on a red allergy-alert wristband. After a risk is identified, additional safety precautions can be implemented to prevent exposure to the offending allergen.**
   c. This may be available but is useless unless the supplies are used appropriately.
   d. This is unnecessary. A person with a latex allergy should not be exposed to latex products.

42. a. **This provides for the safety of patients, staff, and visitors within a hospital. Inadequate lighting causes shadows, a dark environment, and the potential for misinterpreting stimuli (illusions), and is a major cause of accidents in the hospital setting.**
   b. When talking with older adults it is better to lower, not raise, the pitch of the voice. As people age they are more likely to have impaired hearing with higher pitch sounds.
   c. This is not always necessary and therefore could be degrading or promote regression. Sometimes patients' behaviors circumvent nursing care. Not all patients need assistance and many patients who should call for assistance do not.
   d. Although this should be done, furniture and medical equipment are not the only physical hazards that can contribute to falls.

43. a. Water is ineffective against a grease fire. It will scatter the flames and the fire will spread.
   b. **The lid of the frying pan deprives the fire of oxygen. Without oxygen to support combustion, the fire will go out.**
   c. Although this will help to contain the fire to the kitchen, there is a more appropriate intervention to contain the fire to the frying pan.
   d. This is inappropriate. A class A fire extinguisher is designed for fires consisting of paper, wood, upholstery, rags, and ordinary rubbish.

44. a. Aspiration usually is not a risk with bulimia. Bulimia is an insatiable craving for food characterized by episodes of binge eating followed by purging, depression, and self-deprivation.
   b. **When a person is sleepy, sluggish, or stuporous (lethargic) there may be a reduced level of consciousness and diminished reflexes, including the gag and swallowing reflexes. This condition can result in aspiration of food or fluids that can compromise the person's airway and respiratory status.**
   c. A lack of appetite (anorexia) is unrelated to aspiration. The less food or fluid is placed in the mouth, the less the risk for aspiration.
   d. An inflammation of the mucous membranes of the mouth (stomatitis) may result in dysphagia and increase the risk of aspiration. However, of the options offered it does not place a person at the highest risk for aspiration.

45. a. A physical examination requires a patient to assume a variety of positions such as supine, side-lying, sitting, and standing. The nurse should inquire about any positions that are uncomfortable or contraindicated because of past or current medical conditions to prevent complications.
    b. Although this information may be obtained during the course of the physical examination, it is not the priority.
    c. This is not the priority during a physical examination. This might be done to prevent fragmentation of care and ensure continuity of care.
    d. Although this might be done, it is not a priority during a physical examination.

Medication Administration

The following words include English vocabulary, nursing/medical terminology, concepts, principles, or information relevant to content specifically addressed in the chapter or associated with topics presented in it. English dictionaries, your nursing textbooks, and medical dictionaries such as *Taber's Cyclopedic Medical Dictionary* are resources that can be used to expand your knowledge and understanding of these words and related information.

Acromion process
Aerosol
Air-lock technique
Ampule
Apothecary system
Applicator
Asepto syringe
Auditory canal
Automated medication-dispensing system
Blister-pack
Bolus
Cartridge
Cheek
Continuous infusion
Dilute
Diluent
Dispense
Disperse
Dissolve
Dosage
Filtered needle
Five Rights
Gauge
Greater trochanter
Herbs and botanicals
Humerus bone
Infusion
Inject
Injection site grids
Injection sites
   Abdomen
   Deltoid

Dorsogluteal
Rectus femoris
Vastus lateralis
Ventrogluteal
Inner/outer canthus
Instillation
Insulin syringe
Interaction
Intermittent infusion of medication
Label
Lacrimal duct
Lubricate
Mechanism of action
Medication orders
   Single orders
   Standing orders
   Stat orders
   Stop orders
   Telephone order
Medication regimen
Metered-dose inhaler
Metric system
Needle bevel
Orifice
Over-the-counter drugs
Parenteral
Peak level
Pinna of the ear
Posterior superior iliac spine
Potent
PRN orders
Radial nerve
Reconstitution

Routes of administration
   Buccal
   Ear (Otic)
   Epidural
   Eye (Ophthalmic)
   Intradermal
   Intramuscular
   Intrathecal
   Intravenous
   IV push, piggyback
   Nasal cavity
   Rectal
   Subcutaneous
   Sublingual
   Topical
   Transdermal
   Urinary bladder
   Vaginal
Rubber seal
Sciatic nerve
Sharps container
Substance abuse
Syringe
Systemic/local effect
Therapeutic drug level
Titrate
Troche
Trough level
Tuberculin syringe
Unit-dose system
Vial
Weekly pill container
Z-Track

QUESTIONS

1. The nurse evaluates that a patient understands the teaching about taking a sublingual medication when the patient states, "I should place it:
   a. On my skin."
   b. Inside my cheek."
   c. Under my tongue."
   d. In the lower lid of my eye."

2. When administering a bolus dose of a medication via a currently running intravenous infusion, the nurse should first:
   a. Ensure that it is compatible with the solution being infused
   b. Instill it into a 50-cc bag of NS and infuse it via a secondary line
   c. Pinch the tubing above the infusion port while instilling the bolus
   d. Administer it via a volume-controlled device with microdrip tubing

3. To administer a rectal suppository to an adult, the nurse should:
   a. Place the patient in the prone position
   b. Lubricate the medication before insertion
   c. Warm the medication to body temperature
   d. Insert the medication at least 2 inches into the rectum

4. When administering an intradermal injection, the nurse should insert the needle at a:
   a. 15-degree angle
   b. 30-degree angle
   c. 45-degree angle
   d. 90-degree angle

5. A patient who self-administers an aerosol medication by a metered-dose inhaler complains of "the nasty taste of the medication." The nurse should encourage the patient to:
   a. Shake the cartridge longer before using it
   b. Suck on a hard candy after the procedure
   c. Perform oral hygiene before the inhalation of medication
   d. Attach an aerosol chamber to the metered-dose cartridge

6. Which site is least desirable for a 3-ml intramuscular injection?
   a. Deltoid
   b. Dorsogluteal
   c. Ventrogluteal
   d. Vastus lateralis

7. When a patient has difficulty swallowing an aspirin, the nurse should first:
   a. Crush the pill and put it in a teaspoon of applesauce
   b. Dilute the pill in a glass of water and administer it slowly
   c. Call the physician and obtain an order to use a different route
   d. Explain how the medication works and attempt to give it again

8. When placing a cream into the vaginal canal, the nurse should use:
   a. A finger
   b. An applicator
   c. An irrigation kit
   d. A 4×4 gauze pad

9. What should the nurse do first if the medication that is ordered does not have the same name as the medication in the patient's medication draw?
   a. Inform the physician that the medication is unavailable
   b. Direct the pharmacy to deliver the correct medication
   c. Check the medication's generic name
   d. Hold the medication

10. A drug delivered transdermally is:
    a. Inhaled into the respiratory tract
    b. Dissolved under the tongue
    c. Absorbed through the skin
    d. Inserted into the rectum

11. Effective titrating of pain relieving drugs depends upon:
    a. Increasing the dose until conscious sedation is achieved
    b. Altering the dose based on the need to control vomiting and constipation
    c. Changing drugs, doses, times, and routes based on the individual's responses
    d. Administering opiates first, then giving less potent drugs after the pain is under control

12. To limit discomfort when administering injections, the nurse should:
    a. Test for a blood return before injecting the medication
    b. Apply ice to the area before the injection
    c. Pinch the area while inserting the needle
    d. Inject the medication slowly

13. What should the nurse do first when preparing to draw up medication from a vial?
    a. Ensure that the needle is firmly attached to the syringe
    b. Rub vigorously back and forth over the rubber cap with an alcohol swab
    c. Inject air into the vial with the needle bevel below the surface of the medication
    d. Draw up slightly more air than the volume of medication to be withdrawn from the vial

14. To utilize the Z-track technique when administering an injection, the nurse should:
    a. Pinch the site throughout the injection
    b. Massage the site after the needle is removed
    c. Remove the needle immediately after the medication is injected
    d. Change the needle after the medication is drawn into the syringe

15. When administering an intramuscular injection, the nurse should:
    a. Utilize a $1^1/_2$-inch needle
    b. Use a #25-gauge needle size
    c. Insert the needle at a 45-degree angle
    d. Pinch the skin before needle insertion

16. The nurse should instruct the patient to close the eyes after the administration of eye drops to:
    a. Limit corneal irritation
    b. Squeeze excess medication from the eyes
    c. Disperse the medication over the eyeballs
    d. Prevent medication from entering the lacrimal duct

17. Which route is unrelated to the parenteral administration of medications?
    a. Buccal
    b. Z-track
    c. Intravenous
    d. Intradermal

18. How often should "Colace 100 mg q.d." be given?
    a. Three times a day
    b. Four times a day
    c. Every other day
    d. Once a day

19. Which factor related to administration is unique to an intradermal injection?
    a. Utilize the air-bubble technique
    b. Pinch the skin during needle insertion
    c. Insert the needle with the bevel upward
    d. Massage the area after the fluid is instilled

20. The nurse assesses that a patient needs further teaching about the use of a metered-dose inhaler when the patient:
    a. Shakes the cartridge before using it
    b. Blows the nose before the procedure
    c. Presses the cartridge before taking a breath
    d. Exhales completely before pressing the cartridge

21. Which is most essential in the preparation of a reconstituted medication?
    a. Instilling an accurate amount of diluent into the vial
    b. Using a filtered needle when drawing up the medication from the vial
    c. Instilling air into the vial before withdrawing the reconstituted solution
    d. Wiping the rubber seal of the vial with alcohol before and after each needle insertion

22. What is the best method to disperse medication instilled into the ear of an adult?
    a. Press several times on the tragus of the ear
    b. Pull the pinna of the ear backward and downward
    c. Instill the drops into the center of the auditory canal
    d. Roll the patient from the side-lying to the supine position

23. To apply a topical antibiotic to an infected wound, the nurse should:
    a. Use medical asepsis
    b. Apply a thin layer of medication
    c. Rub the medication into the skin surface
    d. Place it on the intact skin around the wound

24. Which is a contraindication for the intake of medications via the p.o. route?
    a. Difficulty swallowing
    b. Gastric suctioning
    c. Unconsciousness
    d. Nausea

25. Which action is inappropriate when administering a rectal suppository to an adult?
    a. Lubricate the tip of the suppository
    b. Place the patient in the left-lateral position
    c. Don a glove when inserting the suppository
    d. Insert the suppository 2 inches into the rectum

26. The site for an intramuscular injection that has the highest risk for injury is the:
    a. Vastus lateralis
    b. Rectus femoris
    c. Ventrogluteal
    d. Dorsogluteal

27. It is most important for the nurse to use a filtered needle when preparing a parenteral medication that:
    a. Has to be reconstituted
    b. Is supplied in an ampule
    c. Appears cloudy in the vial
    d. Is to be mixed with another medication

28. When administering a vaginal suppository, the nurse should:
    a. Irrigate the vagina with normal saline before inserting the suppository
    b. Place the patient in the left-lateral position for the procedure
    c. Insert the suppository along the posterior wall of the vagina
    d. Wear sterile gloves when inserting the suppository

29. Immediately after instilling a liquid medication into an eye, the nurse should:
    a. Apply a sterile eye patch
    b. Keep the lower lid retracted
    c. Wipe toward the inner canthus
    d. Press gently on the inner canthus

30. When administering a transdermal patch, the nurse should:
    a. Use the same area each time to limit skin irritation and excoriation
    b. Rub the area to promote comfort and vasodilation before applying the patch
    c. Shave the area to facilitate adherence of the patch and medication absorption
    d. Remove the old patch 1 hour after applying the new patch to ensure a therapeutic blood level of the drug

31. When administering a subcutaneous injection, the nurse should use a:
    a. 5 ml syringe
    b. #25-gauge needle
    c. Tuberculin syringe
    d. 1$\frac{1}{2}$ inch long needle

32. When instilling nose drops, the nurse should:
    a. Place the patient in the supine position with the head tilted backward
    b. Pinch the nares of the nose together briefly after the drops are instilled
    c. Instruct the patient to blow the nose 5 minutes after the drops are instilled
    d. Insert the drop applicator 1/8 inch into the nose toward the base of the nasal cavity

33. What should the nurse do if a patient is unable to hold a medication cup when administering a pill?
    a. Crush the pill and mix it with applesauce
    b. Obtain a physician's order for the liquid form of the drug
    c. Use the medication cup to introduce the pill into the mouth
    d. Instruct the patient to take the pill from the cup and self-administer the drug

34. What does the nurse want to avoid when administering an intramuscular injection at the dorsogluteal site?
    a. Radial nerve
    b. Humerus bone
    c. Acromion process
    d. Major blood vessels

35. What action should the nurse teach the patient who is self-administering a steroid via a metered dose inhaler?
    a. Rinse the mouth with water after the treatment
    b. Place the lips around the mouthpiece while inhaling
    c. Sit in the semi-Fowler's position with the head supported on a pillow
    d. Distribute the medication by rolling the canister between your hands slowly before administering

36. Which is an inappropriate route for a topical medication?
    a. Intradermal
    b. Bladder
    c. Rectum
    d. Vagina

37. When administering a rectal suppository, the nurse should teach the patient to:
    a. Bear down while the medication is being inserted
    b. Remain flat in bed for at least 3 minutes after the procedure
    c. Assume the right side-lying position with the upper leg flexed
    d. Perform slow thoracic breathing through the nose during insertion

38. What should the nurse do first when drawing up 10 units of Humulin R (regular) insulin and 30 units of Humulin N (NPH) insulin in the same syringe?
    a. Inject 10 units of air into the Humulin R (regular) insulin vial
    b. Inject 30 units of air into the Humulin N (NPH) insulin vial
    c. Draw up 10 units of Humulin R (regular) insulin
    d. Draw up 30 units of Humulin N (NPH) insulin

39. Which action takes priority when medication is to be added to an intravenous fluid bag?
    a. Attaching a completed IV additive label to the bag
    b. Mixing the medication and solution by rotating the bag
    c. Maintaining sterile technique throughout the procedure
    d. Ensuring that the drug and the IV solution are compatible

40. The nurse holds a bottle of liquid medication with the label next to the palm of the hand when pouring a dose to:
    a. Conceal the label from the curiosity of others
    b. Prevent the soiling of the label by spilled liquid
    c. Ensure the accuracy of the measurement of the dose
    d. Guarantee that the label is read before pouring the liquid

41. What should the nurse do when administering a lozenge to a patient's buccal area of the mouth?
    a. Ensure that the medication is dissolved under the tongue
    b. Instruct the patient to take occasional sips of water
    c. Administer the lozenge one hour before meals
    d. Alternate cheeks from one dose to another

42. Which route of drug administration is not considered parenteral?
    a. Epidural
    b. Transdermal
    c. Subcutaneous
    d. Intramuscular

43. Which is most essential when applying a medicated powder to a patient's skin?
    a. Applying a thin layer in the direction of hair growth
    b. Protecting the patient's face with a towel
    c. Dressing the area with dry sterile gauze
    d. Ensuring that the skin surface is dry

44. What should the nurse do first to access an ampule?
    a. Inject the same amount of air as the fluid to be removed
    b. Wipe the constricted neck with an alcohol swab
    c. Break the constricted neck using a barrier
    d. Insert a needle into the rubber seal

45. To limit discomfort when administering medication into the ear of an adult, the nurse should:
    a. Warm the solution to body temperature
    b. Place the patient in a comfortable position
    c. Pull the pinna of the ear upward and backward
    d. Instill the fluid in the center of the auditory canal

46. A patient is instructed to inhale deeply and hold each breath for a second when using a hand-held nebulizer because this action will:
    a. Prolong the treatment
    b. Limit hyperventilation
    c. Disperse the medication
    d. Prevent bronchial spasms

47. Which abbreviation indicates that the physician wants a medication administered twice a day?
    a. p.c.
    b. h.s.
    c. q2h
    d. b.i.d.

48. When administering an intramuscular injection to an morbidly obese patient, the nurse should use:
    a. The Z-track method
    b. An 18-gauge needle
    c. The dorsogluteal site
    d. A needle longer than $1^1/_2$ inches

49. A drug delivered by a suppository is absorbed in the:
    a. Ear
    b. Nose
    c. Mouth
    d. Rectum

50. What is the first thing the nurse should do when administering a vaginal suppository?
    a. Inspect the vaginal orifice
    b. Provide perineal care
    c. Remove the wrapper
    d. Wear sterile gloves

51. To help a patient with short term memory loss to remember to take multiple drugs throughout the day, the nurse should:
    a. Instruct the patient to put medications in a weekly organizational pill container
    b. Design a chart of the medications the patient takes each day during the week
    c. Ask a family member to call the patient when medications are to be taken
    d. Suggest that the patient wear a watch with an alarm

52. What should the nurse do when administering an eye irrigation to the right eye?
    a. Direct the flow of solution from the inner to the outer canthus
    b. Irrigate with an Asepto syringe 2 inches from the eye
    c. Don sterile gloves before beginning the procedure
    d. Position the patient in a right lateral position

53. A medication is delivered by the Z-track method when the nurse:
    a. Uses a special syringe designed for Z-track injections
    b. Pulls laterally and downward on the skin before inserting the needle
    c. Administers the injection in the muscle on the anterior lateral aspect of the thigh
    d. Injects the needle in a separate spot for each dose on a Z-shaped grid on the abdomen

54. When reconstituting a powdered medication the nurse should:
    a. Keep the needle below the initial fluid level as the rest of the fluid is injected
    b. Instill solvent that is consistent with the manufacture's directions
    c. Score the neck of the ampule before breaking it
    d. Shake the vial to dissolve the powder

55. When preparing to administer a tablet to a patient the nurse should remove the p.o. medication from its unit dose package:
    a. Outside the door to the patient's room
    b. When standing next to the patient
    c. In the medication room
    d. At the medication cart

56. When titrating a drug for the patient in pain, which nursing action is most appropriate?
    a. Follow the physician's order exactly for the first 24 hours
    b. Reassess the patient every 8 hours for drug effectiveness
    c. Ask the physician to include a medication order for breakthrough pain
    d. Seek a new order after two doses that do not achieve a tolerable level of relief

57. When the physician orders a troche, the nurse should administer it by placing it in the patient's:
    a. Ear
    b. Eye
    c. Mouth
    d. Rectum

58. What should the nurse do when identifying the left dorsogluteal site for an intramuscular injection?
    a. Locate the lower edge of the acromion and the midpoint of the lateral aspect of the arm
    b. Draw a line from the posterior superior iliac spine to the greater trochanter
    c. Place the heel of the left hand on the greater trochanter
    d. Palpate the anterior lateral aspect of the thigh

59. What action should the nurse teach the patient who has an order for 2 puffs of a bronchodilator via a metered-dose inhaler?
    a. Start breathing in while compressing the canister
    b. Hold the inspired breath for 2–4 seconds
    c. Deliver 2 puffs with each inspiration
    d. Inhale slowly for 8–10 seconds

60. Which is related to an intradermal injection?
    a. 2 ml syringe
    b. 26-gauge needle
    c. 1-inch needle length
    d. 30-degree angle of insertion

ANSWERS AND RATIONALES

1. a. Topical medications are applied on the skin.
   b. A tablet or lozenge given by the buccal route is placed between the cheek and gums.
   c. A sublingual medication is placed under the tongue. It is absorbed quickly through the mucous membranes into the systemic circulation.
   d. A medication placed in the lower conjunctival sac of the eye is administered for its local effect and is considered a topical medication.

2. a. An incompatible solution can increase, decrease, or neutralize the effects of the medication. In addition, an incompatibility may result in a compound or cause a precipitate that is harmful to the patient.
   b. This is done for a medication administered via an intermittent intravenous infusion over a 30- to 90-minute period rather than an intravenous bolus (IV push) dose that is administered over 1 to 5 minutes).
   c. This is not the initial action. This is done immediately before and while instilling the medication to ensure that the medication flows toward the patient rather than in the opposite direction up the tubing.
   d. The volume of fluid of a bolus dose is too small to necessitate a volume-controlled device. In addition, a volume-controlled device does not require microdrip tubing.

3. a. The patient should be placed in the left-lateral or left-Sims' position.
   b. Lubrication eases insertion by reducing friction, which limits tissue trauma and discomfort.
   c. Warming the medication would cause it to melt and it would be impossible to insert. Most rectal suppositories are kept refrigerated until use.
   d. Rectal suppositories should be inserted 4 inches into the rectal canal of an adult.

4. a. An intradermal injection is administered by inserting a needle at a 10- to 15-degree angle through the skin. The small volume of medication instilled just below the epidermis causes the formation of a wheal.
   b. This would be too steep an angle for an intradermal injection and a wheal would not form.
   c. This angle is appropriate for a subcutaneous, not an intradermal, injection.
   d. This angle is appropriate for an intramuscular, not an intradermal, injection.

5. a. This will ensure that the medication is dispersed throughout solution in the cartridge. It will not change the taste of the medication.
   b. This will not prevent the problem from occurring in the first place.
   c. Oral hygiene should be performed after the procedure.
   d. The aerosolized medication enters the aerosol chamber where the larger droplets fall to the bottom of the chamber. The smaller droplets are inhaled deep into the lung rather than falling on the patient's tongue.

6. a. The deltoid, on the lateral aspect of the upper arm, is a small muscle that is incapable of absorbing a large medication volume. This site is more appropriate for a subcutaneous injection.
   b. The dorsogluteal site uses the gluteus maximus muscles in the buttocks, which can absorb larger medication volumes.
   c. The ventrogluteal site uses the gluteus medius and minimus muscles in the area of the hip, which can absorb larger medication volumes.
   d. The vastus lateralis muscle is located on the anterolateral aspect of the thigh, which can absorb larger medication volumes.

7. a. Crushing the tablet produces small particles, which when mixed with applesauce are easier to swallow. The small volume of applesauce minimizes the amount that is swallowed to ensure that the entire dose is taken.
   b. A patient who has difficulty swallowing may not be able to drink an entire glass of water, which would result in not receiving the correct dose.
   c. This may eventually be necessary, but it is not the initial nursing intervention.
   d. Administering it again would be unsafe. Teaching about the medication would not improve the patient's ability to swallow the tablet.

8. a. Either a gloved finger or an applicator is used to insert a vaginal suppository, not a cream.
   b. The consistency of a cream requires that an applicator be used to ensure that the medication is deposited along the full length of the vaginal canal.
   c. The consistency of a cream is too thick to be inserted into the vagina with an irrigating kit.
   d. It is impossible to insert a cream into the vaginal canal with a gauze pad. If attempted, it would traumatize the mucous membranes of the vagina.

9. a. This action is premature.
   b. This eventually may need to be done, but it is not the priority action.
   c. An alternate name for the drug should be determined first. One drug can have several names (chemical, official, trade, and generic names). The generic name is the name assigned by the manufacturer that first develops the drug.
   d. This might ultimately be done, but not until it is determined that it is an inappropriate medication.

10. a. A medication that is aerosolized is inhaled.
    b. A tablet, such as nitroglycerine, is dissolved under the tongue.
    c. A medicated patch or disk can be applied directly to the skin where the medication is released and absorbed over time. This method ensures a continuous therapeutic drug level and reduces fluctuations in circulating drug levels.
    d. Medications in the form of a suppository are inserted into the rectum.

11. a. The purpose of analgesics is to relieve pain, not produce conscious sedation.
    b. Although side effects are considered when titrating a drug, these side effects are manageable. The need for pain relief takes priority.
    c. Titration is the adjustment of drug therapy based

on the patient's response. It manages tolerance while balancing the desired effects and adverse effects.

d. The World Health Organization recommends a three-step sequential approach to managing pain that begins with non-opioid drugs. Strong opioids are on step three and are used as a last resort, alone or in conjunction with non-opioids and adjuvant drugs.

12. a. This prevents injecting medication directly into the circulatory system rather than limiting the discomfort of an injection.
    b. This is contraindicated because it causes vasoconstriction, which would limit absorption of the medication.
    c. Pinching the skin aids in needle insertion when administering a subcutaneous injection. It does not limit the discomfort of injections.
    d. Injecting slowly allows the fluid to be dispersed slowly, which limits tissue trauma and discomfort.

13. a. This will ensure a tight seal and a closed system. If not firmly connected, the hub of the needle could disengage from the barrel of the syringe during preparation or administration of the medication, when internal and external pressures are exerted on the needle and syringe.
    b. The top just needs to be swiped. Rubbing back and forth is a violation of surgical asepsis because it reintroduces microorganisms to the area being cleaned.
    c. This should be avoided because it causes bubbles that could interfere with the drawing up of an accurate volume of solution.
    d. Excess air in the closed system raises pressure in the vial, which may cause bubbles when withdrawing the fluid and result in an inaccurate volume of solution.

14. a. When the Z-track technique is used during an intramuscular injection the skin and subcutaneous tissue are pulled 1 to $1^1/_2$ inches to one side, not pinched.
    b. Massage is contraindicated because it would force medication back up the needle track, which could result in tissue irritation or staining.
    c. Removal of the needle should be delayed 10 seconds to allow the medication to begin to be dispersed and absorbed.
    d. This ensures that medication is not on the outside of the needle, which prevents tracking of the medication into subcutaneous tissue during needle insertion.

15. a. This length needle is required to reach the depth necessary to enter a muscle.
    b. This is too small. Intramuscular injections use a 20- to 22-gauge needle.
    c. This is too shallow an angle for an intramuscular injection. A 90-degree angle is appropriate for an intramuscular injection.
    d. The skin is spread taut, not pinched, for an intramuscular injection.

16. a. Instilling medication into the conjunctival sac prevents the trauma of drops falling on the cornea.

b. Closing the eyes gently, rather than squeezing the lids shut, prevents the loss of medication from the conjunctival sac.
c. Closing the eyes moves the medication over the conjunctiva and eyeball and helps ensure an even distribution of medication.
d. Gentle pressure over the inner canthus for one minute after administration prevents medication from entering the lacrimal duct.

17. a. A parenteral route is one that is outside the gastrointestinal tract. A medication administered by the buccal route dissolves between the cheeks and gums, where it acts on the oral mucous membranes or is swallowed with saliva. The medication is then absorbed through the gastric mucosa and acts systemically.
    b. Z-track is a method for administering an intramuscular injection. The intramuscular route is a parenteral route.
    c. The intravenous route, a parenteral route, instills medication directly into the venous circulation.
    d. The intradermal route, a parenteral route, injects medication just under the epidermis.

18. a. The abbreviation for three times a day is t.i.d. (ter in die).
    b. The abbreviation for four times a day is q.i.d. (quater in die).
    c. The abbreviation for every other day is q.o.d.
    d. The abbreviation for once a day is o.d. (omni die) or q.d. (quaque die).

19. a. The air-bubble or air-lock technique can be used with intramuscular, not intradermal, injections. Its use is controversial particularly with disposable plastic syringes.
    b. Pinching or bunching up tissue is appropriate with subcutaneous, not intradermal, injections.
    c. When medication is injected with the bevel up, a small wheal will form under the skin. This technique is used only with intradermal injections.
    d. Massaging the site of an intradermal injection would disperse the medication beyond the intended injection site.

20. a. Gently shaking the cartridge is desirable because it distributes the medication throughout the solution in the cartridge.
    b. This is desirable because it removes excess secretions from the nasal passages, which ensures a more effective distribution of medication.
    c. This would result in the delivery of less than the desired dose. The cartridge should be pressed at the same time as breathing in through the mouth.
    d. This is desirable because it will ensure a full inspiration, which will deliver an appropriate dose of the medication to the lung.

21. a. The required amount of diluent must be followed exactly in a multiple-strength formulation to ensure accurate dosage preparation. The diluent for a single-dose formulation must be exact so that the

medication is diluted enough not to injure body tissues.

b. A filtered needle should be used when drawing up fluid from an ampule, not a vial.

c. Although this is an advisable practice, it is not as important as administering an accurate dose.

d. The rubber seal must be wiped with alcohol before, not after, needle insertion.

22. **a. Pressing gently on the tragus facilitates the flow of medication toward the eardrum.**

b. This is done to straighten the ear canal of an infant or a young child, not an adult.

c. This can injure the eardrum. Drops should be directed along the wall of the ear canal.

d. This can result in medication flowing out of the ear. The side-lying position with the involved ear on the uppermost side should be maintained for 2 to 3 minutes after the medication is instilled.

23. a. This procedure requires that surgical, not medical, asepsis be used.

b. **A thin layer of medication (cream, lotion, ointment, powder, or paste) is adequate to ensure its action at the site. Excessive medication can cause a buildup of the substance, which may need to be removed before a subsequent application.**

c. Rubbing can traumatize the wound and should be avoided. Ointments can be massaged into intact skin, not infected wounds.

d. The antibiotic needs to be applied directly to the infected wound, not the surrounding skin, to be effective in fighting the infection.

24. a. Nursing interventions such as positioning, mixing a crushed medication in applesauce, and dissolving a medication in a small amount of fluid, can be employed to facilitate the ingestion of medication.

b. Gastric suctioning can be interrupted for 20 to 30 minutes after medication has been instilled via a nasogastric tube.

c. **Nothing that needs to be swallowed should ever be placed into the mouth of an unconscious patient because of the risk for aspiration.**

d. Vomiting, not nausea, is a contraindication for p.o. medications.

25. a. Lubrication is required to limit tissue trauma and ease insertion.

b. The left-lateral position relaxes the external anal sphincter and the suppository follows the natural curve of the rectum downward, promoting retention.

c. Standard precautions should be employed when there is exposure to patients' body fluids.

d. **In an adult, a suppository should be inserted 4 inches to ensure it is beyond the internal sphincter.**

26. a. This site is not near large nerves or blood vessels and the muscle does not lie over a joint. It is a preferred site for all age groups.

b. This site is not near large nerves or blood vessels. It is a preferred site in infants.

c. This site is not near major nerves, blood vessels, or bones. It is a preferred site for adults.

d. **This site has the highest risk for injury because of the close proximity of the sciatic nerve, major blood vessels, and bone.**

27. a. Reconstitution occurs within a closed vial and does not require a filtered needle.

b. **The top of an ampule must be snapped off at its neck to access the fluid. A filtered needle prevents glass particles from being drawn into the syringe.**

c. The majority of medications in vials are clear solutions. Cloudy fluid usually indicates contamination. Seek additional information from a drug guide or pharmacist.

d. It is not necessary to use a filtered needle when mixing medications.

28. a. Perineal care, not a vaginal irrigation, should be performed before inserting a vaginal suppository.

b. The patient should be placed in the supine position with the knees flexed (dorsal recumbent) to facilitate insertion of a vaginal suppository. The left-lateral position is used for an enema.

c. **This facilitates the placement of the vaginal suppository just outside the cervical os so that when it melts it will eventually disperse through the entire vaginal canal.**

d. Medical, not surgical, asepsis is required for the insertion of a vaginal suppository.

29. a. A sterile eye patch usually is not required after the administration of an ophthalmic medication.

b. The retracted lower lid can be released as soon as the medication is instilled.

c. The eye should be wiped from the inner canthus toward the outer canthus.

d. **Gentle pressure exerted on the inner canthus prevents medication from entering the lacrimal duct and being absorbed systemically.**

30. a. Using the same site consistently would cause, not limit, skin irritation and excoriation. The sites for a transdermal patch should be rotated.

b. Both irritation of the skin and vasodilation can result from rubbing the skin and can interfere with absorption of the medication.

c. **A hairless site will ensure that there is effective contact with the skin.**

d. The old patch should be removed at the same time that the new patch is applied.

31. a. A subcutaneous injection should not exceed 3 ml. A 5 ml syringe would be acceptable for an intramuscular injection.

b. **A subcutaneous injection should use a 25- to 29-gauge needle, which delivers a volume appropriate for a subcutaneous injection while minimizing tissue trauma. The diameter of a needle is referred to as its gauge, which ranges from 28 (small) to 14 (large).**

c. The volume of a tuberculin syringe is only 1 ml. For most subcutaneous injections, a syringe that can accommodate up to 3 ml is preferred.

d. This length is appropriate for an intramuscular, not subcutaneous, injection.

32. a. This ensures that gravity will promote the flow of medication to the posterior pharynx.
    b. This is unnecessary and can frighten the patient, who already may be having difficulty breathing.
    c. Blowing the nose should be avoided because it may remove medication from the nose. Five minutes is the length of time the patient should remain in the supine position with the head tilted backward.
    d. Nose drops should be directed toward the midline of the ethmoid bone.

33. a. This is done if the patient has difficulty swallowing.
    b. This is done if the patient has difficulty swallowing a pill even if it is crushed and mixed with applesauce.
    c. **The patient needs assistance. Keeping it in the cup, rather than touching it with the hands, maintains medical asepsis.**
    d. This is unrealistic and unsafe. The patient has demonstrated the need for assistance.

34. a. The radial nerve is at the wrist.
    b. The humerus bone is in the upper arm.
    c. The acromion process is the proximal end of the humerus.
    d. **In addition to other blood vessels, the superior gluteal artery passes through this site. This site may be contraindicated for obese (excessive adipose tissue) and debilitated or older (diminished muscle mass) patients. It is contraindicated in infants and toddlers (muscle mass is not well developed until walking).**

35. a. **Rinsing the mouth removes any remaining medication. This prevents irritation to the oral mucosa and tongue and prevents oral fungal infections.**
    b. This promotes retention of the medication in the oropharynx, where it is swallowed rather than inhaled. This is the correct procedure if an extender (spacer) is attached to the mouthpiece.
    c. The patient should be in an upright (standing, sitting, or high-Fowler's) position to promote lung expansion when inhaling.
    d. This may not mix the medication adequately and result in an inadequate dose. The canister should be shaken several times before use.

36. a. An intradermal injection is inserted below, not on top of, the epidermis.
    b. Medications in the form of solutions can be instilled into the bladder. They are designed to work locally and are considered a topical medication.
    c. Medications in the form of a suppository can be inserted into the rectum and are considered topical medications. Most are designed to work locally, although some are absorbed systemically.
    d. Medications in the form of a suppository, tablet, cream, foam, or jelly can be instilled into the vagina. They are designed to work locally and are considered topical medications.

37. a. This would interfere with the insertion of the suppository. Bearing down before insertion would help identify the opening to the rectum.
    b. This would be too short a length of time. The patient should remain in the left-lateral or supine position for 5 to 30 minutes following insertion of a

suppository to promote retention and facilitate its action.
    c. In this position, the internal anatomy of the intestinal tract would not facilitate the insertion or retention of the suppository. The left side-lying or left Sims' position is preferred.
    d. **Slow thoracic breathing relaxes the rectal sphincter, which facilitates insertion of the suppository.**

38. a. This is unsafe because it may eventually result in a loss of Humulin R insulin from the syringe into the Humulin N insulin vial. This contaminates the long-acting insulin (Humulin N) with the fast-acting insulin (Humulin R) and reduces the dose of Humulin R insulin in the syringe.
    b. **This is the first step because, after the Humulin R insulin is drawn into the syringe, it will only be necessary to withdraw the Humulin N insulin, preventing a possible loss of Humulin R insulin into the Humulin N insulin vial.**
    c. This is difficult to do without first instilling 10 units of air into the vial. It could also result in a loss of Humulin R insulin from the syringe into the Humulin N insulin vial. This contaminates the long-acting insulin (Humulin N) with the fast-acting insulin (Humulin R) and reduces the dose of Humulin R insulin in the syringe.
    d. This could result in Humulin N insulin entering the Humulin R insulin vial, diluting the fast-acting (Humulin R) insulin with the long-acting (Humulin N) insulin.

39. a. Although this is important for safe administration of a medication administered intravenously, it is not the priority.
    b. Although this should be done to ensure distribution of the medication throughout the IV solution, it is not the priority.
    c. Although this is important to prevent infection, it is not the priority.
    d. **An incompatibility could increase, decrease, or neutralize the effect of the medication. It may also cause a compound or precipitate that can harm the patient. This must be done before proceeding with subsequent steps of the procedure.**

40. a. Although patient confidentiality should always be maintained, this is not the reason for holding the label toward the palm of the hand.
    b. **Liquid medication may drip down the side of the bottle and soil the label, which may interfere with the ability to read the label accurately.**
    c. Accuracy of the dose is ensured by using a calibrated cup and measuring the liquid at the base of the meniscus while holding the cup at eye level.
    d. The label should be read before holding it against the palm of the hand.

41. a. This is done with a medication administered via the sublingual, not buccal, route.
    b. Fluid will interfere with the action and absorption of the medication.
    c. It should be administered after or between meals. Food will interfere with the action and absorption of the medication.

d. Alternating cheeks will limit irritation to the mucous membranes in the buccal area.

42. a. A medication to be given via the epidural route is administered through a catheter inserted into the epidural space.
   b. **Parenteral means *outside the digestive system*. However, in health care the parenteral route refers to medications given by injection or infusion. Transdermal medications are absorbed through the skin for a systemic effect.**
   c. A needle is required to reach the subcutaneous tissue, the layer of fat located below the dermis and above muscle tissue.
   d. A needle is required to reach the muscle layer beneath the dermis and subcutaneous tissue.

43. a. This is done with lotions, creams, or ointments.
   b. This is unnecessary. When the powder is sprinkled gently on the site, the powder should not become aerosolized.
   c. This is not a universal requirement. When necessary, a dressing is applied when with a practitioner's order.
   d. **Moisture harbors microorganisms and, when mixed with a powder, will result in a paste-like substance. The site should be clean and dry before medication administration to ensure effective action of the drug.**

44. a. This is done with a vial, not an ampule.
   b. The rubber seal of a vial, not the neck of an ampule, should be wiped with alcohol.
   c. **A barrier, such as a commercially manufactured ampule opener, a sterile 4×4 gauze, or an alcohol swab, should be used to protect the hands from broken glass.**
   d. This is done with a vial, not an ampule.

45. a. **Instilling cold medication into the ear canal is uncomfortable and can cause vertigo and nausea. Holding the bottle of medication in the hand for several minutes warms the solution to body temperature.**
   b. The side-lying position with the involved ear upward must be maintained for 2 to 3 minutes for the instilled medication to disperse throughout the ear canal.
   c. This straightens the ear canal and facilitates the flow of medication toward the eardrum; it does not limit discomfort.
   d. This is contraindicated because the force of the fluid could injure the eardrum.

46. a. There is no advantage in prolonging the treatment.
   b. Slow, deep breathing will limit hyperventilation.
   c. **A pause at the height of inspiration will promote distribution and absorption of the medication before exhalation begins.**
   d. Slow inhalations and exhalations with pursed lips help prevent bronchial spasms.

47. a. The abbreviation for after meals is p.c. (**p**ost **c**ibum).
   b. The abbreviation for hour of sleep is h.s. (**h**ora **s**omni).
   c. The abbreviation for every 2 hours is q2h.
   d. **The abbreviation for twice a day is b.i.d. (bis in die).**

48. a. This technique is used to prevent the flow of medication back up the needle track and is used with medications that are caustic or can stain the tissues.
   b. The diameter of this needle is large to accommodate viscous medications. Its use in relation to the Z-track technique is not routine and depends on the solution being injected.
   c. This site would be the least desirable for a patient who is obese because of the presence of excessive adipose tissue.
   d. **A longer needle is needed to reach the depth required to enter a muscle in this patient.**

49. a. Medicated solutions are administered via drops in the ear.
   b. Medicated solutions are dropped or sprayed in the nose.
   c. Tablets, lozenges, and troches are administered in the mouth.
   d. **Suppositories—semisolid, cone-shaped, or oval-shaped masses that melt at body temperature—are inserted into the rectum.**

50. a. This will eventually be done, but it is not the first priority.
   b. **Perineal secretions should be removed first to ensure effective inspection of the site and to decrease the contamination of the vagina by microorganisms present in the perineal area.**
   c. This is done just before the suppository is lubricated and inserted into the vagina. The wrapper maintains asepsis.
   d. Inserting a vaginal suppository is not a sterile procedure. The nurse wears gloves as part of standard precautions.

51. a. **Pill distribution can be set up once a week. After the medication is taken, the empty section reminds the patient that the medication was taken, which prevents excessive doses. This is a major issue for patients with short-term memory loss.**
   b. This is unrealistic. The chart may be complex, confusing, and require repeated cognitive decisions throughout the day that may be beyond the patient's ability.
   c. This is unrealistic and puts an excessive burden on family members.
   d. This is unrealistic. When the alarm goes off the patient may not remember why it is ringing.

52. a. **This prevents secretions and fluid from entering and irritating the lacrimal ducts.**
   b. A piston syringe should be used because the flow and force of fluid from an Asepto syringe are difficult to control. The irrigating syringe should be held 1 inch, not 2 inches, above the eye.
   c. Medical asepsis, not surgical asepsis, is required for eye irrigations.
   d. The patient should be placed in a sitting or back-lying position with the head tilted toward the affected eye.

53. a. A special syringe is not needed for administering a medication via Z-track. The barrel of the syringe must be large enough to accommodate the volume of solution to be injected (usually 1 to 3 ml) and

the needle long enough to enter a muscle (usually 1½ inches).

b. This creates a zigzag track through the various tissue layers that prevents backflow of medication up the needle track when simultaneously removing the needle and releasing the traction on the skin.

c. The use of the vastus lateralis muscle for a Z-track injection may cause discomfort for the patient. Z-track injections are tolerated better when the well-developed gluteal muscles are used.

d. The needle is inserted into the muscle once for a Z-track injection. The Z represents the zigzag pattern of the needle track that results when the skin traction and the needle are simultaneously removed.

54. a. This will create excessive bubbles that can interfere with complete reconstitution or result in bubbles being drawn into the syringe. Both occurrences can result in an inaccurate dose.

b. Compatibility is necessary so that a compound or precipitate that is harmful to a patient does not result.

c. Reconstitution occurs in a vial (a closed system), not an ampule (an open system).

d. Shaking the vial will create excessive bubbles. The vial should be rotated between the hands to facilitate reconstitution.

55. a. This is unsafe. This exposes the medication to the environment where it could become contaminated or grouped with other medications being administered to the patient, thus interfering with safe administration of one or more of the medications.

b. The medication should be opened and administered immediately to the patient, limiting the potential for contamination. Reading the label immediately before opening the package is an additional safety check. Immediate administration prevents accidental disarrangement of medications that could result in a medication error.

c. This is unsafe. It unnecessarily exposes the medication to the environment because it requires the nurse to carry the medication through the unit to the patient's room. In addition, it can become confused with the medications for other patients.

d. This is unsafe. The medication is exposed unnecessarily to the environment and it can be inadvertently confused with the medications for other patients.

56. a. Although the physician's order should be followed exactly if it is a safe dose, 24 hours is too long a period not to intervene if the medication is not effective.

b. The patient should be assessed every 1 to 2 hours to ensure effectiveness of the drug.

c. This is unnecessary if a titrated drug is the appropriate dose.

d. Two doses is enough time to evaluate the effectiveness of a medication for pain. Patients should not have to endure intolerable levels of pain.

57. a. Medications in the form of a solution are instilled into the ear.

b. Ophthalmic medications in the form of a solution, an ointment, or a disk are administered in the eye.

c. A troche, a lozenge-like tablet, is dissolved slowly in the mouth to provide a localized effect.

d. Medications in the form of suppositories are inserted into the rectum.

58. a. These anatomic landmarks help to identify the deltoid muscle.

b. These anatomic landmarks help to identify the dorsogluteal site. This site contains the well-developed gluteus muscles, particularly the gluteus maximus, in the buttocks.

c. This is the initial placement of the hand when identifying landmarks for the ventrogluteal site.

d. This is associated with the vastus lateralis site. It is between one handbreadth above the knee and one handbreadth below the greater trochanter on the anterior lateral aspect of the thigh.

59. a. This ensures that a maximum amount of the drug is inhaled while the medication is still aerosolized.

b. The breath should be held for 5 to 10 seconds or longer to promote distribution and absorption of the medication.

c. One puff, not 2, should be delivered with each inhalation.

d. The inhalation should start with compression of the canister and continue for another 2 to 3 seconds to ensure distribution of the medication.

60. a. An intradermal injection usually involves a small volume of fluid (e.g., 0.1 ml). A 1 ml syringe, rather than a syringe that can accommodate larger volumes, permits a more precise measurement of a small volume of fluid.

b. A 26-gauge needle has a narrow diameter and short bevel that is conducive to the formation of the wheal associated with an intradermal injection.

c. A 1-inch needle is used for a subcutaneous injection. An intradermal injection is usually administered with a needle that is ½ inch in length.

d. This angle is too extreme and results in an injection that is too deep to form a wheal.

Pharmacology

KEYWORDS

The following words include English vocabulary, nursing/medical terminology, concepts, principles, or information relevant to content specifically addressed in the chapter or associated with topics presented in it. English dictionaries, your nursing textbooks, and medical dictionaries such as *Taber's Cyclopedic Medical Dictionary* are resources that can be used to expand your knowledge and understanding of these words and related information.

Absorption
Adverse effect
Allergic/allergy
American Hospital
   Formulary Service
   Drug Information
Anaphylaxis
Antagonism
Biotransformation
Blood level
Chemotherapy
Compatible
Contraindication
Controlled substance
Dependence
Drug absorption
Drug distribution
Drug Enforcement Agency (DEA)
Drug excretion
Drug metabolism
Drug name
Drug regimen
Food and Drug Administration (FDA)
Generic
Half-life
Herbal remedies
Hypersensitivity
Idiosyncratic effect
Interaction
Local effect
Megadose
Onset—peak—duration
Parenteral route
Pharmacist
Pharmacodynamics
Pharmacokinetics
Physician's Desk
   Reference
Prescription

Prophylactic
Rash
Serum drug level
Side effects
Synergistic
Systemic effect
Target organ
Teratogenic
Therapeutic effect
Tolerance/threshold
Topical
Toxic effect/toxicity
Trade name of drug
United States
   Pharmacopeia
   Drug Information
Urticaria

CLASSIFICATIONS OF DRUGS

Analgesic
Antacid
Antianxiety agents
Antiarrhythmics
Antibacterial
Antibiotic
Anticholinergic
Anticoagulants
Anticonvulsant
Antidepressant
Antidiabetic
Antidiarrheal
Antiemetic
Antifungal
Antihistamine
Antihypertensive
Antineoplastic
Antinflammatory
Antiparkinson
Antipsychotic
Antipyretic

Antiretroviral
Antitussive
Antiulcer
Bronchodilator
Cathartic
Diuretic
Emetic
Expectorant
Hypnotic
Laxative
Lipid-lowering agent
Mucolytic
Narcotic
Skeletal muscle relaxant
Thyroid agents
Vasodilator
Vitamins and minerals

DRUG FORMS

Caplet
Capsule
Elixir
Emulsion
Enteric-coated
Extract
Liniment
Lotion
Ointment
Paste
Pill
Powder
Solution
Suppository
Suspension
Syrup
Tablet
Tincture
Transdermal
Troche (lozenge)

1. Which is the most important nursing action associated with the administration of opioids?
   a. Assess the patient's level of sedation
   b. Have the patient take the opioid with food
   c. Increase the patient's fiber and fluid intake
   d. Administer the patient's medication via the parenteral route

2. A patient who is visiting the clinic is taking liquid Maalox, an antacid agent, for symptoms of indigestion. The most important thing the nurse needs to teach this patient is to:
   a. Keep a log of the location, duration, and character of gastric discomfort
   b. Notify the physician if tarry stools or coffee-ground emesis is observed
   c. Take the drug one hour before meals
   d. Avoid drinking fluids with this drug

3. Which nursing action is important in relation to the administration of most antibiotics?
   a. Assess for constipation
   b. Administer between meals
   c. Encourage foods high in vitamin K
   d. Monitor the volume of urinary output

4. What is the preferred site for an injection of heparin?
   a. Leg
   b. Arm
   c. Buttock
   d. Abdomen

5. Which concept associated with drug therapy and quality of sleep is important to understand to best plan nursing care?
   a. Aggressive pain management intervention will reduce pain but increase insomnia
   b. Abrupt discontinuation of hypnotic drugs can lead to withdrawal symptoms
   c. Sedatives support restful sleep for people experiencing hypoxia
   d. Barbiturates are the drugs of choice for insomnia

6. Which classification of drugs commonly lists diarrhea as an adverse effect?
   a. Sedatives
   b. Narcotics
   c. Antibiotics
   d. Antiemetics

7. Which reaction to a drug has the greatest potential to be life-threatening immediately after administration?
   a. Toxicity
   b. Habituation
   c. Anaphylaxis
   d. Idiosyncratic reaction

8. What time should a blood sample be obtained to determine a trough level for an antibiotic that is administered at 12:00 noon?
   a. 11:00 AM
   b. 11:30 AM
   c. 12:30 PM
   d. 1:00 PM

9. Alternative herbal remedies are:
   a. Required to be labeled with information about their structure
   b. Approved by the Food and Drug Administration
   c. Natural because they are botanical in origin
   d. Safe because they are organic

10. What must the nurse know about a drug to best evaluate whether or not the expected outcome of drug therapy has been achieved?
    a. Side effects
    b. Therapeutic effect
    c. Mechanism of action
    d. Chemical composition

11. Which drug has a daily dose limit?
    a. Motrin
    b. Codeine
    c. Demerol
    d. Morphine

12. The assessment of which vital sign is essential before administering a narcotic?
    a. Pulse
    b. Respirations
    c. Temperature
    d. Blood pressure

13. Which patient adaptation would indicate the need to withhold administering digoxin 0.125 mg?
    a. Diplopia
    b. Tachypnea
    c. Hypertension
    d. Hyperthermia

14. Which assessment is essential before administering an antihypertensive?
    a. Level of consciousness
    b. Apical heart rate
    c. Blood pressure
    d. Respirations

15. Which would be a common nursing diagnosis for patients taking drugs that depress the immune system?
    a. Risk for Infection
    b. Risk for Constipation
    c. Risk for Sensory/Perceptual Alterations
    d. Risk for Ineffective Management of Therapeutic Regimen

16. The ultimate purpose of determining peak and trough levels of a drug is to:
    a. Maintain constant drug levels in the body
    b. Determine the half life of a drug in the body
    c. Establish where biotransformation occurs in the body
    d. Monitor the rate of absorption of the drug in the body

17. Which response is being experienced by a patient who becomes excitable after receiving a narcotic?
    a. Idiosyncratic
    b. Synergistic
    c. Allergic
    d. Toxic

18. Which is the best site for absorption of subcutaneous injections of insulin?
    a. Upper lateral arms
    b. Anterior thighs
    c. Upper chest
    d. Abdomen

19. Which is a good adage to keep in mind when it comes to natural herbal remedies?
    a. "What you don't know will not hurt you."
    b. "There is truth in advertising."
    c. "More is better."
    d. "Buyer beware."

20. Which classification of drugs is commonly used as analgesics when a patient experiences neuropathic pain?
   a. Anticonvulsants
   b. Antidepressants
   c. Antihistamines
   d. Anesthetics

21. The patient at highest risk for toxicity associated with most drugs is the patient with:
   a. Liver disease
   b. Kidney insufficiency
   c. Respiratory difficulty
   d. Malabsorption syndrome

22. The primary reason some oral drugs are administered with food is to:
   a. Prevent drug interactions
   b. Protect the gastric mucosa
   c. Stimulate biotransformation
   d. Reduce the risk of gastric reflux

23. Drugs are absorbed most efficiently when they are administered:
   a. Orally
   b. Rectally
   c. Intravenously
   d. Intramuscularly

24. Which information would be most helpful in determining a patient's physiologic dependence on a drug?
   a. Degree of tolerance
   b. Strength of the dose
   c. Perceived need by the patient
   d. Length of time to achieve the therapeutic effect

25. When evaluating for side effects of a narcotic it is most important for the nurse to assess the patient for:
   a. Nausea
   b. Bradypnea
   c. Tachycardia
   d. Hypertension

26. Which route is generally least desirable for absorption of drugs into the bloodstream?
   a. Oral
   b. Rectal
   c. Intravenous
   d. Subcutaneous

27. A patient with a severe upper respiratory tract infection is being treated with a bronchodilator. The nurse would know that the patient has achieved the therapeutic effect when the patient has less:
   a. Viscous secretions
   b. Difficulty breathing
   c. Respiratory excursion
   d. Bronchovesicular breath sounds

28. A patient admits to taking Milk of Magnesia (MOM) for its laxative effect several times a week. The most important thing the nurse should teach a patient taking MOM is that it:
   a. Can cause dependence and dehydration if taken for more than two weeks
   b. Can cause an accumulation of sodium and potassium ions
   c. Should be accompanied by 2 to 3 glasses of fluid
   d. Should be taken at bedtime

29. What frequency would be most appropriate when administering an antiemetic drug?
   a. q.i.d. when awake
   b. After the patient vomits
   c. 30 minutes before meals
   d. When the patient complains of nausea

30. The nurse understands that oral medications are absorbed more quickly when they are given:
    a. With water
    b. In the morning
    c. On an empty stomach
    d. When the patient is resting

31. What is happening to a patient who develops a rash, urticaria, and pruritus after ingestion of a new drug?
    a. Allergic response
    b. Idiosyncratic effect
    c. Anaphylactic reaction
    d. Synergistic interaction

32. Which fruit should be ingested by a patient who takes a hydrochlorothiazide diuretic daily?
    a. Plum
    b. Orange
    c. Banana
    d. Tangerine

33. Which assessment is essential before administering a drug that is a digitalis derivative?
    a. Pulse rate
    b. Blood pressure
    c. Respiratory rate
    d. Level of consciousness

34. A metered-dose inhaler (MDI) is used to deliver medication to a patient because it:
    a. Provides the patient with a sense of control
    b. Delivers the medication via positive pressure
    c. Directs the medication into the upper respiratory tract
    d. Releases the medication in small particles that can be deeply inhaled

35. The response to medication that occurs more frequently in patients who see a variety of medical specialists because of multiple health problems is drug:
    a. Allergies
    b. Tolerance
    c. Habituation
    d. Interactions

36. Which is the most effective way to achieve and maintain a drug's therapeutic level?
    a. IV push
    b. Sublingual route
    c. Oral administration
    d. Large volume infusion

37. Which is the most effective way to ensure that therapeutic drug levels are maintained?
    a. Ensuring that drugs are ingested two hours before meals
    b. Administering drugs according to physician's orders
    c. Assessing for early signs and symptoms of toxicity
    d. Monitoring the results of serum drug levels

38. Which of these routes of drug administration is the fastest acting?
    a. Buccal
    b. Transdermal
    c. Subcutaneous
    d. Intramuscular

39. Which is the most important action when the nurse discovers that a patient is taking natural herbal remedies?
    a. Learn about the supplement
    b. Think of supplements as drugs
    c. Communicate supplement use to the physician
    d. Include the names and doses of supplements in the health history

40. Which is characteristic of an injection of 5000 units of heparin SC?
    a. 3 ml. syringe
    b. 22-gauge needle
    c. 1½ inch needle length
    d. 90-degree angle of insertion

41. The nurse understands that the advantage of administering a drug via a transdermal patch is that it:
    a. Limits allergic responses
    b. Prevents drug interactions
    c. Delivers the drug over a period of time
    d. Provides a local rather than a systemic effect

42. Physicians generally order hyperlipidemia drug therapy:
    a. Following failure of diet therapy
    b. For patients over 60 years of age
    c. For those who are unable to exercise
    d. After two consecutive months of elevated serum lipid levels

43. The adaptation that indicates that a patient is experiencing a therapeutic response to an antiemetic is a reduction in:
    a. Fever
    b. Anxiety
    c. Vomiting
    d. Coughing

44. When the physician orders ibuprofen (a nonsteroidal anti-inflammatory drug) for a patient with pain, the nurse should teach the patient to:
    a. "Drink at least 3 quarts of fluid a day."
    b. "Monitor your blood pressure every day."
    c. "Eat food when you take this medication."
    d. "Use this medication carefully because it is addictive."

45. When a patient who has a transdermal analgesic patch for cancer experiences breakthrough pain with activity, the nurse should:
    a. Encourage the avoidance of moving
    b. Administer an ordered shorter-acting opiate
    c. Obtain an order for an antianxiety medication
    d. Suggest to the physician that the long-acting opiate be increased

46. Which is the primary purpose of pre-filled, disposable unit-dose intramuscular drug cartridges versus multidose vials? The unit-dose cartridges:
    a. Ensure that the appropriate-length needle is attached
    b. Reduce the incidence of drug interactions
    c. Limit preparation time in emergencies
    d. Ensure the purity of the drugs

47. The nurse recognizes that a presurgical patient has to be weaned from long-term prescribed corticosteroids because sudden discontinuance can contribute to:
    a. Hypothermia
    b. Bleeding
    c. Seizures
    d. Shock

48. The patient has an order for Lomotil, an antidiarrheal agent. The nurse should teach the patient to:
    a. Inform the physician if diarrhea persists for more than 2 days
    b. Be alert to the fact that it may cause hyperactivity
    c. Limit fluid intake to 2000 cc per day
    d. Avoid crushing the tablets

49. An impairment in which organ would be of most concern when assessing a patient's ability to excrete a drug from the body?
    a. Liver
    b. Lungs
    c. Kidneys
    d. Intestines

50. Which patient adaptation would indicate an excessive response to an antihypertensive?
    a. Heart rate of 60 beats per minute
    b. Blood pressure of 90/70 mmHg
    c. Respirations of 24 per minute
    d. Oral temperature of 98° F

51. The patient has an order for Zoloft, an antidepressant. What is the most important nursing intervention?
    a. Monitoring the patient for suicidal tendencies
    b. Advising the patient to engage in psychotherapy
    c. Encouraging the patient to diet because weight gain is common
    d. Teaching the patient to limit alcohol intake to one drink per day

52. The patient is receiving an antipyretic agent. Which would have to be assessed to determine if the medication achieved a therapeutic response?
    a. Intake & output
    b. Pain tolerance
    c. Temperature
    d. Respirations

53. The patient is receiving an antibiotic that has a 4 to 10 mcg/ml therapeutic range, an optimum peak value of 8 to 10 mcg/ml, and a minimum trough level of 0.5 mcg/ml. Which statement is most reflective of a trough level of 0.8 mcg/ml?
    a. It falls within the optimum peak value range
    b. The dose being given is therapeutic
    c. There is a risk for drug toxicity
    d. The level is acceptable

54. Before instituting patient-controlled analgesia (PCA) via a continuous intravenous route for the relief of pain, what is the most important action by the nurse?
    a. Monitoring the patient's analgesic blood levels
    b. Determining the patient's pain tolerance
    c. Assessing the patient's respiratory status
    d. Identifying the patient's pain threshold

55. Which of the following pharmacological terms is correctly matched with the description of a drug classification?
    a. Mucolytic: solidifies tenacious mucus
    b. Expectorant: decreases mucus production
    c. Antitussive: encourages coughing contributing to airway clearance
    d. Bronchodilator: causes relaxation of smooth muscles of respiratory passageways

1. a. Opioids are central nervous system depressants that cause sedation. The patient's level of consciousness must be monitored routinely to prevent an overdose.
   b. Although this might be done because opioids may cause gastric irritation, it is not the priority.
   c. Although this might be done because opioids decrease intestinal motility, it is not the priority.
   d. Opioids are administered by routes other than parenteral, such as oral and transdermal. Parenteral routes include intravenous, subcutaneous, intramuscular, and epidural.

2. a. Although this might be done, it is not the priority.
   b. These are symptoms of gastric bleeding and the physician should be notified immediately. Enzymes act on blood to produce coffee-ground emesis and tarry stools.
   c. Maalox should be taken 1 to 3 hours after a meal and at bedtime to neutralize gastric acid.
   d. This medication should be taken with at least $\frac{1}{2}$ glass of water, particularly with thoroughly chewed tablets to prevent tablets from entering the intestine undissolved.

3. a. Most antibiotics tend to cause diarrhea, not constipation.
   b. Food often interferes with the dissolution and absorption of antibiotics, delaying their action. Food also can combine with molecules of certain drugs, changing their molecular structure, and ultimately inhibiting or preventing their absorption.
   c. Yogurt, not foods high in vitamin K, would be encouraged for a patient receiving antibiotics. Yogurt helps to recolonize the endogenous flora of the GI tract that can be eradicated by antibiotics.
   d. Routine monitoring of urinary output is adequate when antibiotics are being administered.

4. a. The muscles in the legs are not preferred for the administration of heparin because muscle activity associated with walking increases the risk of hematoma formation.
   b. The muscles in the arms are not preferred for the administration of heparin because muscle activity associated with movement of the arms increases the risk of hematoma formation.
   c. The muscles associated with walking are not preferred for the administration of heparin because muscle activity increases the risk of hematoma formation.
   d. The abdomen is the preferred site for the administration of heparin because it lacks major muscles and muscle activity. This site has the least risk for hematoma formation.

5. a. Effective pain management will facilitate rest and sleep, not promote insomnia.
   b. Barbiturate sedative-hypnotics depress the central nervous system and when withdrawn abruptly can cause withdrawal symptoms such as restlessness, tremors, weakness, and insomnia. Long-term use should be tapered by 25% to 30% weekly.
   c. Sedatives, central nervous system depressants, are not advocated for hypoxia because they depress respirations, which would exacerbate the hypoxia.
   d. Barbiturates depress the central nervous system, alter REM and NREM sleep, result in daytime drowsiness, and cause rebound insomnia. For this reason, antianxiety drugs or tranquilizers are preferred.

6. a. Sedatives, used to promote sleep, depress the central nervous system, which may cause constipation, not diarrhea.
   b. Narcotics, opium derivatives used to relieve pain, depress the central nervous system, which may cause constipation, not diarrhea.
   c. Antibiotics can alter the normal flora of the body, resulting in superinfections. Opportunistic fungal infections of the gastrointestinal system may cause a black, furred tongue, nausea, and diarrhea.
   d. Antiemetics, used to prevent or alleviate nausea and vomiting, may cause constipation, not diarrhea.

7. a. Medication toxicity results from excessive amounts of the drug in the body because of overdosage or impaired metabolism or excretion. Most drug toxicity that occurs immediately after administration is preventable through accurate ordering and administration of the medication. Toxicity that occurs through the cumulative effect occurs over time and if recognized early is not life threatening.
   b. Drug habituation is a mild form of psychologic dependence that occurs over time.
   c. Anaphylaxis, a severe allergic reaction, requires immediate intervention (epinephrine, IV fluids, steroids, and antihistamines) because it can be fatal.
   d. An idiosyncratic effect is an unexpected, individualized response to a drug. The response can be an under-response, an over-response, or cause unpredictable, unexplainable symptoms. It is usually not life threatening.

8. a. Eleven AM is too soon. The drug would not be at its lowest concentration in the blood.
   b. Thirty minutes before, and up to, the next scheduled dose is the most appropriate time for a trough blood level to be obtained. The serum level of the drug will be at its lowest.
   c. Peak, not trough, levels are obtained thirty minutes after completion of drug administration.
   d. The blood level of the drug rises once the drug is administered. A value taken at this time will no longer reflect the lowest serum level, which is the purpose of identifying a trough level.

9. a. The Dietary Supplement Health and Education Act of 1994 stipulated that herbs must be labeled with information about their effects on the structure and function of the body. Herbal substances are officially considered food supplements.
   b. The Food and Drug Administration (FDA), a division of the United States Department of Health and Human Services, regulates the manufacture, sale,

and effectiveness of prescription and non-prescription medications, not herbal remedies.

c. Herbs, considered by some to be "natural," are plants that are valued for their medicinal properties. As medicinal substances, they should be viewed by the consumer as drugs.

d. Herbal remedies lack governmental quality standards and regulation. Their safety and efficacy are not guaranteed.

10. a. Side effects are unintended effects other than the therapeutic effect.

b. **Therapeutic effects are the desired, intended effects of the drug. They are the reason for which the drug is prescribed.**

c. Although it is important to know the mechanism of action of a drug (pharmacodynamics), this knowledge is not as important as knowing the physical, mental, behavioral, or emotional responses indicating that a drug is having the desired impact on the patient.

d. Although it is important to know the chemical composition of a drug, this is not as significant as knowing the desired response to the medication.

11. a. **When administered to an adult, ibuprofen (Motrin) should not exceed 3600 mg/day when used as an anti-inflammatory or 1200 mg/day when used as an analgesic or antipyretic. Higher doses do not increase effectiveness and may cause major gastrointestinal and central nervous system adverse effects.**

b. When administered to an adult under the supervision of a practitioner, codeine may exceed the recommended daily dosage of 120 mg.

c. When administered to an adult under the supervision of a practitioner, meperidine (Demerol) may exceed the recommended oral dosage of 1200 mg/day or the IV dose of 15 to 35 mg/hour.

d. Recommended daily doses for morphine vary based on weight of the patient and route of administration. Recommended dosages are routinely exceeded in pain management of patients with chronic, intractable (malignant) pain.

12. a. A narcotic (an opioid analgesic) can cause the side effect of bradycardia, so the pulse should be assessed before administration. However, this assessment is not as essential as another vital sign.

b. **A narcotic depresses the respiratory center in the medulla, which results in a decrease in the rate and depth of respirations. When a patient's respiratory functioning is below acceptable parameters, the drug should be withheld and the practitioner notified.**

c. The side effects and adverse reactions to narcotics do not include alterations in temperature.

d. A narcotic can cause the side effect of hypotension. However, this assessment is not as essential as another vital sign.

13. a. **Digoxin (Lanoxin) can cause sensory changes such as diplopia (double vision), halos, colored vision, blind spots, and flashing lights. If any of these signs of toxicity occur, the medication should be held and a serum digoxin level assessed**

for the drug exceeding its therapeutic range of 0.5 to 2 ng/ml.

b. Tachypnea, an abnormally rapid rate of breathing (usually more than 20 breaths per minute) is not a symptom of digitalis toxicity.

c. Dysrhythmias, not hypertension, are cardiovascular signs of digitalis toxicity.

d. This is unlikely because digoxin does not influence temperature regulation in the body.

14. a. This is unnecessary because antihypertensives do not alter the level of consciousness.

b. The apical heart rate should be assessed before administering cardiac glycosides and antidysrhythmics, not antihypertensives.

c. **Antihypertensives such as β-adrenergic blockers, calcium channel blockers, vasodilators, and ACE inhibitors all act to reduce blood pressure; therefore, the blood pressure should be obtained before and monitored after administration.**

d. Respirations and breath sounds should be assessed before administering bronchodilators and expectorants, not antihypertensives.

15. a. **Drugs that suppress the immune system, such as antineoplastics (destroy stem cells that are precursors to WBCs), steroids (suppress function and numbers of eosinophils and monocytes), and antibiotics (destroy normal body flora), lower the body's ability to fight microorganisms that can cause infection.**

b. These drugs are more likely to cause gastrointestinal disturbances such as anorexia, nausea, vomiting, and diarrhea, not constipation.

c. Most drugs that suppress the immune system frequently do not cause sensory problems. Although some antineoplastic drugs can cause peripheral neuropathy, this response is not as common as gastrointestinal, hematologic, integumentary, and immune system adverse effects.

d. Although this is a potential nursing diagnosis for any patient who must follow a pharmacologic regimen, it is not the most common risk associated with drugs that suppress the immune system.

16. a. **The peak serum level of a drug is the maximum concentration that the drug can reach in the blood (occurs when the elimination rate equals the absorption rate). Trough levels indicate the serum level of a drug just before the next dose is to be administered. The results of these two values determine the dose and time a drug should be administered to maintain a serum level of a drug within its therapeutic range.**

b. Although a drug's half life, the usual amount of time needed by the body to reduce the concentration of the drug by one half, is helpful in determining how frequently a drug should be given initially, it does not reflect an individual patient's response to the drug.

c. Biotransformation, the process of inactivating and breaking down a drug, takes place primarily in the liver. Peak and trough levels may indirectly reflect the rate of biotransformation, not the place it occurs.

d. Peak and trough levels indirectly measure both the

absorption and the inactivation and elimination of a drug from the body. This monitoring is useless without further intervention.

17. **a.** Excitability is an unexpected, unexplainable response to a narcotic. Narcotics are central nervous system depressants that relieve pain and promote sedation, not cause excitability.
    b. A synergistic response associated with a narcotic would be reflected by a lowered level of consciousness and sedation.
    c. Allergic responses frequently manifest as a rash, urticaria, and pruritus.
    d. Toxicity is manifested by sedation, respiratory depression and coma. The antidote naloxone (Narcan) may be necessary.

18.   a. Although insulin can be administered at the deltoid site, it is a small area that is not conducive to injection rotation within the site. The rate of absorption at this site is slower than at the preferred site for insulin administration.
    b. Although insulin can be administered in this site, the tissue of the thighs and buttocks have the slowest absorption rate.
    c. This site is not acceptable for the administration of insulin because of the lack of adequate subcutaneous tissue.
    d. The abdomen is the preferred site for administration of insulin because it is a large area that promotes a systematic rotation of injections and it has the fastest rate of absorption.

19.   a. "What you don't know can hurt you." People should know the ingredients and effects of everything ingested such as fluids, foods, herbal remedies, and medications.
    b. The ultimate purpose of advertising is to sell a product. Advertising may be inaccurate in its statements or inexact by omission of information.
    c. An excess of anything can be deleterious to health. Excess herbs or drugs can result in toxicity.
    d. The manufacture, sale, and effectiveness of herbal remedies are not regulated by the government. The buyer must be responsible for investigating an herbal remedy and making an informed decision about its use.

20.   a. Anticonvulsants do not relieve pain. Anticonvulsants depress abnormal neuronal discharges in the central nervous system, limiting or preventing seizures.
    b. Antidepressant drugs, particularly amitriptylin (Elavil), potentiate the effects of opioids and have innate analgesic properties.
    c. Antihistamines do not relieve pain. Antihistamines block the effects of histamine at the H_1 receptor.
    d. Although anesthetics do block pain, they generally are not used to relieve neuropathic pain. General anesthetics depress the central nervous system sufficiently to allow pain-free invasive procedures (e.g., surgery), and local anesthetics produce brief episodes of decreased nerve transmission when general anesthesia is not warranted.

21.   **a. Drug-metabolizing enzymes in the liver detoxify drugs to a less active form (biotransformation). With liver dysfunction, biotransformation is**

impaired and drugs accumulate, ultimately **reaching toxic levels.**
    b. Although decreased kidney function will adversely affect drug excretion, it does not pose the greatest risk for toxicity.
    c. Most drugs are excreted through the kidneys, not the lungs.
    d. Most drugs are excreted through the kidneys, not the intestines.

22.   a. Drug interactions are not prevented by the presence of food. They occur as long as the modification of a drug occurs in the presence of another drug.
    b. Food protects the gastrointestinal mucosa from being irritated by a drug. Gastrointestinal irritation may result in mucosal erosion and bleeding.
    c. Biotransformation, the detoxification of a drug in the liver, occurs after a drug is absorbed through the gastrointestinal tract. Biotransformation is unrelated to the presence of food when an oral drug is ingested.
    d. The presence of food when an oral drug is administered prevents gastric irritability, not gastric reflux.

23.   a. Food, fluid, and gastric acidity can influence the dissolution and absorption of medications.
    b. The absorption of rectal medications is influenced by the presence of fecal material and is unpredictable.
    c. Intravenous medications enter the bloodstream directly by way of a vein. Intravenous administration offers the quickest rate of absorption and it is within the circulatory system for easy distribution.
    d. The intramuscular route is the second, not the first, most efficient route for absorption of medication.

24.   a. Tolerance is not a reliable indicator of dependence. Tolerance to a drug has occurred when increasing amounts of the drug must be administered to achieve the therapeutic effect.
    b. Strength of a dose is not a reliable indicator of dependence. Factors such as age, weight, gender, and drug tolerance also influence the strength of a dose.
    c. Drug dependence, a form of drug abuse, occurs when a person has an emotional reliance on a drug because there is a craving for the effect or response that the drug produces.
    d. The length of time a drug takes to achieve its therapeutic effect depends on the half-life of the drug and the effectiveness of the drug's ability to alter cell physiology (pharmacodynamics), which is unrelated to dependence.

25.   a. Although nausea and vomiting are common side effects of narcotics, they are not life-threatening and are not as significant as other more dangerous side effects.
    b. A narcotic depresses the respiratory center in the medulla, which results in a decrease in the rate and depth of respirations. Bradypnea is an abnormally slow rate of breathing with a rate less than 12 breaths per minute.
    c. Narcotics may cause bradycardia, not tachycardia.
    d. Narcotics may cause hypotension, not hypertension.

26. a. The oral route is the most common, safe, convenient, efficient, and cost-effective route for delivering medications that are to be absorbed into the bloodstream.
    b. **The rectal route is generally used for the administration of a medication that will act locally. This route is not used routinely for systemic medications because the effectiveness of absorption is unreliable.**
    c. The intravenous route is the primary route for absorption of drugs into the bloodstream because the medication is inserted directly into a vein.
    d. This is the third fastest route for absorption of drugs into the bloodstream after intravenous and intramuscular.

27. a. Mucolytic agents, not bronchodilators, liquefy thick, sticky (viscous) secretions.
    b. **Bronchodilators expand the airways of the respiratory tract, which promotes air exchange and easier respirations.**
    c. The ability of the chest to expand (respiratory excursion) increases, not decreases, the effectiveness of bronchodilators.
    d. Bronchovesicular breath sounds will increase, not decrease, after the administration of a bronchodilator. Bronchovesicular sounds are normal blowing sounds heard over the main stem bronchus. They are blowing sounds that are moderate in pitch and intensity, and equal in length on inspiration and expiration.

28. a. **Prolonged laxative use weakens the bowel's natural responses to fecal distention, resulting in chronic constipation. The osmotic action of magnesium salts in magnesium hydroxide draws water into the intestine, which can cause dehydration and electrolyte imbalances.**
    b. Sodium and potassium are lost from, rather than accumulate in, the body. The magnesium in MOM may be absorbed and result in hypermagnesemia.
    c. Each dose should be followed by a full glass of water to promote a faster effect and help replenish lost fluid. Daily fluid intake should be 2000 to 3000 ml.
    d. This will interrupt sleep. MOM causes bowel elimination 3 to 6 hours after administration.

29. a. This would result in an excessive amount of this type of medication and would not correspond to events that precipitate nausea.
    b. This would be too late. When an antiemetic is administered appropriately, vomiting should not occur.
    c. **Antiemetics should be administered before a meal so that the peak effect of the drug occurs at the time of anticipated nausea.**
    d. This would be too late. Prophylactic administration of an antiemetic will prevent nausea.

30. a. Water will not increase the absorption of medications administered orally. Water will facilitate the swallowing of and the movement of the medication down the esophagus to the stomach.
    b. The time of day does not influence the rate of absorption of medications administered orally.
    c. **Food can delay the dissolution and absorption of**

many drugs; therefore, most oral medications should be administered on an empty stomach. Oral medications should be administered with food only when indicated by the manufacturer's directions.
    d. Physical rest does not influence the rate of absorption of medications administered orally.

31. a. **A drug allergy is an immunologic response to a drug. In addition to integumentary responses, the patient may develop angioedema, rhinitis, lacrimal tearing, nausea, vomiting, wheezing, dyspnea, and diarrhea.**
    b. An idiosyncratic effect is an unexpected, individualized response to a drug. The response can be an under-response, an over-response, or cause unpredictable, unexplainable symptoms.
    c. The early signs of anaphylaxis are shortness of breath, acute hypotension, and tachycardia.
    d. When a drug interaction occurs where the action of one or both drugs is potentiated, it is called a synergistic effect.

32. a. One medium-size plum contains approximately 114 mg of potassium.
    b. One medium-size orange contains approximately 237 mg of potassium.
    c. **Hydrochlorothiazide, by its action in the distal convoluted tubule, promotes the excretion of potassium. Potassium must be replenished because of its vital role in the sodium-potassium pump. One medium-size banana contains approximately 450 mg of potassium.**
    d. One medium-size tangerine contains approximately 132 mg of potassium.

33. a. **Digoxin (Lanoxin) decreases conduction through the SA and AV nodes and prolongs the refractory period of the AV node, resulting in a slowing of the heart rate (negative chronotropic effect). When the heart rate is less than 60 beats per minute or higher than 100 beats per minute the medication should be held and a serum digoxin level assessed for exceeding its therapeutic range of 0.5 to 2 ng/ml.**
    b. Dysrhythmias, not alterations in blood pressure, are cardiovascular signs of digitalis toxicity.
    c. This assessment is unnecessary because a change in respiratory status is not a symptom of digitalis toxicity.
    d. Digitalis toxicity may cause confusion and disorientation, not an altered level of consciousness.

34. a. Although this may be a secondary benefit for some patients, it is not the reason for using an MDI.
    b. Although an MDI delivers the medication via pressure to the patient's mouth, it is the act of the patient's inhalation that delivers the medication to its site of action.
    c. The medication from an MDI is delivered to the lungs, which comprise the lower, not upper, respiratory tract.
    d. **An MDI aerosolizes the medication so that the suspension of microscopic liquid droplets can be inhaled deep in the lung.**

35. a. An allergic reaction results from an immunologic response to a medication to which the patient has been sensitized.
     b. Tolerance occurs when a patient develops a decreased response to a medication and therefore requires an increased dose to achieve the therapeutic response.
     c. Drug habituation is a mild form of psychologic dependence.
     d. **A drug interaction occurs when one drug affects the action of another drug. The effect of one or both drugs increases, decreases, or is negated. The risk for drug interactions increases when multiple drugs are prescribed by multiple practitioners with inadequate communication among the practitioners.**

36. a. An IV push (bolus) is the administration of an undiluted drug directly into the systemic circulation. It is usually administered as a single dose in an emergency. It would achieve the desired level quickly but would not maintain it.
     b. The sublingual route is used intermittently and only when necessary. It is not used to maintain constant therapeutic drug levels.
     c. Although the oral route is the safest, easiest, and most desirable way to administer medications, there are fluctuations in serum blood levels because the medication is administered intermittently one or more times throughout the day.
     d. **With a large volume infusion, a drug is added to an IV container (usually 250 ml, 500 ml, or 1000 ml) and the resulting solution is administered over time. This approach maintains a constant serum drug level.**

37. a. This will not ensure therapeutic drug levels. Although ingesting a drug on an empty stomach might improve dissolution and absorption of some drugs, there are some drugs that should be administered with food to prevent gastric irritation.
     b. A physician's order may or may not maintain therapeutic drug levels.
     c. This would be unsafe because toxicity exceeds therapeutic drug levels.
     d. **The therapeutic dose range reflects the dose that provides the intended response while producing minimal adverse effects. This range is called the therapeutic index. A patient's serum level of a drug should be compared to the therapeutic index to determine if therapeutic levels are being maintained.**

38. a. Medications dissolve between the teeth and gums, mix with saliva, and are swallowed. This route has a slow onset of action.
     b. The transdermal route is noted for its ability to sustain the absorption of medication, not because it produces a rapid response. The absorption of medications administered via the transdermal route is influenced by the condition of the skin, the presence of interstitial fluid, and the adequacy of circulation to the area.
     c. The subcutaneous route is faster-acting than some routes because it is a parenteral route, but slower-

acting than other parenteral routes because it does not have a large blood supply.
     d. **The intramuscular route is the fastest acting route after intravenous because it has a large vascular network that ensures rapid absorption into the blood stream.**

39. a. It is essential for the nurse to be an informed provider of care, but it is not the priority of care for this patient.
     b. Although this should be done, it is not the priority of care for this patient.
     c. **The practitioner should be notified immediately because the herb may interact with prescribed medications or therapies.**
     d. Although this should be done, it is not the priority. Medications or therapies could interact with the herb before the physician reads the information in the health history.

40. a. Most doses of heparin are less than 1 ml. Three milliliters of heparin would be excessive and could result in bleeding.
     b. This gauge needle is too large and can cause unnecessary trauma and bleeding at the insertion site. A 25- or 26-gauge needle is adequate.
     c. This length needle is unnecessarily long and may enter a muscle rather than subcutaneous tissue.
     d. **A 1/2 inch long needle inserted at a 90° angle will ensure that the heparin is inserted into subcutaneous tissue.**

41. a. The composition of the drug, not the route by which it is administered, determines if an allergic response will occur.
     b. The composition of a drug and its molecular reaction with another drug that is concurrently present determines if a drug interaction will occur.
     c. **A transdermal patch placed on the skin gradually releases a predictable amount of medication that is absorbed into the bloodstream for as long as a week. This approach maintains therapeutic blood levels and reduces fluctuations in circulating drug levels.**
     d. Transdermal patches are used for their systemic, not local, effects.

42. a. **Generally, conservative management of hyperlipidemia through dietary modifications and exercise is attempted before resorting to a medication. Lipid-lowering agents have side effects and adverse effects and may interact with other drugs.**
     b. Lipid-lowering agents are ordered for patients who are over 60 years old only when necessary, not because they are over 60 years old.
     c. Exercise is only one factor that influences the patient's lipid status. Factors such as diet, cigarette smoking, stress, concurrent diseases, and family history are additional factors that need to be considered when a pharmacologic regimen is prescribed.
     d. Only people with chronically elevated lipid levels receive antilipidemics because of their significant side effects. Life-style modifications are attempted first.

43. a. Antipyretics, not antiemetics, reduce fever.
    b. Anxiolytics, not antiemetics, reduce anxiety.
    c. **Antiemetics block the emetogenic receptors to prevent or treat nausea or vomiting.**
    d. Antitussives, not antiemetics, reduce the frequency and intensity of coughing.

44. a. This is unnecessary. However, ibuprofen should be taken with a full glass of water to ensure that it enters the stomach and dissolves, which promotes absorption.
    b. This is unnecessary because ibuprofen does not affect the blood pressure. Body temperature should be monitored if ibuprofen is taken for its antipyretic action.
    c. **This is a desirable action because food limits gastric irritation. This drug is irritating to the gastric mucosa and prolongs the bleeding time, which can result in gastrointestinal bleeding.**
    d. Ibuprofen is not addictive.

45. a. This will not promote absorption via the transdermal patch; it could result in the destructive effects of immobility, and may interfere with the quality of life.
    b. **Intermittent episodes of pain that occur despite continued use of an analgesic (breakthrough pain) can be managed by administering an immediate-release analgesic to reduce pain (rescue dosing). This reduces pain during an unanticipated pain episode without unnecessarily raising the dosage of the long-acting analgesic.**
    c. This would be ineffective in this situation. The patient has intractable (malignant) pain that requires an opioid at this time.
    d. This is not the priority. Although this may eventually be necessary, the patient's pain must be relieved immediately.

46. a. Although this is generally true, there are times the attached needle is inappropriate for a particular patient and the nurse must transfer the medication into a standard syringe.
    b. Drug interactions can still occur with pre-filled, disposable cartridges because the drug within the cartridge may alter or be altered by the concurrent presence of another medication.
    c. Although pre-filled cartridges are convenient in an emergency, it is not the primary purpose of having pre-filled cartridges.
    d. **Single dose cartridges prepared by a medication manufacturer or pharmacy ensure the purity of the drug. Vials can be contaminated by glass debris, and multiple-dose vials can be contaminated by rubber debris and microorganisms.**

47. a. Acute adrenal insufficiency may cause hyperthermia, not hypothermia.
    b. Acute adrenal insufficiency is unrelated to hemorrhage.
    c. Acute adrenal insufficiency may cause dizziness and syncope, not seizures.
    d. **Exogenous glucocorticoids cause adrenal suppression. When exogenous steroids are withdrawn abruptly, the adrenal glands are unable to produce adequate amounts of glucocorticoids, thus causing acute adrenal insufficiency and shock.**

48. a. **Diphenoxylate hydrochloride (Lomotil) depresses intestinal motility and effectively controls diarrhea within 24 to 36 hours. If diarrhea persists beyond 48 hours, the physician should be notified.**
    b. Lomotil may depress the central nervous system, which causes drowsiness and sedation, not hyperactivity.
    c. When a patient is experiencing diarrhea fluid should be encouraged, not restricted, to prevent dehydration and electrolyte imbalances.
    d. Lomotil tablets are not enteric-coated and do not have extended-release properties, therefore they may be crushed if necessary.

49. a. The liver is involved with the biotransformation, not excretion, of a drug.
    b. The majority of drugs are not excreted by the lungs, although some drugs, such as general anesthetic agents, are excreted via the respiratory tract.
    c. **The majority of drugs and their metabolites are excreted through the kidneys. Decreased kidney function can result in drug toxicity because of accumulation of the drug within the body.**
    d. The majority of drugs are not excreted through the intestines.

50. a. This heart rate is within the normal range of 60 to 100 beats per minute.
    b. **This blood pressure is less than the average of 120/80 mmHg. The acceptable range for the systolic pressure is 90 to 130 mmHg and the acceptable range for the diastolic pressure is 60 to 90 mmHg. This patient is on the very low side of normal, which would be an excessive drop in a patient who is receiving an antihypertensive.**
    c. Antihypertensives do not directly affect respirations. Respirations may return to the normal range of 12 to 20 breaths per minute when cardiac output improves.
    d. Antihypertensives do not influence body temperature. Normal oral temperatures range between 98° and 98.6° F.

51. a. **When depression lifts during the early stages of antidepressant therapy, the individual has renewed energy that may support the implementation of suicidal ideation. Patient safety is the priority.**
    b. Although this should be done, it is not the priority.
    c. A person will more likely lose, not gain, weight when taking sertraline hydrochloride (Zoloft) because its side effects include anorexia, nausea, and vomiting.
    d. Alcohol should be avoided because it potentiates the central nervous system depressive effects of Zoloft.

52. a. Intake and output is monitored when a patient is taking a diuretic, not an antipyretic.
    b. Pain tolerance is monitored when a patient is taking an analgesic, not an antipyretic.
    c. **Antipyretics lower fever by affecting thermoregulation in the central nervous system and/or inhibiting the action of prostaglandins peripherally.**

d. Respirations are monitored when a patient is taking a central nervous system depressant or bronchodilator, not an antipyretic.

53. a. A trough level does not reflect the peak level. The optimum peak-value range begins at 8 mcg/ml. A peak value of 0.8 mcg/ml would be too low and ineffective.
    b. This is unknown from a trough level. For optimum results, the blood level of the drug should be maintained between 4 to 10 mcg/ml.
    c. This is unknown from a trough level. The risk for drug toxicity occurs when the maximum peak value is reached or exceeded.
    d. **This trough level is acceptable because 0.8 mcg/ml falls above the acceptable minimal trough range of 0.5 mcg/ml.**

54. a. This is unnecessary.
    b. Although this may be done, it is not the priority. Pain tolerance is the highest intensity of pain that the person is willing to endure.
    c. **Analgesics depress the central nervous system; therefore, the respiratory status must be monitored before and routinely throughout administration for signs of respiratory depression.**
    d. Although this may be done, it is not the priority. Pain threshold is the amount of pain stimulation a person requires before it is felt.

55. a. A mucolytic liquefies, not solidifies, tenacious mucus.
    b. An expectorant increases, not decreases, mucus production, so that it promotes the coughing up and removal of mucus from the lungs.
    c. An antitussive relieves, not encourages, coughing.
    d. **Once bronchi and bronchioles relax, their lumens increase in diameter (bronchodilation), causing a decrease in airway resistance.**

Basic Human Needs and Related Nursing Care

5

Hygiene

KEYWORDS

The following words include English vocabulary, nursing/medical terminology, concepts, principles, or information relevant to content specifically addressed in the chapter or associated with topics presented in it. English dictionaries, your nursing textbooks, and medical dictionaries such as *Taber's Cyclopedic Medical Dictionary* are resources that can be used to expand your knowledge and understanding of these words and related information.

Abrasion
Acne
Activities of daily living
Alopecia
Asepsis
Athlete's foot
Back massage
Baths
    Bag bath (towel bath)
    Bed bath (partial/complete)
    Shower (stand-up/shower chair)
    Sitz bath
    Tub bath
    Partial
Bunions
Callus
Cerumen
Circumcised
Conduction
Convection
Corn
Cuticles
Dandruff
Debris
Dental Caries
Dental hygienist

Dentures
Dermatitis
Dermis
Distal
Effleurage
Emery board
Epidermis
Evaporation
Excoriation
Extremities
Flossing
Foot care
Foreskin
Genital
Gingivitis
Glossitis
Glycerin swabs
Grooming
Halitosis
Hard palate
Hirsutism
Integumentary
Kneading
Labia
Maceration
Matted hair

Moisturizing
Mucous membrane
Oral hygiene
Orange stick
Outer/inner canthus
Pediculosis
Penis
Perianal area
Perineal care
Perineum
Periodontal disease
Peripheral neuropathy
Plaque
Proximal
Radiation
Scrotum
Sebaceous glands
Self-care deficit
Shampoo
Smegma
Sordes
Stomatitis
Tangles
Tartar
Toe pleat
Vasodilation

1. The nurse recognizes that draping a patient during a bath prevents heat loss via:
   a. Vasodilation
   b. Conduction
   c. Convection
   d. Diffusion

2. Which is the first assessment the nurse should make when planning to meet the hygiene needs of a patient?
   a. Determine the patient's preferences about hygiene practices
   b. Assess the patient's ability to assist in hygiene activities
   c. Recognize the patient's developmental stage
   d. Collect toiletries needed for the bath

3. The primary purpose of providing hygiene to a patient is to:
   a. Support a sense of well-being by increasing self-esteem
   b. Remove excess oil, perspiration, and bacteria by mechanical cleansing
   c. Promote circulation by stimulating the skin's peripheral nerve endings
   d. Exercise muscles by contraction and relaxation of muscles when bathing

4. Which action is common to a bed bath as well as a tub bath?
   a. Helping the patient wash parts that cannot be reached
   b. Exposing just the part of the body being washed
   c. Obtaining an order from the physician
   d. Ensuring that the call bell is in reach

5. Which defining characteristic would support the nursing diagnosis Self-Care Deficit Bathing/Hygiene?
   a. Presence of joint contractures
   b. Inability to wash body parts
   c. Postoperative lethargy
   d. Visual disorders

6. When assessing a patient with acne, the nurse should understand that acne is caused by:
   a. Dry, flaking skin
   b. An oversecretion of sebum
   c. Microorganisms on the skin
   d. Inadequate hygienic practices

7. Which action best supports a principle associated with asepsis when bathing a patient?
   a. Wearing clean gloves when washing the perineal area
   b. Having the patient void before beginning the bed bath
   c. Replacing the top covers with a clean flannel bath blanket
   d. Washing from the outer canthus to the inner canthus of the eye

8. Which is best when providing oral care to an unconscious patient?
   a. Gauze-wrapped tongue blades with a saline solution
   b. A small amount of non-foaming toothpaste
   c. Half strength mouthwash and saline
   d. Packaged glycerin swabs

9. The most important reason why the nurse washes a patient's extremities from distal to proximal is to:
   a. Decrease the chance of infection
   b. Facilitate removal of dry skin
   c. Stimulate venous return
   d. Minimize skin tears

10. During oral care the nurse softens and removes a patch of dried food and debris stuck to the hard palate of the patient's mouth. When documenting, the nurse identifies this condition as:
    a. Sordes
    b. Plaque
    c. Glossitis
    d. Stomatitis

11. To be effective, brushing the teeth should be done:
    a. 4 times a day
    b. 6 times a day
    c. 3 times a day
    d. 2 times a day

12. When providing hygiene to the patient with peripheral neuropathy, the nurse should:
    a. Seek a physician's order for foot care
    b. File the toenails straight across the nail
    c. Wash the feet with lukewarm water and dry well
    d. Apply moisturizing lotion to the feet, especially between the toes

13. It is most important for the nurse to consider the concept of personal space before which nursing intervention?
    a. Providing a bed bath
    b. Obtaining vital signs
    c. Performing a health history
    d. Ambulating a patient down the hall

14. When bathing a febrile patient, tepid bath water is used to:
    a. Increase heat loss
    b. Remove surface debris
    c. Reduce surface tension of skin
    d. Stimulate peripheral circulation

15. Whether to give a full or partial bed bath would depend upon the:
    a. Physician's order for the patient's activity
    b. Immediate needs of the patient
    c. Time of the patient's last bath
    d. Wishes of the patient

16. Which action describes aseptic technique when making a patient's bed?
    a. Positioning a soiled linen hamper inside the doorway to a patient's room
    b. Containing soiled linen in a pillow case resting on a patient's bedside chair
    c. Washing hands after disposing of a patient's linen in a soiled linen hamper
    d. Using sterile gloves when changing linen soiled by a patient's sanguineous drainage

17. A nursing diagnosis that would be most appropriate for a preoperative patient who is NPO would be Risk for:
    a. Injury
    b. Disuse Syndrome
    c. Impaired Social Interaction
    d. Altered Oral Mucous Membranes

18. The nursing diagnosis of most concern for a patient incontinent of urine and stool would be Risk for:
    a. Disuse Syndrome
    b. Deficient Fluid Volume
    c. Impaired Skin Integrity
    d. Altered Sexuality Patterns

19. When caring for patients who wear eyeglasses the nurse should:
    a. Encourage the use of artificial tears when in the hospital
    b. Dry the glasses with a paper towel after cleaning the lenses
    c. Limit the time that glasses are worn in an effort to rest the eyes
    d. Use warm water to clean the lenses of glasses at least once a day

20. Which is an important action that the nurse should teach patients with diabetes about foot care?
    a. Wear clean stockings or cotton socks each day
    b. Dry your feet vigorously with a towel after bathing
    c. Test the water with your toes before stepping into a bath tub
    d. Use a heating pad rather than a hot water bottle to warm cold feet

21. Which action is most important when providing a patient with a bed bath?
    a. Lower the side rail on the working side of the bed
    b. Ensure that the bath water is at least 110° F
    c. Fold the washcloth like a mitt on the hand
    d. Raise the bed to the highest position

22. What would be the best product to use when giving a back rub?
    a. Rubbing alcohol
    b. Betadine cream
    c. Baby powder
    d. Keri lotion

23. Which is most important when making an unoccupied bed?
    a. Ensure that the hem of the bottom sheet is facing the mattress
    b. Arrange linen in the order in which it is to be used
    c. Shift the mattress up to the headboard of the bed
    d. Check the soiled bed linens for personal items

24. To distribute oil evenly along hair shafts the nurse should:
    a. Brush from the scalp toward the hair ends
    b. Lift opened fingers through the hair
    c. Shampoo the hair once a week
    d. Use a fine-tooth comb

25. Which condition would place a person at the highest risk for self-care toileting and elimination problems?
    a. Amputation of a foot
    b. Early dementia
    c. Fractured hip
    d. Pregnancy

26. The main reason for using mouthwash during oral care is to:
    a. Help reduce offensive mouth odors
    b. Minimize the formation of dental caries
    c. Soften smegma that accumulates in the mouth
    d. Destroy pathogens that are found in the mouth

27. When cleaning a patient's eyes, the nurse should:
    a. Wear sterile gloves
    b. Use a tear-free baby soap
    c. Position the client on the same side as the eye to be cleaned
    d. Wash the eyes with a cotton ball from the outer canthus to the inner canthus

28. What should the nurse do first when planning to shampoo the hair of a patient who has an order for bed rest?
    a. Tape eye shields over both eyes
    b. Brush the hair to remove tangles
    c. Encourage the use of dry shampoo
    d. Wet the hair thoroughly before applying shampoo

29. The patient who would benefit most from soaking the feet as part of a bath would be the patient who:
    a. Has a preference for taking showers
    b. Is ambulating with paper slippers
    c. Has peripheral vascular disease
    d. Is on bed rest

30. Which type of bath would a physician most likely order for a patient who has had perineal surgery?
    a. Sponge bath
    b. Tub bath
    c. Bed bath
    d. Sitz bath

31. Which is most important when making an unoccupied bed?
    a. Position the call bell in reach
    b. Place a pull sheet on top of the draw sheet
    c. Ensure that the bottom sheet is free of wrinkles
    d. Complete one side of the bed before completing the other side

32. When evaluating a patient's oral hygiene practices, the nurse understands that the intervention most effective in removing dental plaque is:
    a. Gargling with mouthwash
    b. Using an abrasive toothpaste
    c. Flossing the teeth with waxed floss
    d. Brushing the teeth with a toothbrush

33. Which is the most appropriate nursing intervention for a patient who has the nursing diagnosis Bathing Self-Care Deficit Related To Impaired Vision?
    a. Provide the patient with liquid bath gel
    b. Give the patient an adapted toothbrush
    c. Ensure that the patient can locate bathing supplies
    d. Monitor the patient's ability to provide self-care through a crack in the curtain

34. The nurse recognizes that teaching about the care of dry skin has been effective when the older adult says, "I should:
    a. Bathe daily with a moisturizing soap."
    b. Wear clothes made of woolen fabrics."
    c. Increase the amount of water that I drink."
    d. Use baby powder rather than lotion on my skin."

35. When providing for the hygiene and grooming needs of an obese patient with a nursing diagnosis of Activity Intolerance, which is the most important nursing intervention?
    a. Maintaining the bed in a high-Fowler's position
    b. Administering oxygen during provision of care
    c. Providing rest periods every 10 minutes
    d. Assessing response to activity

36. Which would be the most appropriate nursing intervention for a hospitalized patient with the nursing diagnosis, Self-Care Deficit Bathing Related to Hemiparesis Secondary to Cerebral Vascular Accident?
    a. Encourage a family member to bathe the patient
    b. Provide minimal supervision during the bath
    c. Give total assistance with a complete bath
    d. Assist with the bath as needed

37. To shave a male patient's facial hair the nurse should:
    a. Shave in the direction of hair growth
    b. Hold the razor at a 90° angle to the skin
    c. Use long, downward strokes with the razor
    d. Wrap the face with a hot wet towel before shaving

38. When providing oral care for a patient with dentures, what is most important for the nurse to do?
    a. Wear sterile gloves when cleaning the dentures
    b. Soak the dentures overnight in a cleansing solution
    c. Apply dental adhesive to the underside of each denture, then insert into the mouth
    d. Rinse both dentures of the soaking solution before reinserting them into the mouth

39. Which is a necessary nursing intervention when meeting the hygiene needs of a patient with cognitive deficits secondary to dementia?
    a. Check the patient every 5 minutes
    b. Encourage attention to each task of bathing
    c. Arrange the bathing equipment within the patient's visual field
    d. Explain in detail everything you will be doing before beginning

40. Which action is most effective in relation to the concept, "Bacteria and enzymes in stool are irritating to the skin"?
    a. Wearing sterile gloves when collecting a patient's stool for culture and sensitivity
    b. Applying a moisture barrier to the perianal area of incontinent patients
    c. Encouraging a patient to drink eight ounces of cranberry juice daily
    d. Toileting a confused patient before each meal

41. Which is most important when making an occupied bed?
    a. Secure top linens under the foot of the mattress and miter the corners
    b. Ensure that the patient's head is always in functional alignment
    c. Fan-fold soiled linens as close to the patient's body as possible
    d. Position the bed in the horizontal position

42. What should the nurse do before bathing the feet of a patient with diabetes?
    a. File the nails straight across with an emery board
    b. Ensure that a physician's order for foot care has been obtained
    c. Teach the patient that daily foot care is essential to healthy feet
    d. Assess for additional risk factors that could contribute to foot problems

43. Which is most important when assisting a female patient with care of the hair?
    a. Ensure that the patient's hair is left dry, not wet
    b. Ask the patient what should be done with her hair
    c. Comb the patient's hair from the proximal to distal end of the hair shaft
    d. Avoid tangles in the patient's hair by using rubbing alcohol as a conditioner

44. The patient who has a fever experienced significant diaphoresis during the night. The patient stated, "I am tired and I just want to sleep." What should the nurse do regarding bathing the patient?
    a. Consult with the physician before providing care
    b. Give a bed bath with complete assistance
    c. Postpone bathing until the afternoon
    d. Wait until the patient feels better

45. The nurse would know that further teaching about correct foot care is needed when an older adult patient says, "I should:
    a. Use hot water to wash my feet."
    b. Cut my toenails straight across."
    c. Apply a water-soluble lubricant."
    d. Wash my feet with mild soap and water."

46. Which action is most important when caring for a patient with an excessively dry mouth?
    a. Swabbing the mouth with a sponge-tipped applicator of lemon and glycerin
    b. Cleansing the mouth four times a day with a water pick
    c. Rinsing the mouth frequently with mouthwash
    d. Providing oral hygiene every two hours

47. The need for oral hygiene would be determined when inspection of a patient's mouth reveals the presence of:
    a. Jaundice
    b. Plaque
    c. Sordes
    d. Tartar

48. When giving a bed bath, which is the best intervention to increase circulation?
    a. Wash the extremities with firm strokes toward the heart
    b. Soak the feet in warm water for at least 10 minutes
    c. Ensure that the water is 115 to 120 degrees F
    d. Expose just the areas that are being washed

49. When providing perineal care to a male patient, the nurse should wash the:
    a. Genital area with hot, sudsy water
    b. Scrotum before washing the glans penis
    c. Shaft of the penis while moving toward the urinary meatus
    d. Penis with one hand while holding it firmly with the other hand

50. When teaching an adolescent about skin care related to acne, the nurse would know that the information was understood when the adolescent says, "I should wash my face:
    a. Every other day with a strong soap."
    b. And then apply an oil-based ointment."
    c. Thoroughly but gently three times a day."
    d. With cool water when I shower in the morning."

51. When providing a bed bath, which part of the body should be washed last?
    a. Face and neck
    b. Arms and hands
    c. Back and perineum
    d. Chest and abdomen

52. The nurse should use a cotton blanket when bathing a patient because air currents increase the loss of heat from the body through the principle of:
    a. Osmosis
    b. Diffusion
    c. Conduction
    d. Vaporization

53. Which is the best intervention to prevent dental plaque?
    a. Rinse the mouth with diluted hydrogen peroxide
    b. Have the teeth cleaned by a dental hygienist once a year
    c. Brush the biting surface of the teeth using a forward and backward motion
    d. Vibrate a toothbrush while holding it at a 45° angle where the teeth meet the gum line

54. The nurse recognizes that additional teaching about skin care is necessary when an older adult says, "I should:
    a. Bathe twice a week."
    b. Rinse well after using soap."
    c. Humidify my home in the winter."
    d. Use a bubble bath preparation when I take a bath."

55. The nurse recognizes that teaching about skin care for a patient who has acne has been effective when the patient states, "I should:
    a. Squeeze the white heads gently and apply a topical antibiotic."
    b. Wash my face several times a day with soap and water."
    c. Wash with an alcohol-based facial cleanser every day."
    d. Use an oil-based cream on my face after washing."

56. When providing fingernail care during a bath the nurse should:
    a. Push the cuticles back with the rounded end of a metal nail file
    b. Clean under the nails with an orange stick
    c. First soak the hands in hot water
    d. Cut the nails in an oval shape

57. When removing a bed pan from under a debilitated patient who has just had a bowel movement, the nurse's first intervention should be to:
    a. Document the results
    b. Provide perineal care
    c. Reposition the patient
    d. Cover the patient with the top linens

58. People on complete bed rest tend to have which common problem with their hair?
    a. Dry hair
    b. Oily hair
    c. Split hair
    d. Matted hair

59. When planning to help a patient dress who is weak on the right side, what should the nurse plan to do?
    a. Put the right sleeve of the gown on first
    b. Keep the patient in an open-backed gown
    c. Encourage the patient to dress independently
    d. Leave the right sleeve off and adjust the tie at the neck

60. A patient is incontinent of loose stools and is mentally impaired. What should the nurse do to help prevent skin breakdown?
    a. Wash the buttocks with strong soap and water
    b. Frequently check the rectal area for soiling
    c. Gently put a pad under the buttocks
    d. Place the call bell in easy reach

1. a. Vasodilation increases blood flow to the surface of the skin, which promotes, not prevents, heat loss.
   b. Conduction is the transfer of heat between two objects in physical contact.
   c. **Convection is the transfer of heat by movement of air along a surface. Using a bath blanket limits the amount of air flowing across the patient, which prevents heat loss.**
   d. Diffusion is the movement of molecules from a solution of higher concentration to a solution of lower concentration.

2. a. **Hygiene is a personal matter determined by individual beliefs, values, and practices. Hygiene practices are influenced by culture, religion, environment, age, health, and personal preferences. When personal preferences are supported, the patient has a sense of control and usually is more accepting of care.**
   b. Although this information is significant in relation to the extent of self-care that may be expected, it is not the first assessment.
   c. The patient's developmental level will influence how the nurse will proceed, but it is not the first assessment.
   d. This is done after several other considerations and just before actually beginning the bath.

3. a. Although a bath is refreshing and relaxing and may improve morale, these are not the primary reasons for bathing.
   b. **The removal of accumulated oil, perspiration, dead cells, and bacteria from the skin limits the environment conducive to the growth of bacteria and skin breakdown. An intact, healthy skin is one of the body's first lines of defense.**
   c. Friction from rubbing the skin increases surface temperature, which increases circulation to the area.
   d. Although range-of-motion exercises may be performed while bathing a patient, it is not the purpose of the bath.

4. a. **Patients can provide self-care within their abilities. When they have limitations, such as an inability to reach a body area, an activity intolerance, a decreased level of consciousness, or dementia, it is the nurse's responsibility to assist the patient regardless of the type of bath.**
   b. This is impossible if the patient is taking a tub bath or shower.
   c. Providing a bed bath is within the scope of nursing practice, so a practitioner's order is unnecessary. An order is necessary for a tub bath or shower because it requires an activity order and is therefore a dependent function.
   d. There is no need for a call bell when a patient is taking a tub bath or a shower because it is unsafe to leave a patient alone.

5. a. This is a *"related to"* factor associated with the nursing diagnosis Impaired Physical Mobility.
   b. **Bathing/Hygiene Self-Care Deficit is a state in which the individual experiences an impaired ability to perform or complete bathing/hygiene activities. Being *unable or unwilling to wash body or body parts* is a defining characteristic for this nursing diagnosis.**
   c. Lethargy and listlessness are defining characteristics associated with the nursing diagnosis Fatigue.
   d. This is a *"related to"* factor associated with the nursing diagnosis Risk for Injury.

6. a. Dry skin is associated with aging, not acne. In the older adult, there is a decrease in sebaceous gland activity and tissue fluid.
   b. **During puberty the sebaceous glands, responding to the influence of androgens, enlarge and increase the production of sebum. The accumulation of sebum can become colonized by bacteria with a resulting inflammatory condition with papules and pustules (acne).**
   c. Microorganisms on the skin play a role in the development of cysts, but microorganisms are not the etiology of acne.
   d. Although inadequate hygienic practices will aggravate the condition, this is not the etiology of the condition.

7. a. **A nurse should use standard precautions when bathing a patient because the nurse may be exposed to body fluids, particularly in the perineal area.**
   b. This action is related to a patient's comfort and elimination needs, rather than asepsis.
   c. A bath blanket promotes privacy and prevents heat loss during a bath and is unrelated to asepsis. A patient's bath blanket can be reused if not soiled.
   d. The eye should always be washed from the inner to the outer canthus to prevent secretions from entering the lacrimal ducts.

8. a. **Unconscious patients often bite down when something is placed in the mouth. Therefore, a padded tongue blade should be placed between the upper and lower teeth to help keep the mouth open during oral care. Other padded tongue blades, wetted with a small amount of saline, should be used to clean the oral cavity.**
   b. Toothpaste should be avoided because it requires flushing the mouth with adequate amounts of water to prevent leaving an irritating residue on the mucous membranes. An unconscious patient usually has a diminished gag reflex and is at risk for aspiration.
   c. Although this is used, it is not the best intervention because mouthwash contains ingredients that can be irritating to the mucous membranes.
   d. Glycerin swabs are not effective in cleaning the oral cavity.

9. a. Friction, regardless of the direction of the washing strokes, in conjunction with soap and water, removes secretions, dirt, and microorganisms that decrease the potential for infection.
   b. Friction, regardless of the direction of the washing strokes, removes dry, dead skin cells.
   c. **The pressure exerted on the skin surface by long, smooth strokes moving from distal to proximal areas also presses on the veins, which promotes venous return.**

d. Long, smooth washing strokes that avoid a shearing force minimize skin tears.

10. a. The accumulation of matter such as food, epithelial elements, dried secretions, and microorganisms (sordes) eventually can lead to dental caries and periodontal disease and therefore must be removed during oral hygiene.
   b. Plaque is an invisible film composed of secretions, epithelial cells, leukocytes, and bacteria that adheres to the enamel surface of teeth.
   c. Glossitis is an inflammation of the tongue.
   d. Stomatitis is an inflammation of the oral mucosa.

11. a. Brushing the teeth after each meal and at bedtime with daily flossing is recommended to stimulate the gums, clean the teeth, and flush the mouth of debris, thus preventing tooth decay and periodontal disease.
   b. Although ideal, brushing the teeth 6 times a day is unrealistic.
   c. This is not often enough to remove debris from the mouth to prevent tooth decay and periodontal disease.
   d. Brushing just 2 times a day is inadequate to prevent tooth decay and periodontal disease.

12 a. A physician's order is unnecessary because providing foot care is within the scope of nursing practice.
   b. When the patient has peripheral neuropathy, this care should be provided by a podiatrist.
   c. Lukewarm water is comfortable and limits the potential for burns. Drying the feet limits moisture that promotes bacterial growth.
   d. Lotion between the toes in the dark moist environment of shoes promotes the growth of bacteria and the development of an infection.

13 a. Touching a patient during a bed bath invades the person's intimate space. When encroaching on a person's intimate space (physical contact to $1\frac{1}{2}$ feet), the nurse should inform the patient when and why it is necessary.
   b. Although the nurse enters a patient's intimate space when obtaining vital signs, it does not involve touching the intimate parts of a patient's body and is therefore less intrusive than many other procedures.
   c. This can be accomplished by remaining in a person's personal space ($1\frac{1}{2}$ to 4 feet) or social space (4 to 12 feet).
   d. Although touching a patient while ambulating invades the person's intimate space it does not involve touching the intimate parts of a patient's body, and is therefore less intrusive than many other procedures.

14. a. Heat is transferred from the warm surface of the skin to the water that is in direct contact with the body. Tepid water is slightly below body temperature, and a person who is febrile has an elevated body temperature.
   b. Friction, not the temperature of the bath water, helps to remove surface debris.
   c. Soap, not the temperature of the bath water, reduces surface tension.
   d. Peripheral circulation is increased by warm water and by rubbing the skin with a washcloth.

15. a. Full or partial bed baths can be administered regardless of the activity order written by the practitioner because it is an independent function of the nurse.
   b. A total patient assessment with an analysis of the data identifies the needs of the patient and the appropriate intervention to meet those needs.
   c. Time has no relevance in relation to identifying what type of bed bath to administer to a patient.
   d. Although this is a consideration, patient teaching should convince a patient what should be done to meet his/her physical needs.

16. a. This violates medical asepsis. A soiled linen hamper should be kept outside the door to a patient's room.
   b. This violates medical asepsis because it contaminates the chair. Soiled linen should be placed immediately into the soiled linen hamper.
   c. The hands should be washed whether or not gloves were worn during the procedure. This prevents the transmission of microorganisms to the nurse and to others. Gloves should be worn if there is potential to be exposed to the patient's excretions or secretions.
   d. Medical, not surgical, asepsis should be followed when changing soiled linen.

17. a. Being NPO is unrelated to the nursing diagnosis Risk for Injury, which is the state in which an individual is at risk for harm because of a perceptual or physiologic deficit, a lack of awareness of hazards, or maturational age.
   b. Being NPO is unrelated to the nursing diagnosis Risk for Disuse Syndrome, which is the state in which an individual is at risk for deterioration of body systems or altered functioning because of prescribed or unavoidable musculoskeletal inactivity.
   c. Being NPO is unrelated to the nursing diagnosis Risk for Impaired Social Interaction, which is the state in which an individual is at risk of experiencing negative, insufficient, or unsatisfactory responses from interactions.
   d. Not drinking anything by mouth can cause dehydration and result in drying of the oral mucous membranes and a coated, furrowed tongue. The nursing diagnosis Risk for Altered Oral Mucous Membranes applies to an individual who is at risk of experiencing disruptions in the oral cavity.

18. a. Incontinence is unrelated to the nursing diagnosis Risk for Disuse Syndrome, which is the state in which an individual is at risk for deterioration of body systems or altered functioning because of prescribed or unavoidable musculoskeletal inactivity.
   b. Incontinence is unrelated to the nursing diagnosis Risk for Deficient Fluid Volume, which is the state in which an individual who is not NPO is at risk of experiencing vascular, interstitial, or intracellular dehydration.
   c. Fecal material contains enzymes that erode the skin, and urine is an acidic fluid that macerates the skin. The nursing diagnosis Risk for Impaired Skin Integrity is the state in which an individual is at risk for altered epidermis and/or dermis.

d. Incontinence is unrelated to the nursing diagnosis Risk for Altered Sexuality Patterns, which is the state in which an individual is at risk of experiencing a change in sexual health.

19. a. This is unnecessary. Not everyone who wears glasses has dry eyes.
    b. A paper towel is coarse and may scratch the lenses of the eyeglasses. A soft nonabrasive cloth or chamois should be used.
    c. Patient preference determines how long eyeglasses can be worn.
    d. Eyeglasses should be cleaned at least once a day because dirty lenses impair vision. Warm, not hot, water is used to prevent distortion of the lens or frame, particularly if it is made of a plastic compound.

20. a. Clean stockings or socks limit exposure to microorganisms and cotton socks absorb moisture, which prevents skin maceration.
    b. Vigorous rubbing with a towel can cause skin trauma in patients with diabetes.
    c. This could result in a burn. Many people with diabetes have peripheral neuropathy with diminished sensation. A bath thermometer should be used to test water temperature.
    d. Warming devices, such as a heating pat or hot water bottle, are contraindicated for patients with diabetes.

21. a. Although this might be done to promote the body mechanics of the nurse, it is not a necessity.
    b. The temperature of bath water should be between 110 and 115 degrees to promote comfort, dilate blood vessels, and prevent chilling. A lower temperature can cause chilling, and a higher temperature can cause skin trauma.
    c. Although a mitt retains water and heat and prevents loose ends from irritating the skin, it is not as essential as other factors that relate to patient safety.
    d. Although the height of the bed should be adjusted to promote the nurse's body mechanics, it is not as essential as other factors that relate to patient safety.

22. a. Rubbing alcohol causes drying of the skin and should not be used.
    b. An antimicrobial cream is inappropriate for a back rub. Betadine stains, irritates, and dries the skin and eliminates the integument's natural flora.
    c. Baby powder mixed with secretions of the skin forms a paste-like substance that supports antimicrobial growth and irritates the skin, which promote skin breakdown.
    d. Keri lotion lubricates the skin and reduces friction between the nurse's hands and the patient's back. Lotion facilitates smooth movement of the hands across the patient's skin, which is relaxing and prevents trauma to the skin.

23. a. Although it is important to provide a smooth surface, it is not the priority.
    b. This is an efficient approach that permits each sheet to be accessible when needed; however, it is not a priority.
    c. Although this is important to ensure that the patient is well supported when the head of the bed is elevated or the knee gatch employed, it is not the priority.
    d. A nurse must take reasonable precautions to ensure that a patient's personal belongings, especially eyeglasses, dentures, and prosthetic devices, are kept safe. Checking for personal belongings before placing soiled linen into a linen hamper is a reasonable, prudent action.

24. a. Brushing the hair from the scalp to the ends of the hair massages the scalp and distributes oils secreted by the scalp down along the length of the hair shaft.
    b. This would provide inadequate hair care. It might be done at the completion of hair care to style the hair.
    c. Shampoos remove, not distribute, oil along the shaft of hair. Shampoos generally contain ingredients that are drying to the hair and scalp.
    d. A fine-tooth comb has pointed ends and should not be used for daily grooming because it can injure the scalp, damage the hair shaft, and split the ends of hair.

25. a. A patient with an amputation can still transfer to a bedside commode or ambulate with crutches to a bathroom.
    b. When a person has early dementia, frequent reminders to perform self-toileting activities or declarative directions about toileting usually are adequate.
    c. Discomfort due to the proximity of the fracture to the pelvic area and the limitations placed on the positioning of, or weight bearing on, the affected leg impact on a patient's ability to use a bedpan or transfer to a commode.
    d. Although the enlarging uterus exerts pressure on the bladder causing urinary frequency and alteration of the person's center of gravity, self-toileting usually is not impaired.

26. a. An offensive odor to the breath (halitosis) can be caused by inadequate oral hygiene, periodontal disease, or systemic disease. Rinsing the mouth with mouthwash will flush the oral cavity of debris and microorganisms, which will reduce halitosis if it is caused by a local problem.
    b. Dental caries are caused by plaque. Therefore, brushing and flossing, not the use of mouthwash, are the most efficient ways to prevent dental caries.
    c. Smegma, a cheesy-like substance secreted by the sebaceous glands, collects under the foreskin of the penis, not the mouth.
    d. Only bactericidal mouthwashes can limit the amount of bacterial flora in the mouth; prolonged or excessive use can result in oral fungal infections.

27. a. Medical, not surgical, asepsis is necessary. Clean gloves are adequate.
    b. Soap is never used around the eyes. The eyes should be washed only with water.
    c. Tilting the head or turning the patient toward the same side as the eye to be washed facilitates the flow of water from the inner to the outer canthus. This prevents secretions from entering the lacrimal ducts.
    d. The eye should be washed from the inner canthus to the outer canthus.

28. a. This is unnecessary. Appropriate positioning will let the water flow by gravity away from the face, and a washcloth can be placed over the eyes.
   b. It is easier and causes less trauma to the hair to brush out tangles when the hair is dry rather then wet.
   c. Dry, powder shampoos can irritate the scalp and dry the hair.
   d. Although this is done, it is not the first intervention.

29. a. This is unnecessary. The feet can be washed thoroughly when taking a shower.
   b. Extra care with the feet is unnecessary because paper slippers provide a barrier between the feet and the floor.
   c. The warm water used to soak the feet promotes vasodilation, which improves circulation to the most distal portions of the feet. Soaking the feet loosens dirt and limits scrubbing, which prevent trauma to the skin. Soaking the feet should be done for just several minutes because prolonged soaking removes natural skin oils, which dries the skin and makes it prone to cracking.
   d. Bed rest does not necessitate soaking the feet during the bed bath.

30. a. A sponge bath is given to reduce a patient's fever through heat loss via conduction and vaporization.
   b. Tub baths are effective for cleaning and rinsing the skin. Tubs are also used for therapeutic baths when medications are added to the water to soothe irritated skin.
   c. A bed bath is indicated for patients with restricted mobility.
   d. A sitz bath immerses a patient from the midthighs to the iliac crests or umbilicus in a special tub, or the patient sits in a basin that fits onto the toilet seat, so the legs and feet remain out of the water. The moist heat to the genital area increases local circulation, cleans the skin, reduces soreness, and promotes relaxation, voiding, drainage, and healing.

31. a. The call bell does not have to be positioned until there is a patient occupying the bed.
   b. A pull sheet is not included in the procedure for an unoccupied bed. In addition, this would create too many layers of linens and wrinkles under a patient. The draw sheet can be used as a pull sheet.
   c. Wrinkles create ridges that exert additional pressure on the skin, promoting discomfort, skin irritation, and the development of pressure ulcers.
   d. Although this is advisable to conserve time and energy, it is not a priority.

32. a. Mouthwash will not remove plaque, the forerunner to dental caries.
   b. Abrasive toothpaste (dentifrice) can harm the enamel of teeth. Non-abrasive toothpaste and a soft toothbrush should be used.
   c. Unwaxed floss is preferred because it is thinner, slides between the teeth more easily, and is more absorbent than waxed floss.
   d. Brushing the teeth involves several techniques: brushing back and forth strokes across the biting surface of teeth; brushing from the gum line to the crown of each tooth; and with the bristles at a 45-degree angle at the gum line vibrating the bristles while moving from under the gingival margin to the crown of each tooth.

33. a. Manipulating a bottle of bath gel may be more difficult than just using a bar of soap.
   b. Adapted toothbrushes are intended for people who have neuromuscular problems that interfere with grasping and manipulating a toothbrush, not for people with impaired vision.
   c. Arranging supplies in relation to the numbers on a clock facilitates the use of equipment by a person with impaired vision and encourages self-care.
   d. This is a violation of patient privacy. Patients have a right to know when they are being assessed.

34. a. Bathing daily, even using a moisturizing soap, is drying to the skin. Two to three times a week is adequate for an older adult who is continent.
   b. Woolen fabrics are coarse and irritate the skin, and therefore should be avoided.
   c. The percentage of body water dramatically decreases with age, and older adults have altered thirst mechanisms that place them at risk for inadequate fluid intake and dehydration. In addition, the skin of older adults is dryer because of a decreased ability to sweat and a decreased production of sebum.
   d. Lotion is preferable to baby powder because lotion lubricates the skin.

35. a. In the high Fowler's position the abdominal organs press on the diaphragm in an obese patient, which limits respiratory excursion. The semi-Fowler's position is preferred.
   b. Administration of oxygen is a dependent function of the nurse and requires a physician's order.
   c. A rest period every 10 minutes may be inadequate or may unnecessarily prolong the bath. This is not individualized to the patient's needs.
   d. Evaluation of a patient's response to care allows the nurse to alter care to meet the patient's individual needs.

36. a. It is not the responsibility of the family to meet the physical needs of a hospitalized relative.
   b. Minimal supervision may result in the completion of an inadequate bath.
   c. This is unnecessary and may lower the patient's self-esteem, precipitate regression, or promote disuse syndrome.
   d. Hemiparesis is a weakness on one side of the body that can interfere with the performance of activities of daily living. Encouraging the patient to do as much as possible will support self-esteem, and assisting when necessary will ensure that hygiene needs are met.

37. a. Shaving in the direction of hair growth limits skin irritation and prevents ingrown hairs.
   b. A safety razor should be held at a 45, not 90, degree angle to the skin.

c. Short, firm but gentle strokes should be used when shaving a patient.

d. A warm, not hot, washcloth applied to the face for several minutes before actually shaving helps to soften the beard.

38. a. Medical, not surgical, asepsis should be followed to protect the nurse from patient secretions.

b. Dentures should not be soaked overnight to prevent corrosion. Follow the package instructions when using commercial products.

c. The nurse should not automatically use dental adhesive. Its use depends on how well the dentures fit and the preference of the patient.

d. Rinsing the dentures with tepid water removes the cleaning agent that could be caustic to the oral mucosa, flushes off debris, and lubricates the dentures (which makes them easier to insert into the mouth).

39. a. This would not be helpful. Patients with dementia do not have the cognitive ability to perform a procedure independently.

b. When progressing through each aspect of the bath give simple, direct statements to limit the amount of incoming stimuli at one time. This will promote comprehension and self-care.

c. The patient has a problem with cognition, not vision.

d. This intervention may precipitate anxiety. The patient does not have the cognitive ability or attention span to understand a detailed explanation before a procedure.

40. a. Clean gloves are adequate; however, sterile equipment and techniques must be followed when obtaining a stool for culture and sensitivity.

b. A skin barrier, such as zinc oxide, protects the skin from the digestive enzymes in feces.

c. Cranberry juice makes urine more alkaline; it does not influence bacteria and enzymes in stool.

d. Patients should attempt to have a bowel movement after a meal to take advantage of the gastrocolic reflex.

41. a. This will promote plantar flexion and should not be done without a toe pleat.

b. Maintaining functional alignment of a patient's head when making an occupied bed promotes comfort and minimizes stress to the respiratory passages and vital anatomy in the neck.

c. Although this is done, it is not the priority.

d. Although this may be done to facilitate tight sheets with minimal wrinkles, it is not the priority. In addition, there are many patients who cannot assume this position.

42. a. A podiatrist should file or cut the toenails of a patient with diabetes. The toenails are usually thickened and hardened, and an inadvertent cut takes a long time to heal.

b. A physician's order is unnecessary. Foot care in relation to hygiene is within the scope of nursing practice.

c. Although this is important, it is not the first priority.

d. A thorough assessment of the patient is the first step of the nursing process. People with diabetes frequently have thick, hardened toenails,

peripheral neuropathy, impaired arterial and venous circulation in the feet, and foot or leg ulcers.

43. a. After shampooing a patient's hair, it may be dried or just toweled dry until it is free of excess moisture.

b. The appearance of one's hair is an extension of self-image. Therefore, the patient's personal preferences should be considered before grooming the hair.

c. Combing or brushing should begin from the ends of the hair, then from the middle to the ends, and finally from the scalp to the ends. This technique limits discomfort and prevents broken ends and damaged hair shafts.

d. Braiding the hair, not the application of alcohol, will help prevent matting and tangles. A small amount of a lubricant, not alcohol, applied to the hair will facilitate the combing out of tangles once they have occurred.

44. a. This is unnecessary. Bathing a patient is within the scope of nursing practice.

b. After explaining the need for the bath, the nurse should administer a bath without the patient's assistance. This will meet the patient's immediate hygiene needs while conserving the patient's energy.

c. This is unsafe. With significant diaphoresis, there is moisture on the patient's skin that can contribute to skin breakdown as well as cause chilling.

d. This is inappropriate because the patient may never feel better. Physical needs can be met while addressing the patient's concerns.

45. **a. Hot water can cause skin trauma in older adults. Older adults tend to have impaired peripheral circulation and diminished peripheral sensation.**

b. This is appropriate care. Cutting straight across prevents splitting and the development of ingrown nails.

c. This is appropriate care. Water-soluble lotions can be applied to the feet to lubricate the skin.

d. This is appropriate care. Mild soap cleans the skin while limiting skin irritation and drying.

46. a. Lemon and glycerin swabs are counterproductive because their use can lead to further dryness of the mucosa and an alteration in tooth enamel.

b. Oral hygiene 4 times a day is inadequate, and a water pick is contraindicated because the force of the water can injure delicate dry mucous membranes.

c. Mouthwash contains astringents that can injure sensitive, delicate dry mucous membranes.

d. Mouth breathing, oxygen use, unconsciousness, and debilitation, among other conditions, can lead to dry oral mucous membranes. The nurse should provide oral hygiene with saline rinses frequently to keep the oral mucosa moist.

47. a. Jaundice, a yellowish discoloration of the skin, mucous membranes, and sclera, is unrelated to the need for additional oral hygiene. Jaundice is related to liver and biliary disease.

b. Plaque, a thin, soft film of secretions, cellular elements, and bacteria, is invisible; its presence cannot be detected by inspection.

c. Sordes is the accumulation of matter, such as remnants of food particles, cellular debris, secretions, and bacteria, in the oral cavity. Sordes can be removed by brushing and flossing the teeth.

d. When plaque remains on the teeth it accumulates at the gum line and becomes hardened and visible (tartar). Dental instruments are needed to remove tartar.

48. a. **The pressure of firm strokes on the skin moving from distal to proximal areas increases venous return. When venous return increases, cardiac output increases.**

b. Prolonged soaking removes the protective oils on the skin; the result is dry, cracked skin that is prone to further injury.

c. This is too hot for bath water because it may cause tissue injury. Bath water should be 110 to 115 degrees Fahrenheit.

d. This prevents chilling, not increases circulation.

49. a. Warm, not hot, water is used to clean the perineal area because the skin and mucous membranes of the genital area are sensitive, and hot water could cause harm.

b. The glans penis, foreskin, and shaft of the penis are cleaned before the scrotum. The scrotum is considered more soiled than the penis because of its proximity to the rectum.

c. When cleaning the shaft of the penis, bathing should start at the glans penis and then proceed down the shaft toward the scrotum.

d. **Stabilizing the penis and holding it firmly facilitates the bathing procedure and usually prevents an erection.**

50. a. Strong soap may irritate fragile skin, and washing every other day is inadequate to cleanse the skin.

b. Oil-based ointments will block sebaceous gland ducts and hair follicles, which will aggravate the condition.

c. **Washing the face with soap and water 3 times a day will remove dirt and oil, which helps prevent secondary infection.**

d. Washing once a day is inadequate to cleanse the skin. Hot, not cool, water is necessary to remove the oily accumulation on the face.

51. a. The face and neck are washed first before soap enters bath water to protect the eyes; soap may be used if it is the patient's preference.

b. Because a bath tends to follow a cephalocaudal progression, the arms and hands would be washed early during a bath.

c. **The perineal area is considered the dirtiest part of the body because of the presence of excretions and secretions. This area is washed last to prevent microorganisms from being transferred to cleaner parts of the body.**

d. As a bath progresses from the head to the toes, the chest and abdomen would be washed during the middle of the bath.

52. a. Osmosis is the movement of water across a membrane from an area of lesser concentration to an area of greater concentration.

b. Diffusion is a process whereby molecules move through a membrane from an area of higher concentration to an area of lower concentration without the expenditure of energy.

c. Conduction is the transfer heat from one molecule to another while in direct physical contact.

d. **Vaporization (evaporation) is the transfer of heat through the conversion of water to a gas. This occurs through perspiration and insensible losses through the skin and lungs.**

53. a. Rinsing the mouth with diluted hydrogen peroxide does not provide the necessary friction needed to remove debris that contributes to the formation of plaque.

b. A dental hygienist will use various dental instruments to remove tartar, which is hardened plaque.

c. Although this is an integral part of dental hygiene, it removes debris from the biting surface of the teeth, not plaque where the teeth and gums meet.

d. **Plaque, composed of bacteria and saliva, forms on the teeth primarily at the gum line. A vibrating toothbrush provides friction that helps to dislodge plaque from the teeth.**

54. a. This is an acceptable practice. Excessive exposure to warm water and soap exacerbates dry skin associated with aging.

b. This is an acceptable practice. Soap removes the protective oils on the skin and soap residue irritates and dries the skin.

c. A humidified environment limits the amount of insensible loss of moisture through the skin, which helps the skin retain fluid and remain supple.

d. **Bubble bath preparations cause irritation and dryness of the skin because they remove essential skin surface oils. Showers are preferable to baths because baths require submersion in warm water, which is detrimental to skin hydration and resiliency.**

55. a. This is contraindicated because it can cause permanent scarring. In addition, infected material within a pustule can spread if squeezed.

b. **This is an acceptable practice because it removes surface oils from sebaceous glands that plug pores, which aggravate the condition.**

c. Alcohol is caustic and drying. Washing the face with soap and hot water several times a day is adequate.

d. This is contraindicated. Oil-based creams will accumulate in pores and aggravate the condition.

56. a. The cuticles should be pushed back with a washcloth or an orange stick.

b. **An orange stick is an implement that is shaped to facilitate removal of debris from under the nails without causing tissue injury. Removal of dirt and debris decreases the risk of infection.**

c. Hot water can cause tissue injury and should be avoided. Warm, not hot, water should be used.

d. Cutting the corners of the nails can cause tissue trauma and promote the development of ingrown nails. The nails should be cut or filed straight across.

57. a. This is done after the patient's immediate needs are met.

b. When rolling a debilitated patient off a bedpan the perianal area is exposed, which permits the nurse to provide immediate perineal hygiene. A bedridden, debilitated patient is incapable of providing self-hygiene after having a bowel movement on a bedpan.

c. This is not the priority after removing a debilitated patient from a bedpan.

d. The top linens should not have been removed during this procedure because they provide privacy and maintain dignity.

58. a. Bed rest does not cause dry hair. Malnutrition, aging, and excessive shampooing cause dry hair.

b. Bed rest does not cause oily hair. Infrequent shampooing causes oily hair.

c. Bed rest does not cause split hair. Excessive brushing, blow drying, and coloring cause split hair.

d. **Bed rest causes matted, tangled hair because of friction and pressure related to the movement of the head on a pillow.**

59. a. **This puts less stress on weak muscles; the stronger side can stretch more easily to dress.**

b. Although this is helpful, the nurse still needs to put the gown on without stressing the joints, tendons, muscles, and nerves of the weak arm.

c. This may be frustrating and tiring and could cause further damage to the weak arm.

d. This is unnecessary. The patient should be dressed appropriately.

60. a. Strong soap can further irritate the skin.

b. **Loose stool contains digestive fluids that are irritating to the skin and should be cleaned from the skin as soon as possible after soiling.**

c. This would not keep stool off the skin.

d. The patient is mentally impaired and is unaware of needs.

Mobility

The following words include English vocabulary, nursing/ medical terminology, concepts, principles, or information relevant to content specifically addressed in the chapter or associated with topics presented in it. English dictionaries, your nursing textbooks, and medical dictionaries such as *Taber's Cyclopedic Medical Dictionary* are resources that can be used to expand your knowledge and understanding of these words and related information.

Alignment
Ambulation
Anterior
Arthroscopy
Atrophy
Axillae
Balance
Base of support
Blanchable erythema
Body mechanics
Bones
Bony prominence
Cane
Cartilage
Contracture
Coordination
Dangle
Deep vein thrombosis
Dermis
Energy
Epidermis
Exercises
   Anaerobic
   Aerobic
   Isometric
   Isotonic
Flaccid
Foot drop
Fracture
Functional alignment
Gait
Gravity
Hemiparesis
Hemiplegia
Hip protector undergarment
Hoyer lift
Hydraulic lift
Ilium
Ischial tuberosities
Joints

Kyphosis
Lateral
Logrolling
Lordosis
Malleolus
Mechanical lift
Misalign
Mobility
Muscles
Occipital
Orthostatic hypotension
Osteoporosis
Paresis
Paraplegia
Pathological fracture
Physical conditioning
Pivot
Popliteal
Positioning devices
   Bed cradle
   Hand-wrist splint
   Hand roll
   Heel and elbow protectors
   Trapeze bar
   Trochanter roll
   Pillow
   Side rail
   Turning and pull sheet
Positions
   Contour
   Dorsal recumbent
   Fowler's (low-, semi-, high-)
   Knee-chest
   Lateral
   Lithotomy
   Orthopnea
   Prone
   Sims'
   Supine
   Trendelenburg

Posture
Pressure relief and reduction devices
   Duoderm
   Mattress overlay
     Air mattress
     Eggcrate mattress
     Dense foam and gel
   Cushions
     Air
     Gel
   Heel and elbow protectors
   Sheepskin
   Specialty beds
Pressure ulcer (Stage I, II, III, IV)
Proprioception
Protracted
Quadriplegia
Range of motion exercises
   Active
   Active-assistive
   Passive
Range of motion movements
   Abduction
   Adduction
   Circumduction
   Flexion
     Dorsal flexion
     Lateral flexion
     Plantar flexion
     Radial flexion
     Ulnar flexion
   Eversion
   Extension
   Hyperextension
   Inversion
   Opposition of thumb
   Pronation
   Rotation
     External
     Internal

<table>
<tr><td>Supination</td><td>Sacral</td><td>Superior</td></tr>
<tr><td>Reactive hyperemia</td><td>Scapulae</td><td>Synovium</td></tr>
<tr><td>Restraints</td><td>Sedentary</td><td>Tendons</td></tr>
<tr><td> Belt</td><td>Shearing force</td><td>Torque</td></tr>
<tr><td> Chest</td><td>Skin integrity</td><td>Transfer</td></tr>
<tr><td> Mitt</td><td>Sling</td><td>Transfer belt</td></tr>
<tr><td> Poncho</td><td>Spasticity</td><td>Turning and positioning</td></tr>
<tr><td> Vest</td><td>Stability</td><td>Venous pooling</td></tr>
<tr><td> Wrist</td><td>Strength</td><td>Zygomatic arch</td></tr>
</table>

QUESTIONS

1. Which nursing action is most dependent on the principle *The wider the base of support the greater the stability*?
   a. Carrying a heavy object
   b. Raising the side rails on a bed
   c. Repositioning a trochanter roll
   d. Transferring a patient from a bed to a chair

2. Which is a basic principle associated with transferring a patient from a bed to a chair using a mechanical lift?
   a. Hook the longer chains on the end of the sling closest to the patient's feet
   b. Ensure that there is a physician's order to use a mechanical lift
   c. Place a sheepskin inside the sling so that it is under the patient
   d. Lead with the patient's feet when exiting the bed

3. Which position should be avoided for a patient at the greatest risk for the development of pressure ulcers?
   a. Low-Fowler's
   b. Side-lying
   c. Supine
   d. Prone

4. Reactive hyperemia over a bony prominence occurs in response to:
   a. Applying a warm soak
   b. Turning a patient off an affected site
   c. Using an effleurage massage technique
   d. Pulling a patient up in bed without using a pull sheet

5. Which motion occurs when the angle is reduced between the palm of the hand and forearm?
   a. Hyperextension
   b. Opposition
   c. Abduction
   d. Flexion

6. Which is a local adaptation to immobility?
   a. Renal calculi
   b. Thrombophlebitis
   c. Muscle contractures
   d. Pathological fracture

7. Which is the greatest potential problem associated with the low-Fowler's position?
   a. Dorsiflexion contractures of the feet
   b. Pressure on the ischial tuberosities
   c. External rotation of the hips
   d. Adduction of the legs

8. What is the best thing the nurse can do to prevent plantar flexion when making the bed?
   a. Tuck in the top linens on just the sides of the bed
   b. Place a toe pleat in the top linens over the feet
   c. Let the top linens hang off the end of the bed
   d. Use trochanter rolls to position the feet

9. Which is a systemic adaptation to immobility?
   a. Plantar flexion contracture
   b. Hypostatic pneumonia
   c. Dependent edema
   d. Pressure ulcer

10. Which stage pressure ulcer would just have partial-thickness skin loss involving the epidermis and dermis?
    a. Stage I
    b. Stage II
    c. Stage III
    d. Stage IV

11. Which is the most important action when assisting a patient to move from the bed to a wheelchair?
    a. Applying pressure under the patient's axillae when standing up
    b. Letting the patient help as much as possible when permitted
    c. Keeping the patient's feet next to each other 1 foot apart
    d. Lowering the bed to below the height of the wheelchair

12. The orthopneic position is used primarily to:
    a. Facilitate respirations
    b. Support hip extension
    c. Prevent pressure ulcers
    d. Promote urinary elimination

13. When doing range-of-motion exercises, moving the thumb so it touches each finger is called:
    a. Flexion
    b. Inversion
    c. Abduction
    d. Opposition

14. An immobilized bedridden patient is placed on a 2-hour turning and positioning program primarily to:
    a. Support comfort
    b. Promote elimination
    c. Maintain skin integrity
    d. Facilitate respiratory function

15. Which is the most important action related to the use of antiembolism hose?
    a. Put them on after the patient's legs have been dependent for several minutes
    b. Monitor the heels for blanchable erythema every eight hours
    c. Apply body lotion before putting them on
    d. Remove and reapply them once a day

16. A major reason injuries occur to nurses when moving patients is because nurses:
    a. Use the longer, rather than the shorter, muscles when moving patients
    b. Place their feet close together when transferring patients
    c. Pull rather than push when turning patients
    d. Misalign their backs when moving patients

17. When positioning a patient on the left side, the nurse should position the:
    a. Right leg resting on top of the left leg
    b. Knees in 90 degrees of flexion
    c. Ankles in plantar flexion
    d. Left shoulder protracted

18. Which motion occurs when the ankle is turned so that the sole of the foot moves medially toward the midline?
    a. Inversion
    b. Adduction
    c. Plantar flexion
    d. Internal rotation

19. What should the nurse do to quickly assess a patient's tolerance to a change in position when transferring the patient from a bed to a wheelchair?
    a. Take the patient's blood pressure
    b. Monitor the patient for bradycardia
    c. Establish whether or not the patient feels dizzy
    d. Allow the patient time to adjust to the change in position

20. To best prevent pressure ulcers when a patient is on bed rest, the nurse should:
    a. Place an air mattress on the bed
    b. Massage bony prominences every shift
    c. Apply a moisture barrier to the sacral area
    d. Raise the head of the bed to the low-Fowler's position

21. Which is a basic principle associated with transferring a patient using a mechanical lift?
    a. Lock the base lever in the open position when moving the mechanical lift
    b. Keep the wheels of the mechanical lift locked throughout the transfer
    c. Ensure that the patient's feet are protected during the transfer
    d. Raise the lift so that the patient is 6 inches off the mattress

22. Which complication of immobility would be of most concern?
    a. Dehydration
    b. Incontinence
    c. Contractures
    d. Hypertension

23. Which stage pressure ulcer would require the nurse to measure the extent of undermining?
    a. Stage 0
    b. Stage I
    c. Stage II
    d. Stage III

24. Which intervention is unnecessary when assisting the patient with active range-of-motion exercises?
    a. Supporting above and below the joint being moved
    b. Positioning the patient in the supine position in bed
    c. Providing on-going encouragement and supervision
    d. Moving the joint through its full range at least three times

25. Which word is most closely associated with nursing care strategies to maintain functional alignment when patients are bedridden?
    a. Endurance
    b. Strength
    c. Support
    d. Balance

26. Which is a localized adaptation to immobility?
    a. Orthostatic hypotension
    b. Muscle atrophy
    c. Osteoporosis
    d. Atelectasis

27. How is the right arm positioned when using the left Sims' position?
    a. On a pillow
    b. Behind the back
    c. With the palm up
    d. In internal rotation

28. Which would be the best example of a discharge goal for a patient with a nursing diagnosis of Impaired Physical Mobility? The patient will:
   a. Understand range-of-motion exercises
   b. Transfer independently to a chair
   c. Be taught ROM exercises
   d. Be kept clean and dry

29. Which assessment reflects a defining characteristic that would support the nursing diagnosis Impaired Physical Mobility?
   a. Exertional fatigue
   b. Sedentary lifestyle
   c. Limited range of motion
   d. Increased respiratory rate

30. Which action is specifically related to the principle, *the greater the base of support, the more stable the body*?
   a. Keeping the back straight when lifting an object
   b. Holding objects close to the body when walking
   c. Locking the wheels of a wheelchair
   d. Using a walker when ambulating

31. Which motion occurs when in the supine position the ankle is bent so that the toes are pointed towards the ceiling?
   a. Supination
   b. Adduction
   c. Dorsal flexion
   d. Plantar extension

32. Which position would contribute most to the formation of a hip flexion contracture?
   a. Semi-Fowler's
   b. Orthopneic
   c. Supine
   d. Sims'

33. The presence of which adaptation is most important to assess before administering passive range-of-motion exercises?
   a. Weakness
   b. Flaccidity
   c. Atrophy
   d. Pain

34. Which medical treatment is specific for a patient with a stage IV pressure ulcer with eschar?
   a. Heat lamp treatment three times a day
   b. Application of a topical antibiotic
   c. Cleansing irrigations every shift
   d. Debridement of the wound

35. Which statement by the patient would indicate immobility-induced thrombophlebitis? "My lower left leg:
   a. Is tingling."
   b. Looks swollen."
   c. Has very dry skin."
   d. Feels cool when I touch it."

36. Raising the arm over the head during range-of-motion exercises is called:
   a. Flexion
   b. Abduction
   c. Supination
   d. Hyperextension

37. Which position places a patient at the greatest risk for pressure on the popliteal space?
    a. Prone
    b. Supine
    c. Contour
    d. Trendelenburg

38. Which new strategy has been demonstrated to reduce the incidence of fractured hips among institutionalized older adults?
    a. Placing bolsters on the sides of a patient's bed
    b. Dressing a patient with a hip protector undergarment
    c. Putting an alarm under a patient's wheelchair cushion
    d. Positioning mats on the floor alongside a patient's bed

39. When a patient with hemiparesis uses a cane, the nurse needs to teach the patient to:
    a. Advance up a step with the weak leg first followed by the strong leg and cane
    b. Adjust the cane height 12 inches lower than the waist
    c. Hold the cane in the strong hand when walking
    d. Look at the feet when walking

40. Logrolling when positioning a patient is most important when the patient has had:
    a. Spinal cord trauma
    b. Abdominal surgery
    c. A long leg cast applied
    d. Cerebral vascular accident

41. Which causes the MOST concern when a person is in the supine position?
    a. Increased cardiac workload
    b. Urinary tract infection
    c. Venous pooling
    d. Sacral pressure

42. Which health problem would place a patient at the greatest risk for complications associated with immobility?
    a. Quadriplegia
    b. Incontinence
    c. Hemiparesis
    d. Confusion

43. When an older adult is afraid of falling, the most common consequence is:
    a. Impaired skin integrity
    b. Occurrence of panic attacks
    c. Self-imposed social isolation
    d. Decreased physical conditioning

44. To best evaluate an ambulating patient's balance, the nurse should assess the patient's:
    a. Posture
    b. Strength
    c. Energy level
    d. Respiratory rate

45. Which safety measure is most important when using a mechanical lift to move a patient from a bed to a wheelchair?
    a. Hook the shorter chains on the sling closest to the patient's feet
    b. Cross the patient's arms across the chest throughout the transfer
    c. Center the sling under the patient from the shoulders to just above the knees
    d. Release the hydraulic valve on the lift swiftly while lowering the patient into a chair

46. Which is a potential problem associated with the supine position?
    a. Flexion of the knees
    b. Pressure on the heels
    c. Pressure on the trochanters
    d. Internal rotation of the hips

47. When lifting a patient, strain to the nurse can be reduced when the nurse:
    a. Moves the patient up against gravity
    b. Uses the large muscles of the legs
    c. Keeps the knees locked
    d. Bends from the waist

48. What should the nurse use to best limit perspiration on dependent skin surfaces of a patient on bed rest?
    a. Ventilated heel protectors
    b. Air-filled rings
    c. Air mattress
    d. Sheepskin

49. Which is the primary reason why immobilized people develop contractures?
    a. Muscles that flex, adduct, and internally rotate are stronger than weaker opposing muscles
    b. Muscle mass and strength decline at a rate of 5 to 10 percent per week
    c. Muscular contractures occur because of excessive muscle flaccidity
    d. Muscle catabolism exceeds muscle anabolism

50. Which action occurs when you turn the palm of the hand downward?
    a. External rotation
    b. Circumduction
    c. Lateral flexion
    d. Pronation

51. Which nursing action is most important after transferring a patient from a bed to a wheelchair?
    a. Ensure that the patient's popliteal areas are not touching the seat edge
    b. Attach the patient's transfer belt to clips on the wheelchair
    c. Place a pillow behind the patient's back
    d. Put the patient's feet flat on the floor

52. The cachectic patient is at highest risk for which skin integrity problem?
    a. Altered tissue perfusion
    b. Perineal excoriation
    c. Reduced sensation
    d. Pressure ulcers

53. Which action is most effective in relation to the concept *Immobility can lead to occlusion of blood vessels in areas where bony prominences rest on a mattress?*
    a. Encouraging the patient to deep breathe 10 times per hour
    b. Placing a sheepskin pad under the patient's sacrum
    c. Performing range-of-motion exercises twice a day
    d. Repositioning the patient every 2 hours

54. Which sites are at the greatest risk for skin breakdown when the patient is sitting in a wheelchair?
    a. Ischial tuberosities
    b. Bilateral scapulae
    c. Trochanters
    d. Malleoli

55. Which nursing action is most dependent on the principle *Moving an object requires less energy if it is not being moved against the force of gravity?*
    a. Flexing the knees and back before lifting something heavy
    b. Placing a patient in body alignment before being turned in bed
    c. Lowering the head of the bed before moving a patient up in bed
    d. Raising the height of the bed to waist level before changing the linens

56. Which describes the placement of a trochanter roll?
    a. Under the small of the back
    b. Behind the knees when supine
    c. Alongside the ilium to midthigh
    d. In the palm of the hand with the fingers flexed

57. Which site is at the greatest risk for skin breakdown when the patient is lying in a lateral position?
   a. Greater trochanter
   b. Ischial tuberosity
   c. Occipital
   d. Scapulae

58. Which would be the earliest assessment that would indicate permanent damage to tissues because of compression of soft tissue between a bony prominence and a mattress?
   a. Nonblanchable erythema
   b. Circumoral cyanosis
   c. Tissue necrosis
   d. Skin abrasion

59. When moving patients up in bed, strain to the nurse can be reduced when the nurse:
   a. Faces the side of the bed while using the arms to move the patient
   b. Keeps the body balanced over a wide base of support
   c. Holds the breath and tenses pelvic muscles
   d. Keeps the elbows and knees straight

60. Which nursing action is important after transferring a patient to a wheelchair?
   a. Applying a vest restraint with the ties attached to the lower frame behind the seat
   b. Supporting the body so that the hip and knees are at 90° angles
   c. Ensuring that the patient is in functional body alignment
   d. Placing the patient in the hall near the nurse's station

ANSWERS AND RATIONALES

1. a. This follows the principle *The closer an object is to the center of gravity the greater the stability and the easier the object is to move.*
   b. Side rails protect patients from falling out of bed and follow the principle *An object in motion stays in motion until it hits an opposing force.*
   c. Trochanter rolls placed lateral to the legs between the iliac crests and knees prevent external hip rotation when the patient is in the supine position. This follows the principle *An object in motion stays in motion until it hits an opposing force.*
   d. When transferring a patient from a bed to a chair both the nurse and patient should have their feet spread the width of their shoulders and with one foot in front of the other. Appropriate body mechanics prevents falls.

2. a. The longer chains go in the holes for the seat support, which keep the legs and pelvis below the upper body. Appropriate placement of the upper and lower chains creates a bucket seat in which a patient is moved safely.
   b. Moving patients with a hydraulic lift is within the scope of nursing practice and a practitioner's order is unnecessary.
   c. This could result in the patient's sliding down and out of the sling during the transfer. Nylon, net, or canvas slings are available.
   d. It does not matter whether the feet or the head exits the bed first as long as functional alignment and safety are maintained.

3. a. Although in the low-Fowler's position the sacral area is at the greatest risk for pressure, the muscles and adipose tissue in the buttocks do provide some protection compared to other vulnerable areas of the body.
   b. In the side-lying position, the majority of the body weight is borne by the greater trochanter. The bone is close to the surface of the skin, with minimal overlying protective tissue.
   c. Although in the supine position the occiput, scapulae, spine, elbows, sacrum, and heels are at risk for pressure, the body weight is distributed more evenly than in some other positions.
   d. Although in the prone position the ears, cheeks, acromion process, anterior superior spinous process, knees, toes, male genitalia, and female breasts are at risk for pressure, the body weight is distributed more evenly than in some other positions.

4. a. Heat causes vasodilation that increases circulation to the area and results in erythema, not reactive hyperemia.
   b. Compressed skin appears pale because circulation to the area is impaired. When pressure is relieved, the skin takes on a bright red flush as extra blood flows to the area to compensate for the period of impeded blood flow.
   c. Effleurage, light stroking of the skin, simulates the peripheral nerves and should not change skin coloration.

   d. This can cause a friction burn or shearing force that can injure blood vessels and tissues.

5. a. Hyperextension of the condyloid joint of the wrist is accomplished by bending the fingers and hand backwards as far as possible.
   b. Opposition of the thumb, which is a saddle joint, occurs when the thumb touches the top of each finger on the same hand.
   c. Abduction of the fingers (metacarpophalangeal joints—condyloid) occurs when the fingers of each hand spread apart.
   d. Flexion of the wrist, a condyloid joint, occurs when the fingers of the hand move toward the inner aspect of the forearm.

6. a. Demineralization of bone is a systemic response to immobility. Without the stress of weight-bearing activity, the bones begin to demineralize and the urine becomes more alkaline. Calcium salts precipitate out as crystals to form calculi.
   b. Thrombophlebitis results from the systemic responses of impaired venous return and hypercoagulability in conjunction with injury to a vessel wall.
   c. A contracture is a localized response to immobility. When muscle fibers are not able to shorten or lengthen, eventually a permanent shortening of the muscles and subsequently of the tendons and ligaments occurs.
   d. Immobility can cause the systemic response of demineralization of bone (disuse osteoporosis) that eventually can result in bone fractures.

7. a. Plantar flexion contractures (foot drop), not dorsiflexion contractures, can occur in the low-Fowler's position.
   b. In the low-Fowler's position, the majority of the body's weight is borne by portions of the pelvis: bony protuberances of the lower portion of the ischium (ischial tuberosities) and the triangular bone at the dorsal part of the pelvis (sacrum).
   c. This is more likely to occur in the supine, rather than the low-Fowler's, position.
   d. Abduction, rather than adduction, of the legs is more likely to occur in the low-Fowler's position.

8. a. Top sheets tucked in along the sides of the bed would still exert pressure on the upper surface of the feet, which may promote plantar flexion. The sides of top sheets, mitered at the foot of the bed, hang feely off the side of the bed.
   b. Making a vertical or horizontal toe pleat at the foot of the bed over the patient's feet leaves room for the feet to move freely and avoids exerting pressure on the upper surface of the feet, thus preventing plantar flexion.
   c. The weight of the top sheets would still exert pressure on the upper surface of the feet, promoting plantar flexion.
   d. Trochanter rolls prevent external hip rotation, not plantar flexion.

9. a. Plantar flexion contracture (foot drop) is a localized response of prolonged extension of the ankle.
   b. Static respiratory secretions provide an excellent media for bacterial growth that can result in hypostatic pneumonia, which is a localized response to immobility.
   c. **Decreased calf muscle activity and pressure of the bed on the legs allow blood to accumulate in the distal veins. The resulting increased hydrostatic pressure moves fluid out of the intravascular compartment into the interstitial compartment, causing edema.**
   d. Prolonged pressure on skin over a bony prominence interferes with capillary blood flow to the skin, which ultimately can result in the localized response of a pressure ulcer.

10. a. In a Stage I pressure ulcer the skin is still intact and presents clinically as reactive hyperemia.
    b. **In a Stage II pressure ulcer the partial-thickness skin loss presents clinically as an abrasion, blister, or shallow crater.**
    c. In a Stage III pressure ulcer there is full-thickness skin loss involving the subcutaneous tissue that may extent to the underlying fascia. The ulcer presents clinically as a deep crater with or without undermining.
    d. In a Stage IV pressure ulcer there is full-thickness skin loss with extensive destruction, tissue necrosis, or damage to muscle, bone or supporting structures.

11. a. This should be avoided because it can injure nerves and blood vessels.
    b. **Encouraging the patient to be as self-sufficient as possible ensures that the transfer is conducted at their pace, promotes self-esteem, and decreases the physical effort expended by the nurse.**
    c. This will provide a narrow base of support and is unsafe.
    d. The bed should be higher, not lower, than the wheelchair so that gravity can facilitate the transfer.

12. a. **Sitting in the high-Fowler's position and leaning forward allows the abdominal organs to drop by gravity, which will promote contraction of the diaphragm. The arms resting on an over-bed table increases thoracic excursion.**
    b. The hips will be in extreme flexion, not extension.
    c. Pressure ulcers can still occur on the ischial tuberosities.
    d. Ambulation is superior to any bed position for promoting urinary elimination.

13. a. Flexion of the metacarpophalangeal joints (condyloid joints) and the interphalangeal joints (hinge joints) occurs by making a fist, which decreases the angles of the joints.
    b. Inversion is turning the sole of a foot medially, which is not a range-of-motion of the hand.
    c. Abduction is moving an arm or a leg away from the midline of the body.
    d. **Opposition occurs when the thumb touches the top of each finger of the same hand.**

14. a. Although turning the patient to a new position every 2 hours provides variety and increased comfort, these are not the primary reasons for this intervention.

   b. Although turning frequently promotes elimination, the upright positions, such as high-Fowler's and sitting, have the greater influence on elimination.
   c. **Compression of soft tissue greater than 32 mmHg prevents capillary circulation and compromises tissue oxygenation in the compressed area. Turning the patient relieves the compression of tissue in dependent areas, particularly those tissues overlying bony prominences.**
   d. Although turning and positioning promotes respiratory functioning, other interventions, such as sitting, deep breathing, coughing, and incentive spirometry, have a greater influence on respiratory status.

15. a. This is unsafe because pressure injures fluid-filled tissue. They should be applied before, not after, the legs are dependent.
    b. **Elastic stockings provide external pressure on the patient's legs to prevent pooling of blood in the veins while not interfering with arterial circulation. Inspecting the skin 3 times a day is adequate.**
    c. When applying elastic stockings, lotion increases friction that can injure tissue. Baby powder can be applied to facilitate application.
    d. This is unsafe. Elastic stockings should be removed for 30 minutes 3 times a day.

16. a. Nurses should use the longer, stronger muscles of the thighs and buttocks when moving patients to protect their weaker back and arm muscles.
    b. Nurses should have a wide base of support when moving patients, to provide better stability.
    c. Nurses should use a pulling motion to turn patients because the muscles that flex, rather than extend, the arm are stronger and pulling, rather than pushing, creates less friction and therefore less effort.
    d. **Misaligning the back when moving patients occurs most often when not facing the direction of the move. Twisting (rotation) of the thoracolumbar spine and flexion of the back place the line of gravity outside the base of support, which can cause muscle strain and disabling injuries.**

17. a. The right leg should be supported on a pillow in front of the left leg.
    b. This excessive flexion can result in flexion contractures of the hip and knee if left in this position extensively.
    c. The ankles should be maintained at 90 degrees.
    d. **In the left lateral (side-lying) position, the left arm is positioned in front of the body with the shoulder protracted. This reduces the pressure on the joint in the shoulder and the acromial process.**

18. a. Inversion, a gliding movement of the foot, occurs by turning the sole of the foot medially toward the midline of the body.
    b. Adduction occurs when an arm or leg moves toward and beyond the midline of the body.
    c. Plantar flexion occurs when the joint of the ankle is in extension by pointing the toes of the foot

downward and away from the anterior portion of the lower leg.

   d. Internal rotation of a leg occurs by turning the foot and leg inward so that the toes point toward the other leg.

19. a. Although a blood pressure reading may indicate the presence of hypotension, the blood pressure should be obtained before and after a transfer to allow a comparison to conclude that the hypotension is orthostatic hypotension.

   b. If the patient is experiencing orthostatic hypotension, the heart rate will increase, not decrease.

   c. Feeling dizzy is a subjective adaptation to orthostatic hypotension. Obtaining feedback from the patient provides a quick evaluation of the patient's response to the transfer.

   d. This is not an assessment. This is a safe intervention for a patient who is experiencing orthostatic hypotension.

20. **a. Air mattresses automatically and rhythmically inflate and deflate, which applies and relieves pressure on various body areas. Capillary beds close at between 12–32 mmHg (capillary closing pressure). Any device that reduces pressure below capillary closing pressure is considered a pressure relief device. Any device that does not consistently reduce pressure below capillary closing pressure is considered a pressure reducing device.**

   b. A bedridden patient is at risk for skin breakdown, and therefore 3 back rubs a day are inadequate.

   c. Moisture barriers prevent skin breakdown when a patient is incontinent of urine or feces; they do not prevent pressure on the skin.

   d. This increases the risk of the patient's sliding down in bed, which may cause shearing force that can injure tissue. In addition, this position increases pressure on the vulnerable sacral area.

21. a. The width of the base depends on the configuration of the bed, objects in the room, and the ultimate destination. The base usually is locked open when lifting or lowering the patient and locked closed when moving the lift.

   b. The wheels must be unlocked to move the lift from under the bed to its ultimate destination.

   c. The legs dangle from the sling and therefore may drag across the linens or hit other objects if not protected.

   d. This is unsafe. The lift should raise the patient high enough to clear the surface of the bed.

22. a. Dehydration is not an adaptation to immobility.

   b. The decreased tone of the urinary bladder and the inability to assume the normal voiding position in bed promotes urinary retention, rather than urinary incontinence.

   c. Contractures result from permanent shortening of muscles, tendons, and ligaments. Contractures are irreversible without surgical intervention.

   d. With immobility, the increased heart rate reduces the diastolic pressure. In addition, there is a decrease in blood pressure related to postural changes from lying to sitting or standing (orthostatic hypotension). This

situation is manageable with a priority on maintaining patient safety.

23. a. There is no Stage 0 in the classification system for staging pressure ulcers.

   b. The skin is still intact and there is no undermining in a Stage I pressure ulcer.

   c. Tissue damage is superficial and there is no undermining in a Stage II pressure ulcer.

   d. In a Stage III pressure ulcer there is full-thickness skin loss involving damage to subcutaneous tissue that may extend to the fascia and there may or may not be undermining, which is tissue destruction underneath intact skin along wound margins.

24. a. Stabilization of body parts ensures that only the joint moves through its full range of motion.

   b. The supine position is more appropriate for performing passive range-of-motion exercises. Active range-of-motion exercises can be performed in any comfortable position.

   c. This promotes motivation and correct completion of the procedure.

   d. Subsequent contraction of muscles tends to be more extensive and efficient, facilitating fuller range of motion.

25. a. Endurance relates to aerobic exercise that improves the body's capacity to consume oxygen for producing energy at the cellular level.

   b. Strength relates to isometric and isotonic exercises, which contract muscles and promote their development.

   c. The line of gravity passes through the center of gravity when the body is correctly aligned; this results in the least amount of stress on the muscles, joints, and soft tissues. Bedridden patients often need assistive devices such as pillows, sandbags, bed cradles, wedges, rolls, and splints to support and maintain the vertebral column and extremities in functional alignment.

   d. Balance relates to body mechanics, and is achieved through a wide base of support and a lowered center of gravity.

26. a. A systemic response to immobility is a decrease in blood pressure related to postural changes from lying to sitting or standing (orthostatic hypotension).

   b. After 24 to 36 hours of inactivity, all the muscles begin to lose their contractile strength, the initial process of atrophy, which is a systemic response to immobility.

   c. Osteoporosis, a systemic response to immobility, is demineralization of bone because of the lack of weight-bearing activity.

   d. The pooling of respiratory secretions that block the bronchioles and the decreased production of surfactant associated with immobility cause the localized effect of atelectasis (collapse of all or part of a lung).

27. **a. In the left Sims' position the patient's right arm and leg are supported on pillows to prevent internal rotation of the shoulder and hip.**

   b. The right arm is positioned in front of, not behind, the back.

c. The right hand is positioned in pronation, not supination.

d. The right arm is positioned to maintain the shoulder in external, not internal, rotation.

28. a. This goal is not measurable as stated. Understanding is not measurable unless parameters are identified.
 b. This goal is patient-centered and measurable.
 c. This is a nursing intervention, not a patient goal.
 d. This is a nursing goal, not a patient goal.

29. a. This is a defining characteristic of the nursing diagnosis Activity Intolerance.
 b. This is a contributing factor for the nursing diagnosis Activity Intolerance.
 c. Limited range of motion is a defining characteristic of the nursing diagnosis Impaired Physical Mobility.
 d. An increased respiratory rate would be an adaptation to activity, not a defining characteristic of the nursing diagnosis Impaired Physical Mobility.

30. a. This follows the principle *Balance is maintained and muscle strain is limited as long as the line of gravity passes through the base of support.*
 b. This follows the principle *The closer an object is held to the center of gravity the greater the stability and the easier the object is to move.*
 c. This follows the principle *An object with wheels that are locked will remain stationary.*
 d. Walkers surround a person on three sides and provide 4 points of contact with the floor. This wide base provides the best support available for assisted ambulation.

31. a. Supination occurs when the hand and forearm rotate so that the palm of the hand is facing upward.
 b. Adduction occurs when an arm or leg moves toward and/or beyond the midline of the body.
 c. Dorsal flexion (dorsiflexion) of the joint of the ankle occurs when the toes of the foot point upward and backward toward the anterior portion of the lower leg.
 d. There is no range of motion called plantar extension. Plantar flexion occurs when the joint of the ankle is in extension by pointing the toes of the foot downward and away from the anterior portion of the lower leg.

32. a. In the semi-Fowler's position the hips are slightly flexed (135 to 165 degrees).
 b. While in the high-Fowler's position the patient is then positioned leaning forward with arms resting on an over-bed table. In the orthopneic position, the hips are extensively flexed at the hips creating an angle less than 90 degrees.
 c. In the supine position, the hips are extended (180 degrees), not flexed.
 d. In the Sims' position, the hip and knee of the upper leg are just slightly flexed.

33. a. Although the extent of weakness should be assessed, it is not the priority.
 b. Although the presence of flaccidity should be assessed, it is not the priority.
 c. Although the degree of atrophy should be assessed, it is not the priority.

d. If the patient is experiencing pain, there will be reluctance to move. An analgesic administered before beginning these exercises will promote acceptance and tolerance of the exercises.

34. a. Heat lamp treatments should not be used because they can cause burns.
 b. Topical antibiotics are used only when the ulcer is infected, not to treat eschar.
 c. Cleansing irrigations are ineffective in removing the thick, fibrin-containing cells of eschar covering the surface of a wound.
 d. Thick, leather-like, necrotic devitalized tissue (eschar) must be removed surgically or enzymatically before wound healing can occur.

35. a. The patient would feel discomfort or pain, not tingling, with thrombophlebitis.
 b. A slowed blood flow and increased viscosity of the blood allow platelets and calcium to settle out against the intimal lining of a vein, which can result in thrombus formation. The inflammatory process causes calf edema, pain, heat, and erythema.
 c. The skin would appear taut and shiny, not dry, with thrombophlebitis.
 d. The area would feel warm, not cool, to the touch with thrombophlebitis.

36. a. The shoulder, a ball-and-socket joint, flexes by raising the arm from a position by the side of the body forward and upward to a position beside the head.
 b. Abduction of the shoulder occurs by moving the arm laterally from a resting position at the side of the body to a side position above the head, with the palm of the hand held facing away from the head.
 c. Supination occurs when the hand and forearm rotate so that the palm of the hand is facing upward.
 d. Hyperextension of the arm occurs by moving an arm from a resting position at the side of the body to a position behind the body.

37. a. In the prone position, there is pressure in front of, not behind, the knees.
 b. In the supine position, the hips and legs are extended, which does not exert pressure on the popliteal space.
 c. In the contour position, the head of the bed and the knee gatch are slightly elevated. The elevated knee gatch puts pressure on the popliteal spaces.
 d. In the Trendelenburg position, the hips and knees are extended, which does not exert pressure on the popliteal space.

38. a. Bolsters prevent arms and legs from becoming entangled in bed rails.
 b. If a padded undergarment is worn when a fall occurs, the padding provides protection for the bony prominences of the pelvis and femurs.
 c. Although this has reduced accidents, not all patients at risk for falls need wheelchairs. The majority of patients who fracture their hips are ambulatory.
 d. Rugs or mats on the floor increase the risk of falls and injury.

39. a. The unaffected leg should be advanced first because

the weight of the body is lifted to the next step on the leg with the greatest strength.

   b. With the tip of the cane placed 6 inches lateral to the foot, the handle should be at the level of the patient's greater trochanter to ensure that the elbow will be flexed 15 to 30 degrees when using the cane.

   c. A cane is a hand-gripped assistive device; therefore, the hand opposite to the hemiparesis should hold the cane. Exercises can strengthen the flexor and extensor muscles of the arms and the muscles that dorsiflex the wrist.

   d. This will cause flexion of the neck, hips or waist that will move the center of gravity outside the line of gravity. Proper body alignment (posture) is essential for balance, stability, and safe ambulation.

40. a. Logrolling turns a patient while keeping the vertebral column, including the head and neck, in straight alignment to prevent twisting (rotation) that can injure the spinal cord.

   b. Pressure of a pillow or the hands held against the abdomen supports an abdominal surgical incision, not logrolling.

   c. This patient does not need to be logrolled. The entire leg from hip to ankle should be supported when turning a patient with a long leg cast.

   d. This patient does not need to be logrolled. The side of the body with hemiparesis or hemiplegia must be supported.

41. a. The supine position increases venous return because the blood does not flow against gravity to return to the heart. An increased venous return increases the workload on the heart by 30 percent, which places the patient at risk for heart failure.

   b. Although prolonged immobility in the supine position can cause urinary stasis that increases the risk for urinary tract infections, it is not the greatest concern.

   c. Venous pooling occurs when the legs are dependent, not when they are level with the heart as they are in the supine position.

   d. Although the supine position causes sacral pressure, it is not the greatest concern.

42. a. Quadriplegia, paralysis of all four extremities, places the patient at greatest risk for pressure ulcers because the patient has no ability to shift the body weight off of bony prominences or change position without total assistance.

   b. Bladder and bowel retraining, incontinence devices, and meticulous skin care limit the potential for skin breakdown when patients are incontinent.

   c. Hemiparesis, muscle weakness on one side of the body, does not prevent a person from shifting or changing position to relieve pressure on the skin.

   d. Confused patients can move independently when uncomfortable or when encouraged and assisted to move by the nurse.

43. a. A person who chooses not to ambulate still has the ability to assume many different sitting or lying-down positions.

   b. Anxiety and ultimately panic that is precipitated by a situation can be prevented by avoiding the situation.

   c. A person who chooses not to ambulate still can socialize.

   d. Most falls occur when ambulating. Fear of falling results in the conscious choice not to place oneself in a position where a fall can occur. Disuse and muscle wasting cause a reduction of muscle strength at the rate of 5 to 10 percent per week so that within 2 months of immobility over 50 percent of a muscle's strength can be lost. In addition, there is a decreased cardiac reserve. These adaptations result in decreased physical conditioning.

44. a. Assessing posture will identify whether the patient's center of gravity is in the midline from the middle of the forehead to a midpoint between the feet and, therefore, balanced within the patient's base of support.

   b. Strength has more to do with the exertion of power, not balance.

   c. Energy has more to do with endurance, not balance.

   d. Assessing respiratory rate establishes a baseline against which to compare respiratory rate after activity to determine tolerance, not balance.

45. a. This will place the lower part of the body level to or above the lower body, which is an unsafe, unstable position because the body is not balanced with the center of gravity in the "seat" of the sling. The shorter chains go in the holes closest to the head, not the feet.

   b. The patient can either cross the arms on the chest or grasp the shorter chains during the transfer.

   c. Centering the sling ensures full support between the shoulders and the knees and with the correct placement of the chains places the center of gravity in the "seat" of the sling. Centering the sling just above the knees prevents pressure on the popliteal space and prevents extension of the lower legs, which would alter the center of gravity and be unsafe.

   d. The hydraulic valve should be opened slowly, not swiftly, because sling movement can be frightening and sudden movement can unbalance the lift.

46. a. The knees are extended, not flexed, when in the supine position.

   b. The supine position is a back-lying position that results in pressure on the heels (calcaneus), which have minimal tissue between the bone and skin, making them vulnerable to the development of pressure ulcers.

   c. There is no pressure on either greater trochanter when in the supine position. Pressure on the greater trochanter occurs when the patient is in a lateral (side-lying) position.

   d. External rotation, not internal rotation, of the hips tends to occur when a patient is in the supine position.

47. a. Muscle strain is reduced when moving patients with gravity, not with the added effort needed to move patients against gravity.

   b. The gluteal and leg muscles should be used rather than the sacrospinal muscles of the back to exert an upward lift. These larger muscles fatigue less quickly, and their use protects the intervertebral disks.

  c. The muscles of the legs are used inefficiently when the knees are kept locked. This increases the strain on the other muscles being used.

  d. Bending from the waist increases the strain on the sacrospinal muscles and intervertebral disks.

48. a. These protect only the heels, not the other dependent areas of the body.

  b. Air-filled rings usually are made of plastic that tends to promote sweating. Air rings are rarely used because they are designed for just the sacral area and often they increase, not decrease, pressure.

  c. Air mattresses usually are made of plastic, which tends to promote sweating.

  d. **The soft tuffs of sheepskin allow air to circulate, thereby promoting the evaporation of moisture that can precipitate skin breakdown.**

49. **a.** **The state of balance between muscles that serve to contract in opposite directions is impaired with immobility. The fibers of the stronger muscles contract for longer periods than do those of the weaker, opposing muscles. This results in a change in the loose connective tissue to a more dense connective tissue and to fibrotic changes that limit range of motion.**

  b. Disuse and muscle wasting cause a reduction in muscle strength at the rate of 5 to 10 percent a week so that within 2 months over 50 percent of a muscle's strength can be lost.

  c. Contractures occur because of muscle spasticity and shortening, not muscle flaccidity.

  d. This is unrelated to contractures. In unused muscles, catabolism exceeds anabolism, and the muscles decrease in size (disuse atrophy).

50. a. External rotation of the shoulder, a ball-and-socket joint, occurs when the upper arm is held parallel to the floor, the elbow is at a 90-degree angle, and the fingers are pointing toward the floor and the person moves the arm upward so that the fingers point toward the ceiling.

  b. Circumduction of the shoulder, a ball-and-socket joint, occurs when an extended arm moves forward, up, back, and down in a full circle.

  c. Lateral flexion of the hand occurs with both abduction (radial flexion) and adduction (ulnar flexion). With the hand supinated, radial flexion occurs by bending the wrist laterally toward the thumb and ulnar flexion occurs by bending the wrist laterally toward the fifth finger.

  d. **Pronation of the hand occurs by rotating the hand and arm so that the palm of the hand is facing down toward the floor.**

51. **a.** **Pressure on the popliteal areas can cause damage to nerves and interfere with circulation and must be avoided.**

  b. Transfer belts should be removed once the patient is transferred.

  c. This would move the patient too close to the front of the seat and would be unsafe.

  d. The patient's feet should be positioned flat on the foot rests of the wheelchair, not the floor, to protect the feet if the wheelchair is moved.

52. a. This is associated with cardiovascular problems.

  b. This is associated with bowel and/or urinary incontinence.

  c. This is associated with the older adult and people with peripheral neuropathy or neurologic diseases.

  d. **Cachexia involves weight loss, muscle atrophy, and decreased subcutaneous tissue, which results in a reduction in the padding between skin and bones, thus increasing the risk of pressure ulcer development.**

53. a. Deep breathing prevents atelectasis and hypostatic pneumonia, not pressure ulcers.

  b. Although sheepskin reduces friction and limits pressure, its main purpose is to allow air to circulate under the patient in order to minimize moisture and maceration of skin.

  c. Range-of-motion exercises help prevent contractures, not pressure ulcers.

  d. **Turning a patient relieves pressure on the capillary beds of the dependent areas of the body, particularly the skin overlying bony prominences, which re-establishes blood flow to the area.**

54. **a.** **When in the sitting position the hips and knees are flexed at 90 degrees and the body's weight is borne by the pelvis, particularly the ischial tuberosities, which are bony protuberances of the lower portion of the ischium. Using a wheel chair results in prolonged sitting unless interventions are used to promote local circulation.**

  b. Pressure to the scapulae occurs in all back-lying positions, such as the supine and Fowler's positions.

  c. Pressure to a trochanter occurs in a side-lying, not the sitting, position.

  d. Pressure to the malleolus (medial and lateral) of the ankle occurs in a side-lying, not a sitting, position.

55. a. The knees can be flexed, but the back should be held in straight alignment to prevent twisting of the spine or straining the muscles in the lower back.

  b. Placing the patient in functional alignment before being turned limits stress or strain on the musculoskeletal system.

  c. **Moving an object along a level surface requires less energy than moving an object up an inclined surface against the force of gravity.**

  d. This follows the principle *Tasks performed close to the center of gravity require less effort.*

56. a. This is unsafe. A trochanter roll placed in the small of the back would be uncomfortable and produce an excessive lumbar curvature.

  b. This is contraindicated because it places unnecessary pressure on the popliteal area.

  c. **A trochanter roll is a rolled wedge, pillow, or sandbag placed by the lateral aspect of the leg between the iliac crest and knees to prevent external hip rotation.**

  d. The diameter of a trochanter roll would be too wide to maintain the hand in functional alignment.

57. a. In the lateral (side-lying) position, the majority of the body's weight is on the greater trochanter of the femur as well as the lateral aspect of the lower scapula and the lateral aspect of the ilium.
    b. The ischial tuberosity, a rounded protuberance of the lower part of the ischium, is at the greatest risk for skin breakdown when the patient is sitting in a chair or lying in a high-Fowler's position.
    c. The occipital area of the head is at the greatest risk for skin breakdown when the patient is lying in the supine position.
    d. The scapulae are at the greatest risk for skin breakdown when the patient is lying in the supine position.

58. a. **Nonblanchable erythema refers to erythema of intact skin that persists when finger pressure is applied. This is the heralding lesion of a Stage I pressure ulcer.**
    b. Circumoral cyanosis is associated with hypoxia, not pressure ulcers.
    c. With necrosis death of cells has occurred. This is a Stage IV, not Stage I, pressure ulcer.
    d. With an abrasion, the superficial layers of the skin are scraped away. This Stage II, not Stage I, pressure ulcer appears reddened and there may be localized serous weeping or bleeding.

59. a. The nurse should face the direction the patient is to be moved to prevent twisting that will move the line of gravity outside of the base of support. In addition, to prevent muscle strain the strong powerful gluteal and leg muscles should be used rather than the muscles of the arms and back.
    b. **When moving a patient the nurse should widen the stance and flex the knees, hip, and ankles. The wide base of support and the lowered center of gravity decrease strain on the nurse.**
    c. Holding the breath (Valsalva maneuver) increases the cardiac workload and decreases coronary artery perfusion and should not be employed when moving patients. The nurse should be exhaling when moving patients. The tensing of the abdominal and gluteal muscles sets the *internal girdle* that protects the intervertebral disks from injury.
    d. The elbows and knees should be slightly flexed, not extended, when moving patients.

60. a. Vest restraints are needed only when a patient's safety is at risk and if there is a physician's order.
    b. The knees do not have to be at 90 degrees. Depending on the needs of the patient, the knees may be supported in the extended position on the wheelchair leg rests.
    c. **After transfer, it is most important that the patient be supported in functional alignment to avoid any strain on neuromusculoskeletal structures of the body.**
    d. This may be necessary only if the patient is confused and needs to be monitored for safety.

Nutrition

KEYWORDS

The following words include English vocabulary, nursing/medical terminology, concepts, principles, or information relevant to content specifically addressed in the chapter or associated with topics presented in it. English dictionaries, your nursing textbooks, and medical dictionaries such as *Taber's Cyclopedic Medical Dictionary* are resources that can be used to expand your knowledge and understanding of these words and related information.

Alcohol abuse
Amino acids
   Essential
   Nonessential
Anabolism
Anorexia
Anorexia nervosa
Anthropometric
   measurements
Atherosclerosis
Basal metabolism
Bolus
Cachectic
Calorie
Calorie count
Catabolism
Cholesterol
Cirrhosis of the liver
Creatinine excretion
Dairy foods
Decaffeinated
Dental carries
Diabetes mellitus
Digestion
Dysphagia
Emulsify
Energy
Enteral
Fiber
Fluoride
Food consistency
   Chopped
   Pureed
   Regular
   Soft
   Liquid
Food Guide Pyramid
Fortified
Gastro-esophageal reflux
   disease (GERD)

Hemoglobin
Hyperglycemia
Ideal body weight
Ingestion
Insoluble fiber
Iron deficiency
Ketones
Ketosis
Kilocalories
Lactulose intolerant
Legumes
Lipids
Malnutrition
Mastication
Metabolic
Morbid obesity
Mottling of teeth
Nausea
Nutrients
   Carbohydrates
   Fats
   Minerals
     Fluoride
     Iodine
     Iron
     Potassium
     Sodium
   Protein
     Incomplete
     Complete
   Water
Obesity
Overweight
Passover
Recommended dietary
   allowances
Serum albumin
Soluble fiber
Stomatitis
Supplements

Swallowing impairment
Synthesis
Tetany
Therapeutic diets
   Clear liquid
   Full liquid
   2 gm sodium
   1200 ADA
   Low residue
   Mechanical soft
Total cholesterol
Transferrin level
Triglycerides
Tube feedings
   Continuous
   Enteral
   Gastrostomy
   Intermittent
   Jejunostomy
   Nasogastric
Underweight
Vegan
Vitamins
   Fat soluble (A, D, E, K)
   Water soluble
     C (ascorbic acid)
     B_1 (thiamine)
     B_2 (riboflavin)
     B_3 (niacin)
     B_6 (pyridoxine)
     B_{12} (cobalamin)
     Biotin
     Folic Acid
     Pantothenic acid
Vomiting
Water soluble fiber

QUESTIONS

1. If you eat 60 gm of fat and a total of 2000 kilocalories, what proportion of your kilocalories would come from fat?
   a. 27%
   b. 20%
   c. 42%
   d. 35%

2. Which food is not permitted on a clear liquid diet?
   a. Strawberry Jell-O
   b. Decaffeinated tea
   c. Strong coffee
   d. Ice cream

3. The best source of fiber is:
   a. White bread
   b. Green beans
   c. Peanut butter
   d. Orange marmalade

4. Over time what happens when the energy expended is greater than the caloric intake?
   a. Fever
   b. Anorexia
   c. Malnutrition
   d. Hypertension

5. Which is an excellent source of vitamin A?
   a. Grapefruits
   b. Tangerines
   c. Bananas
   d. Apricots

6. The best source of protein is:
   a. Milk
   b. Meat
   c. Bread
   d. Vegetables

7. Which dietary source would provide a patient with vitamin D?
   a. Green leafy vegetables
   b. Vegetable oils
   c. Fortified milk
   d. Organ meats

8. Four grams of carbohydrates, 3 grams of protein, and 5 grams of fat furnish how many kilocalories?
   a. 73
   b. 83
   c. 48
   d. 88

9. The laboratory finding that is the best indicator of inadequate protein intake is a:
   a. High hemoglobin
   b. Low serum albumin
   c. Low specific gravity
   d. High blood urea nitrogen

10. A food low in fat that would generally be most desirable to members of an Asian population would be:
    a. Egg rolls
    b. Spareribs
    c. Crispy noodles
    d. Hot and sour soup

11. Which is a source of vitamin C?
    a. Potatoes
    b. Yogurt
    c. Beans
    d. Milk

12. The best source of fiber is:
    a. Apples
    b. Cherries
    c. Apricots
    d. Pineapples

13. Carbohydrates are best known for providing:
    a. Electrolytes
    b. Vitamins
    c. Minerals
    d. Energy

14. What should the nurse do to assist a patient with meals who has dressings over both eyes?
    a. Feed the patient until the dressings are removed
    b. Order finger foods that are permitted on the patient's diet
    c. Encourage eating one food at a time according to the preference of the patient
    d. Explain to the patient where items are located according to the hours of a clock

15. Protein foods are used primarily by the body for:
    a. Energy
    b. Growth
    c. Excretion
    d. Catabolism

16. Which is unrelated to calcium balance?
    a. Osteoporosis
    b. Vitamin D
    c. Tetany
    d. Iron

17. Five grams of protein furnish how many kilocalories?
    a. 20
    b. 15
    c. 60
    d. 45

18. Patients with problems with liver function will have difficulty:
    a. Emulsifying fats
    b. Digesting carbohydrates
    c. Manufacturing red blood cells
    d. Reabsorbing water in the intestines

19. Excessive alcohol intake directly contributes to health problems because it:
    a. Lengthens the passage time of stool through the intestinal tract
    b. Decreases the absorption of many important nutrients
    c. Accelerates the absorption of medications
    d. Interferes with the absorption of glucose

20. A resident of a nursing home who is on a 1200-calorie weight reduction diet has not lost weight in the past month. The nurse should:
    a. Inform the primary care physician of the patient's lack of progress
    b. Instruct the patient to limit intake to 1000 calories per day
    c. Schedule a multidisciplinary team conference
    d. Keep a log of the oral intake for 3 days

21. A food low in fat that would generally be most desirable to the Latino population would be:
    a. Salsa
    b. Pasta
    c. Steamed fish
    d. Refried beans

22. Which is an excellent source of vitamin A?
    a. Blueberry pie
    b. Pumpkin pie
    c. Cherry pie
    d. Pecan pie

23. Which is the best nursing diagnosis for a patient who is anorexic because of stomatitis related to chemotherapy?
    a. Constipation
    b. Risk for Aspiration
    c. Deficient Fluid Volume
    d. Imbalanced Nutrition Less Than Body Requirements

24. How many kilocalories are contained in a 12 gram carbohydrate, 20 gram protein, and 8 gram fat meal?
    a. 160
    b. 152
    c. 360
    d. 200

25. Which vitamin would be most commonly associated with weak bones?
    a. D
    b. K
    c. B
    d. E

26. Which food is the best source of iron?
    a. Eggs
    b. Fruit
    c. Meat
    d. Bread

27. What should the nurse do to encourage the dietary intake of a patient who is eating only 25% of meals?
    a. Suggest that the patient drink between-meal supplements twice a daily
    b. Encourage the patient to engage in light exercise before meals
    c. Teach the patient to avoid fluids and foods that cause flatus
    d. Help the patient with the selection of foods that are liked

28. Which food is permitted on a low-residue diet?
    a. Scrambled eggs
    b. Orange juice
    c. Green beans
    d. Rye bread

29. Which diet would the nurse expect the physician to order for a patient with little or no teeth?
    a. Liquid supplements
    b. Mechanical soft
    c. Pureed
    d. Soft

30. The best source of vitamin C is:
    a. Sunflower seeds
    b. Green peppers
    c. Black beans
    d. Beef liver

31. The food that is the most desirable for a patient on a low-fat diet is:
    a. Eggs
    b. Liver
    c. Cheese
    d. Chicken

32. Which would indicate the greatest need for a gastrostomy feeding tube?
    a. Malabsorption syndrome
    b. Difficulty swallowing
    c. Nausea and vomiting
    d. Stomatitis

33. How many kilocalories are contained in a 12-gram carbohydrate snack?
    a. 48
    b. 96
    c. 72
    d. 118

34. Which is the best source of iodine?
    a. Grapefruit
    b. Salmon
    c. Grains
    d. Beans

35. An excellent food to give to the patient who is confused and disoriented is chicken:
    a. Soup
    b. Salad
    c. Fingers
    d. Casserole

36. When caring for a patient who is practicing Orthodox Judaism, the nurse must remember that:
    a. Coffee and tea are restricted during Passover
    b. Dairy products and eggs are forbidden after sundown on Fridays
    c. Shellfish is permitted but must be prepared according to biblical religious rituals
    d. Dairy foods should not be ingested at the same meal as meats and meat products

37. Which food is a complete protein?
    a. Rye bread
    b. Baked beans
    c. Ground beef
    d. Winter squash

38. What nutrient should the patient be encouraged to eat to facilitate normal blood clotting?
    a. Fish oils
    b. Enriched grains
    c. Green leafy vegetables
    d. Fortified milk products

39. A food that should be avoided when a person has high cholesterol is:
    a. Skim milk
    b. Egg yolks
    c. Turkey burger
    d. Sliced bologna

40. Which is the best behavior modification strategy for controlling food intake?
    a. Asking family members not to bring tempting food into the house
    b. Posting piggy pictures on the refrigerator
    c. Maintaining a daily food intake diary
    d. Avoiding between-meal snacks

41. Two grams of fat furnish how many kilocalories?
    a. 4
    b. 9
    c. 12
    d. 18

42. What nutrient must be ingested for vitamin K to be absorbed?
    a. Carbohydrates
    b. Starches
    c. Proteins
    d. Fats

43. To help prevent atherosclerosis the nurse should encourage the patient to:
    a. Avoid legumes
    b. Drink plenty of fluid
    c. Eat foods rich in soluble fiber
    d. Limit red meat intake to 6 ounces per day

44. Which statement about vitamins is based on a scientific principle?
    a. Eating a variety of foods prevents the need for supplements
    b. Megadoses of vitamins have proven to be most effective in preventing illness
    c. Taking a prescribed vitamin supplement is the best way to ensure adequate intake
    d. Vitamins from more expensive manufacturers are more pure than those from cheaper companies

45. Which situation results in ketosis in a normal person?
    a. Inadequate intake of carbohydrates
    b. Increased intake of protein
    c. Excessive intake of starch
    d. Decreased intake of fiber

46. Which combination is a substitute for a complete protein for a person who is a vegan?
    a. Yogurt and fruit
    b. Bread and cheese
    c. Legumes and rice
    d. Peanut butter and jelly

47. Fat in the diet is unnecessary to absorb:
    a. Vitamin C
    b. Vitamin A
    c. Vitamin E
    d. Vitamin D

48. Which contributing factor most commonly is the cause of obesity?
    a. Sedentary lifestyle
    b. Low metabolic rate
    c. Impaired hormone function
    d. Greater caloric intake than energy expended

49. Which food would best facilitate bone growth?
    a. Orange juice
    b. Peanut butter
    c. Cottage cheese
    d. Baked flounder

50. Which is the best short-term indicator of an improved nutritional status?
    a. Weight gain of 1.5 pounds daily
    b. Increasing transferrin level
    c. Decreasing serum albumin
    d. Appropriate skin turgor

51. How many calories per day would need to be eliminated from the diet to lose 3 pounds in 4 weeks?
    a. 450
    b. 575
    c. 300
    d. 375

52. Which is the major cause of iron deficiency?
    a. Metabolic problems
    b. Inadequate diet
    c. Malabsorption
    d. Hemorrhage

53. Which would best reflect a healthy behavior?
    a. Eating foods low in fat
    b. Wanting to lose 20 pounds
    c. Visiting a physician when ill
    d. Displaying no signs of illness

54. Which adaptation is a common result of fluoride deficiency?
    a. Stomatitis
    b. Dental carries
    c. Bleeding gums
    d. Mottling of the teeth

55. The nurse recognizes that a vegetarian understands the importance of eating kidney beans when the patient says, "Kidney beans are a great source of:
   a. Carbohydrates."
   b. Minerals."
   c. Protein."
   d. Fats."

56. Which is an excellent source of vitamin A?
   a. Sweet potatoes
   b. Red tomatoes
   c. Green beans
   d. Egg plant

57. Which food custom is common to both Islam and Judaism?
   a. Pork is prohibited in the diet
   b. Meat cannot be eaten on Fridays
   c. Special cookware is used for different meals
   d. Meat and dairy products are served at different meals

58. The most common independent nursing intervention to help hospitalized older adults maintain body weight is:
   a. Making meal time a social activity
   b. Taking a thorough nutritional history
   c. Providing assistance with the intake of meals
   d. Encouraging dietary supplements between meals

59. Teaching about a low cholesterol diet is most essential for an adult female patient with a total cholesterol level of:
   a. 200 milligrams per deciliter
   b. 190 milligrams per deciliter
   c. 150 milligrams per deciliter
   d. 100 milligrams per deciliter

60. Which is inappropriate for a healthy weight-reduction diet for an adult female?
   a. Limiting fat to less than 15% of the diet
   b. Maintaining a daily 1200 kilocalorie intake
   c. Including food from the major food groups
   d. Striving for a 2 pound weight loss per week

ANSWERS AND RATIONALES

1. a. Sixty grams of fat × 9 kilocalories per gram = 540 kilocalories. Five hundred and forty kilocalories are 27% of 2000 kilocalories.
   b. This number incorrectly answers the question.
   c. This number incorrectly answers the question.
   d. This number incorrectly answers the question.

2. a. Jell-O is a clear liquid that is a solid when refrigerated and a liquid at room temperature. It is permitted in either form on a clear liquid diet.
   b. Caffeinated or decaffeinated tea is permitted on a clear liquid diet.
   c. Weak or strong and caffeinated or decaffeinated coffee is permitted on a clear liquid diet.
   d. Milk and milk products are not included on a clear liquid diet. Ice cream contains a high solute load, including fat and proteins, which stimulates the digestive process.

3. a. One slice of white bread contains only 0.68 gram of dietary fiber.
   b. One cup of green beans contains 4.19 grams of dietary fiber. Fiber (also called roughage or residue) refers to a diverse group of polysaccharides that provide structure to plants. These insoluble fibers result in a residue in the intestine.
   c. One tablespoon of peanut butter contains only 1.12 grams of dietary fiber.
   d. One tablespoon of orange marmalade contains only 0.14 gram of dietary fiber.

4. a. During the states of malnutrition and starvation, the basal metabolic rate (BMR) decreases because the lean body mass decreases. Fever is associated with an increased, not decreased, BMR.
   b. When energy expended is greater than the caloric intake an individual will experience hunger, not anorexia. Hunger is a dull or acute pain felt around the epigastric area caused by a lack of food. Anorexia is the loss or lack of appetite.
   c. When energy expenditure exceeds caloric intake, eventually body fat and muscle mass breaks down to supply the fuel needed for metabolism. Malnutrition results when the body's cells have a deficiency or excess of one or more nutrients.
   d. When a person is malnourished, eventually the serum protein will be low, which may result in a decreased colloid osmotic pressure and then to the movement of fluid from the intravascular compartment into the peritoneal cavity. When the circulating blood volume decreases, the blood pressure decreases, not increases.

5. a. A serving of ½ grapefruit contains only 162 µgRE of vitamin A.
   b. One medium-sized tangerine contains only 108 µgRE of vitamin A.
   c. One medium-sizex banana contains only 69 µgRE of vitamin A.
   d. Apricots are an excellent source of vitamin A. Three medium-size apricots contain 867 µgRE (Retinol Equivalents) of vitamin A.

6. a. One cup of milk contains only 8 grams of protein.
   b. Food from animal sources (meat, poultry, fish, eggs, and cheese) provides complete proteins and, therefore, are the best sources of protein. Three ounces of meat or poultry contain approximately 19 to 25 grams of protein depending on the type of meat or poultry.
   c. Although a serving of a grain product contains approximately 2 grams of protein, it primarily provides carbohydrates and fiber.
   d. The majority of vegetables provide only 1 to 3 grams of protein.

7. a. Green leafy vegetables are an excellent source of Vitamin K, not D.
   b. Vegetable oils are an excellent source of Vitamin E, not D.
   c. Not many foods contain Vitamin D; therefore, it should be supplemented with fortified food such as milk. One quart of fortified milk contains the Recommended Daily Allowance (RDA) of Vitamin D for children.
   d. The liver is an excellent source of Vitamin K, not D.

8. a. Four grams of carbohydrates equals 16 kilocalories, 3 grams of protein equals 12 kilocalories, and 5 grams of fat equals 45 kilocalories. Sixteen + 12 + 45 = 73 kilocalories.
   b. This is an inaccurate sum of the kilocalories in the various nutrients presented in the question.
   c. This is an inaccurate sum of the kilocalories in the various nutrients presented in the question.
   d. This is an inaccurate sum of the kilocalories in the various nutrients presented in the question.

9. a. Hemoglobin concentration of the blood correlates closely with the red blood cell count. Elevated hemoglobin suggests hemoconcentration from increased numbers of red blood cells (polycythemia) or dehydration.
   b. Serum proteins, particularly albumin, reflect a person's skeletal muscle and visceral protein status. A normal serum albumin level ranges between 3.5 and 5.0 g/dL. Mild depletion ranges between 2.8 and 3.4 g/dL. Moderate depletion ranges between 2.1 and 2.7 g/dL. Severe depletion is less than 2.1 g/dL.
   c. Specific gravity is a urine test that measures the kidney's ability to concentrate urine. A low specific gravity reflects dilute urine that suggests a high urine volume, diabetes insipidus, kidney infections, or severe renal damage with disturbances in concentrating and diluting abilities.
   d. Blood urea nitrogen (BUN) measures the nitrogen fraction of urea, a product of protein metabolism. An elevated BUN suggests renal disease, reduced renal perfusion, urinary tract obstruction, and increased protein metabolism.

10. a. Egg rolls are a fried food. Frying involves cooking food in a solution consisting of saturated or unsaturated fat, which is composed mostly of fatty acids. Fatty acids combine with glycerol to form triglycerides.
    b. Spareribs are high in saturated fat and cooked with sauces that are high in saturated or unsaturated fat.
    c. Crispy noodles are a fried food that should be

avoided. Frying involves cooking food with a saturated or unsaturated fat solution, which is composed mostly of fatty acids. Fatty foods on a low-fat diet should be eaten raw or cooked by broiling, baking, or boiling.

 d. Hot and sour soup contains less fat than the other food choices listed.

11. a. Potatoes are an excellent source of vitamin C (ascorbic acid). One $^1/_2$ pound potato contains approximately 26 mg of vitamin C.
 b. Eight ounces of yogurt contains only 1 mg of vitamin C.
 c. Dry beans (legumes) contain no vitamin C. One cup of green beans contains only 12 mg of vitamin C.
 d. One cup of milk contains only 2 mg of vitamin C.

12. a. Apples are an excellent source of fiber. One medium apple supplies 3.5 grams of dietary fiber.
 b. Ten cherries provide only 1.2 grams of dietary fiber.
 c. Five halves of dried apricots provide only 1.2 grams of dietary fiber.
 d. A $^1/_2$ cup of pineapple provides only 1.1 grams of dietary fiber.

13. a. An electrolyte is a chemical substance that, in solution, dissociates into electrically charged particles. Electrolytes maintain the chemical balance between cations and anions in the body, which is essential for acid-base balance.
 b. Vitamins are organic compounds that do not provide energy, but are needed for the metabolism of energy.
 c. Minerals are inorganic elements or compounds essential for regulating body functions. The major minerals of the body are calcium, phosphorus, sodium, potassium, magnesium, chloride, and sulfur.
 d. Carbohydrates, a group of organic compounds such as saccharides, starch, cellulose, and gum, are the main fuel source for energy. Athletes competing in endurance events often adhere to a diet that increases carbohydrates to 70% of the diet for the last three days before a race (carbohydrate loading) to maximize muscle glycogen storage.

14. a. This does not promote independence and may precipitate feelings of low self-esteem.
 b. This is unnecessary and limits the patient's food choices.
 c. This is unnecessary and may decrease the patient's appetite.
 d. The clock system, which identifies where certain foods are on a plate in relation to where numbers are located on a clock, allows the patient to be independent when eating. Independence with activities of daily living supports self-esteem.

15. a. Carbohydrates, not protein, are the main fuel source for energy. Athletes competing in endurance events often adhere to a diet that increases carbohydrates to 70% of the diet for the last three days before a race (carbohydrate loading) to maximize muscle glycogen storage.
 b. Anabolism, the process by which the body's cells synthesize protoplasm for growth and repair, requires amino acids, which are the essential components of protein.

 c. Although adequate amounts of food from all the food groups are necessary for maintaining healthy functioning systems within the body, it is really effective kidney functioning and an adequate fluid balance that are necessary for excretion. The increased load of nitrogenous wastes associated with an excessive protein intake burden, rather than facilitate, excretion.
 d. Protein is ingested to prevent, not promote, catabolism. Catabolism occurs when complex substances break down into simpler substances, releasing energy.

16. a. Osteoporosis is a disease characterized by a decrease in total bone mass and deterioration of bone tissue that leads to bone fragility and the risk of fractures. Adequate calcium is necessary for building and strengthening bones and preventing osteoporosis.
 b. Vitamin D promotes bone mineralization by producing transport proteins that bind calcium and phosphorus. This increases intestinal absorption, stimulates the kidneys to return calcium to the bloodstream, and stimulates bone cells to use calcium and phosphorus to build and maintain bone tissue.
 c. A decrease in calcium in the blood (hypocalcemia) can eventually lead to tetany, which is characterized by muscle spasms, paresthesias, and convulsions.
 d. Iron is unrelated to calcium balance. Iron is essential for hemoglobin formation.

17. a. One gram of protein is equivalent to 4 kilocalories. Therefore, 5 grams of protein furnish 20 kilocalories.
 b. This number of kilocalories is unrelated to the kilocalorie equivalent for any food nutrient.
 c. This number of kilocalories is equivalent to 15, not 5, grams of protein.
 d. This number of kilocalories is equivalent to 5 grams of fat, not protein.

18. a. Bile is produced and concentrated in the liver and stored in the gallbladder. As fat enters the duodenum, it precipitates the release of cholecystokinin, which stimulates the gallbladder to release bile. Bile, an emulsifier, enlarges the surface area of fat particles so that enzymes can digest the fat.
 b. The liver is not involved with carbohydrate digestion. Ptyalin (secreted by the parotid glands), amylase (secreted by the pancreas), and sucrase, lactase, and maltase (secreted by the walls of the small intestine) digest carbohydrates.
 c. The liver is not involved with red blood cell production. People who are deficient in iron and protein have difficulty with red blood cell production.
 d. The large intestine, not the liver, is involved with reabsorbing water. The majority of the water in chyme is reabsorbed in the first half of the colon, leaving the remainder (approximately 100 cc) to form and eliminate feces.

19. a. Alcohol increases intestinal motility so that it decreases, not increases, the length of time it takes intestinal contents to pass through the body.
 b. Alcohol interferes with vitamin intake,

absorption, metabolism, and excretion. It specifically interferes with the absorption of vitamins A, D, K, thiamin, folic acid, pyridoxine, and B_{12}.

   c. The damaging effects of alcohol decrease, not increase, the efficiency of the process of absorption of medications in the stomach and intestines. However, alcohol can potentiate the action of drugs, such as central nervous system depressants.

   d. Alcohol does not have to be digested. It is absorbed rapidly, 20% from the stomach and 80% from the intestine. Alcohol interferes with the absorption of thiamin, which is essential to oxidize glucose. In addition, the body lacks enzymes to convert non-carbohydrate sources to energy. Therefore, hypoglycemia is associated with alcohol use.

20. a. This is premature. The nurse is abdicating the responsibility to help the patient.

   b. A change in diet requires a practitioner's order. Generally, calories should not be restricted below 1200 cal/day for women or 1500 cal/day for men so that there are adequate amounts of essential nutrients.

   c. This may eventually be done, but it is premature at this time.

   d. When the expected outcome of an intervention is not attained, the situation must be reassessed to determine why and the plan changed appropriately. A record of a dietary intake provides complete objective information about the amounts and types of food consumed. This information provides data about nutrient deficiencies or excesses, eating patterns, behaviors associated with eating, and potential problems and needs.

21. a. Salsa predominantly contains the vegetables tomatoes, onions, and peppers, which are low in fat.

   b. Pasta contains predominantly carbohydrates, not fat. In addition, in the Latino culture, rice and beans are preferred over pasta. Pasta is part of the Italian culture.

   c. Although steamed fish is low in fat, in the Latino culture foods generally are stewed or fried and vegetables, legumes, and meat are preferred.

   d. Refried beans are a fried food that should be avoided on a low-fat diet. Frying involves cooking food with a saturated or unsaturated fat solution, which is composed mostly of fatty acids. Fatty acids combine with glycerol to form triglycerides.

22. a. One piece of blueberry pie contains only 14 µgRE of vitamin A.

   b. Pumpkin is an excellent source of vitamin A. One piece (1/6 of a 9 inch diameter pie) contains 3750 µgRE (Retinol Equivalents) of vitamin A.

   c. One piece of cherry pie contains only 70 µgRE of vitamin A.

   d. One piece of pecan pie contains only 115 µgRE of vitamin A.

23. a. This is not the best nursing diagnosis of the options offered. Although a loss of appetite may contribute to constipation, an increase in fluid intake and an effort to choose high fiber foods can help prevent constipation.

   b. This is not the best nursing diagnosis of the options offered. Although in some patients stomatitis may cause difficulty with swallowing (dysphagia), which may contribute to aspiration, a bland diet soft in consistency will help to minimize dysphagia.

   c. This is not the best nursing diagnosis of the options offered. Ingesting adequate amounts of fluid is generally not a problem as long as acidic fluids are avoided because they irritate the lesions of the mucous membranes.

   d. Stomatitis, inflammation of the mucous membranes of the oral cavity, can be painful. Patients with stomatitis frequently avoid eating and drinking to limit discomfort, which can lead to inadequate nutritional intake.

24. a. This is an inaccurate sum of the kilocalories in the various nutrients presented in the question.

   b. This is an inaccurate sum of the kilocalories in the various nutrients presented in the question.

   c. This is an inaccurate sum of the kilocalories in the various nutrients presented in the question.

   d. Twelve grams of carbohydrates are equal to 48 kilocalories. Twenty grams of protein are equal to 80 kilocalories. Eight grams of fat are equal to 72 kilocalories. Forty-eight + 80 + 72 = 200 kilocalories.

25. a. Vitamin D (also regarded as a hormone) promotes bone mineralization by producing transport proteins that bind calcium and phosphorus, which increases intestinal absorption, stimulates the kidneys to return calcium to the blood stream, and stimulates bone cells to use calcium and phosphorus to build and maintain bone tissue.

   b. Vitamin K promotes blood clotting by increasing the synthesis of prothrombin by the liver; it does not promote strong bones.

   c. The B complex vitamins are related to protein synthesis and cross-linking of collagen fibers, which are essential for integrity of the integumentary system, not to strong bones.

   d. Vitamin E prevents the oxidation of unsaturated fatty acids and thereby prevents cell damage; it does not promote strong bones.

26. a. One egg contains only 1.0 mg of iron.

   b. One serving of fruit contains less than 1.0 mg of iron.

   c. Meat, especially liver, is a good source of iron. Three ounces of meat contain approximately 1.6 to 5.3 mg of iron depending on the type of meat and whether it is a regular or lean cut.

   d. One slice of bread contains only approximately 0.7 to 1.4 mg of iron depending on the type of bread.

27. a. This may further decrease the consumption of food at meal times. Supplements are given in addition to, not to replace, the nutrients that are consumed with meals.

b. Research indicates that exercise decreases appetite and increases the need for calories. Exercise releases beta-endorphin, which results in a state of relaxation and satisfaction with less food.

c. This intervention is premature. It assumes that the inadequate intake is related to discomfort associated with flatus.

d. **A person's cultural, religious, educational, economic, and experiential background influences eating behaviors and food preferences. When familiar, preferred foods are available and personally selected, the patient may feel that the care is individualized and they are in more control, resulting in eating a greater percentage of the meal.**

28. a. **All eggs except fried are permitted on a low-residue diet. A low-residue diet is easily digested and absorbed and limits bulk in the intestines after digestion.**

b. Orange and grapefruit juice contain pulp, a soluble fiber, which is not permitted on a low-residue diet.

c. Green beans contain polysaccharides that provide structure to plants and result in a residual after digestion that is not permitted on a low-residue diet. One cup of green beans contains 4.19 grams of dietary fiber.

d. Whole-grain breads, breads with seeds or nuts, and bread made with bran consist of insoluble fibers that are not permitted on a low-residue diet.

29. a. A person with few or no teeth should be able to meet all daily nutrient requirements without between-meal supplements.

b. **A mechanical soft diet is modified only in texture. It includes moist foods that require minimal chewing and eliminates most raw fruits and vegetables and foods containing seeds, nuts, and dried fruit.**

c. A person with few or no teeth can handle a more substantial diet than pureed foods. A pureed diet is a soft diet blenderized to a semisolid consistency.

d. A person with few or no teeth can handle a more substantial diet than a soft diet. A soft diet is moderately low in fiber and lightly seasoned. A soft diet usually is ordered for patients who are unable to tolerate a regular diet after surgery as a transition between liquids and a regular diet.

30. a. Sunflower seeds contain only trace amounts of Vitamin C.

b. **Green peppers are an excellent source of vitamin C (ascorbic acid). One pepper contains 95 mg of vitamin C.**

c. Black beans contain no vitamin C.

d. Beef liver contains no vitamin C.

31. a. Eggs should be avoided on a low-fat diet. One egg contains 1.7 grams of saturated fat.

b. Liver should be avoided on a low-fat diet. Three ounces of liver contain 2.5 grams of saturated fat.

c. Cheese should be avoided on a low-fat diet. Depending on the cheese, one ounce contains approximately 4.4 to 6.2 grams of saturated fat.

d. **Chicken is permitted on a low-fat diet. Three**

ounces of chicken contains 0.9 gram of saturated fat. A low-fat food should contain less than 1 gram of saturated fat per serving.

32. a. This is not an appropriate therapy for a patient with malabsorption syndrome. A gastrostomy tube permits a formula to be instilled into the stomach, which then progresses to the small intestine where absorption should normally take place. Depending on the etiology, it can cause gastrointestinal irritation, increased intestinal motility, diarrhea, and dehydration.

b. **Difficulty swallowing (dysphagia) that does not respond to dysphagia diets (mechanical soft, soft, blended or puréed liquids) may need the insertion of a gastrostomy tube so that formula feedings can be administered to meet nutritional needs.**

c. Gastric tube feedings are contraindicated in the presence of vomiting because of the potential for aspiration. The cause of the nausea and vomiting should be identified and treated.

d. This is a drastic measure for stomatitis. Stomatitis, an inflammation of the mouth, is usually a temporary problem that responds to pharmacologic therapy and frequent appropriate oral hygiene.

33. a. **Four kilocalories are equivalent to 1 gram of carbohydrates. Therefore, a 12-gram carbohydrate snack furnishes 48 kilocalories.**

b. Twenty-four grams of carbohydrate are equivalent to 96 kilocalories.

c. Eighteen grams of carbohydrate are equivalent to 72 kilocalories.

d. Twenty-nine and a half grams of carbohydrates are equivalent to 118 kilocalories.

34. a. Grapefruit does not contain iodine. Grapefruit is an adequate source of vitamin C (ascorbic acid) and potassium.

b. **Foods naturally high in iodine include saltwater fish, shellfish, and seaweed because it is derived from seawater.**

c. Although some grains contain iodine because of iodated dough conditioners, they are not a rich source. Grains provide carbohydrates and fiber.

d. The iodine in plant sources, such as beans, depends on the mineral content of the soil in which they are grown, and are not rich sources of iodine.

35. a. A confused patient may not know how to manipulate the spoon that is necessary to eat the soup. This could result in spillage and frustration.

b. Eating chicken salad requires the use of a utensil that may be beyond the patient's cognitive ability.

c. **This is a single food item that is usually familiar to most people in the United States. A single familiar food is an easier symbol to decode cognitively than food mixed together on a plate or in a casserole. In addition, the fingers rather than a utensil can handle a piece of chicken.**

d. Eating a casserole requires the use of a utensil that may be beyond the patient's ability. In addition, food mixed together is more confusing than food that is presented individually.

36. a. Leavened bread and cake, not coffee and tea, are forbidden during Passover.
    b. There are no restrictions on dairy products and eggs after sundown on Fridays.
    c. All crustaceans, shellfish, and fish-like mammals such as crab, shrimp, and lobster, scallops, oysters, and clams are forbidden.
    d. **Dairy products and meat/poultry are never served at the same meal or on the same set of dishes. Dairy products are not permitted within 1 to 6 hours after eating meat/poultry. Meat/poultry cannot be eaten for 30 minutes after consuming dairy products. This was practiced so that one food did not contaminate the other.**

37. a. One slice of rye bread contains 2 grams of protein and by itself is not a complete protein.
    b. One cup of baked beans contains approximately 2 grams of protein and by itself is not a complete protein.
    c. **Three ounces of ground beef contain 20 grams of protein. It is an animal source that contains all 8 essential amino acids and is considered a complete protein.**
    d. One cup of winter squash contains 2 grams of protein and by itself is not a complete protein.

38. a. Fish oils contain omega-3 fatty acids that help to decrease triglycerides and total cholesterol, not promote blood clotting.
    b. Grains are unrelated to promoting blood clotting. Grains provide carbohydrates and are an excellent source of fiber. *Enriched* grains have added nutrients that were previously present in the grain, but were removed during processing or lost during storage.
    c. **Green leafy vegetables, such as spinach, lettuce, kale, Brussels sprouts, and cabbage contain vitamin K. Vitamin K plays an essential role in the production of the clotting factors II (prothrombin), VII, IX, and X.**
    d. Milk is unrelated to blood clotting. *Fortified* means that nutrients are added that are not naturally found in the food. Milk is fortified with vitamin D, which is essential for the absorption of calcium.

39. a. One cup of skim milk contains only 18 mg of cholesterol.
    b. **Egg yolks are high in cholesterol and should be avoided by people with high cholesterol. One egg yolk contains 272 mg of cholesterol.**
    c. Three ounces of turkey contain only 45 mg of cholesterol.
    d. Two slices of bologna contain only 31 mg of cholesterol.

40. a. This imposes on family members. A person must learn to cope with temptation because exposure to desirable foods occurs inside and outside the home.
    b. This is degrading and should be avoided. Pictures that reflect a positive outcome are more desirable.
    c. **Behavior modification strategies are most successful when the person has an internal locus of control and is actively involved in self-care. Research demonstrates that self-monitoring of food intake is the single most helpful strategy in weight reduction.**
    d. The rigidity and limitation of avoiding between-meal snacks may cause periods of hypoglycemia, overeating, and noncompliance. Between meal snacks should be calculated into the weight-reduction program to meet both physical and emotional needs.

41. a. This is the number of kilocalories equivalent to 1 gram of protein or 1 gram of carbohydrate.
    b. This number of kilocalories is equivalent to 1 gram of fat.
    c. This number of kilocalories is equivalent to 3 grams of protein or 3 grams of carbohydrates.
    d. **One gram of fat is equivalent to 9 calories. Therefore, 2 grams of fat furnish 18 kilocalories.**

42. a. Carbohydrates are not necessary for the absorption of vitamin K.
    b. Starch is not necessary for the absorption of vitamin K.
    c. Proteins are not necessary for the absorption of vitamin K.
    d. **Vitamin K is one of the fat-soluble vitamins (A, D, E, and K) that are absorbed with fat in chylomicrons, which enter the lymphatic system before circulating in the blood stream. Vitamin K plays an essential role in the production of the clotting factors II (prothrombin), VII, IX, and X.**

43. a. The ingestion of legumes is encouraged, not discouraged, when a person has atherosclerosis because one cup contains 15 grams of protein but only 0.1 to 0.2 gram of saturated fat.
    b. Atherosclerosis is not related to water consumption. Atherosclerosis is caused by excessive lipoproteins that become incorporated into fatty plaques on vessel walls.
    c. **High fiber diets, particularly those rich in soluble fiber, lower total cholesterol and LDL-C levels without lowering HDL-C levels. Adding 6 to 12 grams of soluble fiber to the diet lowers LDL-C levels by 5 to 15%. Cholesterol combines with triglycerides and protein-bound phospholipids to form lipoproteins, which includes LDL-C. Lipoproteins become incorporated into the fatty plaques characteristic of atherosclerosis.**
    d. Red meat is high in saturated fats, and 6 ounces contains 12.6 grams of saturated fat. Lean meats should be limited to less than 5 ounces per day. A low-fat food should contain less than 1 gram of saturated fat per serving.

44. a. **A balanced diet with a variety of foods in moderation from the 5 major food groups in the Food Guide Pyramid (grain, vegetables, fruits, milk, and meat) will provide the recommended daily allowances of essential nutrients without the need for supplements.**
    b. Megadoses of vitamins no longer operate as normal nutritional agents and excesses are detrimental to the body, particularly to the liver and brain.
    c. Vitamins by themselves are useless. Their action contributes to chemical reactions (i.e., they act as catalysts), and they must have their substrate material

to work on, which are carbohydrates, protein, and fats and their metabolites.

d. This may or may not be true.

45. a. When the amount of carbohydrates ingested does not meet the energy requirements of an individual, the body will break down stored fat to meet its energy needs. Ketone bodies are produced during the oxidation of fatty acids.

b. An increased intake of protein helps meet energy demands because when the energy from carbohydrates is depleted, the body converts protein and fatty acids to glucose (gluconeogenesis).

c. Starch is the major source of carbohydrates in the diet and it yields simple sugars on digestion.

d. Fiber is unrelated to ketosis.

46. a. Yogurt, a dairy product, is not included in a vegetarian diet. Pure vegetarians (vegans) eat only plants. Lacto-vegetarians eat vegetables and milk products, lacto-ovovegetarians eat vegetables, milk products, and eggs (some may occasionally eat fish or poultry).

b. Cheese, a dairy product, is not included in a vegetarian diet. Pure vegetarians (vegans) eat only plants.

c. Grains and legumes lack different amino acids. When these foods are combined, they substitute for a complete protein. Complete proteins supply all eight essential amino acids. Essential amino acids are those that cannot be manufactured by the human body and must be obtained from food sources.

d. Peanut butter combined with a grain, not jelly, is a substitute for a complete protein.

47. a. Vitamin C (ascorbic acid) is a water-soluble vitamin. The presence of fat or bile salts are unnecessary for its absorption.

b. Vitamin A is a fat-soluble vitamin that requires fat and bile salts to be absorbed.

c. Vitamin E is a fat-soluble vitamin that requires fat and bile salts to be absorbed.

d. Vitamin D is a fat-soluble vitamin that requires fat and bile salts to be absorbed.

48. a. This is only one theory associated with the cause of obesity.

b. This is only one theory associated with the cause of obesity.

c. This is only one theory associated with the cause of obesity.

d. This is the basis of all weight gain regardless of the etiology. Excess ingested nutrients are stored in adipose tissue (fat) and muscle, which increases body weight. Obesity is body weight 20% or greater than ideal body weight. Glucose is stored as glycogen in the liver and muscle with surplus amounts being converted to fat. Glycerol and fatty acids are stored as triglycerides in adipose tissue. Excess amino acids are used for glucose formation or are stored as fat.

49. a. One cup of orange juice contains only 27 mg of calcium.

b. One tablespoon of peanut butter contains only 5 mg of calcium.

c. Cottage cheese has the highest amount of calcium of all the options and is an excellent source of calcium, which is essential for bone growth. One cup of cottage cheese contains 155 mg of calcium. The NIH Consensus Conference—Optimal Calcium Intake recommends an average intake of 1000 to 1500 mg of calcium daily for an adult depending on various factors.

d. Three ounces of baked flounder contain only 13 mg of calcium.

50. a. A rapid weight gain indicates fluid retention, not nutritional status. One liter of fluid weighs 2.2 pounds.

b. Serum transferrin is a marker for protein status. Because its half-life is 8 days compared to albumin, which is 20 days, serum transferrin levels will provide earlier objective information concerning a person's increasing or decreasing nutritional status.

c. A decreasing serum albumin indicates a deteriorating, not improving, nutritional status. A normal serum albumin level ranges between 3.5 and 5.0 g/dL. Mild depletion values range between 2.8 and 3.4 g/dL. Moderate depletionvalues range between 2.1 and 2.7 g/dL. In severe depletion values are less than 2.1 g/dL.

d. Appropriate skin turgor, fullness, and elasticity that allows the skin to spring back to its previous state after being pinched reflects an adequate fluid, not nutritional, balance.

51. a. This is an inaccurate calculation and is not the correct answer to the question.

b. This is an inaccurate calculation and is not the correct answer to the question.

c. This is an inaccurate calculation and is not the correct answer to the question.

d. One pound of body fat is approximately equivalent to 3500 calories. Three pounds of body fat is equivalent to 10,500 calories. Divide the total calories desired to be lost (10,500) by the number of days of the diet (21) equals the daily reduction in calories needed (375) to meet the goal of losing 3 pounds in 4 weeks.

52. a. Although the inability to form hemoglobin in the absence of other necessary factors, such as vitamin B_{12} (pernicious anemia), can result in iron deficiency, it is not the major cause of iron deficiency.

b. The most common nutrient deficiency in the United States is iron deficiency caused by an inadequate supply of dietary iron. The major condition indicating iron deficiency is anemia.

c. Malabsorption of iron is not the major cause of iron deficiency, although a lack of gastric hydrochloric acid necessary to help liberate iron for absorption and the presence of phosphate or phytate, inhibitors of iron absorption, all can precipitate malabsorption of iron.

d. Although hemorrhage can precipitate iron deficiency, it is not the major etiologic factor.

53. a. A health behavior is an action that promotes a healthy lifestyle. Implementing health-promotion

behaviors is based on the perceived benefits of the actions.

b. This reflects cognition, not behavior.

c. This is a behavior, but it is in response to an illness, not associated with the promotion of health and the prevention of illness.

d. This is one aspect of a person's health status.

54. a. Stomatitis, inflammation of the mucous membranes of the mouth, is most often caused by infectious sources (herpes simplex virus, *Candida albicans*, and hemolytic streptococci), not fluoride deficiency.

b. **Fluroide strengthens the ability of the tooth structure to withstand the erosive effects of bacterial acids on the teeth. The recommended daily intake of fluoride for adults is 1.5 to 4.0 mg.**

c. Bleeding gums is caused by inflammation of the gums (gingivitis), not fluoride deficiency.

d. This is not specifically caused by fluoride deficiency. Yellow, brown, or black discoloration may indicate problems such as staining, a partial or total non-viable nerve, or tetracycline administration during the prenatal period or early childhood.

55. a. Although kidney beans are an excellent source of carbohydrates, a vegetarian diet has many other foods that can be selected to provide this nutrient.

b. Although kidney beans are an excellent source of minerals, especially sodium, potassium, and phosphorus, a vegetarian diet has many other foods that can be selected to provide this nutrient.

c. **Kidney beans are high in protein. One cup of kidney beans contains 15 grams of protein. Complete proteins come from animal sources such as meat, poultry, and fish, but they are not included on a vegetarian diet. Kidney beans combined with a grain are a substitute for a complete protein.**

d. One cup of kidney beans contains only 1 gram of fat.

56. a. **Sweet potatoes are an excellent source of vitamin A. One sweet potato (5 × 2 inches) contains 2488 µgRE (Retinol Equivalents) of vitamin A.**

b. One tomato (2 3/5 inches in diameter) contains only approximately 139 µgRE of vitamin A.

c. One cup of green beans contain only 83 µgRE of vitamin A.

d. One cup of egg plant contains only 6 µgRE of vitamin A.

57. a. **All pork and pork products are prohibited by the religions of Orthodox Judaism and Islam. The dietary laws of Orthodox Judaism are known as The Rules of Kashruth.**

b. This was formerly a practice of Catholicism. This tradition has been relaxed and now meat is prohibited only on certain religious holidays such as Good Friday and Ash Wednesday.

c. In Orthodox Judaism, meat and dairy products cannot be prepared using the same cookware.

d. In Orthodox Judaism, dairy products and meat cannot be eaten at the same meal or prepared and served with the same pots, dishes, or utensils.

58. a. Although this is desirable, it may be impractical or impossible in an acute-care facility. Patient rooms may be private or semiprivate, which would limit exposure to other patients, and patients often are too sick to socialize.

b. Although this can be done, the information will not necessarily improve intake.

c. **Sick older adults often are debilitated, lack energy, and do not feel well. Assistance with meals conserves the patient's energy and demonstrates a caring concern, which may increase the intake of food.**

d. This is a dependent function of the nurse and requires a practitioner's order.

59. a. **A cholesterol level of 200 mg/dl in a woman is on the high side of normal. Acceptable cholesterol levels should be less than 209 mg/dl in women and less than 191 mg/dl in men. Patients should be taught the foods to avoid that are high in cholesterol.**

b. This is an acceptable level of cholesterol for an adult woman.

c. This is an acceptable level of cholesterol for an adult woman.

d. This is an acceptable level of cholesterol for an adult woman.

60. a. This is too low because a certain amount of fat is necessary for metabolism. Although The World Health Organization indicates that fat should supply at least 15% of a person's diet, it is generally accepted that 25% to 30% of the calories in a well-balanced diet should come from fat, with 2/3 being unsaturated (plant sources) and 1/3 being saturated fat (from animal sources).

b. A daily 1200 to 1500 calorie weight reduction diet is reasonable for most adult females. A decrease of 1000 calories a day is needed to lose 2 pounds a week.

c. This is desirable. A balanced diet with a variety of foods in moderation from the 5 major food groups in the Food Guide Pyramid (grain, vegetables, fruits, milk, and meat) will provide the recommended daily allowances of essential nutrients.

d. **A weekly 1- to 2-pound loss is a realistic goal for a weight reduction program for an adult female. This is gradual and attainable while eating sufficient kilocalories to meet energy needs.**

Oxygenation

The following words include English vocabulary, nursing/medical terminology, concepts, principles, or information relevant to content specifically addressed in the chapter or associated with topics presented in it. English dictionaries, your nursing textbooks, and medical dictionaries such as *Taber's Cyclopedic Medical Dictionary* are resources that can be used to expand your knowledge and understanding of these words and related information.

Abdominal thrusts
Accessory muscle use
Activity intolerance
Adventitious breath sounds
Aerosol therapy
Airway clearance
Airway obstruction
Airway resistance
Alveoli
Apical
Apnea
Arterial blood gasses
Artificial airway
Aspiration
Asthma
Atelectasis
Auscultation
Blood coagulability
Breathing, types of
   Abdominal
   Bradypnea
   Deep
   Diaphragmatic
   Pursed-lip
   Tachypnea
   Thoracic
Breath sounds
   Adventitious
     Crackles (rales)
     Gurgles (rhonchi)
     Pleural friction rub
     Stridor
     Wheezes
   Normal
     Bronchial
     Bronchovesicular
     Vesicular
Bronchial spasm
Bronchoscopy
Capillary refill
Cardiac output
Cardiac workload

Cardiopulmonary resuscitation
Cardiovascular
Chest physiotherapy
Chest tube
Chest x-ray
Choking
Chronic bronchitis
Cilia
Circumoral cyanosis
Cough
   Non-productive
   Productive
Cyanosis
Cystic fibrosis
Diffusion
Distal pulses
Dyspnea
Dysrhythmias
Electrocardiogram
Emphysema
Endotracheal tube
Excursion
Exertion
Exhale
Expectorate
Expiration
Extubation
Fatigue
Heimlich maneuver
Hemoglobin saturation
Hemoptysis
Hemorrhage
Humidify
Hypercapnia
Hypertension/hypotension
Hyperventilation/hypoventilation
Hypostatic pneumonia
Hypovolemic shock
Hypoxemia
Hypoxia
Incentive spirometer
Inhale

Inspiration
Intrathorasic pressure
Intubation
Iron deficiency anemia
Laryngeal spasm
Liquefy
Metered-dose inhaler
Mucous membranes
Mucus
Myocardial infarction (MI, heart attack)
Nares
Nebulizer
Oral/nasal pharyngeal airway
Oropharynx
Orthopnea
Orthostatic hypotension
Oxygen delivery systems
   Face mask
   Nasal cannula
   Non-rebreather mask
   Venturi mask
Oxygen liter flow
Oxygen gauge
Oxygen saturation
Oxygen therapy
Pallor
Palpable
Patency
Patent
Percussion
Peripheral
Pneumothorax
Positive pressure ventilation
Postural drainage
Postural hypotension
Productive cough
Prongs
Pulmonary embolus
Pulmonary function tests
Pulse oximetery
Secretions

Sedentary

Sputum

Sternum

Suctioning

  Nasal

  Oropharyngeal

  Tracheal

Systemic

Tenacious secretions

Thoracentesis

Thoracotomy

Thoracic

Thrombophlebitis

Tidal volume

Tissue perfusion

Tracheostomy

Umbilicus

Valsalva maneuver

Vasoconstriction

Vasodilation

Ventilation

Ventilators

Vibration

Viscous secretions

Vital capacity

Xiphoid process

QUESTIONS

1. Which is most reflective of an early adaptation to hypoxia?
   a. Apnea
   b. Cyanosis
   c. Restlessness
   d. Dysrhythmias

2. Which patient adaptation would cause the most concern in the Post-Anesthesia Care Unit?
   a. Pain
   b. Stridor
   c. Lethargy
   d. Diaphoresis

3. After a central venous catheter is inserted into a patient's subclavian vein, the patient has severe dyspnea. The nurse immediately should assess the patient's:
   a. Pulse rate
   b. Anxiety level
   c. Breath sounds
   d. Blood pressure

4. When administering oxygen via a wall-outlet system, the action that would be unnecessary for a low liter flow as opposed to a high liter flow is:
   a. Attaching a flow meter to the wall outlet
   b. Providing oral hygiene whenever necessary
   c. Hanging an *Oxygen in Use* sign outside the patient's room
   d. Humidifying the oxygen before it is delivered to the patient

5. To which position should the nurse assist a patient to assume to use an incentive spirometer?
   a. Sitting
   b. Side-lying
   c. Orthopneic
   d. Low-Fowler's

6. Which would be an appropriate expected outcome for a patient with a nursing diagnosis of Ineffective Airway Clearance?
   a. Respiratory rate remains between 8 and 10 per minute
   b. Presence of bronchovesicular breath sounds
   c. Self-administers oxygen when necessary
   d. Uses pursed-lip breathing

7. Which is the best method for teaching deep breathing and coughing exercises?
   a. Explanation
   b. Demonstration
   c. Video presentation
   d. Brochure with pictures

8. Which is the most important action by the nurse after a patient has a thoracotomy?
   a. Ensure that the patient's intake is at least 3000 cc of fluid per 24 hours
   b. Provide the patient with adequate medication for pain relief
   c. Maintain the integrity of the patient's chest tube
   d. Turn and position the patient every two hours

9. Which complication has most likely occurred when a postoperative patient experiences purulent sputum, dyspnea, and chest pain?
   a. Hypostatic pneumonia
   b. Hypovolemic shock
   c. Thrombophlebitis
   d. Pneumothorax

10. Which reflects the most serious complication of increased blood coagulability precipitated by immobility?
    a. Muscle atrophy
    b. Pain in the calf
    c. Hypotension
    d. Bradypnea

11. Which patient adaptation would indicate respiratory distress?
    a. Respiratory rate of 14 breaths per minute
    b. Productive cough
    c. Sore throat
    d. Orthopnea

12. The nurse identifies that a patient's hands are edematous when attempting to apply a pulse oximetery probe. The priority action should be to:
    a. Attach the probe to one of the patient's toes
    b. Attach the probe to one of the patient's ear lobes
    c. Encourage active range-of-motion exercises of the hand by the patient
    d. Wash the patient's hand with soap and water before attaching the probe to the finger

13. The practitioner's order reads, "6 L Oxygen Via Face Mask." The patient, who has been extremely confused since being in the unfamiliar environment of the hospital, becomes agitated and repeatedly pulls off the mask. The nurse should:
    a. Tighten the strap around the head
    b. Reapply the mask every time the patient pulls it off
    c. Provide an explanation why the oxygen is necessary
    d. Request that the order be changed to a nasal cannula

14. A patient is anxious, has deep rapid breathing, and complains of feeling dizzy and having tingling sensations. The nurse's immediate response should be to:
    a. Have the patient breathe into a paper bag
    b. Place the patient in the supine position
    c. Determine why the patient is upset
    d. Notify the patient's physician

15. Which is the most appropriate expected outcome associated with the use of an incentive spirometer?
    a. Coughing will be stimulated
    b. Sputum will be expectorated
    c. Inspiratory volume will be increased
    d. Supplemental oxygen use will be reduced

16. The reason heat is used instead of cold is that heat:
    a. Minimizes muscle spasms
    b. Prevents hemorrhage
    c. Increases circulation
    d. Reduces discomfort

17. The physician orders chest physiotherapy with percussion and vibration for a newly-admitted patient. The nurse should question this order if when the nurse is performing the admission assessment the patient informs the nurse of a history of:
    a. Emphysema
    b. Osteoporosis
    c. Cystic fibrosis
    d. Chronic bronchitis

18. The nurse knows that teaching about pursed-lip breathing is effective when the patient says its purpose is to:
    a. Precipitate coughing
    b. Help maintain open airways
    c. Decrease intrathoracic pressure
    d. Facilitate expectoration of mucus

19. What should the nurse do first if a patient is choking on food?
    a. Sweep the patient's mouth with a finger
    b. Hit the middle of the patient's back firmly
    c. Determine if the patient can make any verbal sounds
    d. Apply sharp upward thrusts over the patient's sternum

20. To best help liquefy a patient's respiratory secretions the nurse should:
    a. Encourage the patient to increase fluid intake
    b. Teach effective deep breathing and coughing
    c. Change the patient's position every 2 hours
    d. Obtain an order for an antitussive agent

21. Which action would be most effective in meeting the needs of a patient experiencing laryngospasm after extubation?
    a. Ensuring hyperextension of the head
    b. Providing positive pressure ventilation
    c. Instituting cardiopulmonary resuscitation
    d. Administering 60% oxygen via a Venturi mask

22. A patient's hemoglobin saturation via pulse oximetry indicates inadequate oxygenation. What should the nurse do first?
    a. Encourage deep breathing and coughing
    b. Administer oxygen at 3 L per minute
    c. Raise the head of the bed
    d. Call the physician

23. Which diagnostic test would reflect an adaptation to iron deficiency anemia?
    a. Hemoglobin
    b. Platelet count
    c. Serum albumin
    d. Blood urea nitrogen

24. The physiological factor that places the older adult at the greatest risk during surgery is a decrease in:
    a. Skin elasticity
    b. Bladder emptying
    c. Tolerance for pain
    d. Respiratory excursion

25. Which would be an expected outcome for a patient with a nursing diagnosis of Ineffective Peripheral Tissue Perfusion?
    a. Alert and oriented
    b. Palpable distal pulses
    c. Capillary refill longer than 5 seconds
    d. Respirations in the range of 12 to 20 per minute

26. Which is most reflective of an early adaptation to hypoxia?
    a. Increased heart rate
    b. Difficulty breathing
    c. Bradypnea
    d. Pallor

27. Bed rest is used primarily to:
    a. Conserve energy
    b. Maintain strength
    c. Reduce peristalsis
    d. Enhance protein synthesis

28. The nurse recognizes that a patient understands the teaching about how to use an incentive spirometer when the patient:
    a. Maintains a firm seal with the lips around the mouthpiece during inspiration and expiration
    b. Keeps inhaling for several seconds when the visual indicator reaches the inspiratory goal
    c. Blows into the mouthpiece with a long, slow expiration
    d. Begins breathing with a rapid, forceful inspiration

29. The major difference between pursed-lip breathing and diaphragmatic breathing is with diaphragmatic breathing the patient:
    a. Inhales through the mouth
    b. Exhales through pursed lips
    c. Raises both shoulders while breathing deeply
    d. Tightens the abdominal muscles while exhaling

30. The most serious complication of intubation is:
    a. Stomatitis
    b. Atelectasis
    c. Sore throat
    d. Laryngeal spasm

31. A meal tray arrives for a patient who is receiving 24% oxygen via a Venturi mask. To meet this patient's needs, the nurse should:
    a. Request an order to use a nasal cannula during meals
    b. Discontinue the oxygen when the patient is eating meals
    c. Obtain an order to change the Venturi mask to a nonrebreather mask during meals
    d. Arrange for liquid supplements that can be administered via a straw through a valve in the mask

32. Which assessment best indicates a patient's ability to tolerate activity?
    a. Presence of adventitious breath sounds
    b. Vital signs before and after activity
    c. Complaints of weakness
    d. Flexibility of joints

33. When caring for a patient who has a chest tube after thoracic surgery, the nurse should:
    a. Position the collection device on the same plane as the chest
    b. Clamp the tube when providing for activities of daily living
    c. Maintain an air tight dressing over the puncture wound
    d. Empty and measure chest tube drainage every shift

34. When monitoring a patient's pulse oximetry level it is essential that the nurse be aware of the patient's:
    a. Heart rate
    b. Blood pressure
    c. Respiratory rate
    d. Hemoglobin level

35. Which is the most serious complication associated with thrombophlebitis caused by immobility?
    a. Postural hypotension
    b. Blanchable erythema
    c. Dependent edema
    d. Acute chest pain

36. While in a restaurant a pregnant woman is exhibiting a total airway obstruction because of a bolus of food. Which modification of the Heimlich maneuver would be appropriate for this person?
    a. Perform the thrusts with the person in the supine, rather than standing, position
    b. Place the fist with the pinkie finger, rather than the thumb, against the person's body
    c. Thrust against the middle of the sternum rather than between the umbilicus and xiphoid process
    d. Perform thrust gently, rather than forcefully, and discontinue the thrusts after 6 tries if unsuccessful

37. The safest position for an unresponsive patient after oral surgery is the:
    a. Prone position
    b. Supine position
    c. Lateral position
    d. Fowler's position

38. A physician orders chest physiotherapy with percussion and vibration for a patient. After the physician leaves, the patient says, "I still don't understand the purpose of this therapy." The nurse's best reply would be, "It:
    a. Eliminates the need to cough."
    b. Limits the production of bronchial secretions."
    c. Helps clear the airways of excessive secretions."
    d. Promotes the flow of secretions to the base of the lungs."

39. When the head of the bed is elevated to facilitate breathing, the main principle that explains how this action facilitates respiration comes from the science of:
    a. Physics
    b. Biology
    c. Anatomy
    d. Chemistry

40. Which adaptation would be of most concern when assessing pulmonary changes associated with immobility?
    a. Shallow respirations
    b. Oxygen saturation of 96%
    c. Decreased chest wall expansion
    d. Respirations that sound gurgling

41. The nurse recognizes that a patient needs further teaching when a patient using an incentive spirometer:
    a. Inhales slowly and deeply
    b. Tilts the incentive spirometer while breathing in
    c. Raises the inspiratory goal on the spirometer once a day
    d. Takes several normal breaths between using the spirometer again

42. The nurse teaches a patient to make a series of short, forceful exhalations just before actually coughing (huffing). The purpose of this action is to:
    a. Conserve the patient's energy
    b. Liquefy the respiratory secretions
    c. Limit the pain precipitated by coughing
    d. Raise sputum to a level where it can be coughed out

43. Which are the most effective leg exercises to prevent circulatory complications during the postoperative period?
    a. Flexing the knees
    b. Isometric exercises
    c. Dorsiflexion exercises
    d. Passive range of motion

44. Which outcome would best reflect achievement of the goal, "The patient will expectorate lung secretions with no signs of respiratory complications?"
    a. Absence of adventitious breath sounds
    b. Drinking 3000 ml of fluid in the last 24 hours
    c. Deep breathing and coughing nonproductively
    d. Expectorating sputum three times between 3 and 11 PM

45. What should the nurse do first when caring for an infant, a toddler, or a nonverbal patient who is restless, agitated, and irritable?
    a. Administer oxygen
    b. Suction the oropharynx
    c. Reduce environmental stimuli
    d. Determine patency of the airway

46. Which would place a patient at greatest risk for impaired activity tolerance?
    a. Hct of 45%
    b. Hgb of 14 gm/dl
    c. O_2 saturation of 90%
    d. WBC of 7500 cells/mm^3

47. When caring for a patient receiving oxygen via nasal cannula the nurse should:
    a. Reassess the nares, cheeks, and ears for signs of pressure every 2 hours
    b. Apply an oil-based lubricant to the patient's nares during physical hygiene
    c. Loop the tubing over the patient's ears and adjust the tubing firmly under the chin
    d. Alternate the position of the prongs curving upward versus downward every 2 hours

48. The presence of which adaptation would cause the most concern?
    a. Pleural friction rub
    b. Inspirational stridor
    c. Expiratory wheezing
    d. Non-productive cough

49. To increase both the respiratory and the circulatory functions of a patient in a coma, what is the most important thing the nurse should do?
    a. Encourage the patient to cough
    b. Massage the patient's bony areas
    c. Assist the patient with breathing exercises
    d. Change the patient's position every 2 hours

50. When the nurse implements abdominal thrusts during the Heimlich maneuver the nurse is trying to:
    a. Produce a burp
    b. Pump the heart
    c. Push air out of the lungs
    d. Put pressure on the stomach

1. a. Apnea, a complete absence of respirations, is the cause of, not an adaptation to, hypoxia.
    b. Cyanosis, a bluish discoloration of the skin and mucous membranes caused by reduced oxygen in the blood, is a late sign of hypoxia.
    c. **Hypoxia is insufficient oxygen anywhere in the body. An early sign of hypoxia is restlessness, which is caused by the lack of cerebral perfusion of oxygen.**
    d. Dysrhythmia, a pulse with an irregular rhythm, can occur with hypoxia but it is a late adaptation.

2. a. Pain is an expected response to the trauma of surgery and usually can be managed effectively.
    b. **Stridor is an obvious audible shrill, harsh sound caused by laryngeal obstruction. The larynx can become edematous because of the trauma of intubation associated with general anesthesia. Obstruction of the larynx is life-threatening because it prevents the exchange of gases between the lungs and atmospheric air.**
    c. Lethargy, which is drowsiness or sluggishness, is an expected response to anesthesia and narcotic medications because these medications depress the central nervous system.
    d. Although diaphoresis is a cause for concern, it is not as immediately life-threatening as an adaptation in another option. Diaphoresis can be related to a warm environment, impaired thermoregulation, the General Adaptation Syndrome, or shock.

3. a. This is not the priority, although all the vital signs should be obtained eventually.
    b. Although severe dyspnea and anxiety are interrelated, assessment of anxiety is not the priority at this time.
    c. **The subclavian vein is in close proximity to the apex of the lung. If the central venous catheter inadvertently enters the lung, it will cause it to collapse (pneumothorax), resulting is severe shortness of breath (dyspnea), chest pain, cough, hypotension, tachycardia, and anxiety. Auscultation over the site of the collapsed lung will reveal an absence of breath sounds.**
    d. This is not the priority, although all the vital signs should be obtained eventually.

4. a. All oxygen systems should have a flow meter to control and maintain the flow of oxygen gas.
    b. All oxygen is drying to the oral mucosa. Therefore, oral hygiene should be provided frequently to moisten the mucous membranes.
    c. *Oxygen in use* signs should be displayed prominently on the patient's door and bed to alert others that oxygen is in use and safety precautions should be implemented.
    d. **A low-liter flow system administers a volume of oxygen designed to supplement the inspired room air to provide airflow equal to the person's minute ventilation. A high-liter flow system administers a volume of oxygen designed to exceed the volume of air required for the person's minute ventilation. The low-liter flow system is less drying than the high-liter flow system and humidification is unnecessary. A humidifier is a mechanical device that adds water**

vapor to air in a particle size that can carry moisture to the small airways.

5. a. **An upright sitting position in a bed or chair facilitates maximum thoracic excursion because it permits the diaphragm to contract without pressure being exerted against it by abdominal viscera.**
    b. This position is not ideal for the use of an incentive spirometer because it limits thoracic expansion. The side-lying position allows the abdominal viscera to exert pressure against the diaphragm during inspiration and the lung on the lower side of the body is compressed by the weight of the body.
    c. This position raises intra-abdominal and intrathoracic pressures that can limit thoracic excursion.
    d. This position does not maximize the effects of gravity. Gravity could be used to move abdominal viscera away from the diaphragm and thus facilitate the contraction of the diaphragm, both of which promote thoracic expansion.

6. a. This is an unacceptable respiratory rate. The normal range for respirations in an adult is 12 to 20 breaths per minute.
    b. **This is an appropriate expected outcome for the nursing diagnosis Ineffective Airway Clearance, which is the state in which an individual experiences a threat to respiratory status related to an inability to cough effectively. Effective coughing clears the bronchi of secretions, which results in normal bronchovesicular breath sounds.**
    c. This expected outcome is associated with the nursing diagnosis Impaired Gas Exchange, not Ineffective Airway Clearance.
    d. The use of pursed-lip breathing is associated with the nursing diagnosis Impaired Gas Exchange, not Ineffective Airway Clearance.

7. a. This is not the best approach to teach a psychomotor skill. An explanation uses words to describe a behavior that the learner then has to attempt to perform.
    b. **A demonstration is the best strategy for teaching a psychomotor skill. A demonstration is an actual performance of the skill by the teacher who is acting as a role model. A demonstration is usually followed by a return demonstration. The learner can imitate the teacher during a return demonstration, ask questions, and receive feedback from the instructor.**
    c. Although a video provides a realistic performance of the skill, it does now allow for questions or feedback.
    d. A brochure with pictures is too static and unidimensional for teaching a psychomotor skill.

8. a. This is unnecessary. A normal fluid intake of approximately 2000 cc of fluid is adequate.
    b. Although this is extremely important, it is not the priority.
    c. A tension pneumothorax may occur if the integrity of the chest drainage system becomes compromised (e.g., open to atmospheric

pressure, clogged drainage tube, or mechanical dysfunction). **Maintaining respiratory functioning is the priority.**

   d. Although this is done to promote drainage of secretions from lung segments and aeration of lung tissue, it is not the priority.

9. **a. Hypoventilation, immobility, and ineffective coughing that lead to stasis of respiratory secretions and the multiplication of microorganisms cause hypostatic pneumonia. Dyspnea results from decreased lung compliance, chest pain results from coughing and the increased work of breathing, and purulent sputum results from fluid and blood moving from the capillaries into the alveoli.**

   b. Hypovolemic shock is characterized by tachycardia, tachypnea, and hypotension.

   c. Thrombophlebitis is characterized by localized pain, swelling, warmth, and erythema.

   d. Pneumothorax is characterized by a sudden onset of sharp pain on inspiration, dyspnea, tachycardia, and hypotension.

10. a. Although muscle atrophy can occur with immobility, it is unrelated to hypercoagulability. Muscle atrophy is the decrease in the size of a muscle resulting from disuse.

   b. Immobility promotes venous vasodilation, venous stasis and hypercoagulability of the blood, which can precipitate the formation of a clot in a vein of the leg (venous thrombosis) and inflammation of the vein (phlebitis).

   c. Hypotension, an abnormally low systolic blood pressure (less than 100 mmHg), is not related to hypercoagulability precipitated by immobility.

   d. Bradypnea, abnormally slow breathing (less than 10 breaths per minute), is unrelated to hypercoagulability caused by immobility.

11. a. A respiratory rate of 14 in an adult is within the normal range of 12 to 20 breaths per minute.

   b. A productive cough indicates that the person is managing respiratory secretions adequately and keeping the airway patent.

   c. A sore throat indicates posterior oropharyngeal irritation or inflammation. This may or may not progress to respiratory distress.

   d. Orthopnea, the ability to breathe easily only in an upright (standing or sitting) position, is a classic sign of respiratory distress. The upright position permits maximum thoracic expansion because the abdominal organs do not press against the diaphragm and inspiration is aided by the principle of gravity.

12. a. The use of a toe for pulse oximetry can result in inaccurate results because of concurrent problems such as vasoconstriction, hypothermia, impaired peripheral circulation, and movement of the foot.

   b. An ear lobe is an excellent site to monitor pulse oximetry. It is least affected by decreased blood flow, has greater accuracy at lower saturations, and rarely is edematous. This site is used for intermittent, not continuous, monitoring.

   c. The cause of the edema must be identified first

because range-of-motion exercises may be contraindicated.

   d. Soap and water will not resolve the edema. In addition, attaching a pulse oximeter clip sensor to an edematous finger is contraindicated because interstitial fluid interferes with obtaining an accurate oxygen saturation level.

13. a. This is unsafe because it can compress the capillaries under the strap, which may interfere with tissue perfusion and result in pressure ulcers.

   b. This may increase the patient's agitation and it is impractical.

   c. This will probably be useless because an agitated patient often does not understand cause and effect.

   d. Agitated, confused patients generally tolerate a nasal cannula better than a face mask. A nasal cannula (nasal prongs) is less intrusive than masks and masks are oppressive and may cause a patient to feel claustrophobic.

14. **a. Deep, rapid respiration that results in respiratory alkalosis (hyperventilation) can be corrected by rebreathing exhaled carbon dioxide to lower the pH of the blood, which brings the acid-base balance of the body back into the acceptable range (arterial pH of 7.35 to 7.45).**

   b. This will have a negative, not positive, impact on the patient's respiratory status. Anxious people are hypervigilant and cannot lie down without feeling an increase in anxiety. In addition, in the supine position the abdominal organs will press against the diaphragm and interfere with respirations.

   c. This is not the priority at this time. This might be done later to prevent hyperventilation in the future.

   d. This is unnecessary. The patient's needs must be met first and then the patient's condition, the nursing intervention, and the patient's response to the intervention should be documented in the patient's hospital record.

15. a. Although the deep breathing associated with the use of an incentive spirometer may stimulate coughing, this is not the primary reason for its use.

   b. Although sputum may be expectorated after the use of an incentive spirometer, this is not the primary reason for its use.

   c. An incentive spirometer provides a visual goal for and measurement of inspiration. It encourages the patient to execute and maintain a sustained inspiration. A sustained inspiration opens airways, increases the inspiratory volume, and reduces atelectasis.

   d. Patient's who use an incentive spirometer may or may not be receiving oxygen.

16. a. Both cold and heat relax muscles and thus minimize muscle spasms.

   b. Heat promotes, not prevents, bleeding because it causes vasodilation. Cold causes vasoconstriction, which limits bleeding.

   c. Heat raises the skin surface temperature, which promotes vasodilation, which increases blood flow to the area.

   d. Cold reduces discomfort by numbing the area, slowing the transmission of pain impulses, and by

increasing the pain threshold. Heat reduces discomfort by relaxing the muscles.

17. a. These are appropriate interventions for a patient with emphysema. Emphysema is a chronic pulmonary disease characterized by an abnormal increase in the size of air spaces distal to the terminal bronchioles with destructive changes in their walls.
    b. **This intervention provides for patient safety because percussion and vibration with a patient who has osteoporosis may cause fractures. Osteoporosis is an abnormal loss of bone mass and strength.**
    c. These are appropriate interventions for a patient with cystic fibrosis. Cystic fibrosis causes widespread dysfunction of the exocrine glands. It is characterized by thick, tenacious secretions in the respiratory system that block the bronchioles, creating breathing difficulties.
    d. These are appropriate interventions for a patient with chronic bronchitis. Bronchitis is an inflammation of the mucous membranes of the bronchial airways.

18. a. Deep breathing and huff coughing, not pursed-lip breathing, stimulate effective coughing.
    b. **Pursed-lip breathing involves deep inspiration and prolonged expiration against slightly closed lips. The pursed lips create a resistance to the air flowing out of the lungs, which prolongs exhalation and maintains positive airway pressure, thereby maintaining an open airway and preventing airway collapse.**
    c. Pursed-lip breathing increases, not decreases, intrathoracic pressure.
    d. The huff cough stimulates the natural cough reflex and is effective for clearing the central airways of sputum. Saying the word *huff* with short, forceful exhalations keeps the glottis open, mobilizes sputum, and stimulates a cough. The cascade cough is effective in mobilizing secretions when patients have large volumes of sputum. A slow, deep breath is taken and held for 2 seconds while contracting the expiratory muscles. The patient then opens the mouth and performs a series of coughs throughout exhalation.

19. a. This can force the bolus of food further down the trachea and is not done at this time. A sweep of the patient's mouth with a finger is done when the patient becomes unconscious.
    b. This should never be done with an adult because if it is a partial obstruction it interferes with the person's own efforts to clear the airway or can cause the bolus of food to lodge further down the trachea. If it is a total obstruction, slapping the back will be useless and delay the initiation of the abdominal thrust maneuver.
    c. **When a person is choking on food, the first intervention is to determine if the person can speak because the next intervention will depend on if it is a partial or total airway obstruction. With a partial airway obstruction, the person will be able to make sounds because some air can pass from the lungs through the vocal cords. In this situation, the person's own efforts (gagging and coughing) should be allowed to clear the airway. With a total airway obstruction, the person will not be able to make a sound because the airway is blocked and the nurse should immediately initiate the abdominal thrust maneuver (Heimlich maneuver).**
    d. When it is determined that a total airway obstruction exists then five quick sharp abdominal thrusts just below the xiphoid process are delivered to expel the obstruction.

20. a. **A fluid intake of 2500 to 3000 cc is recommended to maintain the moisture of the respiratory mucous membranes. Adequate fluid keeps respiratory secretions thin so that they can be moved by ciliary action or coughed up and spit out (expectorated).**
    b. This will mobilize, not liquefy, respiratory secretions.
    c. This will mobilize, not liquefy, respiratory secretions.
    d. Mucolytics, not antitussives, liquefy respiratory secretions. Antitussives prevent or relieve coughing.

21. a. This will do nothing to correct the obstruction at the glottis (opening through the vocal cords). In addition, tilting the head backward (hyperextension of the neck) elongates the pharynx, reducing airway resistance; however, the tongue will block the airway unless there is also forward pressure applied on the lower angle of the jaw (jaw thrust maneuver).
    b. **Positive pressure will push the vocal cords backward toward the wall of the larynx, opening the glottis (space between the vocal cords), which allows ventilation of the lung.**
    c. This is unnecessary. The patient is having a respiratory, not cardiac, problem.
    d. This is useless because the glottis is obstructed and the oxygenated air will not enter the lung. In addition, the highest percentage of oxygen that can be delivered by a Venturi mask is 40%.

22. a. Although this might be done eventually, it is not the priority at this time. This may or may not help. Inadequate oxygenation can be caused by a variety of problems other than shallow breathing or mucus in the airway.
    b. When administering oxygen in an emergency, the nurse should not exceed 2 L per minute because high oxygen levels can depress respirations in people with chronic obstructive lung diseases. Obtaining and setting up the equipment takes time that can be used for other more appropriate interventions first.
    c. **A nurse can implement this immediate, independent action. Nurses are permitted to treat human responses. Raising the head of the bed facilitates the dropping of the abdominal organs by gravity away from the diaphragm, which permits the greatest lung expansion.**
    d. This is premature. The patient's needs must be met first.

23. a. **Iron is necessary for hemoglobin synthesis. Therefore, reduced intake of dietary iron results in iron deficiency anemia. Hemoglobin is the main component of red blood cells and transports oxygen and carbon dioxide through the blood stream.**

b. Platelets are unrelated to iron deficiency anemia. Platelets (thrombocytes) are nonnucleated, round or oval, flattened, disk-shaped, formed elements in the blood that are necessary for blood clotting.

c. Albumin is unrelated to iron deficiency anemia. Albumin is a protein in the blood that helps to maintain blood volume and blood pressure.

d. Blood urea nitrogen is unrelated to iron deficiency anemia. Blood urea nitrogen (BUN) is a test that measures the nitrogen portion of urea present in the blood. It is an index of glomerular function in the production and excretion of urea.

24. a. Although healing of an incision may take longer in an older adult, it is not as serious as another age-related change. In the older adult, there is atrophy and thinning of both the epithelial and subcutaneous layers of tissue, collagenous attachments become less effective, sebaceous gland activity deceases, and interstitial fluid decreases. These changes lead to decreased skin elasticity.

b. Although there is a greater risk of postoperative urinary complications in older adults, they are not as serious as problems caused by other age-related changes. In the older adult bladder muscles weaken, bladder capacity decreases, the micturition reflex is delayed, emptying of the bladder becomes more difficult, and residual volume increases.

c. Although an incision in an older adult may be painful, it is not as serious as other age-related changes. In addition, in the older adult there is an increased threshold for sensations of pain, touch, and temperature because of age-related changes in the nerves and nerve conduction.

d. **Age-related changes in the older adult include calcification of costal cartilage (making the trachea and rib cage more rigid), an increase in the anterior-posterior chest diameter, and weakening of the thoracic inspiratory and expiratory muscles. These changes decrease respiratory excursion, which can result in multiple life-threatening postoperative complications such as atelectasis and hypostatic pneumonia.**

25. a. This is an appropriate expected outcome for an individual with the nursing diagnosis Acute Confusion, which is a cluster of global, fluctuating disturbances in consciousness, attention, perception, memory, orientation, thinking, sleep-wake cycle, and psychomotor behavior.

b. **This is an appropriate expected outcome for the nursing diagnosis Ineffective Peripheral Tissue Perfusion, which is a decrease in nutrition and respiration at the peripheral cellular level because of a decrease in capillary blood supply. A major defining characteristic of this nursing diagnosis is diminished or absent arterial pulses.**

c. A major defining characteristic of the nursing diagnosis Ineffective Peripheral Tissue Perfusion is a capillary refill greater than 3 seconds. Five seconds indicates a continued problem with peripheral tissue perfusion. After compression, the blanched tissue should return to its original color within 2 seconds (blanch test).

d. This is an appropriate expected outcome for an individual with the nursing diagnosis Ineffective Breathing Patterns, which is an actual or potential loss of adequate ventilation related to an altered breathing pattern.

26. a. **Hypoxia is insufficient oxygen anywhere in the body. To compensate for this lack of oxygen, the heart increases its rate to improve cardiac output, thereby increasing oxygen to all body cells.**

b. Difficulty breathing (dyspnea) is a late, not early, sign of hypoxia.

c. An increase in respirations (tachypnea), not a decrease in respirations (bradypnea), occurs as the body attempts to deliver more oxygen to body cells.

d. Skin color changes are not early adaptations to hypoxia. Pallor is caused by peripheral vasoconstriction that shunts blood away from the skin to the vital organs and occurs with the stress response.

27. a. **Bed rest reduces cardiopulmonary demands, muscle contraction, and other bodily functions. All of this reduces the basal metabolic rate, which conserves energy.**

b. Activity, not bed rest, maintains strength.

c. Although bed rest may limit peristalsis, it is not the most common reason bed rest is ordered.

d. Protein synthesis is enhanced by the intake of amino acids, not bed rest.

28. a. A firm seal around the mouthpiece is necessary during inhalation, but the mouthpiece should be removed during exhalation.

b. **When the visual indicator reaches the preset goal during inhalation, the inhalation should be maintained for 2 to 6 seconds to ensure ventilation of the alveoli.**

c. This is an inappropriate use of an incentive spirometer. The device is used to promote inhalation, not exhalation.

d. This is contraindicated. A rapid, forceful inhalation can collapse the airway. Inspiration should be accomplished through a slow, deep breath.

29. a. Inhalation is through the nose for both diaphragmatic and pursed-lip breathing.

b. Exhalation through pursed lips is performed only with pursed-lip breathing.

c. This action is not part of diaphragmatic or pursed-lip breathing. The use of these accessory muscles of respiration is a compensatory mechanism that helps to increase thoracic excursion when inhaling.

d. **With diaphragmatic breathing, the contraction of abdominal muscles at the end of expiration helps to reduce the amount of air left in the lungs at the end of expiration (residual volume).**

30. a. Although stomatitis—inflammation of the mouth—can occur from irritation caused by the tube used for delivering general anesthesia to a patient during surgery, it is uncommon and not life-threatening.

b. Although atelectasis is serious, it is not as serious as an adaptation in another option. Anesthesia delivered by intubation can interfere with the action of

surfactant, resulting in the collapse of alveoli (atelectasis).

c. Although the tube used for intubation commonly does irritate the posterior oropharynx resulting in a sore throat, it is not as serious as an adaptation in another option.

d. This is a potentially life-threatening complication because it prevents the exchange of gases between the lungs and atmospheric air. Laryngeal spasm can result from irritation caused by the presence of the intubation tube in the glottis (space between the vocal cords) during surgery.

31. a. This intervention will help meet both the nutritional and oxygen needs of the patient. A nasal cannula delivers oxygen via prongs placed in the patient's nares leaving the mouth unobstructed, which promotes talking and eating.

b. This is unsafe because it can compromise the patient's respiratory status while the oxygen is disconnected.

c. A Venturi mask and a nonrebreather mask are both masks that cover the mouth, which interferes with eating.

d. Liquid supplements are unnecessary. The patient should eat the diet ordered by the physician.

32. a. The presence of abnormal breath sounds (adventitious sounds) indicates the presence of a respiratory problem (narrowed airways, presence of excessive respiratory secretions, or pleural inflammation), not a response to activity.

b. Vital signs reflect cardiopulmonary functioning of the body. Vital signs obtained before and after activity provide data that can be compared to determine the body's response to the energy demands of ambulation.

c. Although this may reflect a response to activity, this evaluation is subjective and vague. Measurable, specific outcomes that are objective are the best way to evaluate a patient's physiologic response to an intervention.

d. Flexibility relates to mobility, not one's physiologic capacity to endure activities that require energy.

33. a. The chest drainage system should be kept below the level of the insertion site to promote the flow of drainage from the pleural space and prevent the flow of drainage back into the pleural space.

b. This is contraindicated because clamping a chest tube may cause a tension pneumothorax.

c. An airtight dressing seals the pleural space from the environment. If left open to the environment, atmospheric pressure causes air to enter the pleural space, which results in a tension pneumothorax.

d. This is unnecessary. Chest drainage systems are closed, self-contained systems that have a chamber for drainage. At routine intervals as per hospital policy the date, time, and nurse's initials mark the level of drainage on the drainage collection chamber.

34. a. Although it is important to monitor the heart rate, this is not essential in relation to measuring oxygen

saturation of the blood. The pulse oximeter obtains both the oxygen saturation of the blood and the pulse rate.

b. Although the blood pressure is important to monitor, this is not essential in relation to measuring oxygen saturation of the blood.

c. Although it is are important to monitor respirations, this is not essential in relation to measuring oxygen saturation of the blood.

d. Pulse oximetry is a method of measuring the amount of oxygenated hemoglobin in the blood. Therefore, it is advisable to compare results routinely with the patient's hemoglobin level.

35. a. Postural hypotension is unrelated to phlebitis caused by immobility. Postural hypotension (orthostatic hypotension) is a decrease in blood pressure related to positional or postural changes from the lying down to sitting or standing positions.

b. Blanchable erythema is unrelated to phlebitis caused by immobility. Blanchable erythema (reactive hyperemia) is a reddened area caused by localized vasodilation in response to lack of blood flow to the underlying tissue. The reddened area will turn pale with fingertip pressure.

c. Dependent edema is unrelated to phlebitis caused by immobility. Although fluid will collect in the interstitial compartment (edema) around the phlebitis, it is localized, not dependent, edema. Dependent edema is the collection of fluid in the interstitial tissues below the level of the heart, occurs bilaterally, and is caused usually by cardiopulmonary problems.

d. Immobility promotes venous stasis, which in conjunction with hypercoagulability and injury to vessel walls predisposes patients to thrombophlebitis. These three factors are known as Virchow's triad. A thrombus can break loose from the vein wall and travel through the circulation (embolus) where it eventually obstructs a pulmonary artery or one of its branches causing sudden, acute chest pain, dyspnea, coughing, and frothy sputum.

36. a. This is unnecessary. This is done when the patient is unconscious.

b. When attempting to clear an airway of an obstruction, the thumb side of the hand should always be against the patient's body regardless of the modification in the maneuver.

c. This is the appropriate modification of the abdominal thrust (Heimlich) maneuver for a pregnant woman. This provides thoracic compression while preventing pressure against the uterus that can result in trauma to the woman or the fetus.

d. A gentle thrust will not provide the force necessary to clear the airway. Discontinuing the maneuver before the obstruction is cleared will result in death.

37. a. Although this position allows for drainage from the mouth, it is contraindicated because lying on the side of the face compresses oral tissues, impedes assessment, complicates oral suctioning, and may compromise the airway.

b. This is unsafe. In an unconscious patient, the gag and

swallowing reflexes may be impaired, which increases the risk for aspiration and the tongue falling to the back of the oropharynx and occluding the airway.

 c. This position facilitates the flow of secretions out of the mouth by gravity, keeps the tongue to the side of the mouth maintaining the airway, and permits effective assessment of the oropharynx and respiratory status.

 d. This is unsafe. An unconscious patient is unable to maintain an upright position.

38. a. Chest physiotherapy promotes, not eliminates, the need for coughing

 b. Chest physiotherapy promotes the expectoration of, not limits the production of, bronchial secretions.

 c. The forceful striking of the skin over the lung (percussion, clapping) and fine, vigorous, shaking pressure with the hands on the chest wall during exhalation (vibration) mobilize secretions so that they can be coughed up and expectorated.

 d. Chest physiotherapy mobilizes respiratory secretions so that they can be expectorated, not promotes their flow to the base of the lungs.

39. **a. Raising the head of the bed drops the abdominal organs away from the diaphragm via the principle of gravity, facilitating breathing. Gravity, the tendency of weight to be pulled toward the center of the earth, is a physics principle.**

 b. This is not related to biology. Biology is the study of living organisms.

 c. This is not related to anatomy. Anatomy is the study of the form and structure of living organisms.

 d. This is not related to chemistry. Chemistry is the study of elements, compounds, and atomic relations of matter.

40. a. Although this is a concern, it is not as serious as an adaptation in another option.

 b. This is within the normal range for oxygen saturation, which is 95% or greater.

 c. Although this is a concern, it is not as serious as an adaptation in another option.

 d. Respirations that sound gurgling (gurgles, rhonchi) indicate air passing through narrowed air passages because of secretions, swelling, or tumors. A partial or total obstruction of the airway can occur, which is life-threatening.

41. a. This is the correct way to inhale to maintain an open airway.

 b. The patient is using the incentive spirometer incorrectly and needs further teaching. An incentive spirometer must be held in an upright position. A tilted *flow-oriented* device requires less effort to reach the desired inspiratory volume. A tilted volume-oriented device will not function correctly.

 c. This is an acceptable practice. Inspiratory goals should be progressively increased daily or more frequently depending on the patient's ability to continually maximize the inspiratory volume, which promotes alveoli ventilation.

 d. This is a desirable practice because it prevents hyperventilation and respiratory alkalosis.

42. a. Regardless of the type of cough, coughing uses, not

conserves, energy. However, after the airway is cleared of sputum, the patient's oxygen demands will be met more effectively.

 b. An increased fluid intake, not coughing, liquefies respiratory secretions.

 c. This is not the purpose of huff coughing. Coughing usually is not painful unless the thoracic muscles are strained or the patient has had abdominal or pelvic surgery.

 d. The huff cough stimulates the natural cough reflex and is effective for clearing the central airways of sputum. Saying the word *huff* with short, forceful exhalations keeps the glottis open and raises sputum to a level where it can be coughed up and expectorated.

43. a. Flexing the knee exerts pressure on the veins in the popliteal space; this reduces venous return, which increases, not decreases, the risk of postoperative circulatory complications.

 b. These exercises strengthen muscles; they do not prevent postoperative circulatory complications. Isometric exercises change the muscle tension but do not change the muscle length or move joints.

 c. Alternating dorsiflexion and plantar flexion (calf pumping) alternately contracts and relaxes the calf muscles including the gastrocnemius muscles. This muscle contraction promotes venous return, preventing the venous stasis that contributes to the development of postoperative thrombophlebitis.

 d. Passive range-of-motion exercises are exercises that are done by another person moving a patient's joints through their complete range of movement. This does not prevent postoperative circulatory complications because the power is supplied by a person other than the patient.

44. **a. Adventitious breath sounds are abnormal breath sounds that occur when pleural linings are inflamed or when air passes through narrowed airways or airways filled with fluid. The absence of abnormal sounds is desirable.**

 b. Drinking fluid is an intervention that will liquefy respiratory secretions, facilitating their expectoration. However, just drinking fluid will not ensure that the secretions will be expectorated.

 c. To expectorate secretions, coughing must be productive, not nonproductive. A nonproductive cough is dry, which means that no respiratory secretions are raised and spit out (expectorated) because of coughing.

 d. Although spitting out sputum reflects achievement of the goal in relation to expectorating lung secretions, it does not address the absence of respiratory complications.

45. a. This may or may not be necessary. The need for oxygen administration will depend on the results of other interventions that should be done first.

 b. This is premature. Mucus or sputum may not be the cause of the problem.

 c. This intervention is useless at this time and is not the priority.

 d. Early signs of hypoxia are restlessness, agitation, and irritability due to reduced oxygen to brain

cells. A partial or completely obstructed airway prevents the passage of oxygen into the alveoli and carbon dioxide out of the alveoli. The ABCs of emergency care identify airway as the priority.

46. a. This is within the normal range for hematocrit for men (42 to 52%) and women (36 to 48%).
    b. This is within the normal range for hemoglobin for men (14.0 to 17.4 g/dL or 140 to 174 g/L) and women (12.0 to 16.0 g/dL or 120 to 160 g/L).
    c. An oxygen saturation of 90% is below the normal level of 95% or greater. Adequate oxygen levels are necessary to meet the metabolic demands of activity that requires muscle contraction.
    d. This is within the normal range for white blood cells (WBCs) (5000 to 10,000 cells/mm^3).

47. a. This ensures that tissue irritation or capillary compression does not occur from the nasal prongs, tubing, or elastic strap. The elastic strap should be snug enough to keep the nasal prongs from becoming displaced but loose enough not to compress or irritate tissue.
    b. A water-based, not oil-based, lubricant should be applied to the nares.
    c. This is the correct placement of the tubing; however, it should be secured gently, not firmly, under the chin.
    d. The nasal prongs should always be curving downward to follow the natural curve of the nares. Placing the nasal prongs curving upward does not follow the natural curve of the nasal passage, which can cause tissue injury.

48. a. Although this reflects a problem, it is not as life-threatening as a condition in another option. A pleural friction rub is a grating, rubbing sound that is heard by auscultating over the base of the lung. It is caused by inflamed pleura (pleurisy) rubbing together.
    b. An inspiratory stridor is an obvious audible shrill, harsh sound caused by laryngeal obstruction. Obstruction of the larynx is life-threatening because it prevents the exchange of gases between the lungs and atmospheric air.
    c. Although this reflects a problem, it is not as life-threatening as a condition in another option. Expiratory wheezing is presence of high-pitched musical sounds caused by high-velocity movement of air through narrowed airways. It is associated with asthma, bronchitis, and pneumonia.
    d. Although this reflects a problem, it is not as life-threatening as a condition in another option. A non-productive cough is coughing without mobilizing or expectorating sputum.

49. a. A patient in a coma is unable to respond.
    b. This helps only skin circulation in the small area being massaged.
    c. A patient in a coma is unable to respond.
    d. This helps respirations by preventing fluid from collecting in the lung, which can cause infection; it helps circulation since activity increases circulation, and it relieves local pressure.

50. a. Whatever is causing the obstruction is not caught in the esophagus, which leads to the stomach, but in the respiratory system.
    b. Pressing on the heart (compression) is used in cardiopulmonary resuscitation (CPR).
    c. When trapped air behind an obstruction is forced out, it pushes out what is causing the obstruction.
    d. Whatever is causing the obstruction is not caught in the esophagus, which leads to the stomach, but in the respiratory system.

Urinary Elimination

KEYWORDS

The following words include English vocabulary, nursing/medical terminology, concepts, principles, or information relevant to content specifically addressed in the chapter or associated with topics presented in it. English dictionaries, your nursing textbooks, and medical dictionaries such as *Taber's Cyclopedic Medical Dictionary* are resources that can be used to expand your knowledge and understanding of these words and related information.

24-hour urine collection
Acidic urine
Anuria
Bacteruria
Bladder cues
Bladder irritability
Bladder training
Blood urea nitrogen
Catheter port
Clean catch urine specimen
Commode chair
Condom catheter
Credé maneuver
Cystoscopy
Detrusor muscles
Dysuria
Enuresis
Excretion
Filtration
Foreskin
Fracture bedpan
Glomerular filtration rate
Graduate
Hematuria

Incontinence
   Functional
   Overflow
   Reflex
   Stress
   Total
   Urge
Incontinence pad
Incontinent
Kegel exercises
Ketones
Leg bag
Micturition
Nocturia
Oliguria
Perineal care
Polyuria
Prostate
Pyuria
Reagent strips
Renal calculi
Renal dialysis
Renal perfusion
Residual
Retention

Specific gravity
Suprapubic distention
Trigone
Turbidity
Urea
Ureter
Urethra
Urgency
Urinalysis
Urinary catheters
   Indwelling (Foley)
   Straight catheter
   Suprapubic catheter
   Texas catheter
Urinary diuresis
Urinary diversion
Urinary drainage bag
Urinary hesitancy
Urinary meatus
Urinary obstruction
Urinary output
Urinary tract infection
Urine clarity
Urine specimen from a catheter port
Void

QUESTIONS

1. What should the nurse monitor to best assess a patient's renal perfusion?
   a. Blood pressure every 15 minutes
   b. Urinary output every hour
   c. Body weight every day
   d. I&O every 24 hours

2. Which is a major contributing factor to stress incontinence?
   a. Decreased bladder capacity
   b. Spinal cord dysfunction
   c. Cognitive impairment
   d. Weak pelvic muscles

3. Which is most important when caring for a patient with a urinary retention catheter?
   a. Ensuring that the catheter remains connected to the collection bag
   b. Wearing sterile gloves when accessing the specimen port
   c. Cleansing the urinary meatus with Betadine daily
   d. Increasing fluid intake to 3000 cc per day

4. When assessing for the presence of dysuria, the nurse should ask, "Do you:
   a. Feel that you are able to empty your bladder fully each time you void?"
   b. Have a problem stopping or starting the flow of urine?"
   c. Pass a little urine when you cough or sneeze?"
   d. Experience any pain or burning on urination?"

5. Which adaptation would indicate urinary retention?
   a. Wet bed and undergarments
   b. Burning and pain on voiding
   c. Sudden, overwhelming need to void
   d. Bladder fullness in the absence of voiding

6. An additional nursing diagnosis appropriate for a patient with the nursing diagnoses Bowel Incontinence and Total Incontinence would be Risk for:
   a. Disuse Syndrome
   b. Deficient Fluid Volume
   c. Impaired Skin Integrity
   d. Imbalanced Nutrition Less Than Body Requirements

7. When the nurse documents that the patient has polyuria the nurse is communicating that the patient is:
   a. Excreting excessive amounts of urine
   b. Experiencing pain on urination
   c. Retaining urine in the bladder
   d. Passing blood in the urine

8. Which liquid is unrelated to bladder irritability?
   a. Beer
   b. Coffee
   c. Orange juice
   d. Cranberry juice

9. What is the most common adaptation associated with excessive production of the hormone ADH?
   a. Diuresis
   b. Oliguria
   c. Retention
   d. Incontinence

10. Which nursing intervention would be of the greatest help to most people who need to void for a urine test?
    a. Exerting manual pressure on the abdomen
    b. Encouraging a backward rocking motion
    c. Running water in the sink
    d. Providing for privacy

11. Which is a major contributing factor to overflow incontinence?
    a. Coughing
    b. Mobility deficits
    c. Prostate enlargement
    d. Urinary tract infection

12. The most appropriate way to accurately measure urine output from a urinary retention catheter is via a:
    a. Urinal
    b. Graduate
    c. 30 cc syringe
    d. Urine drainage bag

13. The patient's urine is cloudy, amber, and has an unpleasant odor. The nurse makes the inference that the patient has:
    a. Urinary retention
    b. A urinary tract infection
    c. Ketone bodies in the urine
    d. A high urinary calcium level

14. The intervention that would be most helpful in meeting the needs of a debilitated female patient with nocturia would be:
    a. Encouraging the use of bladder training exercises
    b. Providing assistance with toileting every 4 hours
    c. Positioning a bedside commode near the bed
    d. Teaching the avoidance of fluids after 5 p.m

15. When collecting a urine specimen for culture and sensitivity via a straight catheter, the nurse should:
    a. Use a sterile specimen container
    b. Collect the urine from the catheter port
    c. Inflate the balloon with 10 cc of sterile water
    d. Have the patient void before collecting the specimen

16. Which nursing diagnosis would be the most appropriate for the patient who states, "I can't hold my water once I feel like I have to go."
    a. Reflex Incontinence
    b. Stress Incontinence
    c. Total Incontinence
    d. Urge Incontinence

17. Which action is most important when caring for a patient with a condom catheter?
    a. Providing perineal care every shift
    b. Avoiding kinks in the collection tubing
    c. Ensuring that the Velcro strap is snug, not tight
    d. Retracting the foreskin before the catheter is applied

18. When caring for a patient on bed rest who has a urinary retention catheter, the nurse should:
    a. Irrigate the tubing to ensure patency
    b. Label the tubing with the date that it was inserted
    c. Ensure that the tubing is positioned over the leg
    d. Hang the collection bag on the side rail of the bed

19. Which adaptation best supports the presence of urinary retention?
    a. Nocturia
    b. Hematuria
    c. Bladder contractions
    d. Suprapubic distention

20. Which should be avoided to prevent urinary diuresis?
    a. Narcotics
    b. Caffeine
    c. Activity
    d. Protein

21. The nurse recognizes that additional teaching about fluid intake and urinary incontinence is necessary when the patient said, "If I drink:
    a. Less, I will reduce the risk of loss of bladder control."
    b. More, it will help prevent irritation of my bladder."
    c. Less, it can contribute to a urinary tract infection."
    d. More, I am less likely to become dehydrated."

22. Which constituent, if found in urine, would indicate an abnormality?
    a. Electrolytes
    b. Protein
    c. Water
    d. Urea

23. Which would be the best question to obtain information about a patient's dysuria?
    a. "Tell me about the problems you have been having with urination?"
    b. "How would you describe your experience with incontinence?"
    c. "What are your usual bowel habits?"
    d. "What color is your urine?"

24. Which patient adaptation would cause the most concern?
    a. Anuria
    b. Dysuria
    c. Diuresis
    d. Enuresis

25. A nursing diagnosis most commonly associated with urinary incontinence is:
    a. Deficient Fluid Volume
    b. Disturbed Self-Esteem
    c. Deficient Knowledge
    d. Chronic Pain

26. Which defining characteristic is common to both nursing diagnoses Reflex Incontinence and Total Incontinence?
    a. Urination following an increase in intra-abdominal pressure
    b. Loss of urine without awareness of bladder fullness
    c. Retention of urine with overflow incontinence
    d. Strong, sudden desire to void

27. What action is most important when removing a urinary retention catheter?
    a. Deflate the balloon
    b. Wear sterile gloves
    c. Clean the meatus with soap and water before removal
    d. Dispose of the equipment in an appropriate waste container

28. Which adaptation can the nurse expect when a postoperative patient experiences stress associated with surgery?
    a. Decreased urinary output
    b. Specific gravity of 1.010
    c. Reflex incontinence
    d. Urinary hesitancy

29. What would be the best nursing action to facilitate bladder continence for the patient who is cognitively impaired?
    a. Offer toileting reminders every 2 hours
    b. Provide clothing that is easy to manipulate
    c. Encourage avoidance of fluid between meals
    d. Explain the need to call for the nurse for help with toileting

30. Which nursing intervention takes priority when caring for a bed-bound patient who has Total Incontinence?
    a. Insertion of a retention catheter
    b. Application of an incontinence device
    c. Skin care after episodes of incontinence
    d. Positioning a protective pad under the patient

31. Which is not common to an assessment of both urine and stool?
    a. Constituents
    b. Urgency
    c. Shape
    d. Color

32. Which adaptation indicates that additional assessments are necessary regarding the urinary status of a patient?
    a. Aromatic odor
    b. Pale yellow urine
    c. Specific gravity of 1.035
    d. Output of 50 cc every hour

33. What is a classic indication that a patient has urinary retention with overflow?
    a. Burning with urination
    b. Passing dark yellow urine
    c. Involuntary urination at night
    d. Voiding small amounts of urine frequently

34. Which nursing diagnosis would be most appropriate for the patient who states, "It burns and stings every time I pass urine."
    a. Urinary Retention
    b. Reflex Incontinence
    c. Stress Incontinence
    d. Impaired Urinary Elimination

35. Which is a contributing factor to urinary urgency?
    a. Anesthesia
    b. Full bladder
    c. Dehydration
    d. Urinary obstruction

36. The nurse should encourage an older adult to drink 8 ounces of cranberry juice daily because it:
    a. Dilutes bacterial growth
    b. Promotes an acidic urine
    c. Prevents urinary retention
    d. Stimulates hypoactive detrusor muscles

37. What would be the most appropriate statement the nurse should say to a patient who is about to have a retention catheter removed?
    a. "You may have some temporary incontinence until the bladder reestablishes control."
    b. "You can void into the toilet, but just tell me so I can check it before you flush."
    c. "Bleeding after removal of a catheter is a usual problem so don't be concerned."
    d. "You need to keep track of your fluid intake to avoid a urinary tract infection."

38. A patient with which history would be at highest risk for stress incontinence? A history of:
    a. Lumbar spinal cord injury
    b. Urinary obstruction
    c. Six vaginal births
    d. Confusion

39. What is the most effective nursing intervention to prevent urinary tract infections?
    a. Explain that patients should report burning on urination to the physician
    b. Teach female patients to wipe from the back to the front after urinating
    c. Instruct patients to use bath powder to absorb perineal perspiration
    d. Encourage patients to drink at least 2500 cc every 24 hours

40. Which is the best nursing intervention for a patient with urinary incontinence?
    a. Drying the area well after perineal care
    b. Dusting the perineal area with cornstarch
    c. Providing skin care immediately after soiling
    d. Using a deodorant soap when providing skin care

ANSWERS AND RATIONALES

1. a. Blood pressure measurements do not directly reflect renal perfusion. However, blood pressure measurements reflect cardiac and circulatory functioning and fluid balance, which indirectly provide vague information in relation to renal perfusion.
   b. **Adequate renal perfusion and kidney function are reflected by an hourly urine output of 30 to 50 cc of urine.**
   c. Daily weights reflect fluid balance. One liter of fluid weighs approximately 2.2 pounds.
   d. This is too long a time period to reflect renal perfusion. Intake and output over 24 hours reflects fluid balance.

2. a. This is related to urge incontinence, not stress incontinence.
   b. This is related to reflex incontinence, not stress incontinence.
   c. This is related to total incontinence, not stress incontinence.
   d. **Stress incontinence is an immediate involuntary loss of urine during an increase in intra-abdominal pressure. It is related to weak or degenerated pelvic muscles and structural supports.**

3. a. **Maintaining the connection of the catheter to the drainage bag prevents the introduction of microorganisms that can cause infection. A urinary retention catheter is a closed system that should remain closed.**
   b. Clean, not sterile, gloves should be worn. Surgical asepsis (use of a sterile syringe and alcohol swab) is necessary when accessing the specimen port on a urinary retention catheter.
   c. Betadine is irritating to mucous membranes. Soap and water is adequate.
   d. This is unnecessary. A fluid intake of 2000 to 2500 cc is adequate to promote renal perfusion and urinary tract functioning.

4. a. This question might be asked if there is a concern that the person is retaining urine in the bladder after urinating (residual urine).
   b. This question might be asked if there is a concern that the person is experiencing a difficulty initiating urination (hesitancy) or urge incontinence.
   c. This question relates to stress incontinence, which is the immediate involuntary loss of urine during an increase in intra-abdominal pressure.
   d. **This question relates to painful or difficult urination (dysuria). It is most often caused by bladder or urethral inflammation or trauma.**

5. a. Urine is being passed from, not retained in, the bladder. Voiding in bed at night (nocturnal enuresis) and wet undergarments indicate urinary incontinence.
   b. Painful or difficult urination is called dysuria, not urinary retention.
   c. A sudden, overwhelming need to void is called urgency, not urinary retention.
   d. **With urinary retention urine accumulates in and distends the bladder, resulting in bladder fullness, absence of voiding, and suprapubic distention.**

6. a. These diagnoses are unrelated to Disuse Syndrome, the state in which an individual is experiencing or at risk for deterioration of body systems or altered functioning as a result of prescribed or unavoidable musculoskeletal inactivity.
   b. These diagnoses are unrelated to Deficient Fluid Volume, which is the state in which an individual who is not NPO experiences or is at risk of experiencing vascular, interstitial, or intracellular dehydration.
   c. **With Total Incontinence there is a continuous unpredictable loss of urine and with Bowel Incontinence there is an involuntary passage of stool. Urine is acidic and stool contains digestive enzymes, both of which are irritating to the skin unless removed immediately.**
   d. These diagnoses are unrelated to Imbalanced Nutrition Less Than Body Requirements, which is the state in which an individual who is not NPO experiences or is at risk for inadequate intake or metabolism of nutrients for metabolic needs with or without weight loss.

7. a. **Polyuria is an excessive output of urine. This is associated with problems such as diabetes mellitus, diabetes insipidus, diuresis phase after a burn injury, and reduced antidiuretic hormone.**
   b. This is the definition of dysuria.
   c. This is the definition of urinary retention.
   d. This is the definition of hematuria.

8. a. Beer contains alcohol, which is irritating to the bladder.
   b. Coffee contains caffeine, which is irritating to the bladder.
   c. Orange juice, a citrus fruit, is irritating to the bladder.
   d. **Cranberries have no constituents that irritate the bladder. In addition, it produces a more acidic environment that is less conducive to the growth of microorganisms and prevents bacteria from adhering to the mucous membranes of the urinary tract, promoting their excretion.**

9. a. Diuresis occurs when there is inadequate antidiuretic hormone.
   b. **Antidiuretic hormone (ADH) increases the reabsorption of water by the kidney tubules, decreasing the amount of urine formed. Oliguria is diminished urinary output relative to intake (less than 400 cc in 24 hours).**
   c. With urinary retention urine is formed but it accumulates in the bladder and is not excreted.
   d. Antidiuretic hormone is unrelated to incontinence.

10. a. Manual bladder compression (Credé maneuver) is performed when a patient has bladder flaccidity and is not expected to regain voluntary control.
    b. This rocking motion is used to promote a bowel movement, not voiding.
    c. Although this may be helpful, it is not as important as an intervention in another option.
    d. Few people can void on demand with an

audience. Tending to bodily functions is a personal, private activity in the North American culture. Providing privacy supports patient dignity.

11. a. Coughing, which raises the intra-abdominal pressure, is related to stress incontinence, not overflow incontinence.
    b. Mobility deficits, such as spinal cord injuries, are related to reflex incontinence, not overflow incontinence.
    c. **An enlarged prostate compresses the urethra and interferes with the outflow of urine, resulting in urinary retention. With urinary retention, the pressure within the bladder builds until the external urethral sphincter temporarily opens to allow a small volume (25 to 60 cc) of urine to escape (overflow incontinence).**
    d. Urinary tract infections are related to urge incontinence, not overflow incontinence.

12. a. Although urinals have volume markings on the side, usually they occur in 100 cc increments that do not promote accurate measurements.
    b. **A graduate is a collection container with volume markings usually at 25 cc increments that promote accurate measurements of urine volume.**
    c. This is impractical. A 30 cc syringe is used to obtain a sterile specimen from a Foley catheter.
    d. A Foley collection bag is flexible and balloons outward as urine collects. In addition, the volume markings are at 100 cc increments that do not promote accurate measurements.

13. a. These adaptations do not reflect urinary retention. Urinary retention is evidenced by suprapubic distention and lack of voiding or small, frequent voidings (overflow incontinence).
    b. **The urine appears concentrated (amber) and cloudy because of the presence of bacteria, white blood cells, and red blood cells. The unpleasant odor is caused by pus in the urine (pyuria).**
    c. These adaptations do not reflect ketone bodies in the urine. A reagent strip dipped in urine will measure the presence of ketone bodies.
    d. These adaptations do not reflect excessive calcium in the urine. Urine calcium levels are measured by assessing a 24-hour urine specimen.

14. a. Although this should be done, something must be done to ensure safe urination at night.
    b. This may be too often or not often enough for the patient. A bladder-retraining program should be individualized for the patient.
    c. **The use of a commode requires less energy than using a bedpan or walking to the bathroom. The normal anatomical position uses gravity to empty the bladder fully and thus prevent urinary stasis.**
    d. Fluids may be decreased during the evening or night but they should not be avoided completely. Some fluid intake is necessary for adequate renal perfusion.

15. a. **A culture attempts to identify the microorganisms present in the urine and a sensitivity identifies the antibiotics that are**

effective against the isolated microorganisms. A sterile specimen container is used to prevent contamination of the specimen by microorganisms outside the body (exogenous).
    b. The urine from a straight catheter (single lumen tube) flows directly into the specimen container. Collecting a urine specimen from a catheter port is necessary when the patient has a urinary retention catheter.
    c. A straight catheter has a single lumen for draining urine from the bladder. A straight catheter does not remain in the bladder and therefore does not have a second lumen for water to be inserted into a balloon.
    d. This could result in no urine left in the bladder for the straight catheter to collect. A minimum of 3 cc of urine is necessary for a specimen for urine culture and sensitivity.

16. a. This statement is unrelated to reflex incontinence, which is the involuntary loss of urine occurring at somewhat predictable intervals.
    b. This statement is unrelated to stress incontinence, which is the immediate involuntary loss of urine during an increase in intra-abdominal pressure.
    c. This is unrelated to total incontinence, which is a continuous unpredictable loss of urine without distention or awareness of bladder fullness.
    d. **This statement is related to urge incontinence, which is an involuntary loss of urine associated with a strong, sudden desire to urinate.**

17. a. This is unnecessary. Perineal hygiene should be performed at least once a day and whenever the catheter is changed or replaced.
    b. Although this is important to promote the flow of urine from the patient to the drainage bag, it is not as important as an action in another option.
    c. **The anchoring device (e.g., Velcro, elastic, self-adhesive, inflatable ring) must be snug enough to prevent the condom from falling off but not so tight that it interferes with blood circulation to the penis.**
    d. This is contraindicated. If left in this position, it can constrict the penis and result in edema and tissue injury.

18. a. This is contraindicated because it may introduce microorganisms into the bladder that can cause an infection. Irrigation of a urinary retention catheter is not done prophylactically.
    b. This information should be documented on the patient's hospital record, not the tubing.
    c. **This prevents pressure of the leg on the drainage tube that can interrupt the flow of urine out of the bladder.**
    d. A urine drainage bag should hang on the bed frame. If left on a side rail the catheter may inadvertently be pulled out when the side rail is moved. In addition, it must be kept below the level of the bladder to promote the flow of urine out of the bladder by gravity and prevent a flow of urine back into the bladder from the catheter.

19. a. Excessive urination at night is called nocturia. A person with urinary retention will have small, frequent voidings or dribbling (overflow

incontinence) rather than a complete discharge of urine from the bladder.

b. Hematuria is the presence of red blood cells in the urine. It is associated with bladder inflammation, infection, or trauma, not urinary retention.

c. Urinary retention may produce an atonic bladder rather than bladder contractions.

d. **The bladder lies in the pelvic cavity behind the symphysis pubis. When it fills with urine (600 cc), it extends above the symphysis pubis and when greatly distended (2000 to 3000 cc) it can reach to the umbilicus.**

20. a. Narcotics are central nervous system depressants that can cause urinary retention, not diuresis.

b. **Drinks with caffeine (e.g., coffee, tea, and some carbonated beverages) promote diuresis, which is secretion and excretion of large amounts of urine.**

c. Although activity may increase renal perfusion, which may increase urinary output, the increased fluid lost during activity usually is through insensible losses (e.g., perspiration, moisture in exhaled breaths).

d. Avoiding protein does not prevent diuresis. The presence of protein in the urine indicates that the glomeruli have become too permeable, which occurs with kidney disease. Most plasma proteins are too large to move out of the glomeruli and the small proteins that enter the filtrate are reabsorbed by pinocytosis.

21. a. **The patient needs further teaching. The etiology of urinary incontinence rarely is related to the volume of urine. In addition, if the bladder is not challenged by the presence of fluid, the detrusor muscle loses its tone, promoting incontinence.**

b. This is true. Dilute urine is less irritating to the mucous membranes of the bladder than concentrated urine.

c. This is true. Less fluid intake results in concentrated urine that is more conducive to the growth of bacteria and in less fluid for voiding that could flush microorganisms from the lower urinary tract.

d. This is true. An adequate fluid intake provides enough fluids for biologic processes and urinary and insensible losses. Maintaining fluid balance prevents dehydration.

22. a. Electrolytes are normal constituents of urine, and they fluctuate to help maintain fluid and electrolyte and acid-base balance.

b. **The presence of protein in the urine indicates that the glomeruli have become too permeable, which occurs with kidney disease. Most plasma proteins are too large to move out of the glomeruli and the small proteins that enter the filtrate are reabsorbed by pinocytosis.**

c. Urine normally is composed of 95% water.

d. Urea is a normal constituent of urine. It is formed by liver cells when excess amino acids are broken down (deaminated) to be used for energy production.

23. a. **This open-ended question encourages the patient to talk about the problem from a personal perspective. Follow-up questions can be more specific.**

b. Dysuria is not necessarily related to incontinence.

c. Dysuria is a problem associated with urine, not fecal, elimination.

d. Although an abnormal color of urine may indicate a potential urinary tract infection, which is associated with dysuria, the question is too narrow because it focuses on only one issue.

24. a. **The inability to produce urine (anuria) is a life-threatening situation. If the cause is not corrected, the patient will need dialysis to correct fluid and electrolyte imbalances and rid the body of the waste products of metabolism.**

b. Although this is a concern because it may indicate a urinary tract infection, it is not as serious as an adaptation in another option.

c. The secretion and excretion of large amounts of urine (diuresis) is a concern but it is not as serious as an adaptation in another option.

d. Involuntary discharge of urine after an age when bladder control should have been established (enuresis) is a concern but it is not as serious as an adaptation in another option.

25. a. Deficient Fluid Volume is unrelated to urinary incontinence. Deficient Fluid Volume is the state in which an individual who is not NPO experiences or is at risk of experiencing vascular, interstitial, or intracellular dehydration.

b. **Disturbed Self-Esteem is the state in which an individual experiences or is at risk of experiencing negative self-evaluation about self or capabilities. Incontinence may be viewed by the patient as regressing to child-like behavior and has a negative impact on feelings about the self.**

c. Urinary incontinence may be unpreventable and uncontrollable. Sufficient knowledge may or may not prevent or promote continence. Deficient knowledge is the state in which an individual or group experiences a deficiency in cognitive knowledge or psychomotor skills concerning the condition or treatment plan.

d. Urinary incontinence usually is not related to chronic pain. Chronic pain is the state in which an individual experiences pain that is persistent or intermittent and lasts for longer than 6 months.

26. a. This is related to stress incontinence, which is an immediate involuntary loss of urine during an increase in intra-abdominal pressure.

b. **Involuntary voiding and a lack of awareness of bladder distention are related directly to both nursing diagnoses Reflex Incontinence and Total Incontinence. Reflex Incontinence is the predictable, involuntary loss of urine with no sensation of urge, voiding, or bladder fullness. Total Incontinence is the continuous unpredictable loss of urine without distention or awareness of bladder fullness.**

c. This is related to urinary retention, which is the chronic inability to void followed by involuntary voiding (overflow incontinence).

d. This is related to urge incontinence, which is an involuntary loss of urine associated with a strong, sudden desire to void.

27. a. Deflating the balloon with a syringe ensures that the original amount of fluid instilled is removed. Complete deflation of the balloon prevents trauma to the urethra as the catheter is removed.
   b. Clean, not sterile, gloves should be worn. Medical, not surgical, asepsis is necessary when removing a urinary retention catheter.
   c. This is done after, not before, the catheter is removed.
   d. Although this is an important medical asepsis practice, it is not as important as the action in another option.

28. a. During the General Adaptation Syndrome the posterior pituitary secretes antidiuretic hormone that promotes water reabsorption in the kidney tubules and the anterior pituitary secretes adrenocorticotropic hormone (ACTH) that stimulates the adrenal cortex to secrete aldosterone, which reabsorbs sodium and water
   b. A specific gravity of 1.010, low within the normal range, reflects dilute urine. With the stress response, the urine will be concentrated and the specific gravity will be elevated.
   c. The stress response is unrelated to reflex incontinence. Reflex incontinence is a predictable, involuntary loss of urine with no sensation of urge, voiding, or bladder fullness.
   d. The stress response is unrelated to urinary hesitancy. Hesitancy is the involuntary delay in initiating urination.

29. a. A cognitively impaired person may not be able to receive, interpret, or respond to cues for voiding. Reminding the person to void every 2 hours empties the bladder, which limits episodes of incontinence.
   b. Although this might be done, it is not the most important intervention. A cognitively impaired person may or may not have problems with handling clothing when voiding.
   c. Restriction of fluid intake is an inappropriate way to manage urinary incontinence. The body needs fluids throughout the day to maintain renal perfusion, kidney function, and fluid balance.
   d. A cognitively impaired person may not be able to receive, interpret, or respond to cues for voiding, understand cause and effect, or follow directions.

30. a. This is avoided because it increases the risk of developing a urinary tract infection.
   b. A condom catheter may be used for some male patients but there really are no effective urine collecting incontinence devices for women.
   c. Urine is acidic and contains ammonium chloride, which reacts with bacteria (producing a characteristic ammonia odor). These constituents of urine are irritating to the skin and should be removed immediately.
   d. Although this is advisable, it is done to protect the linens, not the patient, who should be the priority.

31. a. Both urine and stool have normal constituents. Urine has organic constituents (e.g., urea, uric acid, creatinine) and inorganic constituents (e.g., ammonia, sodium, chloride, potassium, calcium). Feces have waste residues of digestion (e.g., bile, intestinal secretions, bacteria) and inorganic constituents (e.g., calcium, phosphorus).
   b. A person can feel an overwhelming need to void as well as defecate.
   c. Only stool can be assessed regarding shape. Stool normally is tubular in shape. Urine is a liquid that assumes the shape of the container in which it is collected.
   d. Both urine and stool can be assessed for color. Normal stool is brown and normal urine is yellow, straw-colored, or amber depending on its concentration.

32. a. This is the normal odor of urine.
   b. Urine normally is pale yellow, straw-colored, or amber depending on its concentration.
   c. Specific gravity is the measure of the concentration of dissolved solids in the urine. The normal range is 1.010 to 1.025.
   d. Adequate renal perfusion and kidney function are reflected by an hourly urine output of 30 to 50 cc of urine.

33. a. This is dysuria. The discomfort is felt as acidic urine flows past inflamed tissue.
   b. This is concentrated urine, which usually is associated with dehydration.
   c. This is nocturnal enuresis.
   d. With urinary retention, the pressure within the bladder builds until the external urethral sphincter temporarily opens to allow a small volume (25 to 60 cc) of urine to escape. As the urine leaves the bladder, the pressure falls and the sphincter closes. This can happen 2 to 3 times an hour with urinary retention.

34. a. This adaptation is not associated with urinary retention, which is the chronic inability to void followed by involuntary voiding (overflow incontinence).
   b. This adaptation is not associated with reflex incontinence, which is the predictable, involuntary loss of urine with no sensation of urge, voiding, or bladder fullness.
   c. This adaptation is not associated with stress incontinence, which is the immediate involuntary loss of urine during an increase in intra-abdominal pressure.
   d. Burning on urination (dysuria) is associated with urgency and frequency. Urgency and frequency are defining characteristics of the nursing diagnosis Impaired Urinary Elimination and usually are caused by bladder or urethral inflammation or trauma.

35. a. Anesthesia is a central nervous system depressant that tends to cause urinary retention, not urgency.
   b. Feeling the need to void immediately (urgency) occurs most often when the urinary bladder is full. In the adult, the bladder normally holds 600 cc of urine, although the desire to urinate can be sensed when it contains as little as 150 to 200 cc. As the volume increases, the bladder wall stretches, sending sensory messages to the sacral spinal cord, and parasympathetic impulses

stimulate the detrusor muscle to contract rhythmically. Bladder contractions precipitate nerve impulses that travel up the spinal cord to the pons and cerebral cortex where the person experiences a conscious need to void.

c. Dehydration causes a decrease in renal perfusion that results in a diminished capacity to form urine (oliguria), not urgency.

d. Urinary obstruction causes suprapubic distention and pain, not urgency.

36. a. Cranberry juice does not dilute bacterial growth. The constituents of cranberries, not the volume of fluid, prevent urinary tract infections (UTIs). Older adults have a greater risk for UTIs because of decreased bladder tone and increased urine residual.

b. Foods that promote an acid urine (e.g., cranberries, prunes, plums, eggs, meat, and whole grain breads) create an environment that is not conducive to the growth of bacteria. Microorganisms grow more readily in an alkaline urine.

c. Cranberry juice does not prevent urinary retention.

d. Cranberry juice does not stimulate hypoactive detrusor muscles.

37. a. Irritation of the internal and external sphincters from when the urinary retention catheter was in place takes time to resolve once the catheter is removed. In addition, because the bladder has been decompressed, it takes time for the cues for voiding (stretch receptors, bladder tone, sphincter functioning) to become responsive.

b. This is unsafe. After a urinary retention catheter is removed, at least the first voided specimen should be measured, assessed, and documented in the patient's medical record.

c. Bleeding is not expected after the removal of a urinary retention catheter. A further assessment is necessary to determine its cause.

d. Although an adequate fluid intake (2000 to 2500 cc) helps to flush microorganisms from the lower urinary tract, just keeping track of the amount of fluid will not prevent infection. Appropriate toileting practices help to prevent urinary tract infections.

38. a. A person with a spinal cord injury will experience reflex incontinence, not stress incontinence.

b. A person with a urinary tract obstruction will experience urinary retention, not stress incontinence.

c. Stress incontinence is an immediate involuntary loss of urine during an increase in intra-abdominal pressure. It is associated with weak pelvic muscles and structural supports resulting from multiple pregnancies, age-related degenerative changes, and overdistention between voiding.

d. A confused person may experience total incontinence, not stress incontinence.

39. a. This will not prevent a urinary tract infection. Burning on urination (dysuria) is an adaptation to acidic urine flowing over inflamed mucous membranes and is a sign of a urinary tract infection.

b. The opposite should be done to prevent microorganisms from the intestines (e.g., *Escherichia coli*) from being drawn from the anus towards the urinary meatus.

c. This should be avoided because it has been implicated as a precipitating cause of gynecological cancer.

d. Drinking 2500 cc of fluid a day produces adequately dilute urine, washes out solutes, and flushes microorganisms out of the distal urethra and urinary meatus.

40. a. Although this is done, it is not the best intervention of the options offered.

b. This should be avoided. Cornstarch can accumulate in folds of the skin and when damp can become like sandpaper and cause friction upon movement.

c. As soon as possible after an incontinence episode, the patient should receive thorough perineal care with soap and water and the area dried well. This action removes urea from the skin, which can contribute to skin breakdown.

d. Plain soap, not deodorant soap, is all that is necessary when providing perineal care after urinary or bowel incontinence.

Intestinal Elimination

QUESTIONS

1. Which word is unique regarding how a soapsuds enema works on the mucosa of the bowel?
   a. Dilating
   b. Irritating
   c. Softening
   d. Lubricating

2. The best time to toilet a patient to encourage bowel training is:
   a. One hour after the patient's meals
   b. Every four hours while the patient is awake
   c. When the patient experiences abdominal fullness
   d. Immediately when a patient has the urge to defecate

3. Which is most important when caring for a patient with a colostomy stoma?
   a. Cleansing the stoma with cool water
   b. Spraying an air-freshening deodorant in the room
   c. Selecting a bag with an appropriate sized stomal opening
   d. Wearing sterile non-latex gloves when caring for the stoma

4. The nursing diagnosis of Perceived Constipation is made when the patient states that a bowel movement is expected every day and:
   a. Inspection of the abdomen reveals distention
   b. Hard, dry stools are defecated daily
   c. Straining is required to pass stool
   d. Laxatives are used excessively

5. Which statement by the patient with diverticulosis would indicate the need for additional health teaching?
   a. "I love to eat strawberries with my morning cereal."
   b. "I sit on the toilet for 10 minutes after breakfast every day."
   c. "I'm going to drink eight glasses of water a day when I get home."
   d. "I like to massage my lower abdomen when I'm trying to have a BM."

6. Which factor could influence the occurrence of diarrhea and constipation?
   a. Increased metabolic rate
   b. High solute tube feedings
   c. Side effects of medications
   d. Inability to perceive bowel cues

7. The nurse recognizes that when compared to other nasogastric tubes used for gastric decompression, a Salem sump tube is uniquely designed to:
   a. Minimize the risk of bowel obstruction
   b. Ensure drainage of the intestines
   c. Prevent gastric mucosal damage
   d. Promote gastric rest

8. What would be the expected color of stool for a patient admitted with a diagnosis of upper GI bleeding?
   a. Red
   b. Pink
   c. Black
   d. Brown

9. Which statement should the nurse use when teaching the patient to avoid foods that have a laxative effect? "You should avoid:
   a. Applesauce."
   b. Chocolate."
   c. Coffee."
   d. Pasta."

10. When administering a small volume hypertonic enema to an adult the nurse should:
    a. Insert the rectal tube 1 to 1.5 inches into the rectum
    b. Maintain pressure on the enema container until after withdrawing the tube
    c. Direct the rectal tube toward the vertebrae as it is inserted into the rectum
    d. Position the enema bottle 12 inches above the level of the patient's rectum

11. Before collecting a stool sample for occult blood, the nurse should:
    a. Wash the patient's perianal area with soap and water
    b. Ask the patient to void before collecting the stool
    c. Plan to collect the first specimen of the day
    d. Secure a sterile specimen container

12. Which is a defining characteristic of the nursing diagnosis Bowel Incontinence?
    a. Frequent, soft stools
    b. Involuntary passage of stool
    c. Impaired rectal sphincter control
    d. Greenish-yellow color to the stool

13. Which question would take priority when collecting a bowel elimination history for a newly admitted patient with a medical diagnosis of possible bowel obstruction?
    a. "Do you use anything to help you move your bowels?"
    b. "When was the last time you moved your bowels?"
    c. "What color are your usual bowel movements?"
    d. "How often do you have a bowel movement?"

14. Which is the most serious adaptation associated with gastric reflux disease?
    a. Diarrhea
    b. Heartburn
    c. Gastric fullness
    d. Esophageal erosion

15. A fracture bedpan should be used for the patient who:
    a. Has a spinal cord injury
    b. Is on bed rest
    c. Has dementia
    d. Is obese

16. Which food works best to increase the bulk in fecal material?
    a. Whole wheat bread
    b. White rice
    c. Pasta
    d. Kale

17. Which statement by a patient with an ileostomy would indicate the need for further education?
    a. "I don't expect to have much of a problem with fecal odor."
    b. "I will have to take special precautions to protect my skin around the stoma."
    c. "I'm going to irrigate my stoma so I have a bowel movement every morning."
    d. "I should avoid gas-forming foods like beans to limit funny noises from the stoma."

18. Which is a major defining characteristic for the nursing diagnosis Diarrhea?
    a. Spastic colon
    b. Impaired sphincter control
    c. Inability to respond to rectal cues
    d. Loose stools more than 3 times a day

19. The nurse discourages straining on defecation primarily because if performed by the patient it could precipitate:
    a. Incontinence
    b. Dysrhythmias
    c. Fecal impaction
    d. Rectal hemorrhoids

20. Mucus in the gastrointestinal tract:
    a. Activates digestive enzymes
    b. Protects the gastric mucosa
    c. Enhances gastric acidity
    d. Emulsifies fats

21. What should the nurse do first when designing and implementing a bowel training program?
    a. Identify factors that hinder defecation
    b. Start the program with a clean bowel
    c. Secure a physician's order
    d. Modify the patient's diet

22. Which would contribute to softening of stool?
    a. Applesauce
    b. Bananas
    c. Cheese
    d. Beans

23. Which independent action by the nurse facilitates defecation of a hard stool?
    a. Applying a lubricant to the anus
    b. Encouraging a sitz bath after defecation
    c. Instilling warm mineral oil into the rectum
    d. Positioning a cold compress against the anus

24. Which action is most important when administering an enema?
    a. Instructing the patient to take deep breaths
    b. Positioning a waterproof pad under the patient
    c. Inserting the enema tube 5 inches into the rectum
    d. Elevating the enema solution container less than 12 inches above the anus

25. The most important action when caring for a nasogastric tube for decompression is:
    a. Using sterile technique when irrigating the tube
    b. Recording the intake and output every 2 hours
    c. Maintaining suction at the prescribed level
    d. Providing oral hygiene every 4 hours

26. Which additional nursing diagnosis would be of most concern for a patient with the nursing diagnosis Diarrhea?
    a. Imbalanced Nutrition Less Than Body Requirements
    b. Risk for Impaired Skin Integrity
    c. Risk for Deficient Fluid Volume
    d. Functional Incontinence

27. What should the nurse do if a colostomy stoma appears pale?
    a. Notify the physician
    b. Listen for bowel sounds
    c. Wash the area with warm water
    d. Gently massage around the stoma

28. A patient with flatulence is concerned about the production of unpleasant odors. This patient should be encouraged to avoid:
    a. Alcohol
    b. Raisins
    c. Coffee
    d. Eggs

29. Which person would be at the highest risk for bowel incontinence? A person who is:
    a. Ninety years old
    b. On a program of sedation for sleep
    c. Disoriented to time, place, and person
    d. Receiving multiple antibiotic medications

30. A nursing diagnosis most commonly associated with prolonged diarrhea is:
    a. Deficient Self-Care
    b. Sexual Dysfunction
    c. Disturbed Body Image
    d. Risk for Impaired Skin Integrity

31. What adaptation would indicate that the patient is experiencing lower gastrointestinal tract bleeding?
    a. Tarry-colored stool
    b. Green-mucoid stool
    c. Orange-colored stool
    d. Bright red–tinged stool

32. Which is detected in a guaiac test of stool?
    a. Bile
    b. Bacteria
    c. Occult blood
    d. Ova and parasites

33. Which action is most essential to ensure accuracy when collecting a specimen for the presence of pinworms?
    a. Press the sticky side of non-frosted cellophane tape across the anus before the patient goes to bed at night
    b. Pass a rectal swab beyond the internal rectal sphincter and rotate gently to collect a specimen
    c. Perform the procedure the first thing in the morning before the first bowel movement
    d. Wash the rectal area gently with soap and water before collecting the specimen

34. Which statement would indicate that the patient understands the need to reestablish normal bowel flora after a week of diarrhea? "I'm going to:
    a. Wean myself off of the antibiotics after my temperature is normal."
    b. Eat a container of yogurt every day for a few days."
    c. Add rice to my diet one meal each day."
    d. Drink eight glasses of water each day."

35. Which type of enema solution works by irritating the intestinal mucosa?
    a. Oil
    b. Soap
    c. Tap water
    d. Normal saline

36. Which adaptation is most significant in indicating the presence of a fecal impaction?
    a. Putrefied odorous flatus
    b. Hard, dry stools that are marble-like in size
    c. Liquid fecal seepage with no passage of stool
    d. Frank red blood surrounding passed hard dry stool

37. The excessive use of laxatives should be avoided primarily because it:
    a. Weakens the natural response to defecation
    b. Results in distention of the intestines
    c. Causes abdominal discomfort
    d. Precipitates incontinence

38. Which is the most appropriate outcome for a hospitalized patient with the nursing diagnosis Diarrhea? "The patient will:
    a. Have no more than 2 bowel movements per day."
    b. Avoid foods that are high in water-soluble fiber."
    c. Take Imodium after each bowel movement."
    d. Drink at least 8 glasses of water per day."

39. Which action is important when assisting a patient with a bedpan?
    a. Position the patient slightly off the back edge of a regular bedpan
    b. Fold the top linen out of the way when putting the patient on the bedpan
    c. Place the flat part of the rim of the fracture bedpan towards the patient's feet
    d. Once on the bedpan raise the head of the bed so that the patient is in the Fowler's position

40. Tarry stools would indicate:
    a. Upper gastrointestinal bleeding
    b. Pancreatic dysfunction
    c. Lactulose intolerance
    d. Inadequate bile salts

41. Which nutrient is best for a patient with diverticulosis?
    a. Tofu
    b. Oatmeal
    c. Corn on the cob
    d. Cucumber spears

42. Which intervention would be most effective in minimizing the use of the Valsalva maneuver?
    a. Positioning the patient in the semi-Fowler's position
    b. Exhaling while contracting the abdominal muscles
    c. Attempting to have a bowel movement every day
    d. Eating rice or pasta several times a week

43. When the nurse uses a cone attached to a colostomy irrigation catheter it works by:
    a. Stopping the outflow of enema solution during the procedure
    b. Dilating the stoma so that the enema tube can be inserted
    c. Facilitating the elimination of drainage from the colon
    d. Preventing prolapse of the bowel during peristalsis

44. Which goal would be most appropriate for a patient with the nursing diagnosis Perceived Constipation? "The patient will:
    a. Defecate every day."
    b. Drink eight glasses of water per day."
    c. Defecate without the use of a laxative."
    d. Verbalize the rationale for the use of laxatives."

45. Which is unrelated to bowel incontinence?
    a. Overdistention of the rectum
    b. Anal sphincter dysfunction
    c. Cognitive impairment
    d. Pain on defecation

46. When the vent of a double-lumen gastric sump tube becomes obstructed, what should the nurse do first?
    a. Instill 10 ml of air into the vent lumen
    b. Position the vent below the level of the stomach
    c. Position the patient in the high-Fowler's position
    d. Withdraw 30 ml of gastric contents from the drainage lumen

47. Which action is most important when teaching patients about the intake of bran to facilitate defecation?
    a. Lean forward when attempting to have a bowel movement
    b. Take a cathartic that will supplement the action of bran
    c. Start with 3 tablespoons of bran each morning
    d. Drink at least eight glasses of fluids each day

48. The nurse recognizes that a large volume tap water enema increases peristalsis by:
    a. Bowel distention
    b. Hypertonic action
    c. Irritating the bowel
    d. The stool's absorbing fluid

49. Which assessment is most indicative of a postoperative ileus?
    a. Passing flatus
    b. Presence of diarrhea
    c. Abdominal distention
    d. Increased intestinal peristalsis

50. A tap water enema is usually given to:
    a. Reduce abdominal gas
    b. Drain the urinary bladder
    c. Empty the bowel of stool
    d. Limit nausea and vomiting

1. a. High-volume (not soapsuds) enemas such as tap-water or saline enemas work by distending (dilating) the lumen of the intestine.
   b. Although a soapsuds enema works by increasing the volume in the colon, its unique attribute is that soap is irritating to the intestinal mucosa. Irritation of the mucosa precipitates peristalsis, which facilitates the evacuation of fecal material.
   c. An oil-retention enema, a small-volume enema, introduces oil into the rectum and sigmoid colon. This softens the feces and lubricates the rectum and anal canal, facilitating defecation.
   d. An oil-retention, not soapsuds, enema lubricates the rectum and anal canal, facilitating the passage of feces.

2. a. Although toileting after eating is often done to take advantage of the gastrocolic reflex, toileting should be done 20 to 30 minutes, not 1 hour, after eating.
   b. This is counterproductive and can lead to frustration. Attempting to defecate should be timed for when the patient normally defecates. Defecation frequently occurs when food or fluid enters the stomach and precipitates the gastrocolic reflex, which stimulates peristalsis.
   c. The feeling of abdominal fullness is related to abdominal distention rather than the need to defecate.
   d. The urge to defecate is associated with mass peristalsis and the pressure of feces in the rectum. When the signals for defecation are ignored, it can result in incontinence or a progressive weakening of the defecation reflex, resulting in constipation.

3. a. This is an acceptable practice. A stoma can be cleaned with water as long as it is not at the extremes of hot or cold.
   b. Although this might be done, it is not the priority.
   c. The opening of the appliance must be large enough to encircle the stoma to within 1/8 to 1/6 inch to protect the surrounding tissue from the enzymes present in the intestinal discharge without impinging on the stoma. Pressure against the stoma can damage delicate mucosal tissue or impede circulation to the stoma, both of which can impair the viability of the stoma.
   d. Clean, not sterile, gloves should be worn when caring for a stoma. Medical, not surgical, asepsis should be practiced. Latex or non-latex gloves can be worn.

4. a. Abdominal distention is a defining characteristic for the nursing diagnosis Constipation, not Perceived Constipation.
   b. The passage of hard, dry stools is a defining characteristic for the nursing diagnosis Constipation, not Perceived Constipation.
   c. Straining at stool is a defining characteristic for the nursing diagnosis Constipation, not Perceived Constipation.
   d. The defining characteristics for the nursing diagnosis Perceived Constipation are the expectation of a daily bowel movement with the resulting overuse of laxatives, enemas, and suppositories and the expected passage of stool at the same time every day.

5. a. This patient needs further teaching because people with diverticulosis should avoid foods with husks and seeds. Strawberries contain tiny seeds that may become lodged in diverticula. Fecal material may combine with these seeds and cause a fecalith that is capable of causing inflammation and perforation of the intestine.
   b. This is an accepted practice. Bowel elimination should follow a familiar routine, and attempting to defecate after breakfast takes advantage of the gastrocolic reflex.
   c. This is desirable for effective bowel function. An adequate intake of fluid ensures that after water is reabsorbed through the large intestines for essential body processes there is enough water left in the intestine to create a soft, formed stool.
   d. This is an accepted practice. Light stroking of the skin (effleurage) reduces abdominal muscle tension, which may facilitate defecation.

6. a. An increased metabolic rate would increase peristalsis and possibly result in diarrhea, not constipation.
   b. A high solute tube feeding has a greater osmotic pressure than surrounding interstitial tissue, which draws fluid into the gastrointestinal tract, which may result in diarrhea, not constipation.
   c. Medications, depending on their physiologic action, side effects, and toxic effects, can cause either constipation or diarrhea.
   d. An inability to perceive bowel cues for defecation results in a lack of response that further weakens the defecation reflex, ultimately causing constipation, not diarrhea.

7. a. Nasointestinal tubes attached to suction remove the fluid that collects behind an intestinal obstruction. They help treat, not prevent, an intestinal obstruction.
   b. All nasogastric tubes attached to suction remove drainage from the stomach, not the intestine. Nasointestinal tubes attached to suction remove fluid from the intestine.
   c. A Salem sump tube is a double-lumen, rather than a single-lumen, tube. The second lumen (blue pigtail) is open to environmental (atmospheric) air, which is drawn into the stomach to equalize the outside pressure with the pressure inside the stomach. This prevents the catheter tip from attaching to the gastric mucosa when the drainage lumen is attached to suction, limiting mucosal damage.
   d. All nasogastric tubes attached to suction empty the stomach contents in an effort to promote gastric and intestinal rest. Gastric glands produce up to 4 to 5 liters of fluid a day that stimulate the intestine unless removed.

8. a. Red-colored stool indicates lower, not upper, gastrointestinal bleeding.
   b. Pink-colored stool, although uncommon, may indicate lower gastrointestinal bleeding mixed with mucus or intestinal fluid.

c. Black (tarry) stool indicates upper gastrointestinal bleeding. Enzymes acting on the blood turn it black. In addition, iron supplements, excessive intake of red meat, and dark green vegetables can cause black stools.

d. Brown is the normal color of stool. This color is caused by the presence of stercobilin and urobilin, which are derived from a pigment in bile (bilirubin).

9. a. Cooked or canned apples do not have the same stimulating effect on the intestines as do raw apples. Applesauce does not have a laxative effect and is permitted on a low-residue diet.

b. Chocolate may cause constipation, not a softer stool.

c. Coffee contains caffeine, which has a laxative effect because it decreases bowel transit time. In addition, a warm liquid beverage stimulates the gastrocolic reflex that precipitates mass peristalsis.

d. Most pasta thickens stool. It does not have a laxative effect and is permitted on a low-residue diet.

10. a. This will not permit safe administration of the enema solution. The rectal tube must be inserted 3 to 4 inches to ensure that the catheter is beyond both the external and internal sphincters.

b. This prevents subsequent suctioning back of the fluid that has just been instilled. In addition, releasing compression on the bottle causes a vacuum at the tip of the nozzle that can injure the mucous membranes of the rectum or anus.

c. This will injure the intestinal mucosa. The catheter should be directed toward the umbilicus, not the vertebrae.

d. A small-volume enema bottle is held directly outside the anus because the solution container is attached to the prelubricated nozzle. The container of a large-volume enema should not exceed a height of 12 inches above the anus.

11. a. This is unnecessary. However, the nurse may assist the patient to perform perineal hygiene after the stool specimen has been obtained.

b. Emptying the urinary bladder before attempting to have a bowel movement prevents accidental contamination of the specimen by urine.

c. This is unnecessary.

d. This is unnecessary. Medical, not surgical, asepsis should be followed.

12. a. This is not a defining characteristic of any nursing diagnosis but it is similar to the defining characteristics for the nursing diagnosis Diarrhea, which are loose, liquid stools and/or increased frequency of stools (more than three times a day).

b. An involuntary passage of stool is a major defining characteristic of the nursing diagnosis Bowel Incontinence, which is the state in which an individual experiences a change in normal bowel habits characterized by involuntary passage of stool.

c. Impaired rectal sphincter control is a pathophysiological related factor, not defining characteristic, for the nursing diagnosis Bowel Incontinence.

d. This is unrelated to the nursing diagnosis Bowel Incontinence. A green or orange color to the stool indicates the presence of an intestinal infection.

13. a. Although this question may be asked, it is not the priority at this time.

b. A cardinal sign of a bowel obstruction is the lack of a bowel movement (obstipation).

c. Although this will be asked, this information relates more to malabsorption, biliary problems, and gastrointestinal bleeding.

d. This is not as valuable as other essential information. Although this will be asked to obtain normal baseline information about intestinal elimination, it is not specific to the presenting physical problem.

14. a. Diarrhea is not associated with GERD.

b. Pain occurring behind the sternum (heartburn) is the predominant symptom of GERD. Although this adaptation is a concern, it is not life-threatening and can be treated.

c. Although feeling full, distended, or bloated can occur with GERD, it is not life-threatening and the patient can be taught interventions to limit its occurrence.

d. With gastroesophageal reflux disease (GERD) a backflow of the contents of the stomach into the esophagus occurs. Gastric juices are acidic (pH less than 3.5), which can cause erosion of the mucous membranes of the esophagus, necessitating surgery.

15. a. A fracture (slipper) bedpan has a low back and is safer to use for a patient with a spinal cord injury because it does not require the patient to lift the buttocks to get on the pan and it provides a more normal alignment of the lower back while on the pan.

b. A fracture pan is unnecessary. A patient on bed rest can use a regular high-back bedpan barring no contraindications.

c. A fracture pan is unnecessary. A patient with dementia can use a toilet, bedside commode, or a regular bedpan depending on the extent of impaired cognitive function.

d. An obese patient can use a toilet, bedside commode, or regular bedpan. A fracture bedpan is too small for an obese person because excess adipose tissue will fill the pan taking the space designed for urine and feces.

16. a. One slice of whole wheat bread contains only 1.5 grams of dietary fiber.

b. A serving of $1/2$ cup of white rice contains only 0.8 gram of dietary fiber.

c. A serving of $3 1/2$ ounces of cooked pasta contains only 1.6 grams of dietary fiber.

d. Kale is an excellent source of dietary fiber. A serving of $3 1/2$ ounces of kale contains 6.6 grams of dietary fiber.

17. a. This is a knowledgeable statement. The odor from drainage is minimal because fewer bacteria are present in the ileum compared to the large intestine. An ileostomy is an opening into the ileum (distal small intestine from the jejunum to the cecum).

b. Cleansing the skin, skin barriers, and a well-fitted appliance to collect the drainage are precautions to protect the skin around an ileostomy stoma. The drainage from an ileostomy contains enzymes that can damage the skin.

   c. This statement is inaccurate in relation to an ileostomy, and indicates that the patient needs more teaching. An ileostomy produces liquid fecal drainage that is constant and cannot be regulated.

   d. This is a correct statement. An ileostomy stoma does not have a sphincter that can control the flow of flatus or drainage, resulting in noise.

18. a. Spastic colon is a pathophysiological related factor, not a defining characteristic, for the nursing diagnosis Diarrhea.

   b. Impaired sphincter control is a pathophysiological related factor for the nursing diagnosis Bowel Incontinence, not Diarrhea.

   c. An inability to recognize, interpret, or respond to rectal cues is a situational related factor for the nursing diagnosis Bowel Incontinence.

   d. The major defining characteristics for the nursing diagnosis Diarrhea are increased frequency of stools (more than three times a day) and/or loose, liquid stools. Diarrhea is the state in which an individual experiences or is at risk for experiencing frequent passage of liquid stool or unformed stool.

19. a. The loss of the voluntary ability to control the passage of fecal or gaseous discharges through the anus (bowel incontinence) is caused by impaired functioning of the anal sphincter or its nerve supply, not straining on defecation.

   b. Straining on defecation requires the person to hold the breath while bearing down (Valsalva maneuver). This maneuver increases the intrathoracic and intracranial pressures, which can precipitate dysrhythmias, brain attack (stroke), and respiratory difficulties, which can be life-threatening.

   c. Fecal impaction is caused by prolonged retention and accumulation of fecal material in the large intestine, not straining on defecation.

   d. Although straining on defecation can contribute to the formation of hemorrhoids, this is not the primary reason straining on defecation is discouraged. Hemorrhoids, although painful, are not life-threatening.

20. a. The presence of fluid or food activates digestive enzymes, not mucus.

   b. Mucus, secreted by mucous membranes and glands, is a viscous, slippery fluid containing mucin, white blood cells, water, inorganic salts, and exfoliated cells. Mucin, a mucopolysaccharide, is a lubricant that protects body surfaces from friction and erosion.

   c. Mucus does not enhance gastric acidity. Gastric acidity enhances digestion.

   d. The low surface tension of bile salts contributes to the emulsification of fats in the intestine.

21. a. Each person is unique. Specific factors that hinder defecation must be identified so that the bowel retraining can be individualized to meet the person's specific needs. Factors such as lack

of fiber in the diet, inadequate fluid intake, a sedentary lifestyle, ignoring the urge to defecate, excessive laxative use, pain on defecation, and lack of toileting privacy can all hinder defecation.

   b. This is unnecessary and impossible.

   c. Teaching a patient about bowel retraining is within the legal practice of nursing.

   d. This may or may not be necessary or possible.

22. a. Applesauce thickens, not softens, stool.

   b. Bananas thicken, not soften stool.

   c. Cheese thickens, not softens, stool.

   d. Beans contain both soluble and insoluble fibers and are second only to bran as the best plant source of fiber. They increase bulk and absorb many times their weight in water to produce a larger, softer stool.

23. a. A lubricant reduces friction, which facilitates the passage of a hard, dry stool through the anus. Nurses are legally permitted to diagnose and treat human responses. Constipation is a human response, and applying a lubricant to the anus is an independent function of the nurse.

   b. A sitz bath requires a practitioner's order and is a dependent, not independent, function of the nurse. A sitz bath will not promote the passage of a hard, dry stool but it may promote hygiene and comfort after the bowel movement.

   c. An oil retention enema softens the feces and lubricates the rectum and anus. However, it requires a practitioner's order and is a dependent, not independent, function of the nurse.

   d. Warm, not cool, compresses may facilitate defecation. Warm compresses may relax the surrounding muscles and the external sphincter, promoting defecation.

24. a. Although this reduces abdominal muscle tension increasing the volume of enema solution that can be tolerated, it is not the priority action.

   b. Although this is an acceptable medical asepsis practice and it promotes patient comfort, it is not the priority action associated with the administration of an enema.

   c. This is unsafe because it can perforate or injure the intestinal wall. A lubricated enema catheter should be inserted 3 to 4 inches in an adult, 2 to 3 inches in a child, and 1 to 1.5 inches in an infant.

   d. This allows the enema solution to flow with a force that is not excessively stimulating so that the integrity of the mucosa is not disrupted and the patient can tolerate a maximal amount of the enema solution. The higher the solution container is held, the faster the solution flows and the greater the force exerted on the colon.

25. a. Medical, not surgical, asepsis is necessary.

   b. It is unnecessary to monitor the intake and output this frequently. The intake and output must be recorded at routine intervals as per hospital policy, usually every 8 and 24 hours.

   c. The level of suctioning is part of the physician's order for nasogastric decompression. Low suction pressure is between 80 and 100 mmHg and high suction pressure is between 100 and

120 mmHg. Suctioning must be maintained continuously with a Salem sump to prevent reflux of gastric secretions into the vent lumen, which will obstruct its functioning and result in mucosal damage.

   d. Oral hygiene should be provided more frequently than this. Because there is no food or fluid to stimulate salivary gland secretion and the tube in the nose may interfere with breathing, precipitating mouth breathing, the mouth becomes dry.

26. a. Although Imbalanced Nutrition Less than Body Requirements may be related to Diarrhea, it is not life-threatening or the priority in comparison to another nursing diagnosis.
   b. Risk for Impaired Skin Integrity is directly related to Diarrhea because the enzymes present in fecal material can erode the skin. However, it is not life-threatening or the priority in comparison to another nursing diagnosis.
   c. Diarrhea is related directly to Deficit Fluid Volume, which is the state in which an individual who is not NPO experiences or is at risk of experiencing vascular, interstitial, or intracellular dehydration. Normally digestive juices of approximately 3.5 to 5 liters are secreted and reabsorbed by the body daily. With diarrhea, the transit time through the intestine is decreased, interfering with the reabsorption of water and resulting in frequent, loose watery stools and dehydration.
   d. Diarrhea is unrelated to the nursing diagnosis of Functional Incontinence, which relates to urinary, not fecal, incontinence. Functional incontinence is the state in which an individual experiences incontinence because of a difficulty or inability to reach a toilet in time.

27. **a. This is an indication that the circulation to the stoma is compromised and viability of tissue is questionable without immediate intervention. The physician should be notified immediately.**
   b. Although this might be done, it is not the priority. Active bowel sounds indicate peristalsis and the presence of flatus in the small intestines, which can occur even if there is an impending problem in the large intestine.
   c. This is inappropriate. This will not improve circulation to the stoma and will waste valuable time.
   d. This is inappropriate. This will not improve circulation and may injure surrounding tissue.

28. a. Alcohol may cause gas but it does not produce an odor.
   b. Raisins may cause gas but they do not produce an odor.
   c. Coffee may have a laxative effect but it does not produce an odor.
   d. Eggs will produce odorous gas and should be avoided. In addition, the patient should be taught to also avoid other odor-producing foods such as asparagus, fish, garlic, green peppers, mustard, onions, radishes, and spicy foods.

29. a. Constipation, not bowel incontinence, is more common in the older adult than other age groups.

Constipation in the older adult is caused by decreased bowel motility, inadequate hydration, inadequate fiber, sedentary life style, abuse of laxatives, and side effects of other medications.
   b. Sedatives depress the central nervous system, which may precipitate constipation, not bowel incontinence.
   c. When a person is disoriented to time, place, and person, the individual may not have the cognitive ability to perceive and interpret the fecal distention and rectal pressure cues to defecate, resulting in bowel incontinence.
   d. Antibiotic medications are known for causing diarrhea, not bowel incontinence.

30. a. Diarrhea is unrelated to Deficient Self-Care, which is the state in which the individual experiences an impaired motor function or cognitive function, causing a decreased ability to perform each of the five self-care activities.
   b. Diarrhea is not related directly to Sexual Dysfunction, which is the state in which an individual experiences or is at risk of experiencing a change in sexual function that is viewed as unrewarding or inadequate.
   c. Diarrhea is not related directly to Disturbed Body Image, which is the state in which an individual experiences or is at risk of experiencing a disruption in the way one perceives one's body image.
   d. Diarrhea is related directly to Risk for Impaired Skin Integrity, which is the state in which an individual experiences or is at risk for damage to the epidermal and dermal tissue. The gastric and intestinal enzymes present in feces are acids capable of eroding the skin.

31. a. Tarry-colored stool indicates upper gastrointestinal bleeding.
   b. Green-mucoid stool indicates the presence of infection.
   c. Orange-colored stool indicates the presence of infection.
   d. Bright red-tinged stool is the cardinal sign of lower gastrointestinal bleeding. When bleeding occurs closer to the anus, enzymes have not digested the blood, so the blood has not turned black.

32. a. Bile is a normal constituent of fecal material and is not detected with the guaiac test.
   b. Bacteria are identified in feces through a stool culture, not the guaiac test.
   c. Testing the feces for occult blood is called the guaiac test or Hemoccult test. This test uses a chemical reagent to detect the presence of the enzyme peroxidase in the hemoglobin molecule.
   d. Ova and parasites are identified through microscopic examination of feces, not the guaiac test.

33. a. Specimen collection is done immediately after awakening from sleep, not before sleep.
   b. This is unnecessary and can injure the anal and rectal mucosa.
   c. This ensures that there will be eggs available for collection at the perianal area. The adult pin worm (*Enterobius vermicularis*) exits the anus at night to lay eggs. The cellophane-tape (Scotch-

tape) test is performed first thing in the morning before a bowel movement or bathing so that these eggs are not disrupted or removed before obtaining a specimen for testing.
d. This will remove any eggs that are present in the perianal area, which will interfere with accurate test results.

34. a. This will not reestablish the normal bowel flora. Discontinuing antibiotics before the full course of therapy is completed can result in a return of the original infection or precipitate the development of a superinfection.
b. **Yogurt is merely milk that is curdled by the addition of bacteria, specifically *Lactobacillus bulgaricus* and *Streptococcus thermophilus*. Eating yogurt helps to restore bacterial balance of the resident flora of the intestine.**
c. Although rice helps to limit diarrhea, it will not reestablish normal bowel flora.
d. Although water is essential for all body processes and to replace fluid lost in the diarrhea, it does not reestablish normal bowel flora.

35. a. Oil lubricates, not irritates, the intestinal mucosa.
b. **Soap irritates the intestinal mucosa and thus stimulates the circular and longitudinal muscles of the intestinal wall, which respond with wave-like movements (peristalsis) that propel intestinal contents toward the anus.**
c. Tap water is a hypotonic solution that exerts a lower osmotic pressure than the surrounding interstitial fluid, causing water to move from the colon into interstitial spaces. In addition, the volume of the fluid distends the lumen of the intestine. These processes stimulate peristalsis and defecation.
d. Normal saline, a solution having the same osmotic pressure of surrounding interstitial fluid (isotonic), works by drawing fluid from interstitial spaces into the colon. This fluid, in addition to the original volume of saline instilled, exerts pressure against the intestinal mucosa, which stimulates peristalsis and defecation.

36. a. Intestinal gas is caused by the decomposition of undigested materials, especially indigestible sugars and fibers. Examples of gas-forming foods are beans, onions, cabbage, and radishes.
b. This is the description of a constipated stool. The longer fecal material remains in the colon, more fluid is reabsorbed, resulting in a hard, dry stool.
c. **Peristalsis above a fecal impaction continues in an attempt to move intestinal contents toward the anus. The liquid portion of feces seeps around the impacted mass.**
d. This is a sign of lower gastrointestinal bleeding caused by trauma to the rectal or anal mucosa when passing a constipated stool.

37. a. **Laxatives cause a rapid transit time of intestinal contents. When used excessively, the bowel's natural responses to fecal distention and rectal pressure weaken, resulting in chronic constipation.**
b. Laxatives increase peristalsis, which helps evacuate the bowel preventing, not promoting, abdominal distention from flatus or intestinal contents.

c. Although excessive laxative use can cause cramping, it is temporary and does not have long-term implications as does the problem in another option.
d. The loss of the voluntary ability to control the passage of fecal or gaseous discharges through the anus (bowel incontinence) is caused by impaired functioning of the anal sphincter or its nerve supply, not excessive laxative use.

38. a. **The defining characteristics for the nursing diagnosis Diarrhea are loose, liquid stools and/or increased frequency of stools (more than three times a day). An appropriate outcome for this nursing diagnosis should relate to a decrease in the number of stools a day and/or the development of a formed stool.**
b. This is an intervention, not an outcome.
c. This is an intervention, not an outcome.
d. This is an intervention, not an outcome.

39. a. This is unsafe and uncomfortable. The patient should be positioned so that the buttocks rest on, not slightly off of, the smooth, rounded rim of a regular bedpan.
b. This is unnecessary. The top linen can be draped over the patient in such a way as to promote placement of the bedpan while maintaining the privacy and dignity of the patient.
c. The opposite is true. A fracture bedpan should be placed with the flat, low end under the patient's buttocks.
d. **Raising the patient to a Fowler's position assumes the familiar, normal position for having a bowel movement. The more vertical position utilizes gravity, and hip flexion raises intra-abdominal pressure, both of which maximize evacuation of feces.**

40. a. **When blood from bleeding in the upper gastrointestinal tract is exposed to the digestive process, the fecal material becomes black (tarry). In addition, exogenous iron, red meat ingestion, and dark green vegetables can make the stool look black.**
b. Pancreatic dysfunction results in impaired digestion of fats (by lipase), protein (by trypsin and chymotrypsin), and carbohydrates (by amylase). Pancreatic dysfunction results in pale, foul-smelling, bulky stools, not tarry stools.
c. A reduction or lack of the secretion of lactase from the wall of the small intestine results in the inability of the body to break down lactose to glucose and galactose. Lactose intolerance causes diarrhea, gaseous distention, and intestinal cramping, not tarry stools.
d. Inadequate bile salts result in less bile entering the intestinal tract. The brown color of stool is caused by the presence of stercobilin and urobilin, which are derived from a pigment in bile (bilirubin). With inadequate bile salts the stool will appear clay-colored.

41. a. Tofu is a soy product that is low in fiber and calories but high in protein and calcium.
b. **One cup of oatmeal contains 2.2 grams of dietary fiber. A high fiber diet is recommended for people with diverticulosis because it produces a**

bulky stool that prevents constipation. Constipation results in straining when defecating, which raises the intra-intestinal pressure and promotes the development of diverticula.

c. Although a $^1/_2$ cup of corn contains 2.9 grams of dietary fiber, it is contraindicated for people with diverticular disease because it contains a husk.

d. Although cucumbers are high in dietary fiber, they are contraindicated for people with diverticular disease because they contain seeds.

42. a. Although the semi-Fowler's position will facilitate a bowel movement by the principle of gravity, it will not prevent the Valsalva maneuver.

b. Exhaling requires the glottis to be open, which prevents the Valsalva maneuver. The Valsalva maneuver is bearing down while holding the breath by closing the glottis.

c. This may result in straining, which employs the use of the Valsalva maneuver.

d. These nutrients thicken stool, which promotes the development of constipation. Constipation may result in straining on defecation, which employs the Valsalva maneuver.

43. **a. The cone advances into the stoma until it effectively fills the opening, which prevents a reflux of solution while the irrigating solution is being instilled. In addition, it helps prevent accidental perforation of the bowel with the rectal catheter.**

b. This is not the purpose of the cone. The catheter is threaded through the center of the cone.

c. The cone is removed before the bowel evacuates its contents.

d. The stoma of a colostomy should never prolapse. If this should occur, the physician should be notified immediately.

44. a. The need to have a bowel movement every day is unnecessary, unrealistic, and a myth. Patterns of bowel elimination vary considerably depending on a multitude of factors.

b. This is an intervention, not a goal. Although desirable for everyone, it does not specifically relate to the nursing diagnosis Perceived Constipation.

c. This is the most appropriate goal for a patient with the nursing diagnosis Perceived Constipation because a defining characteristic of this diagnosis is the excessive use of laxatives to achieve a daily bowel movement.

d. Although knowledge is essential, behavioral outcomes determine if a goal has been achieved.

45. a. An overdistention of the rectum may impair the person's ability to control the external sphincter, resulting in bowel incontinence.

b. Anal sphincter dysfunction is related to bowel incontinence. The internal and external anal sphincters and their nerve supply must be intact to maintain bowel control.

c. People who are cognitively impaired do not perceive or respond to the cues to defecate and as a result experience bowel incontinence.

d. When people experience pain when having a bowel movement, they postpone or ignore the urge to defecate; this results in constipation, not bowel incontinence. As fecal material is retained in the intestines, water continues to be reabsorbed resulting in a hard, dry stool.

46. **a. The only way to reestablish patency of the air vent lumen of a double-lumen nasogastric tube is to instill air into the lumen. The injected air will push the secretions blocking the lumen back into the stomach where the fluid can be removed by the drainage lumen. Keeping the end of the air vent lumen higher than the stomach prevents reflux of gastric contents into the air vent lumen.**

b. This will draw more fluid from the stomach into the air vent lumen by the principle of gravity.

c. This will not reestablish patency of the air vent lumen. The patient is placed in this position as the tube is being inserted to facilitate its passage into the stomach.

d. This will not re-establish patency of the air vent lumen. This is done to ensure that the catheter is in the correct anatomic location.

47. a. This is not specific to the intake of bran. Defecation is facilitated by leaning forward because it increases intra-abdominal pressure.

b. This is counterproductive. Cathartic use will weaken the bowel's natural responses to fecal distention and rectal pressure, resulting in chronic constipation.

c. This is too stimulating for the intestines. Bran use should begin with 1 tablespoon and increased gradually as tolerated because it can cause flatus and distention.

d. Bran is an insoluble fiber that increases bulk in the intestines. Eight glasses of water daily keeps the body well hydrated and the stool soft. Intestinal elimination is dependent on the interrelationship of fiber, water, and activity.

48. **a. A large-volume enema dilates the intestine by exerting pressure against the intestinal wall. This pressure stimulates peristalsis, which propels intestinal contents toward the anus.**

b. The constituents of the enema solution, not its volume, exert a hypertonic or hypotonic action. Hypertonic solutions exert a greater osmotic pressure than the surrounding interstitial fluid, which draws fluid from the interstitial compartment into the colon.

c. A large volume enema stimulates, not irritates, the intestinal mucosa. Castile soap, used with a soapsuds enema, irritates the intestinal mucosa, which precipitates peristalsis and subsequent defecation.

d. Medications, not enemas, influence the relationship between fecal material and water. Emollient/stool-softener laxatives soften and delay the drying of feces, which permit fat and water to penetrate feces. Wetting-agent/stool-softener laxatives lower the surface tension of feces, which helps water to penetrate the feces.

49. a. Flatus, gas in the intestine that is passed through the rectum, requires intestinal motility, not hypomotility, which is seen in postoperative ileus.

b. Diarrhea, the frequent passage of loose, watery stools, is associated with intestinal hypermotility, not hypomotility, which is seen in postoperative ileus.

c. When there is decreased intestinal motility, swallowed air and gastrointestinal secretions accumulate within the intestine causing abdominal distention. A paralytic ileus is the absence of peristalsis, which is most often caused by intestinal manipulation, anesthesia, or hypokalemia.

d. A paralytic ileus (postoperative ileus) is associated with decreased, not increased, intestinal peristalsis.

50. a. A Harris drip (Harris flush) helps get rid of intestinal gas.

b. A urinary catheter (Foley or retention catheter) drains the urinary bladder of urine, not a tap water enema.

c. A tap water enema puts fluid into the large intestine; the pressure and irritation cause the colon to empty of stool.

d. A tap water enema will not affect nausea and vomiting; nothing by mouth or medication can be used to limit nausea and vomiting.

Fluids and Electrolytes

KEYWORDS

The following words include English vocabulary, nursing/medical terminology, concepts, principles, or information relevant to content specifically addressed in the chapter or associated with topics presented in it. English dictionaries, your nursing textbooks, and medical dictionaries such as *Taber's Cyclopedic Medical Dictionary* are resources that can be used to expand your knowledge and understanding of these words and related information.

Acid
Active transport
Aldosterone
Anion
Antidiuretic hormone
Anuria
Atmospheric pressure
Base
Catheter
Cation
Colloid osmotic pressure
Deficient fluid volume
Dehydration
Dependent edema
Diaphoresis
Diffusion
Diluent
Diuretic
Edema
Electrolytes
   Sodium
   Potassium
   Calcium
   Magnesium
   Phosphorus
Filtration

Fluid compartments
   Extracellular
   Intracellular
   Intravascular
   Interstitial
   Third compartment spacing
Fluid restriction
Fluid volume excess
Hydrostatic pressure
Hypercalcemia
Hyperkalemia
Hypermagnesemia
Hyperosmolar
Hypertension
Hypertonic
Hypervolemic
Hypocalcemia
Hypokalemia
Hypomagnesemia
Hypo-osmolar
Hypotension
Hypotonic
Hypovolemic
Icteric
Infiltrate
Infusion port

Insensible fluid loss
Ion
Irrigant
Isotonic
Macro drip
Micro drip
Milliequivalent
Oncotic pressure
Osmolality
Osmolarity
Osmosis
Osmotic pressure
Primary infusion line
Residual
Secondary infusion line
Sensible fluid loss
Skin turgor
Solute
Specific gravity
Tenting
Thirst
Tonicity
Vaporization
Volume controlled device

QUESTIONS

1. Which food should be avoided by a patient who must follow a 2-gm sodium diet?
   a. American cheese
   b. Shredded wheat
   c. Potatoes
   d. Cashews

2. The primary reason tube feedings cause diarrhea are because they are:
   a. Icteric
   b. Isotonic
   c. Hypotonic
   d. Hypertonic

3. Which adaptation wound indicate a potassium deficiency?
   a. Increased blood pressure
   b. Muscle weakness
   c. Chest pain
   d. Dry hair

4. The nurse suspects that a patient may have the nursing diagnosis Excess Fluid Volume when the patient's skin appears:
   a. Dry and scaly
   b. Taut and shiny
   c. Red and irritated
   d. Thin and inelastic

5. The nurse would determine that inflammation of a vein may have occurred at an intravenous insertion site if when touching the area it:
   a. Feels soft
   b. Seems cool
   c. Produces pallor
   d. Causes discomfort

6. When a patient is under extreme stress there is an increased production of antidiuretic hormone (ADH) and aldosterone. Considering the effect of these hormones in the body, the nurse should expect a decrease in the patient's:
   a. Blood pressure
   b. Urinary output
   c. Body temperature
   d. Insensible fluid loss

7. Which fluid would be found on a clear liquid diet?
   a. Ginger ale
   b. Lemon sherbet
   c. Vanilla ice cream
   d. Cream of chicken soup

8. Salt-sensitive people should avoid:
   a. Mayonnaise
   b. Pickles
   c. Eggs
   d. Fish

9. A reduction in fluid intake will contribute to:
   a. A decreased urine output
   b. Incontinence of urine
   c. A retention of urine
   d. Frequent urination

10. Clinical manifestations that are common to both hypokalemia and hyperkalemia are:
    a. Nausea and vomiting
    b. Irritability and confusion
    c. Muscle weakness and dysrhythmias
    d. Increased bowel sounds and diarrhea

11. The best source of calcium is:
    a. Cheese
    b. Lettuce
    c. Peppers
    d. Oranges

12. Which adaptation would most specifically indicate that IV fluid replacement is adequate?
    a. Moist lips
    b. Bounding pulse
    c. Urine output of 50 cc/hr
    d. Blood pressure of 96/60

13. When weighing a patient daily for the purpose of evaluating fluid loss or gain, the nurse should weigh the patient:
    a. Twice a day
    b. One hour before meals
    c. At the same time each day
    d. Before urinating in the morning

14. The nurse suspects that a patient receiving intravenous fluids is experiencing a fluid overload when assessment reveals:
    a. Chills, fever, and generalized discomfort
    b. Dyspnea, headache, and increased blood pressure
    c. Pallor, swelling, and discomfort at the insertion site
    d. A blood return in the tubing close to the insertion site

15. Which would most likely be limited first when a patient has hypertension?
    a. Potassium
    b. Sodium
    c. Protein
    d. Fluids

16. The physician of a critically ill patient should be notified when the patient's hourly urine output first falls below:
    a. 20 cc
    b. 30 cc
    c. 60 cc
    d. 120 cc

17. The nurse understands that excess fluid in the interstitial compartment results from increased:
    a. Oncotic pressure
    b. Diffusion pressure
    c. Hydrostatic pressure
    d. Intraventricular pressure

18. When evaluating fluid intake and output, the fluid intake should be:
    a. About the same as the fluid output
    b. Lower than the urine output
    c. Higher than the fluid output
    d. Equal to the urine output

19. Patients who are taking diuretics must be encouraged to ingest nutrients rich in:
    a. Magnesium
    b. Potassium
    c. Calcium
    d. Sodium

20. The most effective nursing intervention to encourage a confused patient to drink more fluid would be to:
    a. Serve fluid at a tepid temperature
    b. Explain the reason for the desired intake
    c. Offer the patient something to drink every hour
    d. Leave a pitcher of water at the patient's bedside

21. The best source of calcium is:
    a. Rice
    b. Celery
    c. Sardines
    d. Tomatoes

22. When it is determined that an intravenous infusion has infiltrated, the nurse's first action should be to:
    a. Slow the infusion to a "keep the vein open" rate
    b. Clamp the tubing and initiate an incident report
    c. Remove the infusion and start it in another site
    d. Notify the physician of the infiltration

23. The patient on a 2-gram sodium restricted diet should avoid:
    a. Kool-Aid
    b. Club soda
    c. Lemonade
    d. Diet root beer

24. Which assessment is best when monitoring an older adult's fluid and electrolyte status?
    a. Intake and output results
    b. Serum laboratory values
    c. Condition of the skin
    d. Presence of tenting

25. What should be done with the irrigant on an I&O sheet when calculating the fluid balance for a patient with a continuous bladder irrigation?
    a. Add it to the oral intake column
    b. Deduct it from the total urine output
    c. Subtract it from the IV flow sheet as output
    d. Document the intake hourly in the urine output column

26. When patient adaptations include either oliguria or polyuria, which nursing diagnosis would be most likely?
    a. Diarrhea
    b. Impaired Skin Integrity
    c. Deficient Fluid Volume
    d. Imbalanced Nutrition Less Than Body Requirements

27. The best source of potassium is:
    a. Baked potato
    b. Bran flakes
    c. Lean meat
    d. Table salt

28. When discontinuing a patient's intravenous infusion it is essential that the nurse:
    a. Withdraw the catheter along the same angle of its insertion
    b. Wipe the area with an alcohol swab
    c. Flush the line with normal saline
    d. Wear sterile gloves

29. Which food selection by a patient would indicate an understanding regarding an abundant source of calcium?
    a. Bread
    b. Yogurt
    c. Green beans
    d. Peanut butter

30. When a patient is suspected of being hypovolemic, the nurse should further assess the patient for which adaptation?
    a. Decreased heart rate
    b. Thready pulse
    c. Hypertension
    d. Dyspnea

31. A patient is admitted to the hospital for a fever of unknown origin. The nursing assessment reveals profuse diaphoresis, dry, sticky mucous membranes, weakness, disorientation, and a decreasing level of consciousness. The nurse infers that the patient has:
    a. Hyperkalemia
    b. Hypercalcemia
    c. Hypernatremia
    d. Hypermagnesemia

32. Which could the nurse include on a full-liquid diet that is not included on a clear-liquid diet?
    a. Cranberry juice
    b. Ginger ale
    c. Jell-O
    d. Milk

33. A patient becomes hypertensive and short of breath after receiving an intravenous solution that functions as a volume expander. Before notifying the physician, in which position should the nurse place the patient?
    a. Sims'
    b. Supine
    c. Dorsal recumbent
    d. Reverse Trendelenburg

34. The nurse recognizes that the patient understands the importance of eating broccoli when the patient says, "Broccoli is a great source of:
    a. Iron."
    b. Starch."
    c. Calcium."
    d. Potassium."

35. When a patient exhibits an increasing blood pressure and 2-pound weight gain over two days, the nurse should further assess the patient for:
    a. A decrease in heart rate
    b. An increase in skin turgor
    c. An increase in pulse volume
    d. A decrease in pulse pressure

36. Which would be the best way to evaluate the effectiveness of diuretic therapy for a patient with 4+ dependent edema?
    a. Weigh daily
    b. Assess skin turgor
    c. Measure calf girth
    d. Monitor urine specific gravity

37. What is the primary cause of diarrhea in a patient receiving a tube feeding?
    a. A high osmolarity of the feeding
    b. An inadequate volume of the feeding
    c. Failure to test for a residual before the feeding
    d. Lying in the high-Fowler's position during the feeding

38. Which would be most important when assessing adult patients for the effects of vomiting?
    a. Electrolyte values
    b. Mouth condition
    c. Bowel function
    d. Body weight

39. Which problem would place the patient at the greatest risk for hyperkalemia?
    a. Diaphoresis
    b. Vomiting
    c. Diarrhea
    d. Burns

40. When assessing the skin of an older adult, which adaptation would be cause for greatest concern?
    a. Flat, brown-colored spots on the skin
    b. Thin, translucent skin
    c. Tenting of the skin
    d. Dry, flaky skin

41. Which adaptation is common to both excess fluid volume and deficient fluid volume?
    a. Hypotension
    b. Weakness
    c. Agitation
    d. Dyspnea

42. Before administering an intravenous solution containing potassium to a patient, it is essential that the nurse:
    a. Assess the skin turgor
    b. Rate the depth of edema
    c. Obtain the blood pressure
    d. Determine the presence of urinary output

43. Which is the best choice for an appetizer when following a 2-gram sodium diet?
    a. Pigs in a blanket
    b. Stuffed mushrooms
    c. Cheese and crackers
    d. Fresh vegetable sticks

44. An intravenous infusion has infiltrated when inspection of the insertion site appears:
    a. Hard
    b. Inflamed
    c. Reddened
    d. Edematous

45. When caring for a patient who is anorexic, the nurse should understand that liquid supplements:
    a. Should be encouraged with meals
    b. Can be ordered without a physician's order
    c. Can be less filling than foods of equal kilocalories
    d. Should be delivered via tube feeding to be most effective

46. When recording a patient's intake and output, what should be recorded at approximately $1/2$ its volume?
    a. Ice chips given by mouth
    b. A continuous bladder irrigation
    c. A tube feeding of $1/2$ formula and $1/2$ water
    d. Solution used to maintain patency of a tube

47. When patients are taking supplemental calcium, it is important that they be taught to maintain their fluid intake at a minimum of 2500 cc a day to prevent the:
    a. Formation of kidney stones
    b. Occurrence of muscle cramps
    c. Irritation of the bladder mucosa
    d. Mobilization of calcium from bone

48. The nurse evaluates that a patient understands the teaching about foods high in potassium when reviewing the menu for dinner the patient selects:
    a. Baked salmon fillet
    b. Cooked chicken liver
    c. Cream of chicken soup
    d. Lettuce and tomato salad

49. What patient assessment is a major indicator that the patient has the nursing diagnosis Deficient Fluid Volume?
    a. Increased body temperature
    b. Decreased blood pressure
    c. Negative balance of I&O
    d. Shortness of breath

50. The nurse understands that a patient receiving a hypertonic intravenous solution may experience excess fluid in the intravascular compartment as a result of:
    a. Atmospheric pressure
    b. Hydrostatic pressure
    c. Intraocular pressure
    d. Oncotic pressure

ANSWERS AND RATIONALES

1. a. One ounce of American cheese contains 406 mg of sodium and should be avoided on a 2-gram sodium diet.
   b. Two-thirds of a cup of shredded wheat cereal contains 3 mg of sodium and is permitted on a 2-gram sodium diet.
   c. One $^1/_2$ pound baked potato contains approximately 16 mg of sodium and is permitted on a 2-gram sodium diet.
   d. One ounce of natural roasted cashews with no added salt contains approximately 4 mg of sodium and is permitted on a 2-gram sodium diet.

2. a. Icteric is unrelated to tube feeding and fluid shifts. Icteric means pertaining to or resembling jaundice.
   b. Isotonic solutions have the same concentration of solutes as the blood. With isotonic solutions there is no net transfer of water across two compartments separated by a semipermeable membrane.
   c. Hypotonic solutions have a lesser concentration of solutes than does the blood. A hypotonic tube feeding will result in fluid being absorbed from the gastrointestinal tract into the intravascular and intracellular compartments.
   d. Hypertonic solutions have a greater concentration of solutes than does the blood. The high osmolarity of a hypertonic tube feeding exerts an osmotic force that pulls fluid into the stomach and intestine, resulting in intestinal cramping and diarrhea.

3. a. Hypertension is associated with hypervolemia, not a potassium deficiency.
   b. Potassium is an essential component in the sodium-potassium pump, cellular metabolism, and muscle contraction. Patient adaptations associated with a potassium deficiency (hypokalemia) include muscle weakness, fatigue, lethargy, leg cramps, and depressed deep-tendon reflexes.
   c. Chest pain is associated with a myocardial infarction (heart attack) and pulmonary embolus, not a potassium deficiency
   d. Dry hair is associated with malnutrition and hypothyroidism, not a potassium deficiency.

4. a. These are signs of aging and dehydration, not excessive fluid volume.
   b. With excessive fluid volume the increased hydrostatic pressure moves fluid from the intravascular compartment into the interstitial compartment. As fluid collects in the interstitial compartment (edema), the skin appears taut and shiny.
   c. These are signs of the local inflammatory response, not of excessive fluid volume.
   d. These are characteristics of skin in the older adult because of a loss of subcutaneous fat and a reduced thickness and vascularity of the dermis, not of excessive fluid volume.

5. a. The localized edema associated with the inflammatory response causes the affected area to feel firm, not soft.
   b. The localized vasodilation associated with the inflammatory response increases blood flow to the affected area and causes it to feel warm, not cool.
   c. The localized vasodilation associated with the inflammatory response increases blood flow to the affected area and causes erythema, not pallor.
   d. The physiologic response associated with the inflammation of a vein (phlebitis) causes a movement of fluid from the intravascular compartment into the interstitial compartment. Pressure of fluid on the nerve endings causes local discomfort.

6. a. The blood pressure will increase, not decrease, when the circulating fluid volume increases in response to these hormones.
   b. Both hormones are involved with water reabsorption, which conserves fluid and results in a decreased urinary output. With decreased kidney perfusion, the juxtaglomerular cells of the kidneys release angiotensin II, which stimulates the release of aldosterone from the adrenal cortex. Aldosterone promotes the excretion of potassium and reabsorption of sodium, which results in the passive reabsorption of water. As the concentration of the blood (osmolality) increases, the anterior pituitary releases antidiuretic hormone (ADH). ADH causes the collecting ducts in the kidneys to become more permeable to water, promoting its reabsorption into the blood.
   c. ADH and aldosterone do not regulate body temperature.
   d. ADH and aldosterone influence the kidneys to maintain fluid balance. They do not affect insensible fluid loss through the lungs, skin, or intestinal tract.

7. a. Ginger ale is an easily ingested and digested liquid that is permitted on a clear liquid diet. Its short-term objectives are to relieve thirst, prevent dehydration, and minimize stimulation of the gastrointestinal tract.
   b. Sherbet contains milk, which is not permitted on a clear liquid diet.
   c. When ice cream melts, it is not a clear liquid and therefore is not permitted on a clear liquid diet. Milk contains protein and lactose, which stimulates the digestive process; this is undesirable when a patient is receiving a clear liquid diet.
   d. Cream of chicken soup contains milk and small particles of chicken, both of which are contraindicated on a clear liquid diet.

8. a. One tablespoon of mayonnaise contains approximately 80 mg of sodium. This is a lower sodium content than another option.
   b. One dill pickle ($3^3/_4 \times 1^1/_4$ inches) contains approximately 928 mg of sodium and should be avoided by salt-sensitive people.
   c. One egg contains approximately 69 mg of sodium. This is a lower sodium content than another option.
   d. Three ounces of fish contain between 70 mg and 230 mg of sodium, depending on the type of fish. This is a lower sodium content than another option.

9. a. When the serum osmolarity increases because of

309

insufficient fluid intake, antidiuretic hormone (ADH) increases the permeability of the collecting tubules in the kidneys, which increases the reabsorption of water and decreases urine output.

b. Involuntary urination (incontinence) is not associated with a reduced fluid intake.

c. The accumulation of urine in the bladder with an inability to empty the bladder (urinary retention) is unrelated to a decreased fluid intake.

d. Frequent urination occurs with increased, not decreased, fluid intake.

10. a. Anorexia, nausea, and vomiting caused by decreased intestinal motility are associated with hypokalemia, not hyperkalemia.

b. Irritability and confusion are associated with hyperkalemia, not hypokalemia.

c. A deficiency or excess of potassium can cause both muscle weakness and dysrhythmias because of potassium's role in the sodium-potassium pump, cellular metabolism, and muscle contraction.

d. Increased bowel sounds and diarrhea, caused by intestinal hypermotility, are associated with hyperkalemia, not hypokalemia.

11. a. Cheese, a dairy product, is an excellent dietary source of calcium. One ounce of cheese contains approximately 150 mg to 406 mg of calcium depending on the type of cheese.

b. Lettuce is not high in calcium. One cup of shredded loose leaf lettuce contains approximately 38 mg of calcium.

c. Peppers are not high in calcium. One pepper contains approximately 4 mg of calcium.

d. Oranges are not high in calcium. One orange contains approximately 52 mg of calcium.

12. a. This is a nonspecific and too subjective assessment to determine the adequacy of IV fluid replacement.

b. A bounding pulse indicates excessive fluid in the intravascular compartment.

c. The circulating blood volume perfuses the kidneys and produces a glomerular filtrate of which varying amounts are either reabsorbed or excreted to maintain fluid balance. When a person without kidney disease is adequately hydrated, the minimally acceptable urinary output is 30 cc per hour.

d. A blood pressure of 96/60 reflects a decreased circulating blood volume (hypovlemia). The average blood pressure of a healthy adult is 120/80.

13. a. This is unnecessary. In addition, weight varies over the course of the day depending on food and fluids ingested and the weight of clothing being worn. All of these factors obtain information that is not comparable.

b. This is unnecessary. In addition, meal times may vary from day to day, and the information collected will not be comparable.

c. To obtain the most accurate comparable data, patients should be weighed at the same time every day (preferably first thing in the morning), after toileting, wearing the same clothing, and

using the same scale. This controls as many variables as possible to make the daily measurements an accurate reflection of the patient's weight.

d. This would collect information influenced by the volume of urine in the urinary bladder. Weights should always be measured after, not before, voiding to obtain the most accurate, comparable measurements. One liter of fluid is equal to 2.2 pounds.

14. a. These are signs of an infection, not excess fluid volume.

b. IV fluid flows directly into the circulatory system via a vein. Excess intravascular volume (hypervolemia) causes hypertension, pulmonary edema, and headache.

c. These are signs of an IV infiltration, not excess fluid volume.

d. This occurs when the IV bag is held lower than the IV insertion site for several seconds to determine placement and patency of the IV line.

15. a. Potassium restriction is a therapy associated with kidney disease, not hypertension. If diuretics are used to treat a patient's hypertension, potassium supplementation through diet or medications may be employed.

b. In the stepped-care approach to the management of hypertension, sodium intake is restricted in Step I.

c. Protein intake may be restricted when a patient has kidney disease, not hypertension.

d. Fluid restriction is not part of the 4-part stepped-care management of hypertension. Adequate fluids (a minimum of 1500 cc to 2000 cc) are necessary for fluid balance. Fluids may be restricted as an intervention for kidney disease or pulmonary edema, not hypertension.

16. a. The physician should be notified long before the hourly urine output reaches 20 cc.

b. The circulating blood volume perfuses the kidneys, producing a glomerular filtrate of which varying amounts are either reabsorbed or excreted to maintain fluid balance. When a person's hourly urine output is only 30 cc it indicates a deficient circulating fluid volume, inadequate renal perfusion, and/or kidney disease. The physician should be notified.

c. An hourly urine output of 60 cc is close to the normal range of 1400 cc to 1500 cc per 24 hours or 30 cc to 50 cc per hour.

d. The physician does not have to be notified about this. An hourly urine output of 120 cc indicates that there is adequate kidney perfusion. The intake and output should be monitored to ensure that volume depletion does not occur over time.

17. a. Oncotic (colloid osmotic) pressure is the force exerted by colloids (such as proteins) that pull or keep fluid within the intravascular compartment. Oncotic pressure is the major force opposing hydrostatic pressure in the capillaries.

b. Diffusion is a continual intermingling of molecules with movement of molecules from a solution of higher concentration to a solution of lower concentration.

   c. Hydrostatic pressure is the pressure exerted by a fluid within a compartment, such as blood within the vessels. Hydrostatic pressure moves fluid from an area of greater pressure to an area of lesser pressure. Hydrostatic pressure within vessels of the body moves fluid out of the intravascular compartment into the interstitial compartment. Interstitial fluid is extracellular fluid that surrounds cells.

   d. Intraventricular pressure is the pressure that exists in the left and right ventricles of the heart. These pressures do not move fluid from the intravascular compartment to the interstitial compartment.

18. a. The volume and composition of body fluids are kept in a delicate balance (total intake approximately equal to total output) by a harmonious interaction of the kidneys and the endocrine, respiratory, cardiovascular, integumentary, and gastrointestinal systems.

   b. If the total intake is lower than the urine output, the patient will develop a deficient fluid volume.

   c. If the total intake is higher than the total output, the patient will develop an excess fluid volume.

   d. If intake and urine output are equal, the patient will develop a deficient fluid volume because of fluid loss through routes other than the kidneys. In addition to urine output, the body also has insensible fluid loss through the skin, in feces, and as water vapor in expired air.

19. a. Although loop and thiazide diuretics enhance magnesium excretion, which may produce a mild hypomagnesemia, it does not require supplementation.

   b. **Most diuretics affect the renal mechanisms for tubular secretion and reabsorption of electrolytes, particularly potassium. Because of potassium's narrow therapeutic window of 3.5 to 5.0 mEq/L and its role in the sodium-potassium pump and muscle contraction, depleted potassium must be supplemented by increasing the dietary intake of foods high in potassium and/or the administration of potassium drug therapy.**

   c. Serum calcium levels vary depending on the diuretic. Loop diuretics increase calcium excretion, which may produce hypocalcemia. Thiazide diuretics decrease calcium excretion, which may produce hypercalcemia.

   d. Although sodium deficit (hyponatremia) may occur with diuretics, it is usually mild and does not require supplementation.

20. a. Fluids should be administered at the temperature usually associated with the fluid. For example, cool temperatures for juice, soda, and milk and warm temperatures for tea, coffee, and soup. Hot liquids should be avoided for safety reasons.

   b. This probably will be ineffective because a confused person has difficulty understanding cause and effect.

   c. **Frequent smaller volumes of fluid (50 cc to 100 cc per hour) are better tolerated**

physiologically and psychologically than infrequent larger volumes of fluid.

   d. A confused patient, having difficulty understanding cause and effect, may ignore a pitcher of water.

21. a. Rice, regardless of the type, is not high in calcium. One cup of rice contains approximately 5 mg to 33 mg of calcium.

   b. Celery is not high in calcium. One stalk of celery contains approximately 15 mg of calcium.

   c. **Sardines are an excellent source of dietary calcium. Three ounces of sardines contains approximately 371 mg of calcium.**

   d. Tomatoes are not high in calcium. One tomato (2 3/5 inches in diameter) contains approximately 9 mg of calcium.

22. a. This is unsafe because fluid will continue to collect in the interstitial compartment.

   b. Not only should it be clamped, but it also should be removed. An incident report is unnecessary.

   c. **When an IV infiltrates, the IV catheter moves out of the vein and into interstitial tissue (extravasation). The infusion must be discontinued and restarted at another site, preferably another extremity.**

   d. The physician does not have to be notified. However, it does need to be documented in the patient's hospital record.

23. a. Kool-Aid contains no sodium and is permitted on a 2-gam sodium diet.

   b. Club soda contains no sodium and is permitted on a 2-gram sodium diet.

   c. Twelve fluid ounces of lemonade contain approximately 12 mg of sodium and is permitted on a 2-gram sodium diet.

   d. **Twelve fluid ounces of diet root beer contain approximately 170 mg of sodium and should be avoided on a 2-gram sodium diet.**

24. a. This assesses only fluid balance.

   b. **Laboratory studies provide objective measurements of indicators of fluid, electrolyte, and acid-base balance. Common diagnostic tests include arterial blood gases and serum blood studies such as electrolytes (particularly sodium, potassium, chloride, and calcium), osmolarity, and hemoglobin and hematocrit.**

   c. This assesses only fluid balance. In addition, the changes in the integumentary system as a person ages complicate assessment of the skin for fluid balance disturbances in the older adult. Skin changes include loss of dermal and subcutaneous mass (thin and wrinkled), decreased secretion from sebaceous and sweat glands (dry skin), and less organized collagen and elastic fibers (wrinkles, decreased elasticity).

   d. This assesses only fluid balance. *Tenting* occurs when the skin of a dehydrated person remains in a peak or tent position after the skin is pinched together. Caution is advised when assessing an older person because some degree of tenting may occur even when hydrated because of the decrease in skin elasticity and tissue fluid associated with aging. The skin over the sternum is the area that should be tested for tenting.

25. a. The irrigant of a continuous bladder irrigation is instilled into the urinary bladder, not the mouth.
    b. **When a continuous bladder irrigation is in use, drainage from the urinary bladder will consist of both urine and the instilled irrigant. To determine the patient's urinary output, the amount of the irrigant instilled must be deducted from the total urinary output.**
    c. The IV flow sheet should not contain any information regarding intake and output other than the amount and type of fluid that is instilled into the circulatory system.
    d. Intake anywhere in the body should be recorded in the appropriate intake column, not in the urinary output column.

26. a. Frequent, loose, liquid stools, not oliguria or polyuria, are associated with diarrhea.
    b. Oliguria and polyuria are related to fluid balance and kidney functioning, not skin integrity. However, because oliguria may be related to fluid retention and subsequent edema and polyuria may ultimately cause dehydration and dry skin, the patient may eventually be at risk for the nursing diagnosis Impaired Skin Integrity.
    c. **The production of abnormally large amounts of urine by the kidneys without an increase in fluid intake can precipitate a fluid volume deficit. Oliguria, the production of abnormally small amounts of urine by the kidney, is reflected as a negative balance in the intake and output. A negative balance of intake and output is a defining characteristic for the nursing diagnosis Deficient Fluid Volume.**
    d. Oliguria and polyuria are related to fluid balance and kidney functioning, not nutrition. The defining characteristics for the nursing diagnosis Imbalanced Nutrition: Less than Body Requirements are: food intake less than the recommended daily allowance with or without weight loss or actual or potential metabolic needs in excess of intake.

27. a. **This is the best source of potassium of the foods listed. A $\frac{1}{2}$ pound baked potato contains approximately 844 mg of potassium.**
    b. Bran flakes do not contain any potassium.
    c. Depending on the type of meat, 3 ounces of meat contains only 57 mg to 323 mg of potassium and is not the best choice of the options offered.
    d. One teaspoon of salt contains only trace amounts of potassium.

28. a. **Removing a catheter by withdrawing it along the same path of its insertion minimizes injury to the vein and trauma to the surrounding tissue. This action limits seepage of blood and promotes healing of the puncture wound.**
    b. The area should be compressed with a sterile gauze pad. Pressure helps stop the bleeding and prevents the formation of a hematoma. A sterile gauze pad provides for surgical asepsis, which prevents infection.
    c. This is unnecessary.
    d. Clean, not sterile, gloves should be worn by the nurse to prevent exposure to the patient's body fluids.

29. a. Grain products are not high in calcium. One slice of bread contains approximately 20 mg to 49 mg of calcium depending on the type of grain.
    b. **Yogurt is an excellent dietary source of calcium. Eight ounces of yogurt contain 415 mg of calcium.**
    c. Green beans are not high in calcium. One cup of green beans contains approximately 60 mg of calcium.
    d. Peanut butter is not high in calcium. One tablespoon of peanut butter contains approximately 5 mg of calcium.

30. a. When a patient is hypovolemic, the heart rate will increase, not decrease, in an attempt to maintain an effective cardiac output.
    b. **When a patient is hypovolemic there is a reduced volume of circulating blood and less pressure within the vessels, which are reflected in weak, thready peripheral pulses and flattened neck veins.**
    c. When a patient is hypovolemic, there is a reduced volume of circulating blood resulting in hypotension, not hypertension.
    d. Dyspnea is associated with fluid volume excess, not deficit, because of pulmonary congestion.

31. a. Although muscle weakness and lethargy are associated with hyperkalemia, the other adaptations are not.
    b. Although weakness and lethargy are associated with hypercalcemia, the other adaptations are not.
    c. **With profuse diaphoresis the water loss exceeds the sodium loss resulting in hypernatremia. Excess serum sodium precipitates changes in the musculoskeletal (weakness), neurologic (disorientation and decreased level of consciousness), and integumentary (dry, sticky mucous membranes) systems.**
    d. Although muscle weakness, lethargy, and drowsiness are associated with hypermagnesemia, the other adaptations are not.

32. a. Cranberry juice is a clear liquid.
    b. Ginger ale is a clear liquid.
    c. Jell-O is a clear liquid that is a solid when refrigerated and a liquid at room temperature. It is permitted in either form on a clear liquid diet.
    d. **Milk is not on a clear liquid diet. It contains a high solute load, including fat and proteins, which precipitates the digestive process.**

33. a. The Sims' position, a semiprone position, is contraindicated for a patient who is short of breath because it compresses the thoracic cavity and does not permit maximum bilateral lung expansion
    b. The supine position, a horizontal back-lying position, is contraindicated for a patient who is short of breath because the abdominal viscera exerts pressure against the diaphragm, which limits lung expansion.
    c. The dorsal recumbent position, a horizontal back-lying position with flexed knees and hips, is contraindicated for a patient who is short of breath. It increases intra-abdominal pressure, which exerts a force against the diaphragm and thus limits lung expansion.

d. The patient is experiencing a fluid volume excess that is causing an increased workload for the heart and pulmonary edema. The reverse Trendelenburg position keeps the legs and lower part of the body dependent, which limits venous return and minimizes heart and pulmonary congestion.

34. a. One broccoli spear contains only 1.3 mg of iron.
    b. One broccoli spear contains only 8 grams of carbohydrate.
    c. One spear of broccoli contains only 72 mg of calcium.
    d. **Broccoli is an excellent source of potassium. One spear of broccoli contains 491 mg of potassium.**

35. a. With an excess fluid volume the heart rate will increase, not decrease, in an attempt to maintain adequate cardiac output.
    b. In the early stages of an excess fluid volume, a change in skin turgor may not be evident. One liter of fluid is equal to approximately 2.2 pounds.
    c. **With an excess fluid volume the amount of circulating blood volume increases, resulting in full, bounding peripheral pulses.**
    d. The pulse pressure is the difference between the systolic and diastolic pressures of a blood pressure measurement, and the normal range is 30 to 50 mmHg. With an excess fluid volume the pulse pressure increases, not decreases.

36. a. **To obtain the most accurate comparable data, patients should be weighed at the same time every day (preferably first thing in the morning), after toileting, before breakfast, wearing the same clothing, and using the same scale. This controls as many variables as possible to make the daily measurements an objective, accurate reflection of the patient's weight. Approximately 1 kilogram (2.2 lb) of weight gained or lost is equivalent to 1 liter of fluid.**
    b. Although skin turgor is assessed, it is a less accurate assessment because it is based on the nurse's perception and interpretation and is less desirable than an objective assessment.
    c. This assesses the progression or resolution of edema in only a small area of the body, which does not reflect total body fluid losses or gains. Edema generally is not observable until 2.5 to 3.0 liters of fluid have been retained.
    d. This is not an accurate method of assessing the effectiveness of diuretic therapy because it should be considered in relation to other variables, such as urine volume and serum osmolality.

37. a. **A tube feeding formula is usually hypertonic, which exerts an osmotic force that pulls fluid into the stomach and intestine resulting in intestinal cramping and diarrhea.**
    b. This could result in fluid volume deficit and malnutrition, not diarrhea.
    c. This could result in vomiting, not diarrhea. Failure to test for a residual before administering a tube feeding can result in adding more fluid than the stomach can tolerate if there is still fluid remaining from the previous feeding.

d. Placing a patient in the high-Fowler's position during the administration of a tube feeding is done to prevent aspiration of the formula, not diarrhea.

38. a. **Vomiting results in a loss of chloride (greatest amount), sodium (next greatest amount), and potassium (least amount but of greatest importance because it can cause dysrhythmias and cardiac arrest).**
    b. Although oral hygiene is provided, it is performed for comfort, not because there is a life-threatening problem.
    c. This would be done, but it is not the priority.
    d. Although this would be done to assess fluid volume deficit (2.2 pounds equals approximately 1 liter of fluid), it is not as critical as another assessment.

39. a. Sweat is composed of water, potassium, sodium, chloride, glucose, urea, and lactate. Profuse diaphoresis can lead to hypokalemia.
    b. Gastrointestinal fluids are high in potassium. Therefore, vomiting can cause hypokalemia, not hyperkalemia.
    c. Gastrointestinal fluids are high in potassium. Therefore, diarrhea can cause hypokalemia, not hyperkalemia.
    d. **Of the problems listed, a burn is the only one that has an association with hyperkalemia. During the first 24 hours after a burn, potassium is elevated in the blood stream (hyperkalemia) because of oliguria and the destruction of tissue. Eventually during the diuresis phase of a burn, sodium shifts back from the interstitial compartment to the intravascular compartment, secretion and excretion of fluid increase, and the patient becomes hypokalemic.**

40. a. This is an expected integumentary change in the older adult. Brown spots (lentigo senilis) on the skin are caused by a clustering of melanocytes, pigment-producing cells.
    b. A loss of subcutaneous fat and a reduced thickness and vascularity of the dermis that occur with aging results in thin, translucent skin in the older adult.
    c. *Tenting* occurs when the skin of a dehydrated person remains in a peak or tent position after the skin is pinched together. This is a sign of a fluid volume deficit. Care must be taken when assessing an older person because some degree of tenting may occur even when hydrated because of the decrease in skin elasticity and tissue fluid associated with aging; however, in the hydrated patient the tenting will slowly resolve.
    d. A decrease in tissue fluid and sebaceous gland activity associated with aging results in dry, flaky skin.

41. a. A decrease in blood pressure is associated with fluid volume deficit, not excess, because of the decreased circulating blood volume.
    b. **Muscle weakness is a musculoskeletal adaptation to both increased fluid volume and decreased fluid volume because the fluid imbalances alter cellular and body metabolism.**
    c. Agitation and restlessness are neurologic adaptations associated with fluid volume deficit, not excess.
    d. Dyspnea is associated with fluid volume excess, not

deficit, because the fluid overload causes pulmonary congestion.

42. a. This is unnecessary for the administration of potassium. This is part of the assessment of a patient's hydration status, particularly when the patient is at risk for dehydration.
    b. This is unnecessary for the administration of potassium. This is part of the assessment when a patient has a fluid volume excess in dependent tissues where the hydrostatic capillary pressure is high.
    c. Although all the vital signs should be measured when a patient is receiving any fluids or electrolytes, monitoring the heart rate and rhythm are more significant assessments than the blood pressure in relation to the administration of potassium. Both a serum potassium decrease (hypokalemia) and increase (hyperkalemia) cause cardiac dysrhythmias.
    d. **Serum potassium has a narrow therapeutic window (3.5 to 5.0 mEq/L). When kidney function is impaired, potassium can accumulate in the body and exceed the therapeutic level of 5.0 mEq/L, which can cause cardiac dysrhythmias and arrest.**

43. a. One tenth of a pound of frankfurters contains approximately 168 mg of sodium and should be avoided on a 2-gram sodium diet.
    b. Although mushrooms are low in sodium, when stuffed with seasoned bread crumbs ($^1/_3$ cup contains approximately 370 mg of sodium) they should be avoided on a 2-gram sodium diet.
    c. One ounce of cheese contains approximately 106 mg to 400 mg of sodium depending on the cheese. Two crackers contain approximately 44 mg to 165 mg depending on the product. These foods should be avoided on a 2-gram sodium diet.
    d. **As a food group, fresh vegetables have low sodium content. The sodium content of vegetables include 1 cup of broccoli, 17 mg; 1 cup of cauliflower, 20 mg; 1 carrot, 25 mg; 1 pepper, 2 mg; 1 radish, 1 mg; 1 cup of mushrooms, 3 mg; and 6 slices of cucumber, 1 mg.**

44. a. When IV fluid flows into the tissue surrounding a vein (infiltration), the area will feel soft and spongy, not hard.
    b. When the area at the insertion site of an IV appears inflamed, the patient has phlebitis, not an infiltration of an IV.
    c. When the insertion site of an IV is reddened, swollen, warm to the touch, and painful, the patient has phlebitis, not an infiltration of an IV.
    d. **When an IV line moves out of a vein and into subcutaneous tissue, the IV fluid will begin to collect in the interstitial compartment causing swelling (edema).**

45. a. Supplements should be encouraged only between meals, not during meals. Supplements should enhance daily calorie intake, not replace nutrients that are best acquired from a well-balanced diet of daily food intake.
    b. Providing nutritional supplements is a dependent function and requires a practitioner's order.

c. Supplements are nutrient-rich milkshake-type drinks that generally leave a person feeling less full than ingesting the same number of kilocalories and nutrients in food. For this reason, supplements are generally well tolerated by the anorexic patient.
    d. Liquid supplements are equally well absorbed whether delivered by feeding tube or by drinking.

46. a. Ice chips are particles of frozen water that take up more volume when they are frozen than when they melt. When ice chips change from a solid to a liquid, the resulting fluid is approximately $^1/_2$ the volume of the ice chips.
    b. The total amount of the irrigant instilled into the urinary bladder is accounted for as intake. The total volume that was instilled is then deducted from the total urinary output to determine the patient's urinary output.
    c. When a tube feeding solution consists of $^1/_2$ formula and $^1/_2$ water, the final combined volume of the formula plus the water is recorded on the appropriate intake column of the intake and output record.
    d. Whatever volume of solution is instilled into a catheter, the full volume used is recorded when the nurse documents the intervention.

47. a. A high fluid intake increases the volume of urine produced. The resulting frequent urination of dilute urine prevents the formation of renal calculi, which may occur because of the increased precipitation of calcium salts associated with calcium supplementation.
    b. Excessive supplementation of calcium causes hypercalcemia. Muscle tremors and cramps are associated with hypocalcemia, not hypercalcemia.
    c. Neither hypocalcemia nor hypercalcemia irritates the bladder mucosa.
    d. Calcium supplementation and weight bearing, not an increased fluid intake, prevent bone demineralization.

48. a. Three ounces of baked salmon contain only 305 mg of potassium.
    b. One cooked chicken liver contains only 28 mg of potassium.
    c. One cup of cream of chicken soup contains only 273 mg of potassium.
    d. **Lettuce and tomatoes are excellent sources of potassium. One 6-inch diameter head of iceberg lettuce contains 852 mg of potassium, and one 2 3/5-inch diameter tomato contains 255 mg of potassium.**

49. a. A temperature greater than 37.8°C (100°F) orally or 38.8°C (101°F) rectally is a defining characteristic of the nursing diagnosis Hyperthermia, not Deficient Fluid Volume.
    b. A low blood pressure is a defining characteristic of the nursing diagnosis Decreased Cardiac Output, not Deficient Fluid Volume.
    c. **A patient has a negative balance of intake and output when the output exceeds the intake. This is a major defining characteristic of the nursing diagnosis Deficient Fluid Volume.**
    d. Shortness of breath is a minor defining characteristic

of the nursing diagnosis Excess Fluid Volume, not Deficient Fluid Volume.

50. a. Atmospheric pressure is unrelated to excess fluid in the intravascular compartment. Atmospheric pressure is the pressure exerted by the weight of the atmosphere. At sea level, it is approximately 15 pounds per square inch.
    b. Hydrostatic pressure is the pressure exerted by a fluid within a compartment, such as blood within the vessels. Hydrostatic pressure moves fluid out of, not into, the intravascular compartment.
    c. Intraocular pressure does not cause an excess of fluid in the circulatory system. Intraocular pressure is the internal pressure of the eye.
    d. Oncotic (colloid osmotic) pressure is the power of a solution to draw water across a semipermeable membrane. Large molecules within the intravascular compartment will draw fluid from the interstitial compartment into the intravascular compartment.

Pain, Comfort, Rest, and Sleep

QUESTIONS

1. Which nursing diagnosis would be most appropriate for a patient complaining of having racing thoughts at bedtime and insomnia?
   a. Deficient Diversional Activity
   b. Ineffective Individual Coping
   c. Disturbed Thought Processes
   d. Disturbed Sleep Pattern

2. Which statement about a sleep partner would best support a diagnosis of sleep apnea?
   a. "He falls asleep sometimes when he drives so now I do all the driving."
   b. "He kicks and thrashes so much that the bed linen is upside down by morning."
   c. "He has nightmares that are so scary that he wakes me up because he is afraid."
   d. "He snores and gasps all night long, wakes me up and then I can't get back to sleep."

3. Which adaptation is commonly associated with severe acute pain?
   a. Delirium
   b. Vomiting
   c. Confusion
   d. Sleepiness

4. Which adaptation is a result of shortened NREM sleep?
   a. Decreased pain tolerance
   b. Excessive sleepiness
   c. Confusion
   d. Irritability

5. Which statement by a patient experiencing insomnia would indicate the need for further education?
   a. "I like to take a long walk after dinner."
   b. "I always have a small snack just before I go to bed."
   c. "I set my bedroom temperature at 65 degrees at night."
   d. "I drink a few scotch and sodas while I watch TV at night."

6. Which is the shortest acting pain relief method?
   a. Patient controlled analgesia
   b. Intramuscular sedatives
   c. Intravenous narcotics
   d. Regional anesthesia

7. Which concept associated with sleep must the nurse understand to best plan nursing care?
   a. Bedtime routines are associated with an expectation of sleep
   b. Alcohol intake interferes with one's ability to fall asleep
   c. Sleep needs remain consistent throughout the life span
   d. Total time in bed gradually decreases as one ages

8. Which nursing diagnosis associated with sleep deprivation would be most appropriate for a patient who has been in the intensive care unit for two weeks?
   a. Risk for Disturbed Thought Processes
   b. Impaired Gas Exchange
   c. Disuse Syndrome
   d. Powerlessness

9. Which is the most common nursing intervention that will contribute to onset of sleep in the hospitalized patient?
   a. Taking a slow walk around the unit
   b. Providing warm milk before bedtime
   c. Teaching progressive muscle relaxation
   d. Assisting the patient to a position of comfort

10. A concept that is unique to unrelieved chronic pain is that it:
    a. Is generally better tolerated as the duration of exposure increases
    b. Minimally interferes with activities of daily living
    c. Mobilizes the immune response
    d. Is related to current pathology

11. The internal stimulus that most commonly interferes with sleep is:
    a. Buzzing in the ears
    b. Bladder fullness
    c. Hunger
    d. Thirst

12. When giving a back rub, the stroke that is most effective in inducing relaxation at the end of the procedure is:
    a. Percussion
    b. Effleurage
    c. Kneading
    d. Circular

13. Which characteristic of pain is associated with the statement, "The pain moves from my chest down my left arm."
    a. Pattern
    b. Duration
    c. Location
    d. Constancy

14. A concept to teach postoperative patients about pain management is the importance of:
    a. Maintaining a therapeutic serum level of pain medication
    b. Asking for medication once pain is a 7 on a 1-to-10 scale
    c. Using distraction to reduce the pain experience
    d. Assuming a comfortable position

15. Which would best support a nursing diagnosis of Fatigue?
    a. Muscle weakness
    b. Exertional dyspnea
    c. Activity intolerance
    d. Exhaustion unrelieved by rest

16. Which aspect of sleep is most often affected with obstructive sleep apnea?
    a. Amount
    b. Quality
    c. Depth
    d. Onset

17. Which question by the nurse would best assess a patient's pain tolerance?
    a. "Do you take pain medication frequently?"
    b. "How intense on a scale of 1 to 10 is the pain that you feel right now?"
    c. "What activities help distract you so that you don't feel the need for medication?"
    d. "At what point on a scale of 1 to 10 do you feel that you must have pain medication?"

18. Which is the most therapeutic open-ended question the nurse could ask about the quality of a patient's sleep?
    a. "How would you describe your sleep?"
    b. "Do you consider your sleep to be restless or restful?"
    c. "Is the number of hours you sleep at night good for you?"
    d. "Does your bed partner complain about your sleep behaviors?"

19. Which is a common psychological response to pain?
    a. Experiencing fear related to loss of independence
    b. Developing an increased tolerance to the drug
    c. Asking for pain medication to relieve the pain
    d. Verbalizing the presence of nausea

20. The most appropriate goal for an adult who has the nursing diagnosis Disturbed Sleep Pattern Related to Nocturia is, The patient will:
    a. Report fewer early morning awakenings because of a wet bed
    b. Demonstrate a reduction in nighttime bathroom visits
    c. Resume sleeping immediately after voiding
    d. Use an incontinence device at night

21. Which is not a pregnancy-related factor contributing to fatigue?
    a. Increased basal metabolic rate
    b. Changes in hormonal levels
    c. Decreased cardiac output
    d. Low hemoglobin level

22. When meeting patients' sleep and rest needs it is most important for the nurse to:
    a. Teach how sleep and rest promote wellness
    b. Address both the physical and mental components of rest
    c. Encourage at least 8 hours of uninterrupted time for sleep
    d. Recognize that less metabolic energy is expended during illness

23. Which concept associated with rest and sleep must the nurse understand to plan nursing care?
    a. Metabolic rates increase during rest
    b. Energy requirements increase with age
    c. Sleep requirements increase during stress
    d. Catabolic hormones increase during sleep

24. A patient has a total abdominal hysterectomy and debulking for fourth stage ovarian cancer. What should the nurse do first when on the second postoperative day this patient complains of abdominal pain at level 5 of a 1-to-10 pain scale?
    a. Use distraction techniques such as guided imagery
    b. Reposition the patient for personal comfort
    c. Offer a relaxing and comforting back rub
    d. Administer pain medication as ordered

25. Which nursing diagnosis is most important for the nurse to explore when planning care for a patient with narcolepsy?
    a. Disturbed Thought Processes
    b. Self-Care Deficit Syndrome
    c. Risk for Injury
    d. Fatigue

26. The need for additional teaching about how to improve one's sleep pattern would be necessary when the patient says, "I am going to:
    a. Avoid taking a nap in the afternoon."
    b. Take a warm bath in the evening every day."
    c. Set the clock and get up at the same time every day."
    d. Go to bed early, rest, and read a book until I fall asleep."

27. Which adaptation is uniquely associated with shortened REM sleep?
    a. Hyporesponsiveness
    b. Immunosuppression
    c. Irritability
    d. Vertigo

28. Which characteristic of pain is associated with the statement, "It feels like my arm is burning."
    a. Location
    b. Intensity
    c. Quality
    d. Pattern

29. Which sleeping position is best for a person experiencing gastroesophageal reflux disease?
    a. Semi-Fowler's
    b. Right lateral
    c. Supine
    d. Sims'

30. When caring for a patient in pain, the most important thing the nurse must recognize is that:
    a. The extent of pain is directly related to the amount of tissue damage
    b. Administering analgesics for pain will eventually lead to addiction
    c. Behavioral adaptations are congruent with statements about pain
    d. The person experiencing the pain is the authority about the pain

31. Which aspect of sleep is most often affected as a result of anxiety?
    a. Onset
    b. Depth
    c. Stage II
    d. Duration

32. What should the nurse do first when responding to a patient's request for pain medication?
    a. Place the patient in the most comfortable position possible
    b. Use distraction to minimize the perception of pain
    c. Administer pain medication to the patient quickly
    d. Assess the various aspects of the patient's pain

33. With children, which is a major defining characteristic of the nursing diagnosis Disturbed Sleep Pattern?
    a. Hyperactivity
    b. Respiratory disorders
    c. Resisting going to bed
    d. Early morning awakenings

34. Which is a common nursing intervention associated with obstructive sleep apnea?
    a. Teaching the use of devices that support airway patency
    b. Encouraging sleeping in the supine position
    c. Positioning two pillows under the head
    d. Administering sedatives

35. Which statement by the patient would indicate a precipitating factor associated with pain?
    a. "I usually feel a little dizzy and think I'm going to vomit when I have pain."
    b. "I usually have pain after I shower and get dressed in the morning."
    c. "My pain usually comes and goes throughout the night."
    d. "My pain feels like a knife cutting right through me."

36. Which is the most important thing the nurse can do to support a patient's ability to sleep in the hospital setting?
    a. Provide an extra blanket
    b. Limit unnecessary noise on the unit
    c. Shut off lights in the patient's room
    d. Pull curtains around the bed at night

37. One of the most important guidelines associated with providing nursing care to patients with severe chronic pain is:
    a. Determining the level of function that can be performed without pain
    b. Focusing on pain management intervention before pain is excessive
    c. Providing interventions that do not precipitate pain
    d. Asking what is an acceptable level of pain

38. The nurse needs to recognize that when assessing pain:
    a. The lack of expression of pain does not always equate with the pain being experienced
    b. Pain medication can significantly increase a patient's pain tolerance
    c. The majority of cultures value the concept of *suffering in silence*
    d. Most people experience approximately the same pain tolerance

39. Which is the most common cause of sleep deprivation in the hospital setting?
    a. Fragmented sleep
    b. Early awakening
    c. Restless legs
    d. Sleep apnea

40. Which patient statement about pain would cause the most concern?
    a. "At home I take something for pain before it gets too bad."
    b. "They say my pain may get worse and I can't stand it now."
    c. "My pain medication works but I'm afraid of becoming addicted."
    d. "I try to pretend that it is not part of me but it takes a lot of effort."

41. Which most accurately implies physical rest?
    a. Peace of mind
    b. Increased sleep
    c. Decreased movement
    d. Freedom from anxiety

42. Which is a common patient adaptation indicating ICU psychosis associated with sleep deprivation?
   a. Hypoxia
   b. Delirium
   c. Lethargy
   d. Dementia

43. The factor that most commonly interferes with the sleep of people who are hospitalized is:
   a. Napping during the day
   b. Disrupted bedtime rituals
   c. Medication administration
   d. Difficulty finding a comfortable position

44. The patient who poses the greatest challenge to the assessment skills of the nurse when determining a patient's needs for medication in response to acute pain is the patient who is:
   a. Elderly
   b. Confused
   c. Paraplegic
   d. Postoperative

45. Which is a major defining characteristic of the nursing diagnosis Fatigue?
   a. Lacking interest in surroundings
   b. Exhaustion that is relieved by rest
   c. Inability to maintain usual routines
   d. Compromised physical conditioning

46. The action at the painful site that can limit edema and bleeding through vasoconstriction, thereby reducing pain is:
   a. Performing effleurage
   b. Applying a cold pack
   c. Providing massage
   d. Exerting pressure

47. The concept associated with sleep that the nurse must understand to best plan nursing care for the hospitalized patient is:
   a. People require 8 hours of uninterrupted sleep to meet energy needs
   b. Frequency of nighttime awakenings decreases with age
   c. Fear can contribute to the need to stay awake
   d. Bed rest decreases the need to sleep

48. Which word reflects the pattern of pain?
   a. Episodic
   b. Phantom
   c. Moderate
   d. Tenderness

49. Which patient statement about alcohol intake is based on a common physiologic response?
   a. "After I go drinking, I have to urinate during the night."
   b. "When I drink, I get hungry in the middle of the night."
   c. "Falling asleep is hard, but once asleep I sleep great."
   d. "If I drink too much, I oversleep in the morning."

50. When assessing a patient in pain, which defining characteristic is more common in acute pain than in chronic pain?
   a. Self-focusing
   b. Sleep disturbances
   c. Guarding behaviors
   d. Variations in vital signs

51. Preemptive analgesia is used when a nurse medicates the patient:
   a. Before a patient goes to sleep
   b. Equal distant times around the clock
   c. As soon as a patient complains of pain
   d. Before doing a dressing change that has been painful in the past

52. When providing a back massage before bedtime the nurse should:
    a. Use continuous light gliding strokes with finger tips when finishing
    b. Concentrate deep circular motions over the scapulae and sacrum
    c. Knead firmly and quickly over the shoulders and the entire back
    d. Massage gently over the bony prominences of the vertebrae

53. Which nursing diagnosis is most important for the nurse to explore when planning care for a patient diagnosed with chronic fatigue syndrome?
    a. Self-Care Deficit Syndrome
    b. Impaired Physical Mobility
    c. Impaired Gas Exchange
    d. Social Isolation

54. Which sleeping position is best for a person experiencing sleep apnea?
    a. Dorsal recumbent
    b. Semi-Fowler's
    c. Lateral
    d. Supine

55. The most effective intervention to promote sleep that is appropriate for patients in any age group is:
    a. Providing a back rub
    b. Playing relaxing music
    c. Following a bed-time routine
    d. Offering a glass of warm milk

56. When assessing a patient in pain which defining characteristic is more common in chronic pain than in acute pain?
    a. Grunting
    b. Grimacing
    c. Depression
    d. Diaphoresis

57. When caring for patients in pain it is important for the nurse to recognize that patients:
    a. Are able to describe qualities of their pain
    b. Who are in pain will request pain medication
    c. Need to know that the nurse believes what they say about their pain
    d. Will demonstrate vital signs that are congruent with the intensity of pain

58. An adaptation that is a result of shortened NREM sleep is:
    a. Anxiety
    b. Hyperactivity
    c. Delayed healing
    d. Aggressive behavior

59. Which is the most appropriate goal for a patient with a nursing diagnosis of Disturbed Sleep Pattern Related To Pain? The patient will:
    a. Be provided with a back massage every evening before bedtime
    b. Report feeling rested after awakening in the morning
    c. Request less pain medication during the night
    d. Experience 4 hours of uninterrupted sleep

60. Which action is most effective when helping a patient who is experiencing mild pain to get ready for bed?
    a. Obtaining an order for a narcotic
    b. Assisting the patient with relaxing imagery
    c. Encouraging the patient to take a warm shower
    d. Encouraging the patient to be active during the day

61. Which time period is a person most likely to be the most sleepy?
    a. 12 noon to 2 PM
    b. 6 AM to 8 AM
    c. 2 AM to 4 AM
    d. 6 PM to 8 PM

62. A common psychological adaptation to insomnia is:
    a. Vertigo
    b. Fatigue
    c. Headache
    d. Frustration

63. On the day of surgery a postoperative patient states that the pain is unbearable no matter how many times the button is pushed on the patient-controlled analgesia pump. After ensuring the placement of the catheter, the nurse should:
    a. Provide a back massage and reposition the patient for comfort
    b. Ask the physician for IM medication for breakthrough pain
    c. Increase the dosage of medication delivered per hour
    d. Inform the anesthesiologist of the situation

64. Which statement would indicate that the patient is experiencing bruxism?
    a. "I walk around in my sleep almost every night but I don't remember it."
    b. "I annoy the whole family with the loud snoring noises I make at night."
    c. "I occasionally urinate in bed when I am sleeping and it's embarrassing."
    d. "I am told by my wife that I make a lot of noise grinding my teeth when I sleep."

65. Which is a major defining characteristic of the nursing diagnosis Disturbed Sleep Pattern?
    a. Difficulty remaining asleep
    b. Lifestyle disruptions
    c. Mood alterations
    d. Incontinence

ANSWERS AND RATIONALES

1. a. Observations or statements of boredom or depression from inactivity are the major defining characteristics of the nursing diagnosis Deficient Diversional Activity.
   b. Verbalization of an inability to cope, inappropriate use of defense mechanisms, or an inability to meet role expectations are the defining characteristics of the nursing diagnosis Ineffective Individual Coping.
   c. The defining characteristic for Disturbed Thought Processes is inaccurate interpretations of internal or external stimuli.
   d. **Difficulty falling or remaining asleep are the major defining characteristics of the nursing diagnosis Disturbed Sleep Pattern, which is the state in which an individual experiences a change in the quantity or quality of the sleep-rest pattern that causes discomfort or interferes with desired lifestyle.**

2. a. This describes narcolepsy, which is a sudden overwhelming sleepiness (hypersomnia) in the daytime.
   b. This describes sleep terrors, which are episodes of partial awakening accompanied by thrashing, kicking, and rolling movements.
   c. This describes nightmares, which are vivid frightening dreams that occur during REM sleep and awaken the sleeper.
   d. **Episodes of sleep apnea begin with loud snoring followed by silence, during which the person struggles to breathe against a blocked airway. Decreasing oxygen levels cause the person to awaken abruptly with a loud snort.**

3. a. Delirium is not usually a response to severe pain.
   b. **With acute, severe pain, the parasympathetic nervous system is stimulated, causing nausea and vomiting.**
   c. Although patients may respond to severe acute pain by being distracted or withdrawn, confusion is not usually an expected response.
   d. Some patients may sleep through mild pain, but sleep usually is not attainable with severe pain.

4. a. An increased sensitivity to pain is associated with disturbed Rapid Eye Movement (REM) sleep.
   b. **During Non–Rapid Eye Movement (NREM) sleep the parasympathetic nervous system dominates and the vital signs and metabolic rate are low, and growth hormone is consistently secreted, which provides for anabolism. When there is a decrease in these restorative processes, excessive sleepiness results.**
   c. REM sleep is essential for maintaining mental and emotional equilibrium and when interrupted results in confusion, irritability, excitability, restlessness, and suspiciousness.
   d. Irritability, excitability, and restlessness are associated with disturbed REM, not NREM, sleep.

5. a. Activity during the day or early evening stimulates physical functioning and increases mental activity. Activity performed 2 hours before bedtime is appropriate.
   b. A small snack is appropriate because it prevents hunger and promotes sleep if it contains the amino acid L-tryptophan.
   c. Although excessively cold environmental temperatures will cause frequent awakenings, 65 degrees is comfortably cool for sleeping.
   d. **Alcohol shortens sleep onset but its rapid metabolism causes rebound arousal, resulting in shortened REM sleep. It also causes early morning awakenings secondary to a full bladder because alcohol acts as a mild diuretic.**

6. a. Patient-controlled analgesia delivers an intermittent dose of an opioid on demand within safe limitations. Pain relief can be maintained for hours to days.
   b. Intramuscular injections of analgesics usually are effective for 3 to 6 hours.
   c. **Intravenous medications act within 1 to 2 minutes but drug inactivation (biotransformation) also is fast, so there is a short duration of action.**
   d. With regional anesthesia (e.g., nerve block, Bier block, spinal, epidural) an anesthetic agent is instilled around nerves to block the transmission of nerve impulses, thus reducing pain for many hours.

7. a. **An expectation of an outcome of behavior usually becomes a self-fulfilling prophecy. Bedtime rituals include activities that promote comfort and relaxation (e.g., music, reading, praying) and hygienic practices that meet basic physiologic needs (e.g., bathing, brushing the teeth, toileting).**
   b. Alcohol hastens the onset of sleep.
   c. The need for sleep varies and depends on factors such as age, activity level, and health.
   d. The healthy older adult spends more time in bed, spends less time asleep, awakens more often, stays awake longer, and naps more often. REM sleep and Stage IV NREM sleep are reduced, resulting in less restorative sleep. Naps lead to desynchronization of the sleep-wake cycle.

8. a. **Sleep deprivation and dysfunction of the sleep-wake cycle cause ICU psychosis, resulting in Disturbed Thought Processes evidenced by inaccurate interpretations of internal or external stimuli.**
   b. Impaired Gas Exchange relates to problems that interfere with an exchange of oxygen and carbon dioxide between the alveoli of the lungs and the vascular system.
   c. Disuse Syndrome relates to a deterioration of body systems or alteration in function because of prescribed or unavoidable musculoskeletal inactivity.
   d. Sleep deprivation is not related to the nursing diagnosis of Powerlessness, which is the state in which an individual perceives a lack of personal control over certain events or situations that affects outlook, goals, and lifestyle.

9. a. Walking is stimulating and can interfere with the onset of sleep if performed too close to going to bed.
   b. Although milk contains the amino acid L-tryptophan, which promotes sleep, many people do not like milk or avoid fluids before bedtime to limit nocturia.

c. Although progressive muscle relaxation decreases sympathetic nervous system tone, which promotes rest, it is not the most common intervention.

d. Hospital beds can be unfamiliar and uncomfortable. Limited movement, pain, therapeutic equipment, and restrictions on movement may require patients to assume sleeping positions other than their preference. Assisting patients to the most comfortable position possible promotes sleep.

10. a. Persistent chronic pain becomes an unchanging part of life. As the duration of exposure increases, the individual may learn cognitive and behavioral strategies to cope with the pain.

b. Chronic pain can markedly impair activities of daily living.

c. Acute pain and chronic pain both decrease the efficiency of the immune system.

d. Chronic pain may, or may not, have an identifiable cause.

11. a. Although tinnitus can interfere with sleep, it is not the most common problem.

b. Bladder fullness causes pressure in the pelvic area that interrupts sleep. Awakening to void during the night is a common occurrence, particularly in older adult men.

c. Although hunger can interfere with sleep, it is not the most common problem. A light evening snack or glass of milk prevents hunger.

d. Although thirst can interfere with sleep, it is not the most common problem. Thirst is prevented by drinking water as part of the bedtime routine.

12. a. Percussion (tapotement) involves gentle tapping of the skin. Percussion is stimulating and usually is performed during the middle of a back massage.

b. Effleurage involves long, smooth strokes sliding over the skin. When performed slowly with light pressure at the end of a back massage, it has a relaxing, sedative effect.

c. Kneading (petrissage) involves squeezing the skin, subcutaneous tissue, and muscle with a lifting motion. Kneading is stimulating and usually is performed during the middle of a back massage.

d. Circular strokes usually are performed in the area around the buttocks, lower back, and scapulae. They are stimulating and are performed during the beginning of a backrub.

13. a. The pattern of pain refers to time of onset, duration, recurrence, and remissions.

b. Duration refers to how long the pain lasts, which is as aspect of the pattern of pain.

c. This is referred pain, which is pain felt in a part of the body that is a distance from the tissues causing the pain. Referred pain is related to location of pain.

d. Constancy refers to whether the pain is continuous or if there are periods of relief from pain, both of which relate to the pattern of pain.

14. a. Maintaining a therapeutic serum level of an analgesic keeps the patient free from pain and eliminates the peaks and valleys of overmedication and undermedication.

b. This is too long to wait to ask for pain medication. It will take a longer time or a higher dose of medication to return the patient to a pain-free state than if administered earlier.

c. Distraction is usually ineffectual for severe acute pain because of the pain's intensity.

d. A position change alone will be ineffective in relieving severe acute pain because of the pain's intensity.

15. a. One of the major defining characteristics of the nursing diagnosis of Activity Intolerance is exertional fatigue three minutes after stopping activity. Although somewhat related, Fatigue and Activity Intolerance are two separate nursing diagnoses.

b. This is the major defining characteristic of the nursing diagnoses Activity Intolerance and Impaired Gas Exchange

c. Activity Intolerance is a separate nursing diagnosis that relates to a reduction in one's physiologic capacity to endure activities to the degree desired or required.

d. The nursing diagnosis Fatigue is the self-recognized state in which an individual experiences an overwhelming sustained sense of exhaustion and decreased capacity for physical and mental work that is not relieved by rest.

16. a. The amount of time spent sleeping usually is not affected.

b. Sleep apnea is the periodic cessation of breathing during sleep. Episodes occur during REM sleep (interfering with dreaming) and NREM sleep (interfering with restorative sleep), both of which reduce the quality of sleep.

c. Patients still reach the depth of Stage IV NREM sleep.

d. Sleep apnea does not influence the onset of sleep.

17. a. This question focuses on an alleviating factor, medication, rather than on the concept of pain tolerance.

b. This question is determining the patient's perception of the intensity of pain, not pain tolerance.

c. This question focuses on an alleviating factor, distraction, rather than on the concept of pain tolerance.

d. Pain tolerance is the maximum amount and duration of pain that a person is willing to tolerate. It is influenced by psychosociocultural factors and usually increases with age.

18. a. This open-ended question requires patients to explore the topic of sleep as it relates specifically to their own experiences.

b. This direct question gathers information about only one aspect of sleep.

c. This direct question precipitates just a yes or no response.

d. This direct question precipitates just a yes or no response about only one aspect of sleep.

19. a. Psychologic or affective responses to pain relate to feelings and emotional distress. Fear of being dependent on others or loss of self-control are psychological adaptations to pain.

b. Tolerance to a drug is not an adaptation to pain.

Tolerance to a drug can be physiologic and/or psychologic.

c. Requesting pain medication is a behavioral response to pain.

d. Nausea is a physiological response to pain.

20. a. This relates to enuresis, which is recurrent involuntary urination that occurs during sleeping.

b. **This is an appropriate goal for nocturia, which is voluntary urination during the night.**

c. This relates to insomnia, which is difficulty initiating or maintaining sleep.

d. This is an intervention, not a goal.

21. a. The basal metabolic rate rises gradually to an increase of 25%. Normal pregnancy mimics a mild hyperthyroid state to provide the energy required to maintain the pregnancy and promote the development of the fetus.

b. There are major hormonal changes associated with pregnancy. Triiodothyronine (T_3), thyroxine (T_4), cortisol, insulin, parathyroid hormone (PTH), estrogen, progesterone, human chorionic gonadotropin (HCG), relaxin, and human placental lactogen (HPL) increase during pregnancy. Oxytocin is secreted late in pregnancy and prolactin is secreted after birth in response to breastfeeding. Follicle-stimulating hormone (FSH) and luteinizing hormone (LH) cease during pregnancy.

c. **Cardiac output, the amount of blood pumped from the heart in 1 minute, increases by 30 to 50 percent early in the first trimester.**

d. Anemia (low hemoglobin level) associated with pregnancy is called hemodilution of pregnancy. Most of the increased blood volume is plasma causing an imbalance between the ratios of RBCs to plasma and resulting in a decreased hematocrit.

22. a. Although important, this is not as significant as another option.

b. **The mind (psyche) and body (soma) are interrelated and influence each other; therefore, both must be addressed to promote physical and emotional rest.**

c. Although uninterrupted sleep promotes restorative sleep because sleep cycles are not interrupted, the length of time needed is individual.

d. More metabolic energy is expended during illness.

23. a. Metabolic rates decrease by 5 to 25 percent during rest.

b. Energy requirements decrease with age as metabolic processes slow and older adults become more sedentary.

c. **Stress precipitates the sympathetic nervous system increasing cortisone, norepinephrine, and epinephrine, which increase the metabolic rate. Physical and psychic energy expended is restored through rest and sleep.**

d. Catabolic hormones (cortisol and epinephrine) increase with activity, not during sleep. Catabolism is the breaking down of muscle and lean body mass to produce glucose to meet energy needs (gluconeogenesis).

24. a. Guided imagery is more effective for mild pain, not acute, severe pain.

b. Repositioning is effective for mild, not severe, pain.

c. A back massage is ineffective for acute, severe pain; however, it may relax the patient and increase the effectiveness of analgesic medication.

d. **Major abdominal surgery involves extensive manipulation of internal organs and a large abdominal incision that require adequate pharmacologic intervention to provide relief from pain.**

25. a. Narcolepsy is not related to the nursing diagnosis Disturbed Thought Processes, which is the state in which an individual experiences a disruption in mental activities such as conscious thought, reality orientation, problem solving, and judgment.

b. Although the overwhelming daytime sleepiness associated with narcolepsy may interfere with the ability to perform some self-care activities, this is not the major problem related to narcolepsy.

c. **Narcolepsy is excessive sleepiness in the daytime that can cause a person to fall asleep uncontrollably at inappropriate times (sleep attack) and result in physical harm to self or others.**

d. Although a person with narcolepsy may verbalize an overwhelming lack of energy and be unable to maintain usual routines, these are not the primary concerns associated with narcolepsy.

26. a. Naps lead to desynchronization of the sleep-wake cycle and should be avoided.

b. A warm bath may be part of the bedtime ritual because it relaxes muscles, promotes comfort, and facilitates sleep because it raises the core body temperature.

c. Sleep-wake routines should be followed because they support the circadian rhythm associated with sleeping.

d. **When activities other than sleeping are performed in bed, the act of lying down is not specifically associated with the expectation of sleep. Lying down early is counterproductive and may result in frustration.**

27. a. Hyporesponsiveness, withdrawal, apathy, flat facial expression, and excessive sleepiness are physiologic responses associated with a lack of NREM sleep

b. A depressed immune response is a physiologic adaptation to a lack of NREM sleep.

c. **REM sleep is essential for maintaining mental and emotional equilibrium and when interrupted results in irritability, excitability, restlessness, confusion, and suspiciousness.**

d. Shortened NREM sleep can result in vertigo, which is a physiologic response to sleep deprivation.

28. a. The reference to the arm is too general to be related to the location of pain, which is the actual site the pain is felt.

b. Intensity refers to the strength or amount of pain experienced, which often is rated from mild to excruciating.

c. **Quality refers to the description of the pain sensation.**

d. The pattern of pain refers to time of onset, duration, recurrence, and remissions.

29. a. Gastric secretions increase during REM sleep. The semi-Fowler's position limits gastroesophageal reflux because gravity allows the abdominal organs to drop, which reduces pressure on the stomach and results in less stomach contents flowing upward into the esophagus.
    b. This is a horizontal position that increases the pressure of the abdominal organs against the stomach and increases gastric reflux.
    c. This is a horizontal position that increases the pressure of the abdominal organs against the stomach and increases gastric reflux and the risk for aspiration.
    d. This is a horizontal position halfway between lateral and prone. Direct pressure exerted on the stomach, particularly in the left Sims' position, promotes gastric reflux.

30. a. This may or may not be true.
    b. This is not a true statement. The judicious use of narcotics does not necessarily result in addiction. In addition, there are many non-opioid drugs, such as nonsteroidal anti-inflammatory drugs, antidepressants, and anticonvulsants, all of which relieve pain.
    c. This may or may not be true. There may be behavioral signs of pain, such as guarding, grimaces, and clenching the teeth, at the same time that there are no verbal statements indicating the presence of pain. In some cultures, it is unacceptable to complain about pain, or tolerance of pain signifies strength and courage.
    d. Pain is a personal experience. Margo McCaffery, a pain researcher, has indicated that pain is whatever the person in pain says it is and exists whenever the person in pain says it exists.

31. a. Anxiety increases norepinephrine blood levels through stimulation of the sympathetic nervous system, which results in prolonged sleep onset.
    b. Patients with anxiety still reach the depth of Stage IV NREM sleep. However, the number of episodes of and the length of time spent in NREM sleep may be less.
    c. Stage IV, not Stage II, NREM sleep is affected.
    d. The duration of sleep is affected indirectly, not directly, because of the prolonged onset of sleep.

32. a. There is not enough information to indicate that this intervention would be effective. In addition, the position the patient considers most comfortable may be contraindicated based on physician orders or safety issues.
    b. This is premature without information about the intensity of the pain. Distraction is not effective for severe pain.
    c. This is a hasty, impulsive response that may or may not be necessary.
    d. All the factors that affect the pain experience should be assessed, including features such as location, intensity, quality, duration, pattern, aggravating and alleviating factors, and physical, behavioral, and attitudinal adaptations. Assessment must precede intervention.

33. a. Agitation is a minor defining characteristic for the nursing diagnosis of Disturbed Sleep Pattern in an adult, not a child.
    b. Respiratory disorders, such as obstructive sleep apnea, are related factors, not defining characteristics, for the nursing diagnosis of Disturbed Sleep Pattern.
    c. Children may be reluctant to retire at night because of fear, enuresis, or inconsistent adherence to routines by parents.
    d. Early morning awakenings occur with older adults or people who have consumed alcohol.

34. a. A CPAP mask worn over the nose when sleeping keeps the upper airway patent through continuous positive airway pressure.
    b. This increases the episodes of sleep apnea because the structures of the mouth and oropharynx (tonsils, adenoids, mucous membranes, uvula, soft palate, and tongue) drop by gravity and ultimately obstruct the airway.
    c. This flexes the neck, which narrows the upper airway and thus contributes to episodes of sleep apnea. Pillows under the upper shoulders and head or small blocks under the head of the bed may assist in keeping the upper airway open.
    d. Sedatives do not limit episodes of sleep apnea.

35. a. These are physiologic adaptations, not precipitating factors, associated with the pain experience.
    b. Anything that induces or aggravates pain is considered a precipitating factor of pain. For example, precipitating factors may be physical (exertion associated with ADLs, Valsalva maneuver), environmental (extremes in temperature, noise), or emotional (anxiety, fear).
    c. This statement reflects the pattern (onset, duration, and intervals) of the pain experience.
    d. This statement reflects the quality of the pain. Descriptive adjectives, such as knife-like, burning, or cramping, explain how the pain feels.

36. a. Although meeting the basic physiologic need to feel warm is appropriate, a hospital's environment generally is warm, so a top sheet and spread are adequate.
    b. Noise is a major deterrent to sleep in a hospital. Limit environmental noise (paging system, telephones, call light), procedural noise (distributing fluids, providing treatments, rolling drug and linen carts), and staff communication noise.
    c. This is unsafe. Dim the lights or put a night light on to provide enough illumination for safe ambulation to the bathroom.
    d. Although this provides privacy, it does not limit the environmental factors that usually interfere with sleeping in a hospital.

37. a. Although the nurse and patient attempt to do this, there may be unavoidable activities that may precipitate pain.
    b. Administration of analgesics around the clock at regularly scheduled intervals (ATC administration) or by long-acting controlled

release transdermal patches maintains therapeutic blood levels of analgesics, which limit pain at levels of comfort acceptable to patients.

    c. Although the nurse will attempt to do this, there may be significant interventions that must be performed that may precipitate pain.

    d. Although the nurse will ask this question to determine the patient's level of pain tolerance, it is not the priority.

38. a. An obvious response to pain is not always apparent because psychosociocultural factors may dictate behavior. Fear of the treatment for pain, lack of validation, acceptance of pain as punishment for previous behavior, and the need to be strong, courageous, or uncomplaining are factors that influence behavioral responses to pain.

    b. The opposite may be true. As a person experiences relief from pain, the person may be unwilling to endure previously acceptable levels of pain.

    c. This is not a true statement. Although a generalization, many groups such as Jewish, Italian, Greek, and Chinese are able to express their pain.

    d. Pain tolerance varies widely among people and is influenced by experiential, psychologic and sociocultural factors.

39. a. Sleep deprivation occurs with frequent interruptions of sleep because the sleeper returns to Stage I rather than to the stage that was interrupted. There is a greater loss of Stage III and IV NREM sleep, which is essential for restorative sleep.

    b. Although early awakenings often do occur in hospital settings, it is not the most common cause of sleep deprivation in the hospital.

    c. Restless legs syndrome, an intrinsic sleep disorder, is not the most common cause of sleep deprivation in the hospital.

    d. Only 1 to 4 percent of the population has sleep apnea.

40. a. This is desirable because it keeps pain under control before it becomes excessive.

    b. The level of pain tolerance is exceeded. The present pain must be relieved and the patient assured that the future pain also would be controlled.

    c. The concern of addiction is not the priority among these statements. The nurse can respond to this common concern through education and judicious medication administration.

    d. This is not the statement of greatest concern. Nonpharmacologic measures to relieve pain, such as imagery and self-hypnosis, use the mind-body (psyche-soma) connection to reduce pain. The nurse should encourage the use of these measures and validate the energy expended.

41. a. Peace of mind relates to emotional rest because it does not require psychic energy.

    b. The number of hours a person sleeps is not necessarily directly proportional to the amount of physical rest experienced.

    c. Stage IV sleep is the deepest restorative sleep stage where the muscles are completely relaxed

and the person rarely moves and is difficult to arouse.

    d. Freedom from anxiety relates to emotional rest because it does not require psychic energy.

42. a. Hypoxia is associated with obstructive sleep apnea because episodes of upper airway obstruction occur 50 to 600 times a night.

    b. Melatonin, the "hormone of darkness," regulates the circadian phases of sleep. Environmental triggers called synchronizers adjust the sleep-wake cycle to a 24-hour solar day. With ICU psychosis, bright lights and increased sensory input cause disorientation to day and night and interrupt sleep. Interrupted sleep results in lability of mood, irritability, excitability, suspiciousness, confusion, and delirium.

    c. Lethargy and fatigue are earlier signs of sleep deprivation.

    d. Sleep deprivation may cause impaired memory, confusion, illusions, and visual or auditory hallucinations, not dementia.

43. a. The lights, noise, and activity in the hospital environment usually interfere with napping during the day. However, naps when they do occur are usually short and rarely reach Stage IV restorative sleep.

    b. Hospitalized patients can follow their normal bedtime rituals.

    c. Most medications are administered by 10 to 11 PM and should not interfere with sleep.

    d. Patients frequently find hospital beds unfamiliar and uncomfortable. In addition, therapeutic regimens restrict movement or require patients to assume sleeping positions other than their preference.

44. a. Although nurses must recognize that older adults generally have a higher tolerance for pain than younger people do, this is not the greatest challenge in the options presented.

    b. Confused patients have a cognitive deficit that may impair their ability to interpret painful stimuli, report their pain verbally, or fully participate with the nurse in the exploration of their pain. The nurse must use careful assessment, empathy, and knowledge about the patient's problem, especially when caring for cognitively impaired patients in pain.

    c. People with paralyzed lower extremities (paraplegia) do not pose the greatest challenge for pain assessment because they still have sensory functioning, can feel pain, and can communicate with others.

    d. Postoperative pain assessment is not the most difficult situation in which to assess pain because at least one factor is understood, the source of the trauma responsible for the pain.

45. a. This is a minor, not a major, defining characteristic of the nursing diagnosis Fatigue.

    b. Exhaustion relieved by rest relates to the nursing diagnosis Activity Intolerance. The nursing diagnosis Fatigue is related to a sustained sense of exhaustion that is unrelieved by rest.

    c. An inability to maintain usual routines along with

verbalization of distress and an unremitting and overwhelming lack of energy are the major defining characteristics of the nursing diagnosis Fatigue.

d. Compromised physical conditioning caused by factors that compromise oxygen transport relates to the nursing diagnosis Activity Intolerance.

46. a. Effleurage—long, smooth strokes sliding over the skin—reduces pain by using the Gate Control Theory of Pain. Peripheral stimuli transmitted via large-diameter nerves close the gate to painful stimuli that use small-diameter nerves, thereby blocking the perception of pain.

b. **Cold lowers the temperature of skin and underlying tissue and causes vasoconstriction, which reduces blood flow to the area. This controls bleeding and slows the passage of fluid from the intravascular to the interstitial compartment, which limits edema.**

c. Massage is cutaneous stimulation that uses the Gate Control Theory of Pain, not vasoconstriction, to limit pain.

d. Acupressure closes the gate mechanism to pain or stimulates areas near pain fibers leading to the brain, thereby blocking the perception of pain.

47. a. Although uninterrupted sleep is advantageous for restorative sleep, the number of hours depends on the individual.

b. In older adults Stage IV sleep is markedly decreased; they awaken more frequently, and it takes them longer to go back to sleep.

c. **Fear of loss of control, potential death, and the unknown results in the struggle to stay awake, which interferes with the ability to relax sufficiently to fall asleep.**

d. Bed rest does not decrease the need to sleep. The body still needs Stage IV restorative sleep. Often the physiologic problems requiring the bed rest increase the need for sleep.

48. a. **The word episode refers to an incident, occurrence, or time period; therefore, episodic refers here to patterns of pain, and is concerned with time of onset, duration, recurrence, and remissions.**

b. Phantom pain is related to location of pain. Phantom pain is a painful sensation perceived in a body part that is missing.

c. The description of pain as being moderate is related to intensity of pain.

d. Tenderness is a sensory word that describes pain and is related to the quality of pain.

49. a. **Alcoholic beverages are fluids that have a mild diuretic effect. Frequent nighttime awakenings to empty a full bladder are called nocturia.**

b. Excessive drinking usually causes nausea and vomiting rather than hunger.

c. Alcohol hastens, not delays, the onset of sleep.

d. Alcohol disrupts sleep and causes early morning awakenings.

50. a. Self-focusing is associated with chronic, not acute, pain because its unrelenting, prolonged nature interferes with pursuing a normal life. As a result,

there may be changes in family dynamics, sexual functioning, financial status, and self-esteem that result in introspection and depression.

b. Pain is an internal stimulus that can interrupt sleep. Because chronic pain is unrelenting and prolonged, over time interrupted sleep results in sleep deprivation.

c. Guarding behaviors occur in both acute and chronic pain. However, because of the unrelenting prolonged nature of chronic pain, behavioral adaptations such as guarding, stooped posture, and altered gait may become permanent adaptations.

d. **Acute pain stimulates the sympathetic nervous system, which responds by increasing pulse, respirations, and blood pressure. Chronic pain stimulates the parasympathetic nervous system, which resuls in lowered pulse and blood pressure.**

51. a. Hour of sleep (h.s., *hora somni*) medications usually are sedatives that promote rest and sleep.

b. Medications administered *around the clock at regularly scheduled intervals* (ATC) usually maintain therapeutic drug levels regardless of other factors influencing the patient.

c. Medication administered when necessary at the patient's request will have a physician's order that states *p.r.n.* (**p**ro **r**e **n**ata).

d. **The word preemptive means preventive, anticipatory, and defensive. Therefore, preemptive analgesia is administered before activity or interventions that may precipitate pain in an attempt to limit the anticipated pain.**

52. a. **Effleurage involves long, smooth strokes sliding over the skin that have a relaxing, sedative effect. When performed slowly with light pressure at the end of a back massage it is called "feathering off."**

b. Firm, not deep, circular motions are used with back massage.

c. Kneading (petrissage) is not performed over the vertebrae because it is stimulating and traumatic for the vertebral column and spinal cord.

d. Massage over the vertebrae is contraindicated because it is traumatic to the vertebral column and spinal cord. Massage should be performed on either side of the vertebrae.

53. a. **Chronic fatigue syndrome is a condition characterized by the onset of disabling fatigue after an initial viral-like illness. The fatigue is so overwhelming and consuming it interferes with the activities of daily living.**

b. Chronic fatigue syndrome does not impair mobility. The nursing diagnosis Impaired Physical Mobility is the state in which an individual experiences limitation of physical movement but is not immobile.

c. Although fatigue is a minor defining characteristic for the nursing diagnosis Impaired Gas Exchange, the fatigue is caused by hypoxia and is unrelated to chronic fatigue syndrome, which is a very different condition.

d. The fatigue of chronic fatigue syndrome is unrelated to the nursing diagnosis Social Isolation, which is a state in which an individual experiences or perceives a desire for increased involvement with others but is unable to make that contact.

54. a. The dorsal recumbent position is a back-lying position that permits the tongue and soft tissues of the mouth and oropharynx to fall backward by gravity, which obstructs the airway.
  b. The semi-Fowler's position is a back-lying position that permits the tongue and soft tissues of the mouth and oropharynx to fall backward by gravity, which obstructs the airway.
  c. The side-lying position allows the tongue and soft tissues of the mouth and upper respiratory tract to drop away from the oropharynx, promoting an open airway.
  d. The supine position is a back-lying position that permits the tongue and soft tissues of the mouth and oropharynx to fall backward by gravity, which obstructs the airway.

55. a. Back massage is the therapeutic manipulation of muscles and tissues that relaxes tense muscles, relieves muscle spasms, and induces rest or sleep. However, it may be contraindicated, and some people do not like a backrub or consider it an invasion of their personal space.
  b. Music can be relaxing or stimulating depending on the music and the individual.
  c. Following routines provides consistency and comfort in an unfamiliar environment. Bedtime rituals meet basic physiologic needs and usually include physically and emotionally relaxing behaviors.
  d. Although milk contains the amino acid L-tryptophan that promotes sleep, many people do not like milk or avoid fluids before bedtime to limit nocturia.

56. a. Grunting is a minor defining characteristic for acute, not chronic, pain.
  b. Grimacing is a behavioral adaptation associated with acute, not chronic, pain.
  c. Prolonged unrelenting pain interferes with quality of life and is psychologically debilitating, which can result in frustration, depression, and withdrawal.
  d. Diaphoresis is a sympathetic nervous system response to acute, not chronic, pain.

57. a. Patients, particularly children and those who are cognitively impaired, often have problems describing the quality of pain because of difficulty interpreting painful stimuli or having never experienced the sensation before.
  b. Psychosociocultural factors influence patients' lack of request for medication when experiencing pain. Patients may not request medication because they fear the possibility of addiction, consider the pain as punishment for previous behavior, or need to be strong, courageous, or uncomplaining.
  c. Pain is a personal experience, and the nurse must validate its presence and severity as perceived by the patient. This conveys acceptance and respect and promotes the development of trust.
  d. Acute pain increases vital signs because of parasympathetic nervous system stimulation, but chronic pain will not.

58. a. Rapid Eye Movement (REM) sleep is essential for maintaining mental and emotional equilibrium and when interrupted results in anxiety, irritability, excitability, restlessness, confusion, and suspiciousness.
  b. Interrupted REM, not NREM, sleep is associated with hyperactivity, excitability, and restlessness.
  c. During Non-Rapid Eye Movement (NREM) sleep growth hormone is consistently secreted, and provides for protein synthesis, anabolism, and tissue repair.
  d. Interrupted REM, not NREM, sleep is associated with excitability, emotional lability, and suspiciousness. Interrupted NREM sleep is associated with apathy, withdrawal, and hyporesponsiveness.

59. a. This is a planned nursing intervention, not a goal.
  b. Sleep is a sensory experience that restores cerebral and physical functioning. Evaluations related to sleep are based on patient reports because effectiveness of sleep is subjective.
  c. This is a goal for the nursing diagnoses of Acute or Chronic Pain.
  d. Four hours of sleep is not enough for most adults. Most adults require 6 to 8 hours of sleep.

60. a. Narcotics should be a last resort. Nursing interventions or non-narcotic medications are usually effective in limiting mild pain.
  b. Imagery, the internal experience of memories, dreams, fantasies, or visions, uses positive images to distract, which reduces stress, limits mild pain, and promotes relaxation and sleep.
  c. Bathing preferences are highly individual, and the patient may not prefer a shower. In addition, a shower is stimulating and may be contraindicated.
  d. Although daytime activity does promote sleep at night, patients with pain may be reluctant to be active.

61. a. At this time of day, most people are engaged in stimulating activities and generally are not sleepy.
  b. By this time of the normal sleep cycle, most people have had sufficient sleep and are beginning to awaken.
  c. Research has demonstrated that most people experience sleep-vulnerable periods between 2 AM and 6 AM and between 2 PM and 5 PM.
  d. At this time of day, most people are engaged in stimulating activities such as preparing and eating dinner.

62. a. Shortened NREM sleep can result in vertigo, which is a physiologic response to sleep deprivation.
  b. Interrupted REM and NREM sleep can result in fatigue, which is a physiologic response to sleep deprivation.
  c. Shortened NREM sleep can result in headache, which is a physiologic response to sleep deprivation.
  d. Insomnia has a self-perpetuating nature. As the difficulty initiating or maintaining sleep continues, the person becomes more and more concerned, upset, and frustrated with the lack of amount and quality of sleep, further precipitating insomnia.

63. a. These interventions are effective for mild to moderate pain, not severe unbearable pain.
    b. The practitioner may eventually order this, but it is not the nurse's priority intervention.
    c. This is not within the scope of nursing practice.
    d. The pain control plan is ineffective and the physician should be notified to reassess the situation. The analgesic dose may be increased, the analgesic may be changed, or an alternate or additional delivery route selected.

64. a. Somnambulism, sleepwalking, is a parasomnia that occurs during Stage III and IV NREM sleep.
    b. Snoring relates to obstructive sleep apnea, which is a periodic cessation of airflow during inspiration that results in arousal from sleep.
    c. Nocturnal enuresis, bedwetting, is a parasomnia that occurs when moving from Stage III to IV of NREM sleep.
    d. Bruxism, clenching and grinding of the teeth, is a parasomnia that occurs during Stage II NREM sleep. It usually does not interfere with sleep for the affected individual but rather the sleeper's partner.

65. a. Difficulty falling or remaining asleep are the major defining characteristics of the nursing diagnosis Disturbed Sleep Pattern, which is the state in which an individual experiences a change in the quantity or quality of the rest pattern that causes discomfort or interferes with desired lifestyle.
    b. Lifestyle disruptions relate to the definition, not the major defining characteristics, of the nursing diagnosis Disturbed Sleep Pattern
    c. Lability of mood is a minor, not major, defining characteristic of the nursing diagnoses Disturbed Sleep Pattern and Fatigue.
    d. Incontinence is a pathophysiologic related factor, not major defining characteristic, of the nursing diagnosis Disturbed Sleep Pattern.

Perioperative Nursing

The following words include English vocabulary, nursing/medical terminology, concepts, principles, or information relevant to content specifically addressed in the chapter or associated with topics presented in it. English dictionaries, your nursing textbooks, and medical dictionaries such as *Taber's Cyclopedic Medical Dictionary* are resources that can be used to expand your knowledge and understanding of these words and related information.

Abdominal binder
Anesthesia, types
   Epidural
   General
   Local
   Nerve block
   Regional
   Spinal
Anesthesiologist
Anesthetist
Antiembolism stockings
   Elastic
   Sequential compression devices
Bowel preparation
Certified Registered Nurse Anesthetist
Circulating nurse
Collagen production
Conscious sedation
Debridement
Deep breathing and coughing
Drains, types
   Penrose
   Portable wound drainage systems
      Hemovac
      Jackson-Pratt
Dressings, types
   Occlusive dressing
   Dry sterile dressing
   Duoderm and Tegaderm
   Transparent wound barrier: Opsite
   Wet to moist

Granulation
Hypostatic pneumonia
Incision
Informed consent
Intraoperative
Laparoscopic
Latex allergy
Leg exercises
Nasogastric decompression
Negative pressure
NPO status
Pain management
Patient controlled analgesia (PCA)
Perioperative
Postoperative complications
   Aspiration
   Deep vein thrombosis
   Dehiscence
   Evisceration
   Malignant hyperthermia
   Paralytic ileus
   Pneumonia
   Pulmonary emboli
   Wound infection
Positioning
Post-Anesthesia Care Unit
Postoperative
Postoperative protocols
Preoperative
Preoperative check list
Preoperative medication

Radiation safety
Registered Nurse First Assistant
Residual limb
Scrub nurse
Skin preparation
Skin staple
Surgical asepsis
Surgery, purposes of
   Ablative
   Constructive
   Diagnostic
   Palliative
   Reconstructive
   Transplant
Surgery types
   Ambulatory surgery
   Elective surgery
   Urgent surgery
   Emergency surgery
   Minor surgery
   Major surgery
Suture
Tonsillectomy
Turning and positioning
Urinary clearance
Wound
Wound drainage
   Purulent drainage
   Sanguineous drainage
   Serosanguineous drainage
   Serous drainage

1. The difference between a Jackson-Pratt and a Hemovac is:
   a. The size of the collection container
   b. How the pressure within the collection container is reestablished
   c. The type of pressure that promotes drainage to the collection container
   d. Where the collection container should be placed in relation to the insertion site

2. The patient that would be at highest risk receiving general anesthesia would be the patient with:
   a. Gastroesophageal reflux disease
   b. Reduced reflexes
   c. Hypothyroidism
   d. Emphysema

3. Which type of incisional drainage should be expected four hours after surgery?
   a. Serous wound drainage
   b. Purulent wound drainage
   c. Sanguineous wound drainage
   d. Serosanguineous wound drainage

4. Which vitamin is commonly ordered for postoperative patients?
   a. Vitamin A
   b. Vitamin B
   c. Vitamin C
   d. Vitamin K

5. When a patient spikes a temperature during the first postoperative day it usually indicates a potential problem involving the:
   a. Intestines
   b. Bladder
   c. Wound
   d. Lungs

6. Which nursing diagnosis is of most concern while a patient is in the Post-Anesthesia Care Unit?
   a. Acute Pain
   b. Total Incontinence
   c. Disturbed Thought Process
   d. Ineffective Airway Clearance

7. Which nursing action is appropriate when applying a transparent wound barrier (Op-Site, Tegaderm)?
   a. Clean the skin with normal saline before applying the dressing
   b. Stretch the transparent wound barrier snugly over the entire wound
   c. Cover the transparent wound barrier with a gauze 4 × 4 and secure with paper tape
   d. Ensure that reinforcing tape extends several inches beyond the edges of the transparent wound barrier

8. Which is most important when positioning a patient for surgery?
   a. Allowing for skeletal deformities
   b. Preventing pressure on bony prominences
   c. Providing for adequate thoracic expansion
   d. Avoiding stretching of neuromuscular tissue

9. Perioperative nursing care begins when the:
   a. Patient is transferred to the operating room
   b. Decision for surgery is made
   c. Consent form is signed
   d. Patient is anesthetized

10. One hour after surgery for an open reduction and internal fixation for a fractured wrist the nurse notices a centimeter circle of drainage on the patient's cast. What should the nurse do first?
    a. Inform the surgeon immediately
    b. Reinforce the cast with a gauze dressing
    c. Nothing, but continue to monitor the area for expansion
    d. Circle the spot with a pen and date, time, and initial the area

11. Which sudden adaptation on the first postoperative day would indicate a life-threatening event?
    a. Slightly elevated temperature
    b. 2+ edema of the legs
    c. Wound dehiscence
    d. Chest pain

12. The discharge criteria of the Post-Anesthesia Care Unit that is especially specific for the patient with spinal anesthesia is, discharge will occur when:
    a. Oxygen saturation reaches the presurgical baseline
    b. Motor and sensory function returns
    c. Nausea and vomiting are minimal
    d. Headache is considered tolerable

13. A clear liquid diet is ordered on the third postoperative day for a patient who had abdominal surgery primarily because it:
    a. Relieves abdominal distention
    b. Stimulates digestive enzymes
    c. Prevents paralytic ileus
    d. Is easily digested

14. Which nursing action is most important during a patient's stay in the Post-Anesthesia Care Unit?
    a. Monitoring urinary output
    b. Assessing level of consciousness
    c. Ensuring patency of drainage tubes
    d. Suctioning mucus from respiratory passages

15. Which is not a common diagnostic test done prior to surgery for all patients who will be receiving general anesthesia?
    a. Urinalysis
    b. Chest x-ray
    c. Electrocardiogram
    d. Complete blood count

16. Which is the most important nursing action associated with caring for a patient with a Penrose wound drain?
    a. Removing the excess external portion until drainage stops
    b. Removing the soiled dressing carefully
    c. Pinning the drain to the dressing
    d. Maintaining negative pressure

17. Which position is most appropriate for the patient who has received spinal anesthesia?
    a. Prone
    b. Supine
    c. Right lateral
    d. Trendelenburg

18. What nutrient containing vitamin C should the patient be encouraged to eat to facilitate wound healing?
    a. Liver
    b. Cheese
    c. Broccoli
    d. Legumes

19. Which would be most appropriate during the first 24 hours after a tonsillectomy?
    a. Warm pudding
    b. Milk shake
    c. Soft toast
    d. Ice pops

20. To best assess a patient's gastrointestinal status postoperatively, the nurse should:
    a. Identify the time of the first bowel movement
    b. Monitor for tolerance of a clear liquid diet
    c. Palpate for abdominal distention
    d. Auscultate for bowel sounds

21. Four days after abdominal surgery, while being transferred from a bed to a chair, a patient says to a nurse, "My incision felt funny all of a sudden." What should the nurse do first?
    a. Take the patient's vital signs
    b. Apply an abdominal binder immediately
    c. Place the patient in the low-Fowler's position
    d. Encourage the patient to deep breathe and relax

22. When admitting a patient who is to receive general anesthesia in the morning for ambulatory surgery, it is most important for the nurse to ask, "Did you:
    a. Void this morning?"
    b. Eat or drink anything after midnight last night?"
    c. Have a bowel movement within the last 24 hours?"
    d. Practice your deep breathing and coughing exercises yesterday?"

23. A patient should be placed in a semi-Fowler's position after abdominal surgery primarily to:
    a. Support ventilation
    b. Facilitate the passing of flatus
    c. Encourage urinary elimination
    d. Promote drainage in the wound drainage system

24. Which would cause the greatest risk for postoperative nausea and vomiting after receiving general anesthesia?
    a. Obesity
    b. Inactivity
    c. Hypervolemia
    d. Unconsciousness

25. On the second postoperative day after an above-the-knee amputation the patient's elastic dressing accidentally comes off. What should the nurse do first?
    a. Wrap the residual limb with an elastic compression bandage
    b. Apply a saline dressing to the residual limb
    c. Elevate the limb on two pillows
    d. Notify the physician

26. Which action is most effective in preventing postoperative urinary tract infections?
    a. Dietary roughage
    b. Adequate fluid intake
    c. Sitz baths twice a day
    d. Intake of citrus fruit juices

27. After patients have received conscious sedation they are:
    a. Unresponsive and pain-free
    b. At risk for malignant hyperthermia
    c. Sleepy but arousable for several hours
    d. Positioned in the supine position to prevent headache

28. A portable wound drainage system should be emptied:
    a. After it is full
    b. Every 2 hours
    c. When it is half full
    d. At the end of each shift

29. Which patient having emergency surgery would the nurse anticipate to be at highest risk for postoperative mortality?
    a. Chronic alcoholic
    b. Older adult
    c. Epileptic
    d. Infant

30. Which is the best way to prevent postoperative thrombophlebitis?
    a. Elevation of the legs on two pillows
    b. Utilization of compression stockings at night
    c. Deep breathing and coughing exercises daily
    d. Leg exercises 10 times per hour when awake

31. Vitamin C is often ordered by the physician for a postoperative patient to:
    a. Improve digestion
    b. Support collagen production
    c. Encourage growth of red blood cells
    d. Minimize the formation of deep vein thrombosis

32. After a patient has abdominal surgery, the nursing diagnosis that would cause the most concern would be:
    a. Constipation
    b. Urinary Retention
    c. Self-Care Deficient Syndrome
    d. Ineffective Breathing Pattern

33. Which is the most important information that the nurse needs to know when a patient arrives in the Post-Anesthesia Care Unit?
    a. Type and extent of the surgery
    b. Anxiety level before the surgery
    c. Special requests that were verbalized by the patient
    d. Type and amount of IV fluids administered during surgery

34. An adaptation that would indicate a risk for wound dehiscence is:
    a. Pain along the incision line the second postoperative day
    b. Discomfort along the incision line the first postoperative day
    c. Slight crusting along the incision line the fourth postoperative day
    d. Serosanguineous drainage along the incision line the sixth postoperative day

35. The nurse understands that a central venous catheter inserted into a peripheral vein is preferable to a central venous catheter inserted into a subclavian vein because a peripheral catheter will:
    a. Be in the superior vena cava
    b. Never cause a pneumothroax
    c. Always prevent the development of an infection
    d. Allow large volumes of fluid to be administered

36. Evidence of a postoperative wound infection usually is not apparent before the:
    a. Fifth day
    b. Third day
    c. Ninth day
    d. Seventh day

37. Which patient adaptation is most common after spinal anesthesia?
    a. Headache
    b. Neuropathy
    c. Lower back discomfort
    d. Increased blood pressure

38. A hospitalized patient who has been receiving medications via a variety of routes for several days is scheduled for surgery at 10:00 AM. On the day of surgery the nurse should plan to:
    a. Use an alternate route for the oral medications
    b. Withhold all the previously ordered medications
    c. Withhold the oral medications and administer the other drugs
    d. Obtain directions from the physician regarding the medications

39. Which is the most common diet ordered after surgery?
    a. Clear liquids
    b. Full liquids
    c. Low fiber
    d. Regular

40. Which adaptations would best support the decision to discharge the patient from the Post-Anesthesia Care Unit?
    a. SaO₂ of 95%, vital signs stable for 30 minutes, active gag reflex
    b. Afebrile, presence of adventitious breath sounds, ability to cough
    c. Urinary output of 30 cc per hour, awake, turning from side to side
    d. Tolerable pain, ability to move all extremities, dry, intact dressing

41. The most important aspect associated with general anesthesia is:
    a. Ensuring the loss of pain sensation
    b. Providing for adequate ventilation
    c. Observing for reflex activity
    d. Monitoring the heart rate

42. A patient has a right abdominal incision. When giving instructions on how to get out of bed, the nurse should teach the patient to:
    a. Exit from the left side of the bed
    b. Ask the nurse to apply an abdominal binder
    c. Hold a pillow on the abdomen with both hands
    d. Use the right elbow to assist in lifting the body to a sitting position

43. Which complication has occurred when a postoperative patient experiences tachycardia, sudden chest pain, and a low blood pressure?
    a. Pulmonary embolus
    b. Hemorrhage
    c. Heart attack
    d. Pneumonia

44. Which is the most effective nursing action to help the postoperative patient manage abdominal discomfort in the absence of bowel sounds?
    a. Encouraging frequent ambulation
    b. Ensuring adequate fluids by mouth
    c. Providing sufficient fiber in the diet
    d. Administering p.r.n. pain medication

45. Which patient adaptation would indicate altered renal perfusion during the postoperative period?
    a. Oliguria
    b. Cachexia
    c. Yellow sclera
    d. Suprapubic distention

46. When is an oral airway removed after general anesthesia?
    a. As soon as the patient arrives in the Post-Anesthesia Care Unit
    b. Upon completion of a head to toe assessment of the patient
    c. When the patient tries to eject the airway from the mouth
    d. Once the patient exhibits restlessness

47. When evaluating the effectiveness of interventions for meeting the nutrient needs of patients during the first days after abdominal surgery, which outcome is most important?
    a. Nausea and vomiting has not occurred
    b. Fluid and electrolytes are balanced
    c. Wound healing is progressing
    d. Oral intake is reestablished

48. After assessing a postoperative patient for a patent airway, which is the next most important assessment to be made by the nurse?
    a. Condition of drains
    b. Cardiovascular status
    c. Level of consciousness
    d. Location of surgical dressing

49. Which nursing diagnosis would be the priority for a patient in the Post-Anesthesia Care Unit?
    a. Acute Pain R/T Tissue Trauma
    b. Nausea R/T Effects of Anesthesia
    c. Risk for Aspiration R/T Reduced Level of Consciousness
    d. Deficient Fluid Volume R/T Excessive Loss Through Indwelling Catheters and Drains

50. When changing an abdominal dressing it is noticed that the wound edges are separated and several loops of the patient's bowel are protruding from the wound. What should the nurse do first?
    a. Take the patient's vital signs
    b. Notify the physician immediately
    c. Apply a sterile saline dressing to the patient's wound
    d. Place the patient in a 10 degree Trendelenburg position

51. Which action is most important when applying antiembolism stockings?
    a. Ensuring that the toe window is properly positioned
    b. Applying the stockings after the patient is out of bed
    c. Flexing the knee as the stocking is pulled over the knee
    d. Removing the stocking once every 24 hours for 30 minutes

52. Which nutrients are the best in supporting collagen production?
    a. Whole grain breads
    b. Yellow vegetables
    c. Citrus fruits
    d. Red meat

53. An important action by the nurse when caring for a patient recovering from abdominal surgery that would facilitate ventilation would be:
    a. Preventing abdominal distention
    b. Positioning in the side-lying position
    c. Monitoring respiratory status every hour
    d. Providing passive range-of-motion exercises

54. A patient undergoing perineal surgery should be placed in the:
    a. Sims' position
    b. Supine position
    c. Lithotomy position
    d. Trendelenburg position

55. The nurse identifies that 4 hours after surgery a patient's portable wound drainage system contains only a small amount of drainage. The nurse's initial action should be to:
    a. Inspect the site of the incision
    b. Check the drainage system tubing for kinks
    c. Open the collection container and reestablish pressure
    d. Move the collection container below the level of the insertion site

1. a. A Hemovac is designed to accommodate 100, 400, or 800 ml of drainage depending on the system used, while a Jackson-Pratt accommodates volumes under 100 ml of drainage.
   b. Both create a vacuum by closing the air vent while compressing the device.
   c. Both work by gentle negative pressure that draws fluid from the tissues to the collection chamber.
   d. Both collection chambers should be placed below the site of insertion to allow gravity to work in conjunction with the negative pressure within the self-contained systems.

2. a. This is not a problem with general anesthesia because of interventions such as NPO status for at least 8 hours before surgery, use of a cuffed endotracheal tube, and positioning.
   b. Although this is significant to know when monitoring a patient throughout the surgical experience, it does not place a patient at the highest risk.
   c. Although a decreased metabolism is taken into consideration when monitoring reflexes during the induction, maintenance, and reversal phases of anesthesia, hypothyroidism does not place a patient at the highest risk.
   d. **Respiratory problems complicate the administration of inhalation anesthesia. Emphysema is characterized by destruction of alveoli, loss of elastic recoil, and narrowing of bronchioles, which results in alveolar hyperinflation and increased airflow resistance.**

3. a. Serous exudate is a clear, watery fluid consisting mainly of serum. It is the exudate expected before final wound healing.
   b. Purulent exudate is a thick drainage known as pus, which consists of leukocytes, liquefied dead tissue debris, and bacteria. This is unexpected and indicates the presence of a wound infection. Wound infections become apparent 2 to 11 days postoperatively.
   c. Sanguineous (hemorrhagic) exudate consists of large amounts of red blood cells and is associated with open wounds or hemorrhage.
   d. **Serosanguineous exudate, a combination of serous and sanguineous drainage, consists of plasma and red blood cells and is pale red and watery. This is the initial drainage expected after surgery.**

4. a. Although vitamin A is associated with epithelial tissue, it usually is not ordered individually but rather as part of a multivitamin.
   b. Although the B complex vitamins are related to protein synthesis and cross-linking of collagen fibers, they usually are not ordered individually but rather as part of a multivitamin.
   c. **Vitamin C (ascorbic acid) is essential for collagen formation, the single most important protein of connective tissue. The recommended daily dose is 60 mg; however, a postoperative patient may need up to 1000 mg of vitamin C for tissue repair, necessitating supplementation.**
   d. Although vitamin K promotes blood clotting by increasing the synthesis of prothrombin by the liver,

it usually is not ordered individually unless the patient has liver disease or a bleeding tendency.

5. a. The absence of intestinal motility (paralytic ileus), not infection, is the intestinal adaptation that can occur during the first 24 to 36 hours after surgery. Abdominal distention and absent bowel sounds, not a fever, indicate this problem.
   b. Postoperative bladder infection usually is related to urinary catheterization. A bladder infection would not be apparent during the first 24 hours after catheterization because microorganisms take 24 to 72 hours to multiply sufficiently to present symptoms.
   c. Microorganisms introduced into the incision at the time of surgery take 24 to 72 hours to multiply sufficiently to present symptoms.
   d. **When postoperative pneumonia (an inflammation of the lung with consolidation and exudation) occurs, patient symptoms are evident usually any time within 36 hours after surgery.**

6. a. Although this is important for patient comfort, it is not life-threatening.
   b. Patients may become incontinent while or after receiving anesthesia; however, it is not life-threatening. In addition, this does not occur often because of preoperative bowel preparation and the temporary insertion of a urinary catheter.
   c. Although this can occur as a short-term response to anesthesia, it is not life-threatening.
   d. **Anesthesia causes a loss of the pharyngeal, laryngeal, and gag reflexes; these losses interfere with the protective mechanisms of coughing and swallowing. Because the patient is unable to clear the airway, oral secretions in the oropharynx and trachea may compromise a patent airway. In addition, occlusion of the airway may occur because of decreased muscle control of the tongue and jaw.**

7. a. **This removes exudate and ensures adhesion of the dressing. Transparent adhesive films are nonabsorbent semipermeable (which allows oxygen exchange) dressings that are impermeable to water and bacteria.**
   b. This restricts mobility and may exert undue pressure on the surface of the wound. The dressing should be laid gently over the wound and the edges pressed against the skin to ensure adherence.
   c. This defeats one of the purposes of a transparent dressing, wound visualization.
   d. A transparent dressing is self-contained, and reinforcing tape usually is not necessary.

8. a. Although this is always taken into consideration when positioning a patient during the intraoperative period, it is not the priority.
   b. It is impossible to prevent all pressure on bony prominences during the intraoperative period. Specific positions are necessary to allow exposure and access to the operative area. Positioning devices and padding are used to minimize trauma.
   c. **Facilitating respirations is always the priority because permanent brain damage can result from cerebral hypoxia in as little as 4 to 6 minutes.**

d. Although stretching of neuromuscular tissue is avoided during the intraoperative period, it is not the priority.

9. a. The nurse would be negligent if nursing care began at this point in the surgical experience. This is the intraoperative phase of the perioperative experience.
b. **The surgical experience begins as soon as the decision for surgery is made. Perioperative nursing responsibilities begin immediately and continue throughout the preoperative, intraoperative, and postoperative phases.**
c. Significant nursing care must be provided before this point in time. The operative consent form is signed during the preoperative phase of the perioperative experience.
d. The nurse would be negligent if nursing care were to begin only at this point in the surgical experience. This is the intraoperative phase of the perioperative experience.

10. a. This is premature, because some drainage occurs with an incision.
b. This is undesirable, because it impedes the ability to assess the site in the future.
c. This is undesirable, because the determination of expansion will be a subjective assessment without objective parameters.
d. **This determines objectively the time and extent of the bleeding and the person who performed the assessment. The extent of progression of the bleeding can be established objectively using the original circle as a standard.**

11. a. A slight elevation of body temperature is expected after surgery because of the body's response to the stress of surgery.
b. Dependent edema indicates problems such as a fluid and electrolyte imbalance, impaired kidney function, or decreased cardiac output. All are serious, but generally manageable.
c. Dehiscence, separation of the wound margins, is more likely to occur between the fifth and eighth postoperative days, and it is not life-threatening.
d. **An acute onset of chest pain within 24 hours of surgery may indicate myocardial infarction in response to the stress of surgery. It can also be caused by a pulmonary embolus, although this is more likely to occur between the seventh and tenth postoperative days. Both of these complications are life-threatening.**

12. a. The respiratory status of all postoperative patients should be stable and adequate regardless of the type of anesthesia used.
b. **The ability to move and feel sensations in all four extremities is especially important after receiving spinal anesthesia (subarachnoid block) because it indicates that nerve damage has not occurred because of the lumbar puncture necessary for the introduction of the anesthetic agent into the subarachnoid space.**
c. Nausea and vomiting are associated with general, not spinal anesthesia.
d. This is unrealistic. Although a headache is associated with spinal anesthesia (subarachnoid block), it may

manifest after discharge from the Post-Anesthesia Care Unit and persist for several days until the cerebrospinal fluid pressure returns to normal.

13. a. A clear liquid diet is contraindicated in the presence of abdominal distention because gas has accumulated in the intestines because of a lack of intestinal motility.
b. This is not the purpose of a clear liquid diet. A full liquid diet or food would more likely stimulate gastric enzymes.
c. A clear liquid diet is administered after a paralytic ileus resolves, not to prevent its occurrence.
d. **The molecules in clear liquids are less complex and easier to ingest, tolerate, and digest than those in a full liquid diet or food.**

14. a. Although this is done to ensure that the minimal hourly urine output is 30 cc, it is not the priority.
b. Although this is part of the routine assessment of a patient recovering from anesthesia, particularly conscious sedation and general anesthesia, it is not the priority.
c. Although tubes and equipment are always monitored and maintained, the patient is the priority.
d. **Maintaining a patent airway is always the priority to prevent respiratory distress and hypoxia.**

15. a. This is necessary to determine urine composition and possible abnormalities associated with kidney function, glucose metabolism, or urinary tract infection.
b. This is necessary to evaluate respiratory status and heart size.
c. **An electrocardiogram (ECG) is done to monitor or identify pre-existing cardiac problems or disease. It usually is required for surgical patients with previously identified cardiac problems or who are 40 years of age or older.**
d. This is necessary to determine the oxygen carrying capacity of the blood (RBCs, Hct, and Hgb), the status of the immune system (WBCs), and risk for bleeding (coagulation studies).

16. a. A Penrose drain, a small pliable, flat latex tube extends beyond the insertion site by approximately 2 inches. This prevents it from being lost inside the wound and allows its placement between gauze dressings to absorb drainage. As a drain is shortened, it is withdrawn approximately 1 inch and cut to maintain the same 2-inch length outside the body. Although this is done, it is not the priority action associated with a Penrose drain.
b. **This is necessary to prevent inadvertent removal of the Penrose drain because it is placed between several layers of gauze dressings to absorb drainage.**
c. This is not done to avoid inadvertently removing the drain during a dressing change.
d. A Penrose drain functions by gravity, not negative pressure.

17. a. This position limits respiratory excursion, increases the work of breathing, and does not exert pressure on the needle insertion site, which is desirable.
b. **Patients who have received spinal anesthesia (subarachnoid block) are placed in the supine**

position to limit leakage of cerebrospinal fluid from the needle insertion site. Bed rest in the supine position, pressure against the infusion site, and hydration limit a headache associated with spinal anesthesia.

c. This position does not exert pressure on the insertion site, which is necessary to minimize leakage of spinal fluid from the puncture site. This is the position used while the lumbar puncture is performed.

d. This increases the pressure within the cranial vault, which would increase, not decrease, a headache.

18. a. Although liver (1 portion equals $6^{1}/_{2} \times 2^{3}/_{8} \times {}^{3}/_{8}$ inches) contains approximately 23 mg of vitamin C, it is noted for being a source of niacin (nicotinic acid) and vitamin D.

b. Cheese does not contain vitamin C; it is noted for containing calcium.

c. **One medium-size spear of broccoli contains 113 mg (cooked) or 141 mg (raw) of vitamin C, which is essential for the formation of collagen. Collagen is a protein substance that adds tensile strength to a healing wound.**

d. Legumes do not contain vitamin C, they are noted for containing protein and phosphorus.

19. a. Warm liquids and food are contraindicated during the first several days after a tonsillectomy because they cause vasodilation, which may increase bleeding from the vascular mucous membranes of the oropharynx.

b. Milk and milk products are avoided during recovery from oral surgery because some health professionals believe milk increases the consistency of phlegm.

c. Toast would be a mechanical irritant to the operative site that could disrupt the healing process and precipitate bleeding.

d. **An ice pop is a frozen clear liquid that promotes vasoconstriction and limits bleeding from the operative site. Flavors that have a red color are contraindicated because they complicate assessing for bleeding.**

20. a. A bowel movement would occur long after the first signs of intestinal motility were evident.

b. Administration of fluids before intestinal motility has returned is unsafe and contraindicated. A clear liquid diet is not administered until there are definitive signs of intestinal motility.

c. Although this is done, it is not the best assessment for paralytic ileus. Abdominal distention can be caused by problems other than paralytic ileus, such as hemorrhage, peritonitis, and urinary retention.

d. **Bowel sounds are high-pitched gurgling sounds that vary in frequency, intensity, and pitch; they are caused by the propulsion of intestinal contents through the lower alimentary tract. These sounds are the first indication that intestinal motility is returning.**

21. a. This should be done eventually, but it is not the priority.

b. An abdominal binder may be used in high-risk patients to prevent, not treat, dehiscence and evisceration.

c. The low-Fowler's position, a back-lying position,

permits inspection of the operative site and promotes retention of abdominal viscera by gravity if dehiscence has occurred. Slight flexion of the hips reduces tension on the abdominal musculature.

d. This is contraindicated because deep breathing increases intra-abdominal pressure, which could cause evisceration.

22. a. Although this may be asked, it is not the priority. The patient will be instructed to void just before being taken to surgery. Urinary retention may occur 6 to 8 hours after surgery.

b. **Fasting 8 hours before surgery leaves the gastrointestinal tract relatively empty of food content, so that the risk of vomiting and aspirating emesis are minimized. Minimizing risks to airway obstruction is the priority.**

c. Although this may be asked, it is not the priority. Paralytic ileus may develop within 24 to 36 hours after surgery.

d. Although this may be asked, it is not the priority. After surgery, patients may develop atelectasis during the first 24 hours or pneumonia any time during the first 36 hours.

23. a. **In the semi-Fowler's position, the abdominal organs drop by gravity, which permits maximum thoracic excursion. In addition, slight flexion of the hips reduces abdominal muscle tension, which limits pressure on the suture line and facilitates diaphragmatic (abdominal) breathing.**

b. Resting in bed in any position promotes flatus retention. Ambulation promotes intestinal motility, which promotes the passage of flatus.

c. Inactivity results in decreased detrusor muscle tone, incomplete bladder emptying, and urinary stasis. The high-Fowler's position and ambulation use gravity to promote urinary elimination.

d. This position does not facilitate drainage via a portable wound drainage system. Negative pressure creates the vacuum that draws fluid into a portable wound drainage system.

24. a. **Obese people have excess adipose tissue that exerts pressure on the abdominal cavity, which raises intra-abdominal pressure. Increased intra-abdominal pressure exerts pressure on the gastrointestinal tract, raising the risk of nausea and vomiting.**

b. Although inactivity delays recovery of intestinal motility after surgery, a diligent activity and ambulation schedule should prevent paralytic ileus and its related nausea and vomiting.

c. Intestinal hypomotility, not hypervolemia, is related to postoperative nausea and vomiting. Hypervolemia is an increase in intravascular blood volume.

d. Unconsciousness is not directly related to postoperative nausea and vomiting.

25. a. **Gentle compression is desirable because it prevents bleeding and promotes molding and shrinkage of the residual limb.**

b. This is unsafe because soaking promotes the breakdown of connective tissue fibers (maceration), which impedes wound healing by primary intention.

c. This is unsafe because it promotes hip flexion contractures.

d. This would be done eventually, but caring for the patient is the immediate priority.

26. a. Dietary roughage prevents constipation, not urinary tract infections.

b. **Adequate (approximately 2000 to 3000 ml/day) fluid intake promotes a dilute urine and more frequent emptying of the bladder, both of which limit the development of a urinary tract infection. The stasis of concentrated urine promotes microbial growth.**

c. A sitz bath can promote the development of a urinary tract infection if medical aseptic techniques are not followed.

d. The ingestion of citrus juice causes an alkaline urine, which provides a favorable environment for the multiplication of microorganisms and the development of a urinary tract infection.

27. a. This occurs with general anesthesia, not conscious sedation.

b. Life-threatening malignant hyperthermia is a rare, autosomal dominant–inherited syndrome that is precipitated by anesthetic inhalation agents and neuromuscular blocking medications used to induce general anesthesia, not conscious sedation.

c. **Conscious sedation involves the use of intravenous opioids and sedatives to decrease the level of consciousness to a degree where the person can still maintain an airway and respond to verbal commands.**

d. Patients who have received spinal anesthesia (subarachnoid block), not conscious sedation, are placed in the supine position to limit leakage of cerebrospinal fluid from the needle insertion site. Bed rest in the supine position, hydration, and pressure against the infusion site limit headache associated with spinal anesthesia.

28. a. This is undesirable because of the reduced effectiveness of the system's negative pressure. The power of the suction decreases as the collection chamber fills.

b. Depending on the amount of drainage, this may be unnecessary or not often enough to maintain adequate suction. Opening the device increases the risk of infection and should be done only when necessary.

c. **The force of the vacuum within the system reduces as the collection chamber fills. Therefore, the collection chamber should be emptied when it is half-full to ensure the effectiveness of suction.**

d. Although this is done at specified intervals for an accurate intake and output record, it may not be adequate if there is moderate to large amounts of drainage.

29. a. **Chronic alcoholism disrupts the structure and function of the liver. A decrease in the synthesis of bile salts prevents the absorption of vitamin K, which is essential for the production of clotting factors II, VII, IX, and X. Therefore, these patients are at risk for hemorrhage. In addition,**

malnutrition results in decreased protein synthesis, anemia, and vitamin deficiencies, all which interfere with fluid and electrolyte balance and wound healing.

b. Although older adults are a higher surgical risk than younger adults because of the physiologic changes associated with aging (such as prolonged healing and decreased cardiac functioning, homeostatic capacity, and respiratory excursion), they are not at the highest risk for postoperative mortality as another option.

c. Although patients with epilepsy have their own unique problems that must be considered, they are not at the highest risk for postoperative mortality as another option.

d. Although infants have a greater surgical risk than children and young to middle-aged adults because they have a lower total blood volume, larger percentage of body fluid, and difficulty maintaining body temperature as a result of an immature shivering reflex, they are not at the highest risk for postoperative mortality as another option.

30. a. This is undesirable because pressure on the popliteal space constricts the vessels, which impedes venous return, promotes venous stasis, and injures tissues. Vessel injury, venous stasis, hypercoagulability, and dehydration all contribute to thrombophlebitis.

b. Although helpful, this will promote venous return for a limited amount of time (approximately 8 hours). The patient will be at risk for the remaining time in the day (approximately 16 hours).

c. This helps to prevent atelectasis and pneumonia, not thrombophlebitis; these should be performed hourly when awake.

d. **Leg exercises are an active intervention by the patient that contracts the muscles of the legs. This rhythmically compresses the veins, which promotes venous return and prevents venous stasis.**

31. a. Vitamin C does not improve digestion.

b. **Vitamin C (ascorbic acid) promotes collagen production, an essential component of the proliferative phase of wound healing. In addition, vitamin C enhances capillary formation, decreases capillary fragility, increases the tensile strength of the wound, and provides a defense against infection because of its role in the immune response.**

c. Vitamin B_{12} (cobalamin), folic acid, and iron promote red blood cell production, not vitamin C.

d. Vitamin C promotes the strength of capillaries, not large veins. Ambulation, leg exercises, and hydration prevent deep vein thrombosis.

32. a. Although constipation is a concern, it is not life-threatening.

b. Although urinary retention is a concern, it is not life-threatening.

c. Although a person may experience impaired motor or cognitive functioning, they are not life-threatening.

d. **After abdominal surgery, patients frequently have shallow respirations because when the diaphragm contracts with a deep breath it increases intra-abdominal pressure, which causes pain at the operative site.**

33. a. This is significant information because there are unique stressors and expected adaptations to various types of surgery that may direct the plan of care for the patient.
    b. Although this information may be communicated, the physiologic needs of the patient are the priorities in the immediate postoperative period.
    c. Although reasonable requests are honored, the status of the patient or the environment may prohibit them.
    d. Although this information is important and will be communicated, it is only one aspect of the patient's care.

34. a. This is an expected response to surgery, particularly during the first 48 hours after surgery.
    b. Pain, not discomfort, along the incision line is expected during the first 24 hours after surgery.
    c. The inflammatory phase of wound healing begins immediately after injury and lasts 3 to 6 days. It involves the formation of a fibrin matrix that acts as the structural framework for further cellular repair. Cellular debris and serosanguineous exudate cause what looks like a crust along the incision as the scab forms; this is an expected part of wound healing.
    d. This indicates that the incision's edges may not be intact and are vulnerable for dehiscence and evisceration. By the sixth postoperative day the exudate should be serous, not serosanguineous.

35. a. Both entry sites place the catheter in the superior vena cava.
    b. A pneumothorax is not a concern with a peripherally inserted central venous catheter. Pneumothorax is a complication of a central venous catheter inserted into a subclavian vein because of its close proximity to the apex of the lung.
    c. Both entry sites carry a risk of infection because the first line of defense, the skin, has been pierced.
    d. Both entry sites allow for the administration of large volumes of fluid because the distal ends of their catheters are both in the superior vena cava.

36. a. A wound infection is less likely to occur at this time because the proliferative or reconstructive phase of wound healing begins approximately 4 days after tissue damage. By the fifth postoperative day the wound has filled with highly vascular fibroblastic connective tissue that protects the body from microorganisms.
    b. Microorganisms introduced into a surgical site take 24 to 72 hours to multiply and present local adaptations of pain, swelling, erythema, warmth, and purulent discharge and systemic adaptations of fever and tachycardia.
    c. A wound infection is less likely to occur at this time because by the second postoperative week there is progressive collagen accumulation and the formation of the basic structure of the scar, which protect the body from microorganisms.
    d. A wound infection is less likely to occur at this time because by the seventh postoperative day the surface epithelium has a normal thickness and the subepithelial layers are bridged, which protect the body from microorganisms.

37. a. Leakage of cerebrospinal fluid from the needle insertion site reduces cerebrospinal fluid pressure, which causes a headache.
    b. Neuropathy, inflammation or degeneration of the peripheral nerves, is not a response to spinal anesthesia.
    c. Although the needle insertion site may feel uncomfortable in some people, it is not a common adaptation after spinal anesthesia.
    d. Anesthetic agents cause a decrease, not increase, in blood pressure.

38. a. This action is beyond the scope of the legal practice of nursing.
    b. Withholding medications without a significant reason is unsafe. These medications may be essential to maintain the patient's physical or emotional status.
    c. It is unsafe to withhold medications without an important reason. The withheld medications may be essential to maintain the patient's physical or emotional equilibrium.
    d. This intervention meets the patient's needs and adheres to the laws that govern the practice of nursing. A change in the route of medication delivery requires an order from a practitioner because medication administration is a dependent function of the nurse.

39. a. The molecules in clear liquids are less complex and easier to ingest, tolerate, and digest than those in a full liquid diet or food.
    b. This is not the most common diet ordered postoperatively, although a full liquid diet frequently precedes solid food.
    c. A low fiber diet is ordered for specific problems such as intestinal inflammation or infection. When able to be tolerated postoperatively, dietary fiber promotes intestinal motility and prevents constipation.
    d. This is not the most common diet ordered postoperatively, although most initial postoperative diets eventually progress to a regular diet.

40. a. These adaptations are essential for discharge from the Post-Anesthesia Care Unit because they reflect the body's vital functions, such as airway, breathing, and circulation.
    b. The lack of a fever is not a criterion for discharge from the Post-Anesthesia Care Unit because a low-grade fever is an expected response to the stress of surgery. The other listed adaptations are desirable for discharge.
    c. A postoperative patient may not be able to turn from side to side, but the patient should be able to move all extremities. The other listed adaptations are desirable for discharge.
    d. A dry dressing may be unrealistic. Some drainage from a surgical incision is expected in the immediate postoperative period. The other listed adaptations are desirable.

41. a. Although this is essential to proceed with the surgery, it is not as high a priority as another option.
    b. During stage III surgical anesthesia the patient experiences a loss of the pharyngeal, laryngeal, and gag reflexes, as well as spontaneous

respirations (apnea). Maintaining a patent airway and ventilation are the priorities.

c. Although the reflexes are assessed as the patient progresses through the induction, maintenance, and reversal stages of anesthesia, it is not as high a priority as another option.

d. Although the heart rate is monitored throughout the surgical experience, it is not as high a priority as another option.

42. a. When exiting from the left side of the bed, the left lateral side of the abdomen will be compressed against the bed by body weight. The left, not right, side of the abdomen will absorb the majority of the muscular strain exerted by the transfer.

b. Although this might be done for patients at high risk for dehiscence, abdominal binders are not used routinely because they increase intra-abdominal pressure; this exerts a force against the diaphragm that impedes maximum respiratory excursion.

c. This is unsafe. At least one upper extremity should be used to help raise the body to a sitting position and promote balance during the transfer out of bed.

d. This places an unnecessary strain on the abdominal muscles in the area of the incision.

43. a. These are the classic signs of a pulmonary embolus. Chest pain results from local tissue hypoxia, tachycardia from systemic hypoxia, and hypotension from decreased cardiac output. A pulmonary embolus is caused by a thrombus lodging in a vessel in the pulmonary circulation and occluding blood supply to the capillary side of the alveolar-capillary membrane.

b. Although tachycardia and hypotension occur with hemorrhage, chest pain does not.

c. Although tachycardia and chest pain occur with a myocardial infarction (heart attack), the blood pressure would probably increase, not decrease. The blood pressure decreases eventually if cardiogenic shock occurs.

d. Pneumonia, inflammation of the lung with consolidation and exudation, is associated with tachycardia and chest discomfort. However, it does not have a sudden onset and the blood pressure will increase, not decrease.

44. a. Abdominal cramping with the absence of bowel sounds indicates trapped, nonmoving gas. Ambulation is an active exercise that improves gastrointestinal tone and promotes intestinal motility. Intestinal motility moves gas towards the rectum where it is expelled.

b. Oral fluids are contraindicated in the absence of bowel sounds. They would remain in the stomach and cause discomfort, nausea, and vomiting. Vomiting raises the risk for aspiration.

c. Food is contraindicated in the absence of bowel sounds because it would remain in the stomach and intestines, which would result in discomfort, nausea, and vomiting.

d. Narcotic analgesics decrease, not increase, intestinal motility because of their depressant effects.

45. a. Oliguria is diminished urine secretion in relation to fluid intake, which is indicated by a negative balance in the intake and output record or hourly urine outputs of less then 30 cc. Oliguria is caused by decreased renal perfusion or kidney disease.

b. This is not an adaptation related to altered renal perfusion. Cachexia is malnutrition and emaciation associated with serious diseases such as cancer.

c. Yellow sclera indicates jaundice. Jaundice is the accumulation of bile pigments in tissue, which is associated with liver or biliary problems, not altered renal perfusion.

d. Suprapubic distention indicates urinary retention, which is an inability of the bladder to empty, not a problem with renal perfusion. If it occurs, it usually becomes evident 6 to 8 hours after surgery.

46. a. This is unsafe unless certain critical parameters in the patient's status have been attained.

b. This is unsafe unless certain critical parameters in the patient's status have been attained.

c. Generally, a postoperative patient will spit out an oral airway when the gag reflex returns. The airway should remain out at this time because persistent gagging will induce vomiting, which increases the potential for aspiration.

d. This is unsafe unless certain critical parameters in the patient's status have been attained.

47. a. This is an unrealistic expectation considering all the stressors that can contribute to these problems. Essential nutrient needs can be met despite the presence of nausea and vomiting.

b. Fluid is the most basic nutrient of the body and it contains compounds such as electrolytes. Electrolytes help maintain fluid balance, contribute to acid-base balance, and facilitate enzyme and neuromuscular reactions. The narrow safe limits of the volumes and composition of fluid compartments are essential for the life-sustaining processes of nutrition, metabolism, and excretion.

c. Wound healing takes time and it is difficult to evaluate during the inflammatory phase, which lasts approximately 1 to 4 days.

d. Oral intake should not be reestablished until intestinal motility returns, which may take several days.

48. a. Although this ultimately will be assessed, the physiologic status of the patient is the priority.

b. Assessment in acute situations always follows the ABCs: Airway, Breathing, Circulation. Once a patent airway and ventilation are ensured, then the cardiovascular status is assessed.

c. Although this eventually will be assessed, it is not the priority at this time.

d. Both the location and status of the dressing should be assessed, but not until more critical assessments are completed.

49. a. Although the physical trauma of surgery causes pain and it must be relieved, it is not the priority.

b. Although anesthesia can cause nausea, nausea is not a nursing diagnosis. In addition, nausea is not the priority problem in the Post-Anesthesia Care Unit.

c. With an altered level of consciousness, the pharyngeal, laryngeal, and gag reflexes may be impaired. The inability to cough or swallow can result in aspiration of oral secretions.

d. Excessive fluid loss precipitates a deficient fluid volume, but the nurse generally has time to safely meet this need.

50. a. This should be done eventually, but it is not the priority.

b. The physician should be notified after the patient's safety is ensured.

c. After appropriate positioning, a sterile dressing soaked in sterile normal saline should be applied to keep the viscera moist until the abdominal incision is resutured.

d. This would compromise the patient's respiratory status. The patient should be placed in the low-Fowler's position or supine position with the knees slightly flexed to reduce tension on the abdominal musculature.

51. a. The toe window should be positioned over the toes or sole of the feet depending on the manufacturer. This ensures that the stocking is aligned correctly and the distal portion of the foot can be accessed to perform the blanch test to assess for peripheral circulation.

b. The stockings should be applied before, not after, the patient gets out of bed. If stockings are applied after getting out of bed, they will compress edematous tissues and cause injury.

c. Flexion impedes and extension promotes application of an antiembolism stocking. Most antiembolism stockings are knee high rather than thigh high.

d. This is inadequate. Antiembolism stockings should be removed every 8 hours for 30 minutes. This permits inspection and physical hygiene.

52. a. Whole grains contain trace amounts or none of the vitamin necessary for collagen production. Whole grains are noted primarily for containing vitamin E and potassium.

b. Yellow vegetables are noted for being a major source of vitamin A, which is not the vitamin most responsible for collagen production.

c. Citrus fruits are the best sources of vitamin C. Vitamin C promotes collagen production, which is essential in the proliferative and maturation phases of wound healing.

d. Red meat contains trace amounts or none of the vitamin necessary for collagen formation with the exception of liver (1 portion equals $6^{1}/_{2} \times 2^{3}/_{8} \times^{3}/_{8}$ inches), which contains 23 mg of vitamin C.

53. a. Abdominal distention raises the pressure within the abdominal cavity, which exerts pressure against the diaphragm, impeding its contraction and limiting thoracic excursion.

b. This should be avoided. When in a side-lying position, aeration of the dependent side of the lung is limited because of pooling of secretions and the weight of the body compressing the dependent part of the body.

c. This is not an active intervention to facilitate respirations, but it is an important assessment to evaluate the patient's response to surgery and interventions used to facilitate respirations.

d. Passive range-of-motion exercises do not facilitate respirations; they help prevent contractures.

54. a. The Sims' position is not used during the intraoperative period.

b. The supine position is the most common position for surgery, particularly abdominal, not perineal, surgery.

c. The lithotomy position, back lying with the hips and knees flexed and the legs supported in stirrups, provides optimal visualization of and access to the area related to perineal surgery.

d. A patient's legs are adducted when in the Trendelenburg position, which does not permit visualization of or access to the perineal area.

55. a. Although this will be done, it is not the initial action when monitoring the effectiveness of a portable wound drainage system.

b. Anything that interferes with the force of negative pressure from the device to the surgical site (kinks in tubing, compression of the tubing, blood clots or debris in the tubing) will result in ineffective drainage. The amount of drainage should be greatest during the first 24 to 48 hours after surgery.

c. This may be unnecessary. Opening the air vent increases the risk of infection and should be done only to empty the device or reestablish pressure.

d. The device should already be below the level of the insertion site.

Alternate Question Formats

In 1994, the National Council of State Boards of Nursing (NCSBN) initiated computer adaptive testing as its method of administering NCLEX examinations. Computer adaptive testing provides an individualized testing experience because each subsequent question on the test is determined by the test taker's performance on the previous question while adhering to a detailed test plan. This approach provides an excellent opportunity for the test taker to demonstrate competence. Before April 2003, all of the questions on NCLEX examinations were multiple-choice items. After April 2003, item formats on NCLEX examinations include questions other than multiple-choice items. The NCSBN calls these items "Alternate NCLEX Item Formats."

Innovative item formats use the benefits of computer technology to assess knowledge via methods other than the four-option, multiple-choice item. Alternate formats include questions that require test takers to fill in the blanks, identify multiple answers, perform a mathematical calculation or respond to a question in relation to a graphic image, picture, chart, or table. This chapter includes 25 questions that use formats other than the multiple-choice question. Creativity was employed to develop these items based on the information provided by the NCSBN. As the NCLEX examinations incorporate these questions, statistical analyses will facilitate refinement of these new formats. As alternate item formats progress beyond their infancy, the NCSBN will be able to provide additional information for test takers, nursing students, and faculty.

1. When a patient who had a total abdominal hysterectomy six days ago is being ambulated, she complains of dyspnea and stabbing chest pain on inspiration. Assessment reveals a pulse of 110 and respirations of 35. While many of the following actions may be implemented, which three take priority?
   - (a) _____ Administer oxygen
   - (b) _____ Assess breath sounds
   - (c) _____ Take vital signs every 30 minutes
   - (d) _____ Return the patient to bed by wheelchair
   - (e) _____ Monitor the patient's oxygen saturation
   - (f) _____ Place the patient in the Fowler's position

2. The nurse is caring for a surgical patient four days after surgery. The patient had 3 ounces of apple juice, 1 soft-boiled egg, and 4 ounces of tea for breakfast. She voided 450 ml of urine before lunch and vomited 100 ml at 11:00 AM. She did not want lunch but she did suck on 8 ounces of ice chips between 12:00 noon and 4 PM. She voided 600 ml at 3:00 PM. At 4:00 PM, the Jackson-Pratt drain was emptied of 35 ml of serosanguineous drainage. What is the patient's total output during 8 AM to 4 PM?
   Answer: _____

3. Which data would the nurse need to know to ensure that the correct IV solution is running? Check only the data that apply.
   - (a) _____ The tubing drop factor
   - (b) _____ The drip rate per minute
   - (c) _____ The solution indicated on the IV bag
   - (d) _____ The volume of solution in the IV bag
   - (e) _____ The solution ordered by the physician

4. Which bony prominence would be at the greatest risk for a pressure ulcer when lying in the right lateral position? Mark an X over the area.

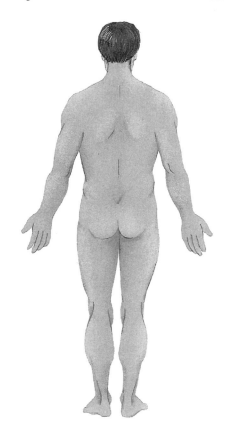

5. Which data would the nurse need to know to make the determination that an IV is "on time." Check only the data that apply.
   (a) ____ The drip rate per minute
   (b) ____ The time the bag was hung
   (c) ____ The solution indicated on the IV bag
   (d) ____ The volume of solution in the IV bag
   (e) ____ The milliliters per hour ordered by the physician

6. The nurse needs to calculate the patient's intake during the 8 AM to 4 PM shift. The patient had a scrambled egg, 4 ounces of orange juice, and 6 ounces of tea for breakfast at 8:00 AM. The patient voided 300 cc at 10:00 and vomited 200 cc at 11:00. For lunch, the patient had 60 cc of broth and sucked on 4 ounces of ice chips. The patient voided another 500 cc at 2:00 and had 4 ounces of Italian ice at 3:00. The patient had 2 piggy backs at 100 cc each during the shift. Calculate the patient's fluid intake.
   Answer: _____

7. Identify the common signs and symptoms of the Local Adaptation Syndrome (LAS) associated with a laceration of the thumb. Indicate all that apply.
   (a) ____ Pain
   (b) ____ Heat
   (c) ____ Erythema
   (d) ____ Increased heart rate
   (e) ____ Decreased blood pressure
   (f) ____ Elevated blood glucose level

8. What angle of insertion should be used when performing a subcutaneous injection using a syringe with a needle that is $1/2$ inch long?
   Answer: _____

9. Identify the common adaptations to hemorrhage (blood volume deficit of 30-40%). Indicate all that are relevant.
   (a) ____ Bradypnea
   (b) ____ Tachycardia
   (c) ____ Flushed skin
   (d) ____ Bounding pulse
   (e) ____ Delayed capillary refill
   (f) ____ Decreased urinary output

10. The primary care practitioner orders an antidysrhythmic medication of 2g IV per 1000 mL D_5W at 4 mg per minute. At what rate should the nurse set the infusion pump?
    Answer: _____

11. Which postoperative complication will ambulation help to prevent? Select all that apply.
    (a) ____ Hypovolemia
    (b) ____ Constipation
    (c) ____ Dehiscence
    (d) ____ Atelectasis
    (e) ____ Infection

12. Identify the colostomy site along the large intestines that would produce the most liquid stool, thereby placing the patient at greatest risk for skin breakdown. Select site a, b, c, or d.
    (a) ____
    (b) ____
    (c) ____
    (d) ____

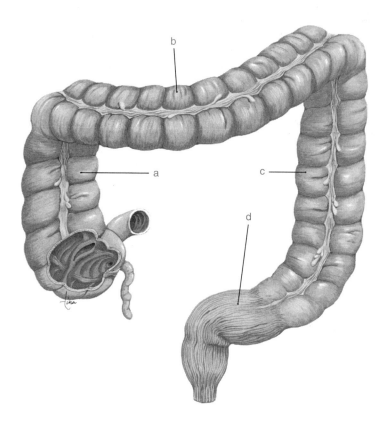

13. Which 2 patients should the nurse attend to first?
    (a) ____ A 5 day post-surgical patient who states, "Something feels very strange in my belly."
    (b) ____ A patient admitted for hypertension who would like pain medication for a headache.
    (c) ____ A patient who is anxious to have an IV removed after being informed by the physician that it can be discontinued.
    (d) ____ A patient who is awaiting to be escorted to the lobby after being discharged.
    (e) ____ A patient who got dizzy when the Nursing Assistant was transferring the patient from a wheel chair to the bed.

14. What was the patient's temperature on June 7th at 4 PM?
    Answer: _____

Room No. __104__   Hosp. No. __427396__

JUNE

Day of Month	5				6				7				8				9				10				11			
Day in Hospital	1				2				3				4				5				6				7			
	A M		P M		A M		P M		A M		P M		A M		P M		A M		P M		A M		P M		A M		P M	
Hour	4	8	12	4	8	12	4	8	12	4	8	12	4	8	12	4	8	12	4	8	12	4	8	12	4	8	12	4	8	12	4	8	12	4	8	12	4	8	12	4	8	12

Medication

TEMPERATURE — 106° 105° 104° 103° 102° 101° 100° 99° Normal 98° 97° 96°

15. A patient is learning self-care in relation to a 2-gram sodium diet. The nurse knows that further teaching is necessary when the patient selects which foods high in sodium? Check all that apply.
    (a) ____ Apple juice
    (b) ____ Corned beef
    (c) ____ Canned soup
    (d) ____ Broccoli spears

16. The primary care provider orders an antibiotic of 400,000 units IM qid. The medication vial contains 1,000,000 units with the following directions. Add 4.6 mL of diluent to yield a concentrated solution of 200,000 units per mL. How much solution of the antibiotic should the nurse administer?
    Answer: _____

17. Check each therapeutic intervention that involves the principle of gravity.
    (a) ____ Foley catheter
    (b) ____ Penrose drain
    (c) ____ Hemovac drain
    (d) ____ Tap water enema
    (e) ____ Gastric decompression

18. Mark an X where the nurse should place a stethoscope when assessing for placement of a nasogastric tube.

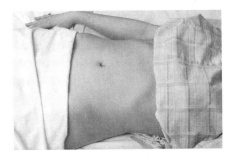

19. Which actions reflect principles of surgical asepsis? Check all that apply.
    - (a) ____ Washing hands
    - (b) ____ Keeping the sterile field dry
    - (c) ____ Holding sterile objects above the waist
    - (d) ____ Wearing personal protective equipment
    - (e) ____ Considering the outer $1/2$ inch of sterile field as contaminated
    - (f) ____ Adding contents to field holding the package 2 inches above the field

20. A patient states, "The only reason I smoke and drink is because I am a high strung person and I use them to help me relax." Which defense mechanism is being used by this patient?
    Answer: _____

21. Which tasks can the nurse delegate to a Nursing Assistant? Check all that apply.
    - (a) ____ Helping a patient who is constipated choose foods from a diet menu
    - (b) ____ Teaching a patient how to walk with a walker
    - (c) ____ Applying Duoderm to unbroken skin
    - (d) ____ Weighing a patient using a bed scale
    - (e) ____ Emptying a Foley collection bag

22. The nurse moves a patient's leg through range of motion demonstrated in the figure. What is this joint movement known as?
    Answer: _____

23. The primary care provider orders a calorie count for a malnourished patient. Over a 24-hour period the patient consumes 30 grams of fat, 80 grams of carbohydrates, and 40 grams of protein. What is the calorie count for this patient?
    Answer: _____

24. A dying patient states, "The worst part of dying is that I'll never see my children marry or enjoy grandchildren." This statement reflects which stage of grieving according to Kübler-Ross?
    Answer: _____

25. The nurse receives the following information about patients at the change-of-shift report. Although all the patients should be assessed, indicate which 2 patients should be assessed first.
    - (a) ____ A patient who just was informed of having cancer
    - (b) ____ A patient who was complaining of feeling nauseated
    - (c) ____ A patient receiving a titrated medication via an infusion pump
    - (d) ____ A patient who received an analgesic by mouth for pain immediately before report
    - (e) ____ A patient whose vital signs included an irregular a pulse and labored respirations

1. **(a)** The patient most likely experienced a pulmonary embolus. Administering oxygen is essential to facilitate gas exchange.
   (b) While important, this is not one of the three actions that take priority.
   (c) Vital signs should be taken more frequently than every 30 minutes in this situation.
   (d) Using a wheelchair limits muscle activity. Activity can contribute to more emboli and increase the demand on the heart and lungs.
   (e) Same as #b.
   (f) The high-Fowler's position facilitates thoracic expansion and ventilation, which are necessary for this patient.

2. 450 cc of urine before lunch
   100 cc of vomitus at 11:00 AM
   600 cc of urine at 3:00 PM
     35 cc of serosanguineous drainage—from Jackson-Pratt drain at 4:00 PM

   _____

   1185 cc total output

3. **(a)** This is necessary to know to calculate the IV drip rate, not to determine if the correct IV solution is running.
   (b) The drip rate per minute will tell you the current rate at which the IV is running, not whether the correct IV solution is running.
   (c) The nurse needs to have two pieces of data to determine if the correct IV solution is running. First, what is the solution the physician ordered and then what solution is in the IV bag? These solutions must be identical to administer ordered IV solutions safely.
   (d) Same as #a.
   (e) The administration of IV fluids is a dependent function of the nurse. The solution ordered by the physician must be verified.

4. This site is at risk because it is dependent when lying in a right lateral position; the majority of body mass overlies this area and it bears a greater part of the body's weight.

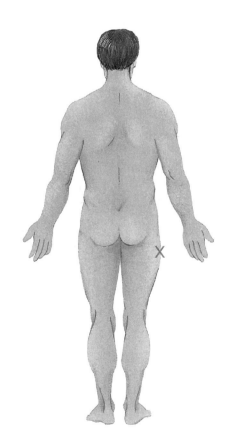

5. **(a)** This is not necessary to know when determining whether an IV is "on time."
   (b) This is one of three pieces of data that the nurse needs to know to determine whether an IV is "on time." The nurse needs to identify how many minutes/hours the IV has been running and then multiply this number by the milliliters of solution ordered by the physician per minute/hour. This volume is then deducted from the original volume in the IV bag. The actual volume that is in the bag should be compared to the volume that should be in the bag. If the volumes match, the IV is "on time," if there is more fluid than should be in the bag then the IV is "behind schedule," if there is less fluid than should be in the bag then the IV is "ahead of schedule."
   (c) This is necessary to know to ensure that it is identical to the solution ordered by the physician, not to determine whether an IV is "on time."
   (d) Same as #b.
   (e) Same as #b.

6. One ounce of fluid equals 30 cc of fluid.
   120 cc of orange juice
   180 cc of tea
     60 cc of broth
     60 cc of ice water (1 ounce of ice chips is equal to
       15 cc)
   120 cc Italian ice (Italian ice becomes a liquid at room
       temperature)
   <u>200 cc of piggy-back solution</u>
   740 cc total intake

7. **(a)** **Pain is caused by irritation of nerve tissue by chemical substances and the pressure of fluid congestion in the area of local trauma.**
   (b) **Heat is caused by an increased blood flow in response to the release of histamine at the site of local trauma.**
   (c) **Erythema is caused by an increased blood flow in response to the release of histamine and an increased capillary permeability in response to kinins at the site of local trauma or infection.**
   (d) This is unrelated to the Local Adaptation Syndrome (LAS). An increased heart rate is associated with activation of the sympathetic nervous system seen in the General Adaptation Syndrome (GAS).
   (e) This is unrelated to the LAS. An increased, not decreased, blood pressure is associated with activation of the sympathetic nervous system seen in the GAS.
   (f) This is unrelated to the LAS. An elevated blood glucose level occurs in response to the secretion of glucocortcoids in the GAS.

8. **90°.**

9. (a) Tachypnea, not bradypnea, occurs in response to sympathetic nervous system stimulation as the body attempts to deliver more oxygen to body tissues.
   (b) **This occurs in response to sympathetic nervous system stimulation as the body attempts to deliver more oxygen to body tissues.**
   (c) The skin becomes pale and cold, not flushed, in response to hemorrhage as peripheral vasoconstriction occurs in an attempt to shunt blood to vital organs of the body.
   (d) This is reflective of fluid overload (hypervolemia), not hypovolemia associated with hemorrhage.
   (e) **This occurs in response to peripheral vasoconstriction in an attempt to shunt blood to vital organs.**
   (f) **When fluid needs to be retained in the body as is seen in hemorrhage, antidiuretic hormone (ADH) is released and water is reabsorbed in the kidneys; the result is a decrease in urinary output.**

10. The nurse has to calculate how many milliliters to administer per minute to deliver 4 mgs per minute. Solve for x using ratio and proportion after converting 2 grams to its equivalent of 2000 milligrams.
$$\frac{\text{Desired}}{\text{Have}} \quad \frac{4 \text{ mg}}{2000 \text{mg}} = \frac{x \text{ mL}}{1000 \text{ mL}}$$

$$2000x = 4000$$
$$x = 4000 \div 2000$$
$$x = 2\text{ml}$$

The hourly volume to be infused is calculated by multiplying the milliliters per minute (2) by the number of minutes (60). Therefore, the infusion pump should be set at **120 cc per hour.**

11. (a) Ambulation will not prevent blood loss that results in hypovolemia.
    (b) **Ambulation promotes intestinal peristalsis that results in a bowel movement.**
    (c) Supporting the incisional site during coughing and deep breathing helps to prevent dehiscence.
    (d) **Ambulation promotes deep breathing that helps the alveoli to expand.**
    (e) The use of sterile technique and handwashing will help prevent infection.

12. **(a)** **This site is the ascending colon, which contains the most liquid stool because it is at the beginning of the large intestine. As stool moves through the large intestine, fluid is reabsorbed and stool becomes more dry and formed.**
    (b) Stool in the transverse colon is pasty.
    (c) Stool in the descending colon is formed but soft.
    (d) Stool in the sigmoid colon is formed and firm.

13. **(a)** **This may indicate evisceration (protrusion of viscera through separated wound edges), which needs immediate action to prevent extension of the wound separation and to limit invasion of microorganisms.**
    (b) **The headache may indicate that the blood pressure is too high, which could precipitate a brain attack (stroke).**
    (c) Although this needs to be done, it is not life-threatening and can wait.
    (d) Same as #c.
    (e) Orthostatic hypotension is a common occurrence when moving from a sitting to standing position. The patient is safe in bed at this time. This concern can be addressed later after patients who need immediate attention receive care.

14. Find the box in the top left that indicates "Day of Month." Read towards the right across the row until you see the box with the 7 (indicating the 7th day of the month). Look two rows down below the box with the 7 until you see the box with PM. Now look below the PM box for the box with the 4. Guide your eye down the column until you find a dot on a line. From the dot on the line guide your eye left across the row until you reach the numbers running along the left end of the graph. The nearest dark line below the row with the dot that indicates a full degree of temperature is 101. The dot in the 4 PM column is one light colored line above the 101 line indicating 2 tenths of a degree of temperature. Therefore, the dot in the 4 PM column indicates a temperature of **101.2 °F.**

15. (a) Apple juice contains approximately 7 mg of sodium per cup and is permitted on a 2-gm sodium diet.

Room No. __104__   Hosp. No. __427396__

JUNE

Day of Month	5			6			7			8			9			10			11		
Day in Hospital	1			2			3			4			5			6			7		
	A M		P M	A M		P M	A M		P M	A M		P M	A M		P M	A M		P M	A M		P M	
Hour	4 8 12	4 8 12		4 8 12	4 8 12		4 8 12	4 8 12		4 8 12	4 8 12		4 8 12	4 8 12		4 8 12	4 8 12		4 8 12	4 8 12	
Medication																					

TEMPERATURE graph with markings at 106°, 105°, 104°, 103°, 102°, 101°, 100°, 99° (Normal), 98°, 97°, 96°

(b) Corned beef contains approximately 800 mg of sodium per 3 ounces and should not be included in a 2-gm sodium diet.

(c) Most canned soups contain between 800 and 1000 mg of sodium per cup and are contraindicated on a 2-gm sodium diet.

(d) One broccoli spear contains approximately 20 mg of sodium and is permitted on a 2-gm sodium diet.

16. Solve for x using ratio and proportion.

$$\frac{\text{Desired}}{\text{Have}} \quad \frac{400{,}000}{200{,}000} = \frac{x \text{ mL}}{1 \text{ mL}}$$

$$200{,}000\, x = 400{,}000$$
$$x = 400{,}000 \div 200{,}000$$
$$x = \textbf{2 mL of the antibiotic solution}$$

17. (a) Gravity is the force that pulls mass toward the center of the earth. Urine flows by gravity out of the bladder through a tube (Foley catheter) into a collection bag.

(b) A Penrose drain is a flexible collapsible tube with a potential diameter of approximately 1 inch that drains fluid from inside a surgical site to a dressing via gravity.

(c) A Hemovac, is a closed wound drainage system, that uses negative pressure, not gravity, to drain secretions from an incisional site.

(d) Enema fluid flows from a container through a rectal tube into the large intestine via gravity. The force of the flow is regulated by raising or lowering the height of the enema bag in relation to the rectum. Raising the bag increases the force; lowering the bag decreases the force.

(e) A nasogastric tube removes fluid from the stomach via negative pressure, not gravity.

18. Auscultating over the **left upper quadrant slightly to the left of the midsternal line** will detect whooshing, gurgling, or bubbling sounds in the stomach as air is instilled through a nasogastric tube.

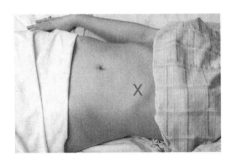

19. (a) This is a principle of medical, not surgical, asepsis.

(b) Moisture contaminates a sterile field by facilitating the movement of microorganisms from the un-sterile surface below the field to the sterile field by capillary action.

(c) Sterile items, including sterile gloved hands, held below the waist are considered contaminated.

(d) This protects the caregiver and is a principle of medical, not surgical, asepsis.

(e) A one, not $^{1}/_{2}$, inch border is considered contaminated.

(f) Sterile items should be dropped onto the field from a 6-inch, not 2-inch, height to avoid accidentally contaminating the field.

20. The patient is using **rationalization** to justify certain behaviors to make them appear reasonable.

21. (a) This is outside the scope of practice of a Nursing Assistant. It requires knowledge about foods, fiber, and teaching principles.
    (b) Patient teaching is an independent role of the nurse, not a Nursing Assistant. This task requires an understanding of anatomy and principles of physics and teaching.
    (c) Duoderm is a type of dressing. Applying dressings is a dependent function of the nurse and requires a physician's order or facility protocol. Assessment of the area and correct application of Duoderm is within the scope of nursing practice.
    (d) This is within the scope of practice of the Nursing Assistant.
    (e) Same as d.

22. **External rotation** occurs when the entire leg is rolled outward from the body so that the toes point away from the other leg.

23. Fat contains 9 calories (cal) per gram, and carbohydrates and proteins each contain 4 calories per gram. To compute the total caloric intake, multiply the grams of food consumed by the appropriate amount of calories per gram. Therefore, 30 grams of fat $\times$ 9 cal = 270 cal; 80 grams of carbohydrates $\times$ 4 cal = 320 cal; and 40 grams of protein $\times$ 4 cal = 160 cal. The product of adding 270 + 320 + 160 is 750. The total caloric intake for this patient is **750 calories.**

24. This patient is in the **stage of depression.** In this stage, people grieve over what has happened and what cannot be.

25. (a) This information may have precipitated a crisis for this patient. Psychosocial needs of patients are as important as physiologic needs.
    (b) This is not a life-threatening adaptation. Other patient situations are a greater priority.
    (c) Although they should be monitored, infusion pumps deliver fluid volumes safely. Other patient situations are a greater priority.
    (d) An analgesic by mouth takes approximately 20 to 30 minutes to be effective. This patient's response to the medication can be evaluated after other patients' needs are met.
    (e) These vital signs are outside the normal range; therefore, this patient should be assessed first because these adaptations may indicate a life-threatening situation.

Glossary of English Words Commonly Encountered on Nursing Examinations

Abnormality — defect, irregularity, anomaly, oddity

Absence — nonappearance, lack, nonattendance

Abundant — plentiful, rich, profuse

Accelerate — go faster, speed up, increase, hasten

Accumulate — build up, collect, gather

Accurate — precise, correct, exact

Achievement — accomplishment, success, reaching, attainment

Acknowledge — admit, recognize, accept, reply

Activate — start, turn on, stimulate

Adequate — sufficient, ample, plenty, enough

Angle — slant, approach, direction, point of view

Application — use, treatment, request, claim

Approximately — about, around, in the region of, more or less, roughly speaking

Arrange — position, place, organize, display

Associated — linked, related

Attention — notice, concentration, awareness, thought

Authority — power, right, influence, clout, expert

Avoid — keep away from, evade, let alone

Balanced — stable, neutral, steady, fair, impartial

Barrier — barricade, blockage, obstruction, obstacle

Best — most excellent, most important, greatest

Capable — able, competent, accomplished

Capacity — ability, capability, aptitude, role, power, size

Central — middle, mid, innermost, vital

Challenge — confront, dare, dispute, test, defy, face up to

Characteristic — trait, feature, attribute, quality, typical

Circular — round, spherical, globular

Collect — gather, assemble, amass, accumulate, bring together

Commitment — promise, vow, dedication, obligation, pledge, assurance

Commonly — usually, normally, frequently, generally, universally

Compare — contrast, evaluate, match up to, weigh or judge against

Compartment — section, part, cubicle, booth, stall

Complex — difficult, multifaceted, compound, multipart, intricate

Complexity — difficulty, intricacy, complication

Component — part, element, factor, section, constituent

Comprehensive — complete, inclusive, broad, thorough

Conceal — hide, cover up, obscure, mask, suppress, secrete

Conceptualize — to form an idea

Concern — worry, anxiety, fear, alarm, distress, unease, trepidation

Concisely — briefly, in a few words, succinctly

Conclude — make a judgment based on reason, finish

Confidence — self-assurance, certainty, poise, self-reliance

Congruent — matching, fitting, going together well

Consequence — result, effect, outcome, end result

Constituents — elements, component, parts that make up a whole

Contain — hold, enclose, surround, include, control, limit

Continual — repeated, constant, persistent, recurrent, frequent

Continuous — constant, incessant, nonstop, unremitting, permanent

Contribute — be a factor, add, give

Convene — assemble, call together, summon, organize, arrange

Convenience — expediency, handiness, ease

Coordinate — organize, direct, manage, bring together

Create — make, invent, establish, generate, produce, fashion, build, construct

Creative — imaginative, original, inspired, inventive, resourceful, productive, innovative

Critical — serious, grave, significant, dangerous, life-threatening

Cue — signal, reminder, prompt, sign, indication

Curiosity — inquisitiveness, interest, nosiness, snooping

Damage — injure, harm, hurt, break, wound

Deduct — subtract, take away, remove, withhold

Deficient — lacking, wanting, underprovided, scarce, faulty

Defining — important, crucial, major, essential, significant, central

Defuse — resolve, calm, soothe, neutralize, rescue, mollify

Delay — hold up, wait, hinder, postpone, slow down, hesitate, linger

Demand — insist, claim, require, command, stipulate, ask

Describe — explain, tell, express, illustrate, depict, portray

Design — plan, invent, intend, aim, propose, devise

Desirable — wanted, pleasing, enviable, popular, sought after, attractive, advantageous

Detail — feature, aspect, element, factor, facet

Deteriorate — worsen, decline, weaken

Determine — decide, conclude, resolve, agree on

Dexterity — skillfulness, handiness, agility, deftness

Dignity — self-respect, self-esteem, decorum, formality, poise

Dimension — aspect, measurement

Diminish — reduce, lessen, weaken, detract, moderate

Discharge — release, dismiss, set free

Discontinue — stop, cease, halt, suspend, terminate, withdraw

Disorder — complaint, problem, confusion, chaos

Display — show, exhibit, demonstrate, present, put on view

Dispose — to get rid of, arrange, order, set out

Dissatisfaction — displeasure, discontent, unhappiness, disappointment

Distinguish — to separate and classify, recognize

Distract — divert, sidetrack, entertain

Distress — suffering, trouble, anguish, misery, agony, concern, sorrow

Distribute — deliver, spread out, hand out, issue, dispense

Disturbed — troubled, unstable, concerned, worried, distressed, anxious, uneasy

Diversional — serving to distract

Don — put on, dress oneself in

Dramatic — spectacular

Drape — cover, wrap, dress, swathe

Dysfunction — abnormal, impaired

Edge — perimeter, boundary, periphery, brink, border, rim

Effective — successful, useful, helpful, valuable

Efficient — not wasteful, effective, competent, resourceful, capable

Elasticity — stretch, spring, suppleness, flexibility

Eliminate — get rid of, eradicate, abolish, remove, purge

Embarrass — make uncomfortable, make self-conscious, humiliate, mortify

Emerge — appear, come, materialize, become known

Emphasize — call attention to, accentuate, stress, highlight

Ensure — make certain, guarantee

Environment — setting, surroundings, location, atmosphere, milieu, situation

Episode — event, incident, occurrence, experience

Essential — necessary, fundamental, vital, important, crucial, critical, indispensable

Etiology — assigned cause, origin

Exaggerate — overstate, inflate

Excel — to stand out, shine, surpass, outclass

Excessive — extreme, too much, unwarranted

Exhibit — show signs of, reveal, display

Expand — get bigger, enlarge, spread out, increase, swell, inflate

Expect — wait for, anticipate, imagine

Expectation — hope, anticipation, belief, prospect, probability

Experience — knowledge, skill, occurrence, know-how

Expose — lay open, leave unprotected, allow to be seen, reveal, disclose, exhibit

External — outside, exterior, outer

Facilitate — make easy, make possible, help, assist

Factor — part, feature, reason, cause, think, issue

Focus — center, focal point, hub

Fragment — piece, portion, section, part, splinter, chip

Function — purpose, role, job, task

Furnish — supply, provide, give, deliver, equip

Further — additional, more, extra, added, supplementary

Generalize — to take a broad view, simplify, to make inferences from particulars

Generate — make, produce, create

Gentle — mild, calm, tender

Girth — circumference, bulk, weight

Highest — uppermost, maximum, peak, main

Hinder — hold back, delay, hamper, obstruct, impede

Humane — caring, kind, gentle, compassionate, benevolent, civilized

Ignore — pay no attention to, disregard, overlook, discount

Imbalance — unevenness, inequality, disparity

Immediate — insistent, urgent, direct

Impair — damage, harm, weaken

Implantation — to put in

Impotent — powerless, weak, incapable, ineffective, unable

Inadvertent — unintentional, chance, unplanned, accidental

Include — comprise, take in, contain

Indicate — point out, sign of, designate, specify, show

Ineffective — unproductive, unsuccessful, useless, vain, futile

Inevitable — predictable, to be expected, unavoidable, foreseeable

Influence — power, pressure, sway, manipulate, affect, effect

Initiate — start, begin, open, commence, instigate

Insert — put in, add, supplement, introduce

Inspect — look over, check, examine

Inspire — motivate, energize, encourage, enthuse

Institutionalize — to place in a facility for treatment

Integrate — put together, mix, add, combine, assimilate

Integrity — honesty

Interfere — get in the way, hinder, obstruct, impede, hamper

Interpret — explain the meaning of, to make understandable

Intervention — action, activity

Intolerance — bigotry, prejudice, narrowmindedness

Involuntary — instinctive, reflex, unintentional, automatic, uncontrolled

Irreversible — permanent, irrevocable, irreparable, unalterable

Irritability — sensitivity to stimuli, fretful, quick excitability

Justify — explain in accordance with reason

Likely — probably, possible, expected

Logical — using reason

Longevity — long life

Lowest — inferior in rank

Maintain — continue, uphold, preserve, sustain, retain

Majority — the greater part of

Mention — talk about, refer to, state, cite, declare, point out

Minimal — least, smallest, nominal, negligible, token

Minimize — reduce, diminish, lessen, curtail, decrease to smallest possible

Mobilize — activate, organize, assemble, gather together, rally

Modify — change, adapt, adjust, revise, alter

Moist — slightly wet, damp

Multiple — many, numerous, several, various

Natural — normal, ordinary, unaffected

Negative — no, harmful, downbeat, pessimistic

Negotiate — bargain, talk, discuss, consult, cooperate, settle

Notice — become aware of, see, observe, discern, detect

Notify — inform, tell, alert, advise, warn, report

Nurture — care for, raise, rear, foster

Obsess — preoccupy, consume

Occupy — live in, inhabit, reside in, engage in

Occurrence — event, incident, happening

Odorous — scented, stinking, aromatic

Offensive — unpleasant, distasteful, nasty, disgusting

Opportunity — chance, prospect, break

Organize — put in order, arrange, sort out, categorize, classify

Origin — source, starting point, cause, beginning, derivation

Pace — speed

Parameter — limit, factor, limitation, issue

Participant — member, contributor, partaker, applicant

Perspective — viewpoint, view, perception

Position — place, location, point, spot, situation

Practice — do, carry out, perform, apply, follow

Precipitate — to cause to happen, to bring on, hasten, abrupt, sudden

Predetermine — fix or set beforehand

Predictable — expected, knowable

Preference — favorite, liking, first choice

Prepare — get ready, plan, make, train, arrange, organize

Prescribe — set down, stipulate, order, recommend, impose

Previous — earlier, prior, before, preceding

Primarily — first, above all, mainly, mostly, largely, principally, predominantly

Primary — first, main, basic, chief, most important, key, prime, major, crucial

Priority — main concern, giving first attention to, order of importance

Production — making, creation, construction, assembly

Profuse — a lot of, plentiful, copious, abundant, generous, prolific, bountiful

Prolong — extend, delay, put off, lengthen, draw out

Promote — encourage, support, endorse, sponsor

Proportion — ratio, amount, quantity, part of, percentage, section of

Provide — give, offer, supply, make available

Rationalize — explain, reason

Realistic — practical, sensible, reasonable

Receive — get, accept, take delivery of, obtain

Recognize — acknowledge, appreciate, identify, aware of

Recovery — healing, mending, improvement, recuperation, renewal

Reduce — decrease, lessen, ease, moderate, diminish

Reestablish — reinstate, restore, return, bring back

Regard — consider, look upon, relate to, respect

Regular — usual, normal, ordinary, standard, expected, conventional

Relative — comparative, family member

Relevance — importance of

Reluctant — unwilling, hesitant, disinclined, indisposed, adverse

Remove — take away, get rid of, eliminate, eradicate

Reposition — move, relocate, change position

Require — need, want, necessitate

Resist — oppose, defend against, keep from, refuse to go along with, defy

Resolution — decree, solution, decision, ruling, promise

Resolve — make up your mind, solve, determine, decide

Response — reply, answer, reaction, retort

Restore — reinstate, reestablish, bring back, return to, refurbish

Restrict — limit, confine, curb, control, contain, hold back, hamper

Retract — take back, draw in, withdraw, apologize

Reveal — make known, disclose, divulge, expose, tell, make public

Review — appraisal, reconsider, evaluation, assessment, examination, analysis

Ritual — custom, ceremony, formal procedure

Rotate — turn, go around, spin, swivel

Routine — usual, habit, custom, practice

Satisfaction — approval, fulfillment, pleasure, happiness

Satisfy — please, convince, fulfill, make happy, gratify

Secure — safe, protected, fixed firmly, sheltered, confident, obtain

Sequential — chronological, in order of occurrence

Significant — important, major, considerable, noteworthy, momentous

Slight — small, slim, minor, unimportant, insignificant, insult, snub

Source — basis, foundation, starting place, cause

Specific — exact, particular, detail, explicit, definite

Stable — steady, even, constant

Statistics — figures, data, information

Subtract — take away, deduct

Success — achievement, victory, accomplishment

Surround — enclose, encircle, contain

Suspect — think, believe, suppose, guess, deduce, infer, distrust, doubtful

Sustain — maintain, carry on, prolong, continue, nourish, suffer

Synonymous — same as, identical, equal, tantamount

Thorough — careful, detailed, methodical, systematic, meticulous, comprehensive, exhaustive

Tilt — tip, slant, slope, lean, angle, incline

Translucent — see-through, transparent, clear

Unique — one and only, sole, exclusive, distinctive

Universal — general, widespread, common, worldwide

Unoccupied — vacant, not busy, empty

Unrelated — unconnected, unlinked, distinct, dissimilar, irrelevant

Unresolved — unsettled, uncertain, unsolved, unclear, in doubt

Utilize — make use of, employ

Various — numerous, variety, range of, mixture of, assortment of

Verbalize — express, voice, speak, articulate

Verify — confirm, make sure, prove, attest to, validate, substantiate, corroborate, authenticate

Vigorous — forceful, strong, brisk, energetic

Volume — quantity, amount, size

Withdraw — remove, pull out, take out, extract

Index

Page numbers followed by t refer to tables; and page numbers in *italics* refer to illustrations. *Specific questions and answers have not been indexed.*